P9-CJH-894

AMOUNT OF CREAM TO DISPENSE

Rule of nines

For t.i.d. application—9 gm of cream
covers 9% of skin area daily.

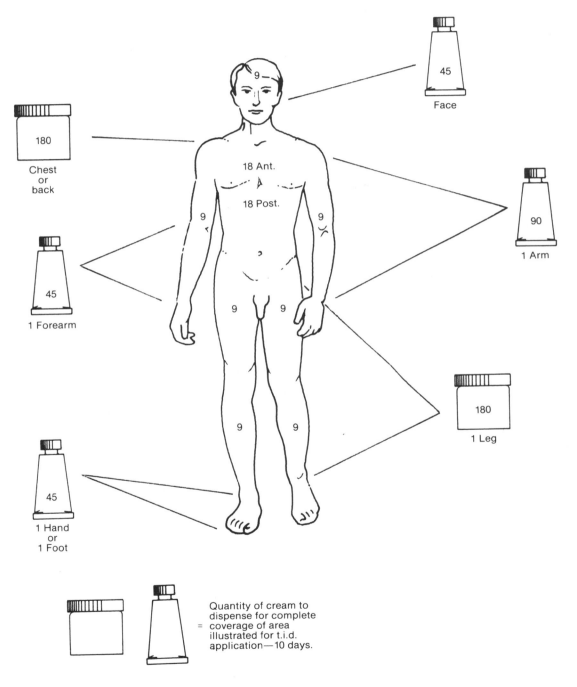

Face

Chest
or
back

18 Ant.

18 Post.

1 Arm

1 Forearm

1 Leg

1 Hand
or
1 Foot

= Quantity of cream to
dispense for complete
coverage of area
illustrated for t.i.d.
application—10 days.

Clinical Dermatology

A Color Guide to Diagnosis and Therapy

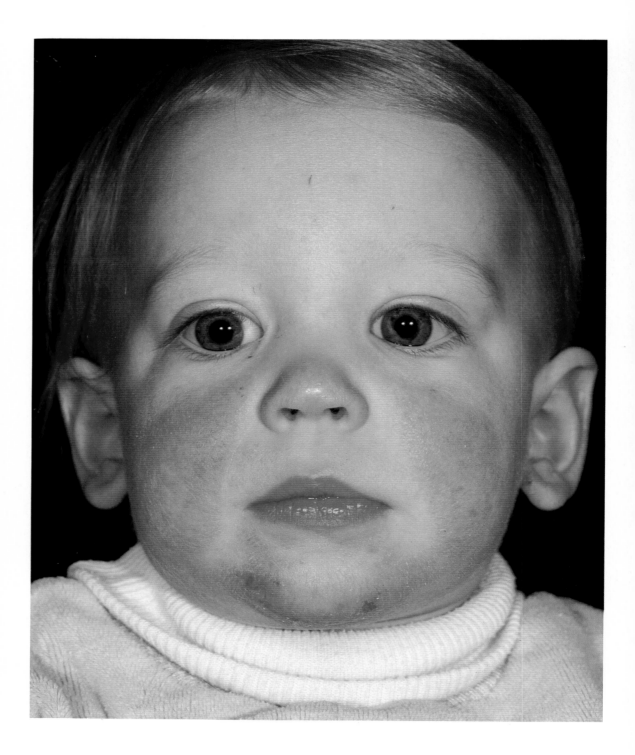

Clinical Dermatology

A Color Guide to Diagnosis and Therapy

Thomas P. Habif, M.D.

Adjunct Assistant Professor of
Clinical Medicine (Dermatology),
Dartmouth Medical School

With **768** illustrations

including **719** in color

The C. V. Mosby Company

ST. LOUIS · TORONTO · PRINCETON   1985

MOSBY

A TRADITION OF PUBLISHING EXCELLENCE

Editor: Carol Trumbold
Assistant editor: Anne Gunter
Project coordinator: Mary Espenschied
Manuscript editors: Daphna Gregg, Jerie Jordan, Atlanta, Ga.
Design: Kathleen A. Johnson
Production: Jeanne Genz, Teresa Breckwoldt
Index: Melvin J. DuPont

Composed by Academia Typographers Limited, St. Louis,
in Helvetica with Bauhaus display lines

Four-color separations film was scanned by Colorific Litho, Inc.,
St. Louis, on a Crossfield Magnascan 645IM with a 175-line screen
ruling, utilizing a round dot for maximum detail

Printed by Walsworth Publishing Company, Marceline, Mo.,
on 70# Warrenflo

Copyright © 1985 by The C.V. Mosby Company

All rights reserved. No part of this publication may be reproduced,
stored in a retrieval system, or transmitted, in any form or by any
means, electronic, mechanical, photocopying, recording, or otherwise,
without prior written permission from the publisher.

Printed in the United States of America

The C.V. Mosby Company
11830 Westline Industrial Drive, St. Louis, Missouri 63146

Library of Congress Cataloging in Publication Data

Habif, Thomas P.
   Clinical dermatology, a color guide to diagnosis
and therapy.

   Includes bibliographies and index.
   1. Dermatology—Atlases. I. Title. [DNLM:
1. Dermatology—atlases. WR 17 H116c]
RL81.H3 1985   616.5′022′2   84-14899
ISBN 0-8016-2233-6

AC/W/W 9 8 7 6 5 4 3 2   02/A/257

To my wife
Dorothy
who makes everything happen
and my sons
Tommy and David

Preface

My objective in writing this book was to provide a thoroughly illustrated text that included practical therapeutic information for practicing physicians who see dermatologic problems in their offices. When designing this book, I constantly kept in mind that it was necessary to combine the best features of a picture book and a therapeutic manual to create the kind of practical resource a busy practicing physician needs.

The classic method of organizing skin diseases is used. A discussion of the most up-to-date standard therapeutic practice follows the description of each disease. Common diseases such as acne, fungal infections, viral infections, and psoriasis are covered in depth. Care was taken to include the classic examples of these disorders and to incorporate photographs of variations seen at different stages. Rare diseases such as pemphigus and mycosis fungoides are discussed for purposes of differential diagnosis and because they are mentioned frequently in the literature. Basic dermatologic surgical techniques are covered in detail. Highly specialized techniques such as Mohs' chemosurgery are described so that the primary physician can be better prepared to suggest referral.

The photographs, taken specifically for this project, were made with a large-format camera that produced 6- by 7-cm negatives. Transparencies of this size require little enlargement and thus preserve maximum detail and full color saturation. The "point source" lighting technique was used to minimize glare and enhance detail.

I spoke with several authors before beginning this project. One author mentioned that his favorite part of a book was its preface because he enjoyed reading about another author's suffering and sacrifice during its preparation. Although this project required a great deal of time, the suffering was minimal—I enjoyed writing it.

My special thanks go to the following people who contributed to the quality of this publication:

Barry M. Austin, M.D., Alan N. Binnick, M.D., Richard D. Baughman, M.D., William E. Clendenning, M.D., Robert L. Diamond, M.D., Leanor D. Haley, Ph.D., Thomas Hokanson, P.A., Warren M. Pringle, M.D., Cameron L. Smith, M.D., and Steven K. Spencer, M.D., for medical photographs.

Cameron L. Smith, M.D., John M. Shearman, M.D., Patricia C. Adams, M.D., Richard G. Attenborough, M.D., and Sue Stone, M.D., for manuscript review. Patricia Habif and Susan Lohmeyer for editorial assistance. N. Parker Prescott for illustrations. Jean E. McGee and Margaret A. McNicholas for literature search–Medline. Michele G. Mathieu, Donna F. Garvin, and Gail E. Marshall for manuscript preparation and word processing. Allen J. Habif, Esq., David V. Habif, M.D., David V. Habif, Jr., M.D., Janet W. Prescott, Kathleen C. Scanlon, Charles L. Thayer, M.D., Gerald F. Giles, Esq., and William A. Nolen, M.D., for technical advice.

Photographs of some of the more unusual conditions were made possible through the consideration of the following physicians, who referred patients to me for photography: Stanley W. Machaj, M.D., Steven D. Paul, M.D., Charles C. Pinkerton, M.D., Ira S. Schwartz, M.D., Gerald B. Shattuck, M.D., and Henry L. Sonneborn, M.D.

I wish to thank the entire staff of The C.V. Mosby Company for their smooth coordination of this project. I am most grateful to Mary Espenschied for supervising the text editing, to Jeanne Genz for her skill in designing the layout and format of each page, to Jerry Wood for supervising the color reproduction and printing, and to the editor, Carol Trumbold, who from the beginning influenced every aspect of this text.

Thomas P. Habif

Acknowledgments

The inclusion in this text of such a large number of four-color photographs printed at high resolution would not have been possible without generous educational grants from the following individuals and corporations:

Joan T. Baldwin

Mr. and Mrs. Donald R. Baldwin

American Dermal Corporation

Dermik Laboratories, Inc.

Herbert Laboratories

Ortho Pharmaceutical Corporation

Owen Laboratories

Portsmouth Hospital

Schering Corporation

Serono Laboratories, Inc.

Syntex Laboratories, Inc.

Contents

Chapter Fifteen
Vesicular and Bullous Diseases, 325

Chapter Sixteen
Connective Tissue Diseases, 341

Chapter Seventeen
Hypersensitivity Syndromes and Vasculitis, 366

Chapter Eighteen
Light-Related Diseases and Disorders of Pigmentation, 382

Chapter Nineteen
Benign Skin Tumors, 403

Clinical Dermatology

A Color Guide to Diagnosis and Therapy

Chapter One

Anatomy and Principles of Diagnosis

The Diagnosis of Skin Disease

What could be easier than the diagnosis of skin disease? The pathology is before your eyes! Why then do nondermatologists have such difficulty interpreting what they see?

There are three reasons. To begin with, there are literally hundreds of cutaneous diseases. Secondly, a single disease entity can vary in appearance. A common seborrheic keratosis, for example, may have a smooth, rough, or eroded surface and a border that is either uniform or as irregular as a melanoma. Thirdly, skin diseases are dynamic and change in morphology. Many diseases, such as herpes simplex, undergo an evolutionary process: they may begin as a red papule, evolve into a blister, and then become an ulcer that heals with scarring. If hundreds of entities can individually vary in appearance and evolve through several stages, it is necessary that one recognize thousands of permutations in order to diagnose cutaneous diseases confidently. What at first glance appeared to be simple to diagnose may now appear to be simply impossible.

Dermatology is a morphologically oriented specialty. As in all specialties the medical history is important; however, the ability to interpret the findings is even more important. The diagnosis of skin disease must be approached in an orderly and logical manner, and the temptation to make rapid judgments after hasty observation must be controlled. The recommended approach to the patient with skin disease is as follows:

- Obtain a brief history from the patient, noting duration, rate of onset, location, symptoms, previous episodes, family history, allergies, occupation, and previous treatment.
- Determine the extent of the eruption by having the patient disrobe completely.
- Determine the primary lesion. Examine the lesions carefully; a hand lens is a valuable aid for studying skin lesions.
- Determine the nature of any secondary or special lesions.
- Determine the distribution of the skin disease.
- Formulate a differential diagnosis.
- Obtain a skin biopsy and perform laboratory tests, such as potassium hydroxide examination for fungi, skin scrapings for scabies, Gram stain, fungal and bacterial cultures, cytology (Tzanck test), Wood's light examination, patch tests, dark field examination, and blood studies.

Primary lesions

Most skin diseases begin with a basic lesion that is referred to as a primary lesion. Identification of the primary lesion is the key to accurate interpretation and description of cutaneous disease. Its presence provides the initial orientation and allows the formulation of a differential diagnosis. Definitions of the primary lesions and their differential diagnoses are given in Table 1-1. Vesicles and bullae are discussed in Chapter 15.

TABLE 1-1

PRIMARY SKIN LESIONS

Description	Differential diagnosis	

Macule

A circumscribed flat discoloration, which may be brown, blue, red, or hypopigmented

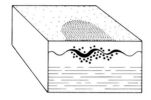

Brown
  Beckers nevus
  Cafe-au-lait spot
  Erythrasma
  Fixed drug eruption
  Freckle
  Junction nevus
  Lentigo
  Lentigo maligna
  Melasma
  Photoallergic drug eruption
  Phototoxic drug eruption
  Stasis dermatitis
  Tinea nigra palmaris
Blue
  Ink (tatoo)
  Maculae caeruleae (lice)
  Mongolian spot
  Ochronosis

Red
  Drug eruptions
  Juvenile rheumatoid arthritis (Still's disease)
  Rheumatic fever
  Secondary syphilis
  Viral exanthems
Hypopigmented
  Idiopathic guttate hypomelanosis
  Piebaldism
  Postinflammatory (psoriasis)
  Radiation dermatitis
  Nevus anemicus
  Tinea versicolor
  Tuberous sclerosis
  Vitiligo

Papule

An elevated solid lesion up to 0.5 cm in diameter; color varies; papules may become confluent and form plaques

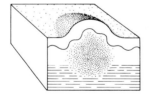

Flesh colored, yellow, or white
  Adenoma sebaceum
  Basal cell epithelioma
  Closed comedone (acne)
  Flat warts
  Granuloma annulare
  Lichen nitidus
  Lichen sclerosis et atrophicus
  Molluscum contagiosum
  Milium
  Nevi (dermal)
  Neurofibroma
  Pearly penile papules
  Pseudoxanthoma elasticum
  Sebaceous hyperplasia
  Skin tags
  Syringoma
Brown
  Dermatofibroma
  Keratosis follicularis
  Melanoma
  Nevi
  Seborrheic keratosis
  Urticaria pigmentosa
  Warts

Red
  Acne
  Atopic dermatitis
  Cholinergic urticaria
  Chondrodermatitis nodularis chronica helicis
  Eczema
  Folliculitis
  Insect bites
  Keratosis pilaris
  Leukocytoclastic vasculitis
  Miliaria
  Polymorphic light eruption
  Psoriasis
  Pyogenic granuloma
  Scabies
  Urticaria
Blue or Violaceous
  Angiokeratoma
  Blue nevus
  Lichen planus
  Lymphoma
  Kaposi's sarcoma
  Melanoma
  Mycosis fungoides
  Venous lake

TABLE 1-1, cont'd

PRIMARY SKIN LESIONS

Description	Differential diagnosis	
Plaque A circumscribed, elevated, super-ficial, solid lesion more than 0.5 cm in diameter, often formed by the con-fluence of papules	Eczema Mycosis fungoides Papulosquamous (papular and scaling) Discoid lupus erythematosus Lichen planus Pityriasis rosea Psoriasis Seborrheic dermatitis Syphilis (secondary) Tinea corporis Tinea versicolor	

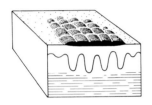

Nodule A circumscribed, elevated, solid le-sion more than 0.5 cm in diameter; a large nodule is re-ferred to as a tumor	Basal cell epithelioma Erythema nodosum Furuncle Hemangioma Kaposi's sarcoma Keratoacanthoma Lipoma Lymphoma Melanoma	Metastatic carcinoma Mycosis fungoides Neurofibromatosis Prurigo nodularis Sporotrichosis Squamous cell carcinoma Warts Xanthoma

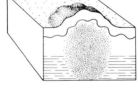

Wheal A firm edematous plaque resulting from infiltration of the dermis with fluid; they are tran-sient and may last only a few hours	Angioedema Dermographism Hives Insect bites Urticaria pigmentosa (mastocytosis)	

Continued.

TABLE 1-1, cont'd

PRIMARY SKIN LESIONS

Description	Differential diagnosis	
Pustule A circumscribed collection of leukocytes and free fluid that varies in size	Acne Candidiasis Dermatophyte infection Dyshidrosis Folliculitis Gonococcemia Hidradenitis suppurativa	Herpes simplex Herpes zoster Impetigo Psoriasis Pyoderma gangrenosum Rosacea Varicella

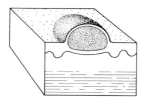

Vesicle*
A circumscribed collection of free fluid up to 0.5 cm in diameter

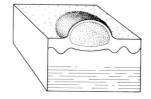

Bulla*
A circumscribed collection of free fluid more than 0.5 cm in diameter

*Vesicles and bullae are discussed in Chapter 15.

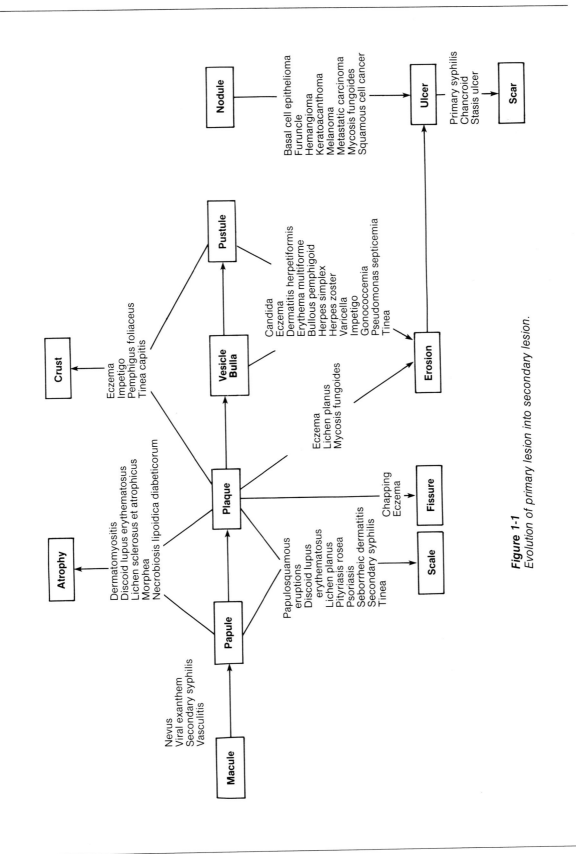

Figure 1-1
Evolution of primary lesion into secondary lesion.

Secondary lesions

Secondary lesions develop during the evolutionary process of skin disease or are created by scratching or infection (Table 1-2). They may be the only type of lesion present, in which case the primary disease process must be inferred. The evolution of primary lesions into secondary lesions is illustrated in Figure 1-1.

TABLE 1-2

SECONDARY SKIN LESIONS

Description	Differential diagnosis

Scales
Excess dead epidermal cells that are produced by abnormal keratinization and shedding
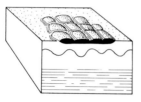
	Fine to stratified
	  Erythema craquele
	  Ichthyosis (quadrangular)
	  Lupus erythematosus (carpet tack)
	  Pityriasis rosea (collarette)
	  Psoriasis (silvery)
	  Scarlet fever (fine on trunk)
	  Seborrheic dermatitis (greasy)
	  Syphilis (secondary)
	  Tinea (dermatophytes)
	  Tinea versicolor
	  Xerosis (dry skin)
	Scaling in sheets
	  Scarlet fever (hands and feet)
	  Staphylococcal scalded skin syndrome

Crusts A collection of dried serum and cellular debris; a scab 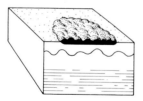	Acute eczematous inflammation Atopic (face) Impetigo (honey colored) Pemphigus foliaceus Tinea capitis
Erosions A focal loss of epidermis; they do not penetrate below the dermal-epidermal junction and therefore heal without scarring 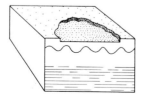	Candidiasis Dermatophyte infection Eczematous diseases Intertrigo Perlèche Senile skin Toxic epidermal necrolysis Vesiculobullous diseases

TABLE 1-2, cont'd

SECONDARY SKIN LESIONS

Description	Differential diagnosis

Ulcers

A focal loss of epidermis and dermis; they heal with scarring

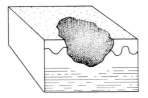

Aphthae
Chancroid
Decubitus
Factitial
Ischemic
Necrobiosis lipoidica diabeticorum
Neoplasms
Pyoderma gangrenosum
Radiodermatitis
Syphilis (chancre)
Stasis ulcers

Fissure

A linear loss of epidermis and dermis with sharply defined, nearly vertical walls

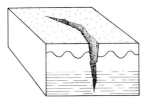

Chapping (hands, feet)
Eczema (fingertip)
Intertrigo
Perleche

Atrophy

A depression in the skin resulting from thinning of the epidermis or dermis

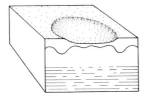

Aging
Dermatomyositis
Discoid lupus erythematosus
Lichen sclerosis et atrophicus
Morphea
Necrobiosis lipoidica diabeticorum
Radiodermatitis
Striae
Topical and intralesional steroids

Scar

An abnormal formation of connective tissue implying dermal damage; when following injury or surgery they are initially thick and pink but with time become white and atrophic

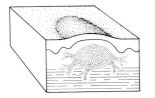

Acne
Burns
Herpes zoster
Hidradenitis suppurativa
Porphyria
Varicella

TABLE 1-3

SPECIAL SKIN LESIONS

Description	Differential diagnosis
Excoriation An erosion caused by scratching; are often linear	—
Comedone A plug of sebaceous and keratinous material lodged in the opening of a hair follicle; the follicular orifice may be dilated (blackhead) or narrowed (whitehead or closed comedone)	—
Milia A small, superficial keratin cyst with no visible opening	—
Cyst A circumscribed lesion having a wall and a lumen; the lumen may contain fluid or solid matter	—
Burrow A narrow, elevated, tortuous channel produced by a parasite	—
Lichenification An area of thickened epidermis induced by scratching; the skin lines are accentuated so that the surface looks like a washboard	—

Telangiectasia
Dilated superficial blood vessels
	Actinicly damaged skin
	Adenoma sebaceum
	Ataxia-telangiectasia
	Basal cell carcinoma
	Bloom's syndrome
	CREST syndrome
	Hereditary hemorrhagic telangiectasia
	Keloid
	Lupus erythematosus
	Necrobiosis lipoidica diabeticorum
	Of the proximal nail fold
	    Dermatomyositis
	    Lupus erythematosus
	    Scleroderma
	Poikiloderma
	Radiodermatitis
	Rosacea
	Scleroderma
	Vascular spiders
	    Pregnancy
	    Cirrhosis
	Xeroderma pigmentosum

Petechiae A circumscribed deposit of blood less that 0.5 cm in diameter **Purpura** A circumscribed deposit of blood greater than 0.5 cm in diameter	Gonococcemia Leukocytoclastic vasculitis Meningococcemia Platelet abnormalities Progressive pigmentary purpura Rocky Mountain spotted fever Scurvy Senile (traumatic)

Special lesions

A certain number of unique structures and changes called special lesions occur (Table 1-3).

Examination technique

The skin should be examined methodically, rather than merely visually scanning wide areas. It is most efficient to mentally divide the skin surface into several sections and carefully study each section. For example, when studying the face, examine the area around each eye, the nose, the mouth, the cheeks, and the temples.

Approach to treatment

Most skin diseases can be managed successfully with the numerous agents and techniques available. Do not prescribe medications, particularly topical steroids, if a diagnosis has not been established. Some physicians are tempted to experiment with various agents and, if the treatment fails, refer the patient to a specialist. This is not a logical or efficient way to practice medicine.

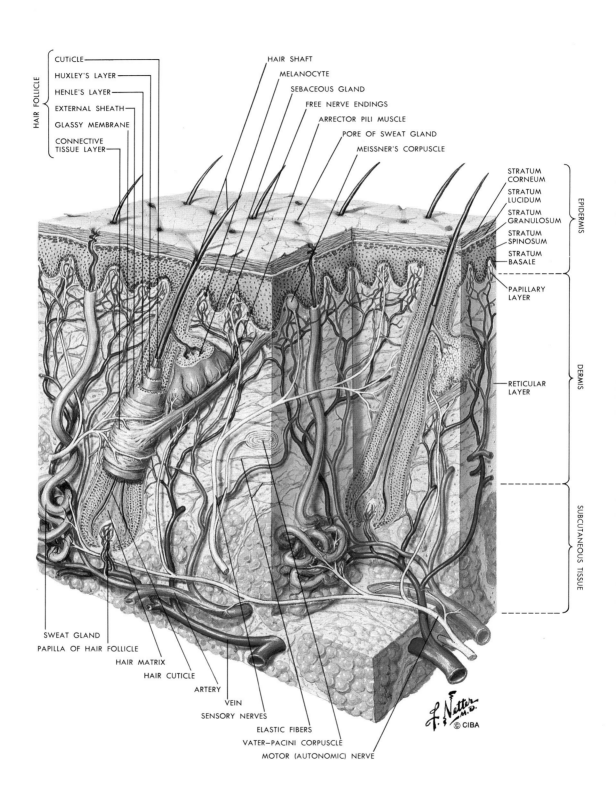

HAIR FOLLICLE
CUTICLE
HUXLEY'S LAYER
HENLE'S LAYER
EXTERNAL SHEATH
GLASSY MEMBRANE
CONNECTIVE TISSUE LAYER

HAIR SHAFT
MELANOCYTE
SEBACEOUS GLAND
FREE NERVE ENDINGS
ARRECTOR PILI MUSCLE
PORE OF SWEAT GLAND
MEISSNER'S CORPUSCLE

STRATUM CORNEUM
STRATUM LUCIDUM
STRATUM GRANULOSUM
STRATUM SPINOSUM
STRATUM BASALE

EPIDERMIS

PAPILLARY LAYER

RETICULAR LAYER

DERMIS

SUBCUTANEOUS TISSUE

SWEAT GLAND
PAPILLA OF HAIR FOLLICLE
HAIR MATRIX
HAIR CUTICLE
ARTERY
VEIN
SENSORY NERVES
ELASTIC FIBERS
VATER–PACINI CORPUSCLE
MOTOR (AUTONOMIC) NERVE

F. Netter M.D.
© CIBA

Skin Anatomy

The skin (Figure 1-2) is divided into three layers: the epidermis, the dermis, and the subcutaneous tissue. The skin is thicker on the dorsal and extensor surfaces than on the ventral and flexor surfaces.

Epidermis

The epidermis, which is the outermost part of the skin, is stratified squamous epithelium. The thickness of the epidermis ranges from 0.05 mm on the eyelids to 1.5 mm on the palms and soles. The complex microscopic anatomy of the epidermal-dermal junction is discussed in Chapter 15, "Vesicular and Bullous Diseases." The innermost layer of the epidermis consists of a single row of columnar cells called basal cells that divide and form keratinocytes (prickle cells), which comprise the spinous layer. The cells of the spinous layer are connected by intercellular bridges or spines that histologically appear as lines between the cells. The keratinocytes synthesize insoluble protein, which remains in the cell and will eventually become a major component of the outer layer (the stratum corneum). The cells continue to flatten and their cytoplasm appears granular (stratum granulosum); they finally die as they reach the surface to form the stratum corneum. There are three types of branched cells in the epidermis: the melanocyte, which synthesizes pigment (melanin); the Langerhans' cells, which serves as a frontline element in immune reactions of the skin; and the Merkel cell, the function of which is not clearly defined.

Dermis

The dermis varies in thickness from 0.3 mm on the eyelid to 3.0 mm on the back and is composed of three types of connective tissue: collagen, elastic tissue, and reticular fibers. The dermis is divided into two layers: the thin upper layer (the papillary layer) is composed of thin, haphazardly arranged collagen fibers; the thicker lower layer (the reticular layer) extends from the base of the papillary layer to the subcutaneous tissue and is composed of thick collagen fibers arranged parallel to the surface of the skin. Histiocytes are wandering macrophages that accumulate hemosiderin, melanin, and debris created by inflammation. Mast cells, locate primarily around blood vessels, manufacture and release histamine and heparin.

Dermal nerves and vasculature

The sensations of touch and pressure are received by the Meissner's and Vater-Pacini corpuscles. The sensations of pain, itching, and temperature are received by unmyelinated nerve endings in the papillary dermis. Stimulation created by inflammation at low intensity causes itching whereas high intensity stimulation causes pain. Therefore, scratching converts the intolerable sensation of itching to the more tolerable sensation of pain and eliminates pruritus. The autonomic system supplies the motor innervation of the skin. Adrenergic fibers innervate the blood vessels (vasoconstriction), hair erector muscle, and apocrine glands. Autonomic fibers to eccrine sweat glands are cholinergic. Sebaceous glands are regulated by the endocrine system and are not innervated by autonomic fibers. The anatomy of the hair follicle is described in Chapter 23.

ADDITIONAL READINGS

Ackerman AB: Development, morphology and physiology. In Moschella SL, Pillsbury DM, and Hurley HJ, editors: Dermatology, Philadelphia, 1975, W.B. Saunders Co.

Breathnach AS, Wolff K: Structure and development of the skin. In Fitzpatrick TB, Eisen AZ, Wolff K, Freedberg IM, Austen KF, editors: Dermatology in general medicine, New York, 1979, McGraw-Hill Book Company.

Ebling FJ: The normal skin. In Rook A, Wilkinson DS, Ebling FJG, editors: Textbook of dermatology, third edition. Oxford, 1979, Blackwell Scientific Publications.

Montagna W: The structure and function of the skin. New York, 1962, Academic Press.

Epidermis

Matoltsy AG: Keratinization. J Invest Dermatol **67**:20, 1976.

Montagna W, et al, editors: Special issue on the epidermis: proceedings of the 24th annual symposium on the biology of skin. J Invest Dermatol **65**:1, 1975.

Dermis

Montagna W, et al, editors: Special issue on the cells of the dermis: proceedings of the 27th annual symposium on the biology of skin. J Invest Dermatol **71**:1, 1978.

Wuepper KD, et al, editors: Structural elements of the dermis: proceedings of the 31st annual symposium on the biology of skin. J Invest Dermatol **79**:15s, 1982.

Figure 1-2 (opposite)
Skin anatomy. (© Copyright 1967, CIBA Pharmaceutical Company, Division of CIBA-GEIGY Corporation. Reprinted with permission from Clinical Symposia illustrated by Frank H. Netter, M.D. All rights reserved.)

Chapter Two

Topical Therapy and Topical Corticosteroids

Topical Therapy

A wide variety of topical medications are available for treating cutaneous disease. Specific medications are covered in detail in the appropriate chapters. Basic principles of topical treatment will be discussed here.

The skin is an important barrier that must be maintained in order to function properly. Any insult that removes water, lipids, or protein from the epidermis alters the integrity of this barrier and will compromise its function. Restoration of the normal epidermal barrier is accomplished with the use of mild soaps and emollient creams and lotions. One should observe an old and often-repeated rule: "If it is dry, wet it; if it is wet, dry it."

Dry diseases. Dry skin or dry cutaneous lesions have lost water and, in many instances, the epidermal lipids and proteins that help contain epidermal moisture. These substances are replaced with emollient creams and lotions.

Wet diseases. Exudative inflammatory diseases release serum that leaches the complex lipids and proteins from the epidermis. A wet lesion is managed with wet compresses that suppress inflammation, debride crust and serum, and then dry. Once the wet phase of the disease has been controlled, the lipids and proteins must be restored through emollient creams and lotions.

Emollient creams and lotions

Emollient creams and lotions restore water and lipids to the epidermis. The preparations listed in Table 2-1 accomplish this goal. Preparations containing urea or lactic acid have special lubricating properties and may be more effective. Creams are thicker and more lubricating than lotions. Petroleum jelly and mineral oil contain no water; water should be applied to the skin before application. Emollients should be applied as frequently as necessary to keep the skin soft. Chemicals such as menthol and phenol are added to lubricating lotions to control pruritus (Table 2-2).

TABLE 2-1

EMOLLIENTS AND SOAPS FOR RESTORING WATER AND LIPIDS TO THE EPIDERMIS

Creams	Lotions	Soaps and cleansers
Aquacare, 2% urea*	Aquacare, 2% urea	Alpha Keri soap
Aquacare/HP, 10% urea	Aquacare, 10% urea	Basis, superfatted bar soap
Carmol, 20% urea	Complex-15, phospholipids	Basis, glycerin bar soap
Complex-15, phospholipids	Keri	Cetaphil lotion
Dermatology formula	Keri Light	Dove
Keri	Jeri-Lotion	Neutrogena dry-skin soap
Lubriderm	Lacticare, 5% lactic acid	Nivea Creme soap
Nivea Moisturizing	Lubraderm	Oilatum soap
	Moisturel	Purpose brand soap
Nutraplus, 10% urea	Nivea Moisturizing	Shephard's Moisturizing soap
Purpose Dry Skin, lactic acid	Nutraderm	
Shephard's	Nutraplus, 10% urea	
	Shephard's	
	Ultra-Mide 25	
	Wondra	

*Preparations containing phospholipid, lactic acid, and urea have special lubricating properties.

TABLE 2-2

ANTIPRURITIC LOTIONS

Sarna
  0.5% menthol, 0.5% phenol, 0.5% camphor in an emollient base
Schamberg
  0.25% menthol, 1.5% phenol, 8.25% zinc oxide, 30% cotton seed oil, 15% olive oil

TABLE 2-3

DISEASES TREATED WITH WET COMPRESSES

Acute eczematous inflammation (poison ivy)
Ezematous inflammation with secondary infection (pustules)
Bullous impetigo
Herpes simplex and herpes zoster (vesciular lesions)
Infected exudative lesions of any type
Insect bites
Intertrigo (groin or under breasts)
Nummular eczema (exudative lesions)
Stasis dermatitis (exudative lesions)
Stasis ulcers
Sunburn (blistering stage)
Tinea pedis (vesicular stage or macerated web infections)

TABLE 2-4

APPLICATION OF WET DRESSINGS

1. Obtain clean, soft cloth such as bedsheeting or shirt material. The cloth need not be new or sterilized. Compress material must be washed at least once daily if it is to be used repeatedly.
2. Fold the cloth so that there are four to eight layers and cut to fit an area slightly larger than the area to be treated.
3. Wet the folded dressings by immersing in the solution and wring out to the point of sopping wet (neither running nor just damp).
4. Place the wet compress on the affected area and leave in place for 30 minutes to 1 hour. Do not pour solution onto a wet dressing to keep it wet since this practice will increase the concentration of the solution and may cause irritation. Remove the compress and replace it with a new one.
5. Dressing are left in place for 30 minutes. Dressings may be used 2 to 4 times a day or continuously. Discontinue the wet compress when the skin becomes dry. Excessive drying causes cracking and fissures.

TABLE 2-5

WET DRESSING SOLUTIONS

Solution	Preparation	Indications
Burow's solution (aluminum sulfate and calcium acetate) Bluboro powder Domeboro powder and tablets	One packet or tablet in a pint of water produces a modified 1:40 Burow's solution	Mildly antiseptic; for acute inflammation
Silver nitrate, 0.1%-0.25%	Supplied as a 50% aqueous solution. A 0.25% solution is made by the pharmacist by adding 1 tsp of the stock solution to 1000 ml of water. Stains skin dark brown and metal black.	Bactericidal; for exudative infected lesions (e.g., stasis ulcers and stasis dermatitis)
Acetic acid, 1%-2.5%	Vinegar is 5% acetic acid. Make 1% solution (approximate) by adding ½ cup of vinegar (white or brown) to 1 pint of water.	Bactericidal; for certain gram-negative bacteria (e.g., *Pseudomonas aeruginosa*), otitis externa, *Pseudomonas* intertrigo
Water	Tap water does not have to be sterilized.	Poison ivy, sunburn, any noninfected exudated or inflamed process

Wet dressings

Wet dressings, or compresses, are a valuable aid in the treatment of exudative (wet) skin diseases (Table 2-3). Their importance in topical therapy cannot be overstated. The technique for wet compress preparation and application is described in Table 2-4. Wet compresses provide the following benefits:

- Antibacterial action: Different chemicals may be added to the water to provide an antibacterial effect (Table 2-5).
- Wound debridement: A wet compress macerates vesicles and crust, helping to debride these materials when the compress is removed.
- Inflammation suppression: Compresses have a strong antiinflammatory effect. The evaporative cooling causes constriction of superficial cutaneous vessels, thereby decreasing erythema and the production of serum. Wet compresses control acute inflammatory processes such as acute poison ivy faster than both topical and orally administered corticosteroids.
- Drying: Wet dressings cause the skin to dry. Wetting something to make it dry seems paradoxical, but the effects of repeated cycles of wetting and drying are observed in chapped lips caused by licking, irritant hand dermatitis resulting from repeated washing, and the soggy sock syndrome in children.

The temperature of the compress solution should be cool when an antiinflammatory effect is desired and tepid when attempting to debride an infected, crusted lesion. Covering a wet compress with a towel or plastic inhibits evaporation, promotes maceration, and increases skin temperature, which facilitates bacterial growth.

Topical Corticosteroids

Topical corticosteroids are a powerful tool for treating skin disease. Understanding the correct use of these agents will result in the successful management of a variety of skin problems. Several corticosteroid products are available, and new ones appear almost monthly. Pharmaceutical companies have responded to the great demand for these agents with an increasing number of products, but all these preparations have basically the same antiinflammatory properties. They differ only in strength, base, and price.

Strength

The antiinflammatory properties of topical corticosteroids result in part from their ability to induce vasoconstriction of the small blood vessels in the upper dermis. This property is used in an assay procedure to determine the strength of each new product. These products are subsequently tabulated in seven groups, with Group I the strongest and Group VII the weakest (Table 2-6).[1] The treatment sections of this book will recommend topical steroids by group number rather than by generic or brand name, since the agents in each group are essentially equivalent in strength. When a new topical corticosteroid appears on the market, ask to which group it belongs and add it to the list in Table 2-6. The concentration of steroid listed on the tube cannot be used to compare its strength with other steroids. Some steroids are much more powerful than others, and only small concentrations are needed to produce maximum effect. Nevertheless, it is difficult to convince patients that Lidex cream 0.05% (Group II) is more potent than hydrocortisone 1.0% (Group VII).

It is unnecessary to learn many steroid brand names. Familiarity with one preparation from Groups II, V, and VII gives one the ability to safety and effectively treat any steroid-responsive skin disease. Most of the topical steroids are fluorinated (that is, a fluorine atom has been added to the hydrocortisone molecule). Fluorination increases potency but also the possibility of side effects. Recent products such as Westcort Cream increase potency without fluorination. As yet, it is uncertain whether the incidence of side effects will be reduced by the elimination of the fluorine atom.

Avoid having the pharmacist prepare or dilute topical steroid creams. The active ingredient may not be dispersed uniformly, resulting in a cream of variable strength. The cost of pharmacist preparation is generally higher because of the additional labor required. High quality steroid creams such as triamcinolone (Kenalog, Aristocort) are available in large quantities at a low cost.

TABLE 2-6

ORDER OF POTENCY OF TOPICAL STEROID PREPARATIONS

Group*	Brand name	Generic name	Tube size (gm)
I	Diprolene Ointment 0.05%	Betamethasone dipropionate in a propylene glycol ointment base	15, 45
II	Cyclocort Ointment 0.1%	Amcinonide	15, 60
	Diprosone Ointment 0.05%	Betamethasone dipropionate	15, 45
	Florone Ointment 0.05%	Diflorasone diacetate	15, 30, 60
	Halog Cream 0.1%	Halcinonide	15, 30, 60, 240
	Lidex Cream 0.05%	Fluocinonide	15, 30, 60, 120
	Lidex Gel 0.05%	Fluocinonide	15, 30, 60, 120
	Lidex Ointment 0.05%	Fluocinonide	15, 30, 60, 120
	Maxiflor Ointment 0.05%	Diflorasone diacetate	15, 30, 60
	Topicort Cream 0.25%	Desoximetasone	5, 15, 60
	Topicort Ointment 0.25%	Desoximetasone	5, 15, 60
III	Aristocort Cream 0.5%	Triamcinolone acetonide	15, 75, 240
	Diprosone Cream 0.05%	Betamethasone dipropionate	15, 45
	Florone Cream 0.05%	Diflorasone diacetate	15, 30, 60
	Kenalog Ointment 0.5%	Triamcinolone acetonide	20
	Maxiflor Cream 0.05%	Diflorasone diacetate	15, 30, 60
	Valisone Ointment 0.1%	Betamethasone valerate	5, 15, 45
IV	Aristocort Ointment 0.1%	Triamcinolone acetonide	15, 75, ½ lb.
	Benisone Gel 0.025%	Betamethasone benzoate	15, 60
	Cordran Ointment 0.05%	Flurandrenolide	15, 30, 60, 225
	Cyclocort Cream 0.1%	Amcinonide	15, 60
	Fluonid Ointment 0.025%	Fluocinolone acetonide	15, 60
	Kenalog Ointment 0.1%	Triamcinolone acetonide	15, 60, 425
	Synalar Ointment 0.025%	Fluocinolone acetonide	15, 30, 60, 120
	Topicort LP Cream 0.05%	Desoximetasone	15, 60
	Uticort Gel 0.025%	Betamethasone benzoate	15, 60
V	Aristocort A Cream 0.1%	Triamcinolone acetonide	15, 60
	Cloderm Cream 0.1%	Clocortolone pivalate	15, 45
	Cordran Cream 0.05%	Flurandrenolide	15, 30, 60, 225
	Diprosone Lotion 0.05%	Betamethasone dipropionate	20, 60
	Fluonid Cream 0.025%	Fluocinolone acetonide	15, 60
	Kenalog Cream 0.1%	Triamcinolone acetonide	15, 60, 80, 240, 5.25 lb.
	Kenalog Lotion 0.1%	Triamcinolone acetonide	15, 60
	Locoid Cream 0.1%	Hydrocortisone butyrate	15, 45
	Synalar Cream 0.025%	Fluocinolone acetonide	15, 30, 60, 120
	Synemol Cream 0.025%	Fluocinolone acetonide	15, 30, 60, 120
	Topicort LP 0.05%	Desoximetasone	15, 60
	Tridesilon Ointment 0.05%	Desonide	15, 60
	Valisone Cream 0.1%	Betamethasone valerate	5, 15, 45
	Valisone Lotion 0.1%	Betamethasone valerate	20, 60
	Westcort Cream 0.2%	Hydrocortisone valerate	15, 45, 60, 120
VI	Locorten Cream 0.03%	Flumethasone pivalate	15, 60
	Synalar Solution 0.01%	Fluocinolone acetonide	20, 60
	Tridesilon Cream 0.05%	Desonide	15, 60
VII	Topicals with hydrocortisone, dexamethasone, prednisolone		
	Hytone Cream 1%	Hydrocortisone	15, 120
	Hytone Cream 2.5%	Hydrocortisone	15, 120

Courtesy Richard B. Stoughton, M.D.
*Group I is the most potent; Group VII is the least potent. Preparations within each group have similar potency.

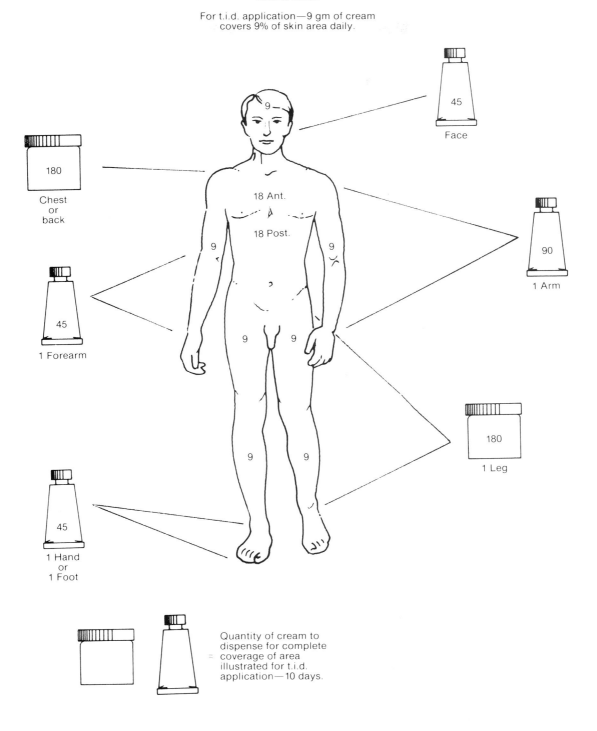

Rule of nines

For t.i.d. application—9 gm of cream covers 9% of skin area daily.

9

18 Ant.

18 Post.

9   9

9   9

9   9

45
Face

180
Chest
or
back

90
1 Arm

45
1 Forearm

180
1 Leg

45
1 Hand
or
1 Foot

= Quantity of cream to dispense for complete coverage of area illustrated for t.i.d. application—10 days.

Figure 2-1
Amount of cream to dispense.

Vehicle

The vehicle or base is the substance in which the active ingredient is dispersed. The base determines the rate at which the active ingredient is absorbed through the skin.[2,3] Components of some bases may cause irritation or allergy.

Creams. The cream base is a mixture of several different organic chemicals (oils) and water, and it usually contains a preservative. Creams have the following characteristics:

- White color and somewhat greasy texture
- Components that may cause irritation, stinging, and allergy
- High versatility (i.e., may be used in nearly any area), therefore the base most often prescribed
- Cosmetically most acceptable, particularly new emollient bases (e.g., Lidex-E, Topicort, and Cyclocort)
- Possible drying effect with continued use, therefore best for acute exudative inflammation
- Most helpful for intertriginous areas (e.g., groin, rectal area, and axilla)

Ointments. The ointment base contains a limited number of organic compounds consisting primarily of greases such as petroleum jelly with little or no water. Many ointments are preservative-free. Ointments have the following characteristics:

- Translucent (looks like petroleum jelly)
- Greasy feeling; persists on skin surface
- More lubrication than creams, thus desirable for dryer lesions
- Greater penetration of medicine than creams and therefore enhanced potency (see Table 2-6, Synalar Cream in Group V and Synalar Ointment in Group IV)
- Too occlusive for acute (exudative) eczematous inflammation or intertriginous areas such as the groin

Gels. Gels are greaseless mixtures of propylene glycol and water, some also containing alcohol. Gels have the following characteristics:

- A clear base with a jelly-like consistency
- A sticky, unpleasant feeling, sometimes irritating; not prescribed as frequently
- Useful for acute exudative inflammation such as poison ivy and in scalp areas where other vehicles mat the hair

- Alcohol gels (Benisone, Uticort) are drying and cooling and are best suited for acute exudative pruritic eruptions such as poison ivy; they aggravate dry cracked and fissured lesions by producing more dryness
- Nonalcohol gels (Topsyn) are more lubricating and are well suited to dry scaling lesions in the scalp

Solutions and lotions. Solutions may contain water and alcohol as well as other chemicals. Solutions have the following characteristics:

- Clear or milky appearance
- Most useful for scalp because they penetrate easily through hair leaving no residue
- May result in stinging and drying when applied to intertriginous areas such as the groin

Aerosols. Aerosols are composed of steroids suspended in a base and delivered under pressure by isobutane or propane propellant. Aerosols have the following characteristics:

- Useful for scalp (long probe attached to the can may be inserted through the hair to deliver medication more easily to the scalp)
- Useful for moist lesions such as poison ivy
- Convenient for patients who lack mobility and have difficulty reaching the lower legs

Steroid-antibiotic mixtures

Several products contain a combination of antibiotic and corticosteroid. Neomycin-steroid products such as Mycolog and Neo-synalar are commonly prescribed. Presently dermatologists disagree about the desirability of these combination products.[4,5] The majority of steroid-responsive skin diseases can be managed successfully without topical antibiotics. Oral antibiotics have demonstrated more effectiveness than topical antibiotics. Neomycin is a sensitizer and may complicate an already prolonged and difficult-to-control problem such as stasis dermatitis. Present governmental guidelines for welfare recipients prohibit reimbursement for steroid-antibiotic mixtures.

Amount of cream to dispense

The amount of cream dispensed is very important. Patients do not appreciate being prescribed a $22.00 60-gm tube of cream to treat a small area of hand dermatitis. Unrestricted use of potent steroid creams can lead to side effects. Patients rely on the judgement of the physician to determine the correct amount of topical medicine. If too small a quantity is prescribed, patients will conclude that the treatment did not work. It is advisable to allow for a sufficient amount of cream and then set limits on duration and frequency of application. A few steroids (e.g., triamcinolone and hydrocortisone) are available in generic form. They are purchased in bulk by the pharmacist and can be dispensed in large quantities at considerable savings.

The amount of cream required to cover a certain area can easily be calculated by remembering that 1 gm of cream covers 10 cm $\times$ 10 cm or 100 cm^2 of skin.[6] Thirty grams of cream will cover the entire skin surface of the average-size adult.

The "rule of nines" can be used to estimate the percentage of surface to be treated. Simply calculate the percentage of the total surface area involved and multiply by 30 gm to determine the number of grams required for a single application. The calculations for twice daily application for a 10-day course are illustrated in Figure 2-1.

Application
Frequency

Tachyphylaxis refers to the decrease in responsiveness to a drug as a result of enzyme induction. The term is used in dermatology in reference to acute tolerance to the vasoconstrictive action of topically applied corticosteroids. Experiments have revealed that vasoconstriction decreased progressively when a potent topical steroid was applied to the skin 3 times daily for 4 days.[7] The vasoconstrictive response returned 4 days after termination of therapy. These experiments support years of complaints by patients about initial dramatic responses to new topical steroids, which diminish with constant use. It would, therefore, seem reasonable to instruct the patient to apply creams on an interrupted schedule (e.g., 2 days of treatment followed by 2 days without treatment). However, this method of therapy is not generally advocated at the present time. Most dermatologists recommend 2 to 4 times daily application until the disease clears. In most cases this schedule produces adequate results.

Methods

Simple application. Creams and ointments should be applied 2 to 4 times a day in a thin layer. A uniformly thin application can be achieved if small quantities are applied about 2 or 3 inches apart and smoothly rubbed together. Patients should be informed that it is unnecessary to wash before each application. Patients must be encouraged to continue treatment until the lesion is clear. They will often decrease the frequency of application or stop entirely when lesions appear to be improving quickly. Other patients are so impressed with the efficacy of these agents that they continue treatment after the disease has resolved in order to prevent recurrence. Adverse reactions may follow this practice.

Different skin surfaces vary in their ability to absorb topical medicine. The thin eyelid skin heals quickly with Group VI or VII steroids, while thicker skin on palms and soles offers a greater barrier to the penetration of topical medicine and requires more potent therapy. Intertriginous (skin touches skin) areas (e.g., axilla, groin, rectal area, and underneath the breasts) will respond more quickly with weaker strength creams. The apposition of two skin surfaces performs the same function as an occlusive dressing, which greatly enhances penetration. The skin of infants and young children is more receptive to topical medicine and will respond quickly to weaker creams. A baby's diaper has the same occlusive effect as covering with a plastic dressing. Penetration of steroid creams is greatly enhanced; therefore, only Group V, VI, or VII preparations should be used under the diaper. Inflamed skin absorbs topical medicines much more efficiently. This explains why red inflamed areas generally have such a rapid initial response when treated with weaker topical steroids.

Occlusion. Occlusion with a plastic dressing (e.g., Saran Wrap) is an effective method for enhancing absorption of topical steroids. The plastic dressing holds perspiration against the skin surface, which hydrates the top layer of the epidermis (stratum corneum). Topical medication penetrates through a moist stratum corneum from 10 to 100 times more effectively than through dry skin.[8] Lesions respond much faster than with simple application. Eruptions that are resistant to simple application may heal quickly with the introduction of a plastic dressing. Nearly any area can be occluded; the entire body may be occluded with a vinyl exercise suit, available at most sporting goods stores.

Discretion should be used with occlusion. Do not occlude moist areas. This could result in the rapid development of infection.[9] Creams rather than ointments are generally occluded, but ointments may be covered if the lesions are particularly dry. Weaker, less expensive products (e.g., triamcinolone cream, 0.1%) will provide excellent results. Large quantities of this medicine may be purchased at a substantial saving.

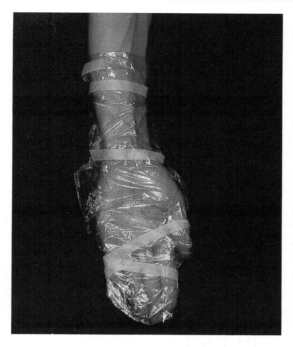

Figure 2-2
Occlusion of the hand. A plastic bag is pulled on and pressed against the skin to expel air. Tape is wound snugly around the bag. A sock may be worn to hold the plastic against the foot.

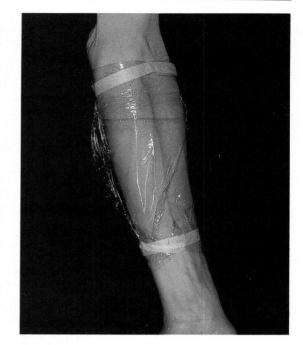

Figure 2-3
Occlusion of the arm. A plastic sheet (e.g., Saran Wrap) is wound about the extremity and secured at both ends with tape. A plastic bag with the bottom cut out may be used as a sleeve and held in place with tape or an Ace bandage.

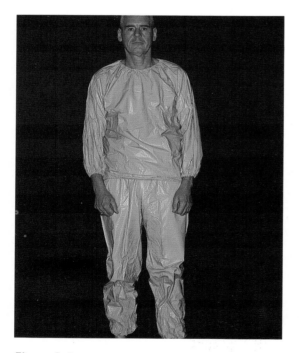

Figure 2-4
Occlusion of the entire body. A vinyl exercise suit is a convenient way to occlude the entire body.

Method. Clean the area with mild soap and water. Antibacterial soaps are unnecessary. Gently rub the medicine into lesions. Cover the entire area with plastic (e.g., Saran Wrap, Handi-Wrap, plastic bags, or gloves) (Figures 2-2 to 2-4). Secure the plastic dressing with tape so that the plastic is close to the skin and the ends are sealed. An airtight dressing is unnecessary. The plastic may be held in place with an Ace bandage or a sock. Best results are obtained if the dressing remains in place for at least 2 hours. Many patients find that bedtime is the most convenient time to wear a plastic dressing and will therefore wear it for 8 hours. More medicine is applied shortly after the dressing is removed and while the skin is still moist.

Dressings should not remain on the area continuously because infection or follicular occlusion may result. If an occluded area suddenly becomes worse or pustules develop, infection, usually with staphylococci, should be suspected (Figure 2-5). Oral antistaphylococcal antibiotics should be given (e.g., cephalexin 500 mg twice daily). Tetracycline is generally ineffective.

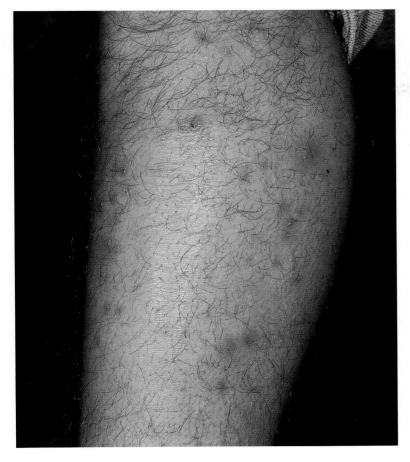

Figure 2-5
*Infection following occlusion.
Pustules have appeared
at the periphery of an eczematous
lesion. Plastic dressing had
been left in place for 24 hours.*

TABLE 2-7

REPORTED ADVERSE REACTIONS TO TOPICAL CORTICOSTEROIDS

Rosacea, perioral dermatitis, acne
Skin atrophy with telangiectasia, stellate pseudoscars (arms), purpura, stria (from ana-
   tomical occlusion, e.g., groin)
Tinea incognito, impetigo incognito, scabies incognito
Ocular hypertension, glaucoma, cataracts
Allergic contact dermatitis
Systemic absorption
Burning, itching, irritation, dryness caused by vehicle (e.g., propylene glycol)
Miliaria and folliculitus following occlusion with plastic
Skin blanching from acute vasoconstriction
Rebound phenomenon (e.g., psoriasis becomes worse after treatment is stopped)
Nonhealing leg ulcers; steroids applied to any leg ulcer retard healing process
Hypopigmentation
Hypertrichosis of face

A reasonable occlusion schedule is twice daily for a 2-hour period or 8 hours at bedtime, with simple application once or twice during the day.

Occluded areas will often become dry, and the use of lubricating cream or lotion should be encouraged. This may be applied shortly after medicine is applied, when the plastic dressing is removed, or at other convenient times.

Adverse reactions

Because information concerning the potential dangers of potent topical steroids has been so widely disseminated, some physicians have abandoned their use. Topical steroids have been used for approximately 30 years with an excellent safety record. They do, however, have the potential to produce a number of adverse reactions. Once these are understood, the cream of the most appropriate strength can be prescribed confidently. Table 2-7 lists the reported adverse reactions to topical steroids. A brief description of some of the more important adverse reactions is presented in the following pages.

Steroid rosacea. Steroid rosacea[10] is a side effect frequently observed in fair-skinned, middle-aged women who initially complain of erythema with or without pustules, called the "flusher blusher complexion." In a typical example, the physician prescribes a mild topical steroid, which initially gives pleasing results. Tolerance (tachyphylaxis) occurs and a new, more potent topical steroid is prescribed to suppress the erythema and pustules that have reappeared after the use of the weaker preparation. This progression to more potent creams may continue until Group I or II steroids are applied several times each day. Figure 2-6, A, shows a middle-aged woman who has applied a Group V steroid cream once every day for 5 years. Intense erythema and pustulation occurs each time attempts are made to discontinue topical treatment (Figure 2-6, B and C).

Management. Strong topical steroids must be discontinued. Tetracycline (250 mg 4 times daily) or erythromycin (250 mg 4 times daily) may reduce the intensity of the rebound erythema and pustulation that predictably occur during the first 10 days (Figure 2-7). Occasionally, cool, wet compresses with or without 1% hydrocortisone cream will be necessary if the rebound is intense. Thereafter, mild noncomedogenic lubricants (those that do not induce acne, such as Nutraderm lotion) may be used for the dryness and desquamation that will occur. Erythema and pustules will generally be present at a low grade level for months.[11] Low doses of tetracycline or erythromycin (250 mg 2 or 3 times a day) may be continued until the eruption clears. The pustules and erythema eventually subside, but some telangiectasia and atrophy may be permanent.

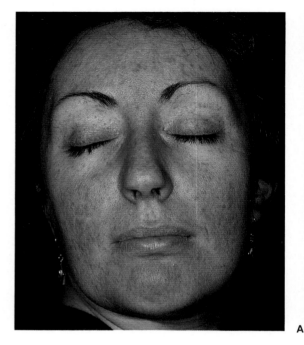

A

Figure 2-6
Steroid rosacea. **A,** Numerous red papules formed on the cheeks and forehead with constant daily use of a Group V topical steroid. **B,** Ten days after discontinuing use of Group V topical steroid. **C,** Two months after discontinuing use of topical steroids. Telangiectasia has persisted; rosacea has improved with oral antibiotics.

Figure 2-7 (opposite)
Steroid rosacea. **A,** Intense erythema and pustulation appeared 10 days after discontinuing use of a Group V topical steroid. The cream had been applied every day for one year. **B,** Patient shown in **A** 24 days after discontinuing the Group V topical steroid. Pustules have cleared without any treatment. Gradual improvement followed over the next several months.

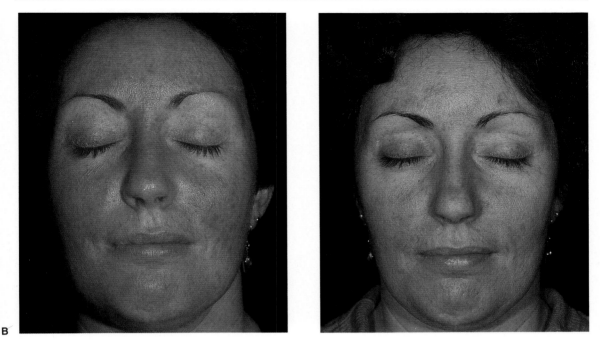

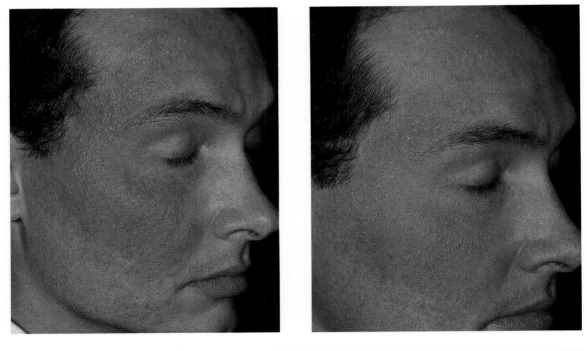

Atrophy. Long-term use of strong topical steroids in the same area may result in thinning of the epidermis and regressive changes in the connective tissue in the dermis. The affected areas are often depressed slightly below normal skin and usually reveal telangiectasia, prominence of underlying veins, and hypopigmentation. Purpura and ecchymosis result from minor trauma. The face (Figure 2-8), dorsa of the hands (Figure 2-9), extensor surfaces of the forearms and legs and the intertriginous areas are particularly susceptible. In most cases atrophy is reversible and may be expected to disappear in several months. Diseases (such as psoriasis) that respond slowly to strong topical steroids require weeks of therapy. Some atrophy may subsequently be anticipated (Figure 2-10).

Occlusion will enhance penetration of medicine and accelerate the occurrence of this adverse reaction. Patients are frequently familiar with this side effect and must be assured that the use of strong topical steroids is perfectly safe when used as directed for 2 to 3 weeks. They must also be assured that, if some atrophy does appear, it will in most cases resolve when therapy is discontinued.

Atrophy in the rectal and vaginal areas may appear much more quickly than in other areas.[12] The thinner epidermis offers less resistance to the passage of corticosteroids into the dermis. These are intertriginous areas where the apposition of skin surfaces acts in the same manner as a plastic dressing, retaining moisture and greatly facilitating absorbtion. These delicate tissues become thin and painful and sometimes exhibit a susceptibility to bleeding with scratching or intercourse. The atrophy seems to be more enduring. Therefore, careful instruction about duration of therapy must be given (e.g., twice a day for 10 days). If the disease does not resolve quickly with topical therapy, reevaluation is necessary.

Atrophy may appear very rapidly after intralesional injection of corticosteroids (e.g., for treatment of acne cysts or in attempting to promote hair growth in alopecia areata). The side effect of atrophy is utilized to reduce the size of hypertrophic scars and keloids. When injected into the dermis, 5 mg/ml of Kenalog may produce atrophy; 10 mg/ml of Kenalog will almost always produce atrophy. For direct injection into the skin, stronger concentrations should probably be avoided.

Long-term use (over months) of even weak topical steroids on the upper inner thighs or in the axillae will result in striae analogous to those on the abdomen of pregnant women (Figure 2-11). These changes are irreversible. Pruritus in the groin area is common, and patients are considerably relieved by the less potent steroids. Symptoms often recur after treatment is terminated; it is a great temptation to continue topical treatment on an as needed basis.

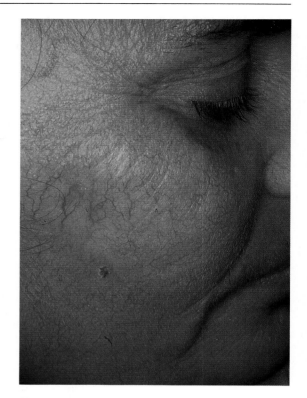

Figure 2-8
Atrophy and telangiectasia after continuous use of a Group IV topical steroid for 6 months.

Every attempt must be made to determine the underlying process and discourage long-term use.

Alteration of infection. Cortisone creams applied to cutaneous infections may alter the usual clinical presentation of those diseases and produce unusual atypical eruptions.[13,14] Cortisone cream suppresses the inflammation that is attempting to contain the infection and allows unrestricted growth. Tinea of the groin is characteristically seen as a localized, superficial plaque with a well-defined scaly border (Figure 2-12). A Group II corticosteroid applied for 3 weeks to this common eruption produced the rash seen in Figure 2-13. The fungus rapidly spread to involve a much wider area, and the typical sharply defined border is gone. Untreated tinea rarely produces such a florid eruption in temperate climates. This altered clinical picture has been called tinea incognito.

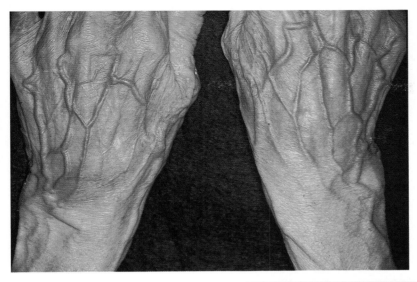

Figure 2-9
Severe steroid atrophy after continuous occlusive therapy over several months.

Figure 2-10
Steroid atrophy. Atrophy with prominence of underlying veins and hypopigmentation following use of Cordran Tape applied daily for 3 months to treat psoriasis. Note that small plaques of psoriasis still persist.

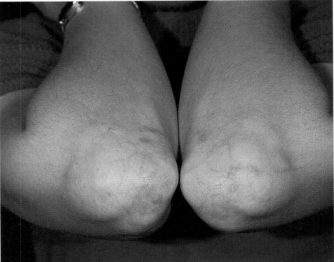

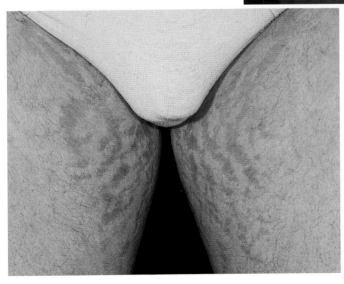

Figure 2-11
Striae of the groin after long-term use of Group V topical steroids for pruritus.

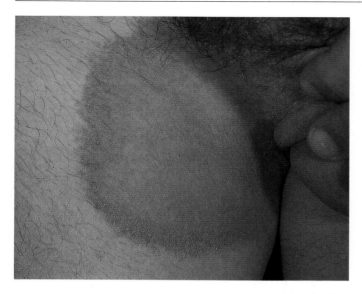

Figure 2-12
Typical presentation of tinea of the groin before treatment.

Figure 2-13
Tinea incognito. A bizarre pattern of inflammation created by applying a Group II topical steroid twice daily for 3 weeks to an eruption similar to that seen in Fig. 2-12. A potassium hydroxide preparation showed numerous fungi.

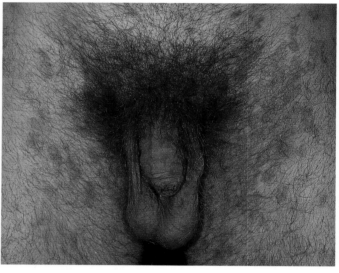

Figure 2-14 shows a young girl who applied a Group II cream daily for 6 months to treat "eczema." The large plaques retain some of the characteristics of certain fungal infections by having well-defined edges. The red papules and nodules are atypical and are usually observed exclusively with an unusual form of follicular fungal infection seen on the lower legs. Figure 2-15 shows another example of tinea incognito.

Boils, folliculitis, rosacea-like eruptions, and diffuse fine scaling have been reported from treating tinea with topical steroids. If a rash has failed to respond after a reasonable length of time or if the appearance changes, consider tinea, bacterial infection, or allergic contact dermatitis from some component of the steroid cream.

Scabies and impetigo may likewise initially improve as topical steroids suppress inflammation. Consequently, both diseases become worse when the creams are discontinued (or, possibly, continued). Figure 2-16 shows numerous pustules on the leg, which are characteristic of staphylococcal infection resulting from treatment of an exudative plaque of eczema with a Group V topical steroid.

Figure 2-16 (opposite)
Impetiginized eczema with satellite pustules after treatment of exudative eczema with a Group V topical steroid.

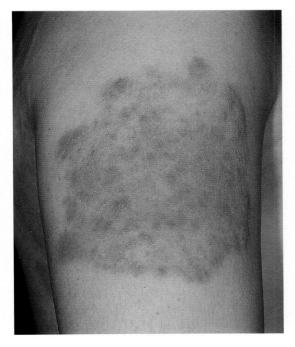

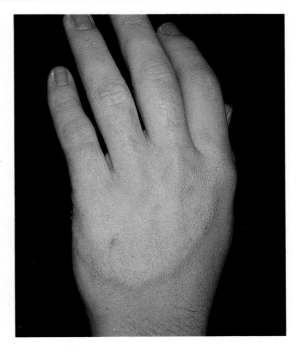

Figure 2-14
Tinea incognito. A plaque of tinea initially diagnosed as eczema was treated for 6 months with a Group II topical steroid. Red papules have appeared where only erythema was once present.

Figure 2-15
Tinea incognito. A marked reduction in erythema has occurred after treatment of this cutaneous fungal infection with a Group IV topical steroid.

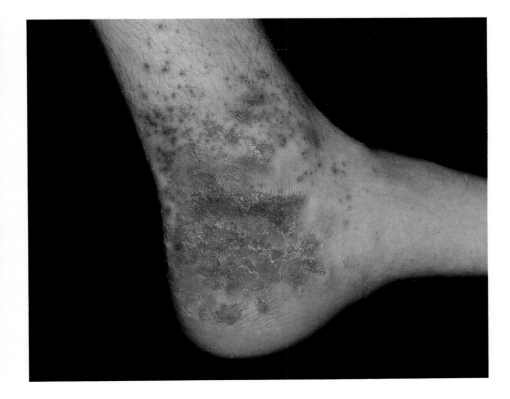

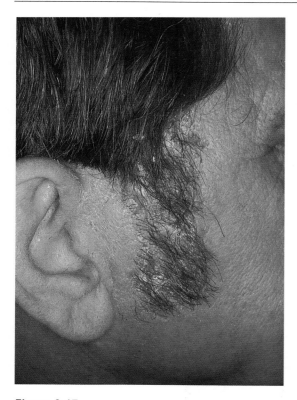

Figure 2-17
Acute contact allergy to a preservative in a Group II steroid gel.

Contact dermatitis. Topical steroids are the drug of choice for allergic and irritant contact dermatitis, but occasionally topical steroids cause such dermatitis.[15] Allergic reactions to various components of steroid creams, such as preservatives (parabens), vehicle (lanolin), antibacterials (neomycin), and perfumes (Mycolog cream), have all been documented. Figure 2-17 shows allergic contact dermatitis to a preservative in a Group II steroid gel. The cream was prescribed to treat seborrheic dermatitis. Allergic reactions may not be intense. Inflammation created by a cream component (such as a preservative) may be suppressed by the steroid component of the same cream, and the eruption simply smoulders, neither improving nor worsening, presenting a very confusing picture.

If inflammation improves and then suddenly becomes worse during treatment with a topical steroid, then allergic contact dermatitis to some component of that cream should be considered.

Systemic absorption. The possibility of producing systemic side effects from absorption of topical steroids concerns all physicians who use these agents. Several case reports in the past 20

years have documented systemic effects after topical application of glucocorticoids for prolonged periods. Cataracts, retardation of growth,[16] failure to thrive, and Cushing's syndrome[17] have all been reported.

The physician attempting to avoid complications chooses the weaker preparations; these all too frequently fall short of expectation and fail to give the desired antiinflammatory effect. The disease does not improve, but rather becomes worse because of the delay imposed in choosing the weaker, "safer" cream. Pruritus continues, infection may set in, and the patient becomes frustrated. Hydrocortisone cream 0.5% for intense inflammation is a waste of time and money. In general, a topical steroid of adequate strength should be used several times daily for a specific length of time, such as 7 to 10 days, in order to obtain rapid control. Adrenal suppression may result even during this short interval when Group II and III steroids are used to treat wide areas of inflamed skin. This suppression of the hypothalamic-pituitary-adrenal axis is generally reversible in 24 hours and is unlikely to produce side effects characteristic of long-term systemic use.[18]

Children. Many physicians worry about systemic absorption and will not use any topical steroids stronger than 1% hydrocortisone on infants. One study revealed that stronger creams can be used safely.[19] Infants (7 to 96 months) with severe atopic dermatitis were treated with triamcinolone acetonide ointment 0.1% (Kenalog ointment) applied 4 times each day for 6 weeks. The total quantities of ointment used during the 6-week period were large, varying from 414 to 1191 gm. No patient showed suppression of the hypothalamic-pituitary-adrenal axis. The author concluded that the tendency to abandon the use of fluorinated steroids such as triamcinolone acetonide 0.1% in infants and children was not justified, nor is the use of placebo concentrations of hydrocortisone.

The author who reviewed the use of fluorinated topical steroids in infants concluded that one need not take refuge in homeopathic doses of hydrocortisone when confronted with a case of eczema, seborrheic dermatitis, or psoriasis in an infant.[20] The relative safety of moderately strong topical steroids and their relative freedom from serious systemic toxicity despite widespread use in the very young has been clearly demonstrated. Patients should be treated for a specific length of time with a medication of appropriate strength. Steroid creams should not be used continuously for many weeks and those patients not responding in a predictable fashion need reevaluation.

Adults. Table 2-8 lists the degree of adrenal suppression that can be expected from different treatment schedules using topical steroids.[18] Suppression may occur during short intervals of treatment

TABLE 2-8

DEGREE OF ADRENAL SUPPRESSION WITH VARIOUS TOPICAL STEROIDS

Steroid group	Frequency	Body surface treated (%)	Duration	Occlusion	Suppression*
II†	b.i.d.	50	5 days	No	None
II†	b.i.d.	50	5 days	Yes	Yes
II	b.i.d.	30	5 days	No	Immediate, but decreases during treatment
II	b.i.d.	30	5 days	Yes	Marked; persists throughout treatment period
V	b.i.d.	30	5 days	No	Mild decrease
V	b.i.d.	30	5 days	Yes	Moderate decrease
II	t.i.d.	5-50	4-6 wks.	No	Little or none
V	t.i.d.	5-50	4-6 wks.	No	None

Modified from Gomez EC, Kaminester L, Frost P: Topical halcinonide cream and betamethasone valerate: effects on plasma cortisol. Arch Dermatol 113:1196, 1977.
*Adrenal suppression was rapidly reversible in all cases.
†Normal skin.

with Group I, II, III, IV, or V topical steroids, but recovery is rapid when treatment is discontinued. Physicians may prescribe strong agents when appropriate, but the patient must be cautioned that use should be only for a specific length of time.

Glaucoma. There are isolated case reports of glaucoma occurring after the long-term use of topical steroids around the eyes.[21] Glaucoma induced by prolonged use of steroid-containing eyedrops instilled directly into the conjunctival sac is encountered more frequently by the ophthalmologist. The mechanism by which glaucoma develops from topical application is not understood, but presumably cream applied to the lids seeps over the lid margin and into the conjunctival sac. It also seems possible that enough steroid could be absorbed directly through the lid skin into the conjunctival sac to produce the same results. This problem almost certainly occurs more frequently than is reported. Inflammation around the eye is a common problem. Offending agents that cause inflammation may be directly transferred to the eyelids by rubbing with the hand or may be applied directly, as with cosmetics. Women who are sensitive to a favorite eye makeup will often continue using that makeup on an interrupted basis, not suspecting the obvious source of allergy. Patients have been seen who alternate topical steroids with a sensitizing makeup. It appears that these patients are likely to develop glaucoma. Unsupervised use of over-the-counter hydrocortisone cream might also induce this type complication.

No studies have yet determined what quantity or strength of steroid cream is required to produce glaucoma. It would, therefore, seem prudent to restrict the use of these agents to a 2- to 3-week period and use only Group VI and VII preparations.

REFERENCES

1. Stoughton RB: A perspective of topical corticosteroid therapy. In Farber E and Cox A, editors: Psoriasis: Proceedings of the second international symposium, New York, 1976, Yorke Medical Books.
2. Stoughton RB: Bioassay systems for formulations of topically applied glucocorticoids. Arch Dermatol **106:** 825, 1972.
3. McKenzie AW: Percutaneous absorption of steroids. Arch Dermatol **86:**911, 1972.
4. Leyden JJ, Kligman AM: The case for topical antibiotics. Prog Dermatol **10**(4), 1976.
5. Rasmussen JE: The case against topical antibiotics. Prog Dermatol **11**(1), 1977.
6. Schlagel CA, Sanborn ED: The weights of topical preparations required for total and partial body inuction. J Invest Dermatol **42:**252, 1964.
7. duVivier A: Tachyphylaxis to topically applied steroids. Arch Dermatol **112:**1245, 1976.
8. Sulzberger MD, Witten VH: Thin pliable plastic films in topical dermatologic therapy. Arch Dermatol **84:**1027, 1961.
9. Maibach HI, Stoughton RB: Topical corticosteroids. Med Clin North Am **57:**1253, 1973.

10. Leyden JJ, Thew M, Kligman AM: Steroid rosacea. Arch Dermatol **110:**619, 1974.
11. Sneddon IB: The treatment of steroid-induced rosacea and perioral dermatitis. Dermatologica **152**(suppl 1):231, 1976.
12. Goldman L, Kitzmiller KW: Perianal atrophoderma from topical corticosteroids. Arch Dermatol **107:**611, 1973.
13. Ive FA, Mark SR: Tinea incognito. Br Med J **3:**149, 1968.
14. Burry J: Topical drug addiction: adverse effects of fluorinated corticosteroid creams and ointments. Med J Austr **1:**393, 1973.
15. Goin JD: Contact sensitivity to topical corticosteroids. J Am Acad Dermatol **10:**773, 1984.
16. Munto DD: Percutaneous absorption in humans with particular reference to topical steroids and their systemic influence, doctoral dissertation, London, 1975, University of London.
17. May P, Stein EJ, Ryter RJ, Levy P: Cushing's syndrome from percutaneous absorption of triamcinolone cream. Arch Intern Med **136:**612, 1976.
18. Gomez EC, Kaminester L, Frost P: Topical halcinonide cream and betamethasone valerate: effects on plasma cortisol. Arch Dermatol **113:**1196, 1977.
19. Rasmussen JE: Percutaneous absorption of topically applied triamcinolone acetonide in children. Arch Dermatol **114:**1165, 1978.
20. Rasmussen JE: Percutaneous absorption in children. In Year book of dermatology, Chicago, 1979, Year Book Medical Publishers, Inc.
21. Brubaker RF, Halpin JA: Open angle glaucoma associated with topical administration of flurandrenolide to the eye. Mayo Clin Proc **50:**320, 1975.

Chapter Three

Eczema and Hand Dermatitis

Eczema (eczematous inflammation) is the most common inflammatory skin disease. Although the term *dermatitis* is often used when referring to an eczematous eruption, the word means inflammation of the skin and should not be used by itself to designate an eczematous process. Recognizing a rash as eczematous rather than psoriasiform or lichenoid, for example, is of fundamental importance if one is to be effective in diagnosing skin disease. Here as with other skin diseases it is important to look carefully at the rash and determine the primary lesion.

It is essential to recognize the quality and characteristics of the components of eczematous inflammation (erythema, scale, and vesicles) and to determine how these differ from other rashes with similar features. Once familiar with these features, the experienced clinician can recognize a process as being eczematous even in the presence of secondary changes produced by scratching, infection, or irritation. With the diagnosis of eczematous inflammation established, a major part of the diagnostic puzzle has been solved.

There are three stages of eczema: acute, subacute, and chronic. Each represents a stage in the evolution of a dynamic inflammatory process. Clinically, an eczematous disease may start at any stage and evolve into another. Most eczematous diseases, if left alone (that is, neither irritated, scratched, nor medicated), would resolve in time without complication. This ideal situation is almost never realized; scratching, irritation, or attempts at topical treatment are almost inevitable. Itching to some degree is a cardinal feature of eczematous inflammation.

Stages of Eczematous Inflammation

Acute eczematous inflammation

Poison ivy dermatitis is the classic example of acute eczematous inflammation.

Physical findings. The degree of inflammation varies from moderate to intense. A bright red swollen plaque with a pebbly surface evolves in hours. Close examination of the surface reveals tiny clear serum-filled vesicles (Figure 3-1). The eruption may not progress further or it may go on to develop blisters. The vesicles and blisters may be confluent and are often linear. Linear lesions result from dragging the offending agent across the skin with the finger during scratching. The degree of inflammation in cases caused by allergy is directly proportional to the quantity of antigen deposited on the skin. Excoriation predisposes to infection and causes serum, crust, and purulent material to accumulate.

Symptoms. Acute eczema itches intensely. Patients scratch the eruption even while sleeping. A hot shower temporarily relieves itching because the pain produced by hot water is better tolerated than the sensation of itching.

Course. Lesions may begin to appear from hours to 2 to 3 days after exposure and may continue to appear for a week or more. These later occurring, less inflammatory lesions are confusing to the patient, who cannot recall additional exposure. Lesions produced by small amounts of allergen are slower to evolve. They are not produced, as is generally thought, by contact with the serum of ruptured blisters, since the blister fluid does not contain the offending chemical. Acute eczematous inflammation evolves into a subacute stage before resolving.

Etiology. Inflammation is caused by contact with specific allergens such as Rhus (poison ivy, oak, or sumac) and chemicals. In the id reaction vesicular reactions occur at a distant site during or after a fungal infection, stasis dermatitis, or other acute inflammatory processes.

Treatment

Cool wet dressings. The evaporative cooling produced by wet compresses causes vasoconstriction and rapidly suppresses inflammation and itching. Burow's powder, available in a 12-packet box, may be added to the solution to suppress bacterial growth. A clean cotton cloth is soaked in cool water, folded several times, and placed directly over the affected areas (see Table 2-4). Evaporative cooling produces vasoconstriction and decreases serum production; therefore wet compresses should not be held in place and covered with towels or plastic wrap since this prevents evaporation. The wet cloth macerates vesicles and, when removed, mechani-

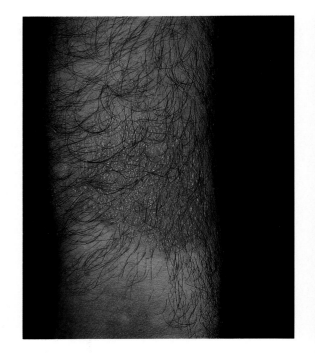

Figure 3-1
Acute eczematous inflammation. Numerous vesicles on an erythematous base. The vesicles may become confluent with time.

cally debrides the area and prevents serum and crust from accumulating. Wet compresses should be removed after 30 minutes and replaced with a freshly soaked cloth. Although it is tempting to leave the drying compress in place and rewet it by pouring solution onto the cloth, irritation may occur from the accumulation of scale, crust, and serum and the increased concentration of aluminum sulfate and calcium acetate, the active ingredients in Burow's powder.

Oral corticosteroids. Oral corticosteroids such as prednisone are useful for controlling intense or wide-spread inflammation and may be used in addition to wet dressings. Prednisone (20 mg twice daily for 7 to 14 days in adults) will control most cases of poison ivy, but prednisone may be started at 20 mg 3 times a day or higher and maintained at that level for 3 to 5 days when treating intense or generalized inflammation. Sometimes 21 days of treatment are required for adequate control. The dosage should not be tapered for these relatively short courses because lower doses may not give the desired anti-inflammatory effect. Inflammation may reappear as diffuse erythema and possibly may be more exten-

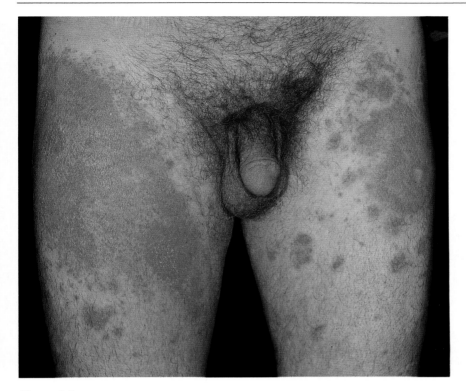

Figure 3-2
*Subacute eczematous inflammation. Erythema
and scaling is present, the surface is dry, and the
borders are indistinct.*

sive if the dose is either too low or tapered too rapidly. Avoid commercially available steroid dose packs because they taper the dosage and treat for too short a time. Topical corticosteroids are of little use in the acute stage because the cream will not penetrate through the vesicles.

Antihistamines. Antihistamines, such as diphenhydramine (Benadryl) and hydroxyzine (Atarax), do not alter the course of the disease, but they relieve itching and provide enough sedation so patients can sleep. They are given every 4 hours as needed.

Antibiotics. The use of oral antibiotics may greatly hasten resolution of the disease if signs of superficial secondary infection such as pustules, purulent material, and crusts are present. Staphylococcus is the usual pathogen and cultures are not routinely necessary. Deep infection (cellulitis) is rare with acute eczema. Oral administration for 6 to 10 days of erythromycin, cephalexin, dicloxacillin, or oxacillin is effective. Topical antibiotics are much less effective.

Subacute eczematous inflammation

Physical findings. Erythema and scale are present in various patterns, usually with indistinct borders. The redness may be faint or very intense (Figure 3-2). Psoriasis, superficial fungal infections, and eczematous inflammation may have a similar appearance. The borders of the plaques of psoriasis and superficial fungal infections are well defined. Psoriatic plaques have a deep rich red color and silvery white scales.

Symptoms. Symptoms vary from no itching to intense itching.

Course. Subacute eczematous inflammation may be the initial stage or it may follow acute inflammation. Irritation, allergy, or infection can convert a subacute process into an acute one. Subacute inflammation will resolve spontaneously without scarring if all sources of irritation and allergy are withdrawn. Excess drying created from washing or continued use of wet dressings will cause cracking and fissures. If excoriation is not controlled, the subacute process can be converted to a chronic one. The differential diagnosis of subacute eczematous inflammation is listed in Table 3-1.[1]

TABLE 3-1

DIFFERENTIAL DIAGNOSIS OF SUBACUTE ECZEMATOUS INFLAMMATION[1]

Allergic contact dermatitis
Asteatotic eczema
Atopic dermatitis
Chapped fissured feet (sweaty sock dermatitis)
Circumileostomy eczema
Diaper dermatitis
Exposure to chemicals

Intertrigo
Irritant contact dermatitis
Irritant hand eczema (Figure 3-3)
Nipple eczema (nursing mothers)
Nummular eczema (Figure 3-4)
Perioral lick eczema
Stasis dermatitis

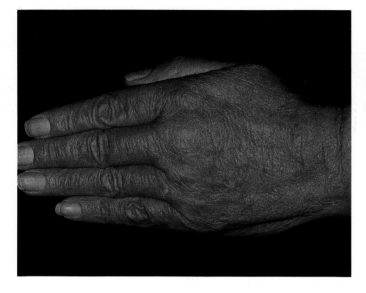

Figure 3-3
Subacute eczematous inflammation of irritant contact dermatitis. Erythema and scaling caused by repeated immersion of the hands in soap and water.

Figure 3-4
Subacute eczematous inflammation. Erythema and scaling in a round or nummular pattern.

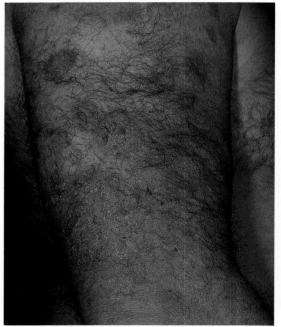

Treatment. It is important to discontinue wet dressings while acute inflammation evolves into subacute inflammation. Excessive drying creates cracking and fissures that predispose to infection.

Topical corticosteroids. These agents are the treatment of choice (see Chapter 2). Creams may be applied 2 to 4 times a day with or without occlusion. Ointments may be applied 2 to 4 times a day for drier lesions. Subacute inflammation requires Groups III through V corticosteroids for rapid control. Occlusion with creams will hasten resolution, and the less expensive, weaker products such as triamcinolone cream 0.1% (Kenalog) will give excellent results.

Lubrication. This is a simple but essential part of therapy. Inflamed skin becomes dry and is more susceptible to further irritation and inflammation. Resolved dry areas may easily relapse into subacute eczema if proper lubrication is neglected. Lubricants are best applied a few hours after topical steroids and should be continued for days or weeks after the inflammation has cleared. Frequent application 3 or 4 times a day should be encouraged. Applying lubricants directly after a shower seals in moisture. Lotions or creams with or without the hydrating chemicals urea and lactic acid may be used. Bath oils are helpful if used in amounts sufficient to make the skin feel oily when the patient leaves the tub.

Lotions. Keri, Lacticare (10% lactic acid), Nutraderm, Nutraplus (10% urea), Shepard's, and Wondra lotions are useful (see Table 2-1).

Creams. Creams such as Nutraderm, Nutraplus (10% urea), Keri, Neutrogena, Nivea, Purpose (4% lactic acid), Eucerin, and Shepard's may be used (see Table 2-1).

Mild soaps. Frequent washing with drying soaps such as Ivory delays healing. Infrequent washing with mild or superfatted soaps, e.g., Dove, Keri, Purpose, Basis (see Table 2-1), should be encouraged. It is usually not necessary to use hypoallergenic soaps or to avoid perfumed soaps. Although allergy to perfumes is possible, the incidence is low.

Antibiotics. Eczematous plaques that remain bright red during treatment with topical steroids may be infected. Infected subacute eczema should be treated with appropriate systemic antibiotics, which are usually those active against staphylococci. Systemic antibiotics are more effective than topical antibiotics or antibiotic-steroid combination creams.

Chronic eczematous inflammation

Physical findings. Chronic eczematous inflammation is a clinical-pathologic entity and does not indicate simply any long-lasting stage of eczema. If scratching is not controlled, subacute eczematous inflammation can be modified and converted to chronic eczematous inflammation. The inflamed area thickens and surface skin marking may become more prominent. Thick plaques with deep parallel skin marking ("washboard lesion") are said to be lichenified (Figure 3-5). The border is well defined but not as sharply as in psoriasis (Figure 3-6). The sites most commonly involved are those areas that are easily reached and associated with habitual scratching (e.g., dorsal feet, lateral forearms, anus, and occipital scalp), areas where eczema tends to be long-lasting (e.g., the lower legs, as in statis dermatitis), and the crease areas (anticubital and popliteal fossa, wrists, and ankles) in atopic dermatitis.

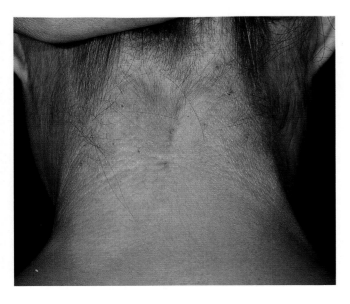

Figure 3-5
Chronic eczematous inflammation. Erythema and scaling are present, and the skin lines are accentuated.

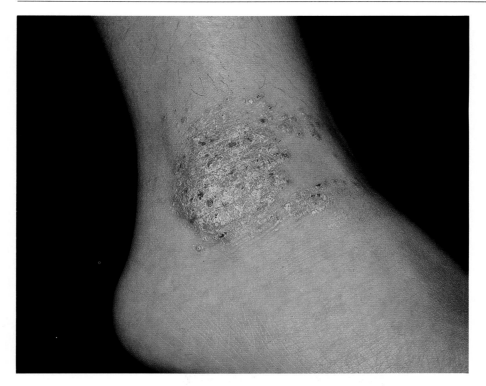

Figure 3-6
Chronic eczematous inflammation. A plaque of lichen simplex chronicus created by excoriation is present. Accentuated skin lines and eczematous papules beyond the border help to differentiate this process from psoriasis.

Symptoms. There is moderate to intense itching. Scratching at times becomes violent, leading to excoriation and digging, and ceases only when pain has replaced the itch. Patients with chronic inflammation scratch while asleep.

Course. Scratching and rubbing become habitual and are often done unconsciously. The disease then becomes self-perpetuating. Scratching leads to thickening of the skin, which itches more than before. It is this habitual manipulation that causes the difficulty in eradicating the disease. Some patients enjoy the feeling of relief that comes from scratching and may actually desire the reappearance of their disease after treatment.

Etiology. Chronic eczematous inflammation may follow subacute inflammation or it may be caused by lichen simplex chronicus or prurigo nodularis.

Treatment. Chronic eczematous inflammation is resistant to treatment and requires potent steroid therapy.

Topical steroids. Groups II to V topical steroids are used with occlusion each night until clear—

usually 1 to 3 weeks. Group I or II topical steroids should be applied 2 to 4 times daily by simple application in areas where occlusion is difficult.

Intralesional injection. Intralesional injection (Kenalog, 10 mg/cc) is an effective mode of therapy. Lesions that have been present for years may completely resolve after one injection or a short series of injections. The medicine is delivered with a 27-gauge needle and the entire plaque is infiltrated until it blanches white. Resistant plaques require additional injections given at 3- to 4-week intervals.

Excision. Although rarely necessary, excision should be considered if multiple intralesional injections fail and if the lesion is very hypertrophic.

Prurigo nodularis is resistant to treatment. Intralesional steroids, excision, or cryosurgery with liquid nitrogen may be considered.

Hand Eczema

Inflammation of the hands is one of the most common problems encountered by the dermatologist. Hand dermatitis causes discomfort and embarrassment and, because of its location, interferes significantly with normal daily activities. Hand dermatitis is common in industrial occupations: it can threaten job security if inflammation cannot be controlled. The diagnosis and management of hand eczema is a challenge. Not only are there many

TABLE 3-2

HAND DERMATITIS: DIFFERENTIAL DIAGNOSIS AND DISTRIBUTION

Location	Redness and scaling	Vesicles	Pustules

Back of hand	Atopic dermatitis
	Irritant contact dermatitis
	Lichen simplex
	   chronicus
	Nummular eczema
	Psoriasis
	Tinea
		Id reaction
		Scabies (web
		   spaces)
			Bacterial infection
			Psoriasis
			Scabies (web
			   spaces)
			Tinea

Palmar surface	Fingertip eczema Hyperkeratotic eczema Keratolysis exfoliativa Psoriasis Tinea	Allergic contact dermatitis Dyshidrosis	Bacterial infection Dyshidrosis Psoriasis

patterns of eczematous inflammation (Table 3-2), but there are other disease entities, such as psoriasis, that may appear eczematous. The original primary lesions and their distribution become modified with time by irritants, excoriation, infection, and treatment. All stages of eczematous inflammation may be encountered in hand eczema.

Irritant contact dermatitis

Irritant hand dermatitis (housewives' eczema, dishpan hands, detergent hands) is the most common type of hand inflammation. Some people can withstand long periods of repeated exposure to various chemicals and maintain normal skin. At the other end of the spectrum, there are those who develop chapping and eczema from simple hand washing. Those patients whose hands are easily irritated may have the atopic diathesis.

Pathophysiology. The stratum corneum is the protective envelope that prevents exogenous material from entering the skin and body water from escaping. The stratum corneum is composed of dead cells, lipids (from sebum and cellular debris), and water-binding organic chemicals. The stratum corneum of the palms is thicker than the dorsa and is more resistant to irritation. The pH of this surface layer is slightly acidic. Environmental factors or elements that change any component of the stratum corneum will interfere with its protective function and expose the skin to irritants. Factors such as cold winter air and low humidity promote water loss. Substances such as organic solvents and alkaline soaps extract water-binding chemicals and lipids. Once enough of these protective elements have been extracted, eczematous inflammation may occur.

Clinical presentation. The degree of inflammation depends on factors such as strength and concentration of the chemical, individual susceptibility, site of contact, and time of year. Allergy, infection, scratching, and stress will modify the picture.

Stages of inflammation. Dryness and chapping are the initial changes of irritant hand dermatitis (Figure 3-7). Extremely painful cracks and fissures

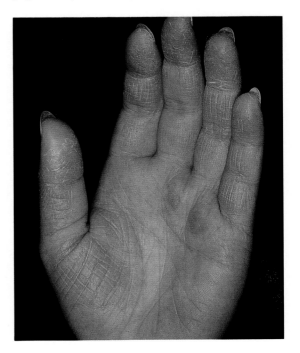

Figure 3-7
Early irritant hand dermatitis with dryness and chapping.

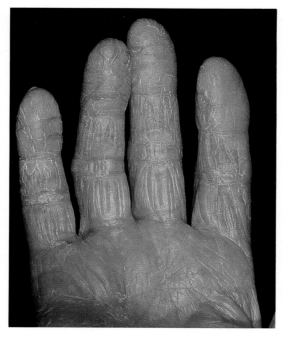

Figure 3-8
Irritant hand dermatitis. Subacute eczematous inflammation with severe drying and splitting of the fingertips.

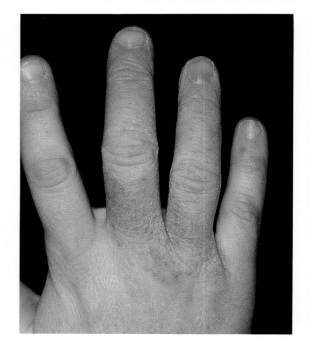

Figure 3-9
Irritant hand dermatitis. Subacute eczematous inflammation appeared on the dry, chapped third and fourth fingers.

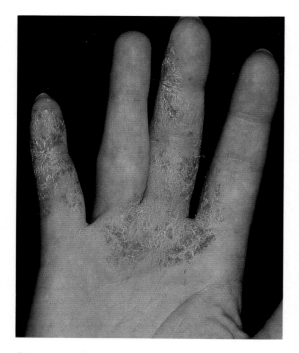

Figure 3-10
Irritant hand dermatitis. Numerous tiny vesicles suddenly appeared on these chronically inflamed fingers.

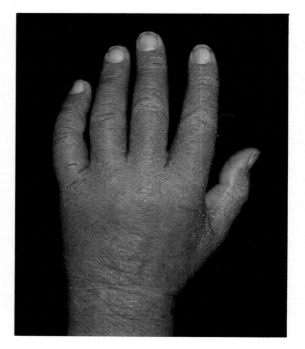

Figure 3-11
Severe irritant dermatitis. Numerous vesicles are present on all surfaces of the hand. The skin is red, infected, and oozes serum.

TABLE 3-3

IRRITANT HAND DERMATITIS: INSTRUCTIONS FOR PATIENTS

1. Wash hands as infrequently as possible. Ideally, soap should be avoided and hands simply washed in lukewarm water.
2. Shampooing must be done with rubber gloves or by someone else.
3. Avoid direct contact with household cleaners and detergents. Wear cotton, plastic, or rubber gloves when doing housework.
4. Do not touch or do anything that causes burning or itching (e.g., wool; wet diapers; peeling potatoes or handling fresh fruits, vegetables, and raw meat).
5. Wear rubber gloves when irritants are encountered. Rubber gloves alone are not sufficient because the lining collects sweat, scales, and debris and can become more irritating than those objects to be avoided. Dermal white cotton gloves should be worn next to the skin under unlined rubber gloves. Several pairs of cotton gloves should be purchased so they can be changed frequently. Try on the rubber gloves over the white cotton gloves at the time of purchase to make sure of a comfortable fit.

occur, particularly in joint crease areas and around the fingertips. Then the backs of the hands become red, swollen and tender. The palmar surface, especially the fingers, becomes red and continues to be dry and cracked. A red, smooth, shiny, delicate surface that splits easily with the slightest trauma may develop. These are subacute eczematous changes (Figures 3-8 and 3-9).

Acute eczematous inflammation occurs with further irritation causing vesicles to ooze and crust. Itching intensifies and excoriation leads to infection (Figure 3-10). Finally, necrosis and ulceration followed by scarring will occur if the irritating chemical is too caustic (Figure 3-11).

Patients at risk. Individuals at risk include mothers with young children (changing diapers), individuals whose jobs require repeated wetting and drying (e.g., surgeons, dentists, dishwashers, bartenders, fishermen), industrial workers whose jobs require contact with chemicals (e.g., cutting oils), patients with scabies who use Kwell repeatedly, and patients with the atopic diathesis.

Treatment. The inflammation is treated as outlined earlier in this chapter under Stages of Eczematous Inflammation. Lubrication and avoidance of further irritation aids in preventing recurrence. A program of irritant avoidance should be carefully outlined for each patient (Table 3-3).[2]

Atopic hand dermatitis

Hand dermatitis may be the most common form of adult atopic dermatitis (see Chapter 5, Atopic Dermatitis). Patients susceptible to this type of dermatitis have a lower threshold for developing eczematous inflammation when exposed to irritants. The backs of the hands, particularly near the finger webs, are affected (Figure 3-12). The dermatitis be-

gins as a typical irritant reaction with chapping and erythema. Atopic dermatitis in the form of subacute and chronic eczematous inflammation with lichenification appears and is intensified by scratching. Atopic hand eczema is managed like irritant hand eczema.

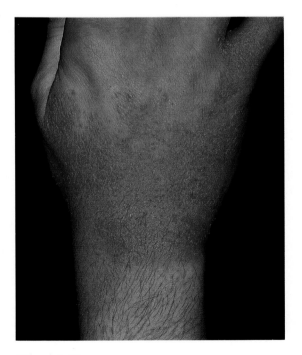

Figure 3-12
Irritant hand dermatitis in a patient with the atopic diathesis. Irritant eczema of the backs of the hands is a common form of adult atopic dermatitis.

Allergic contact dermatitis

Allergic contact dermatitis of the hands is not as common as irritant dermatitis. However, allergy as a possible cause of hand eczema, no matter what the pattern, should always be considered in the differential diagnosis; it may be investigated by patch testing in appropriate cases. The incidence of allergy in hand eczema was demonstrated by patch testing in a study of 220 patients with hand eczema.[3] In 12% of the 220 patients, the diagnosis was established with the aid of a standard screening series now available in a modified form from the American Academy of Dermatology.[4] Another 5% of the cases were diagnosed as a result of testing with additional allergens. The hand eczema in these two groups (17%) changed dramatically after identification and avoidance of the allergens found by patch testing. Table 3-4 lists some possible causes of allergic hand dermatitis.[5]

Physical findings. The diagnosis of allergic contact dermatitis is obvious when the area of inflammation corresponds exactly to the area covered by the allergin (e.g., a round patch of eczema under a watch or inflammation in the shape of a sandal strap on the foot). Similar clues may be present with hand eczema, but in many cases allergic and irritant hand eczemas cannot be distinguished by their clinical presentation. Hand inflammation, whatever the source, is modified by further exposure to irritating chemicals, washing, scratching, medication, and infection. Inflammation of the dorsum of the hand is more often irritant or atopic than allergic.

Treatment. Allergy may be seen as acute, subacute, or chronic eczematous inflammation and is managed accordingly.

Nummular eczema

Eczema that appears as one or several coin-shaped plaques is called nummular eczema. This pattern often occurs on the extremities but may appear as hand eczema. The plaques are usually confined to the backs of the hand (Figure 3-13). The number of lesions may increase, but once established they tend to remain the same size. The inflammation is either acute, subacute, or chronic and itching is moderate to intense. The cause is unknown. Thick chronic scaling plaques of nummular eczema look like psoriasis. The disease is treated as acute, subacute, or chronic eczema.

Lichen simplex chronicus

A localized plaque of chronic eczematous inflammation that is created by habitual scratching is called lichen simplex chronicus or localized neurodermatitis. The back of the wrist is a typical site. The plaque is thick with prominent skin lines (lichenification) and the margins are fairly sharp. Once established, the plaque does not usually increase in area. This is treated in the same manner as chronic eczematous inflammation.

Keratolysis exfoliativa

Keratolysis exfoliativa is a common chronic asymptomatic noninflammatory bilateral peeling of the palms of the hand and soles of the feet of unknown cause (Figure 3-14). The eruption is most common during summer months and is often associated with sweaty palms and soles.[6] Some people experience this phenomenon only once, whereas others have repeated episodes. Scaling starts simultaneously from several points on the palms or soles with 2 to 3 mm of round scale that appears to have originated from a ruptured vesicle; however, these vesicles are never seen. The scale continues to peel and extend peripherally, forming larger roughly circular areas that resemble ringworm, while the central area becomes slightly red and tender. The scaling borders may coalesce. The condition resolves in 1 to 3 weeks and requires no therapy other than lubrication.

TABLE 3-4

ALLERGIC HAND DERMATITIS: SOME POSSIBLE CAUSES

Allergens	Sources
Nickel	Door knobs, handles on kitchen utensils, scissors, knitting needles, industrial equipment, hair dressing equipment
Potassium dichromate	Cement, leather articles (gloves), industrial machines, oils
Rubber	Gloves, industrial equipment (hoses, belts, cables)
Fragrances	Cosmetics, soaps, lubricants, topical medications
Formaldehyde	Wash and wear fabrics, paper, cosmetics, embalming fluid
Lanolin	Topical lubricants and medications, cosmetics

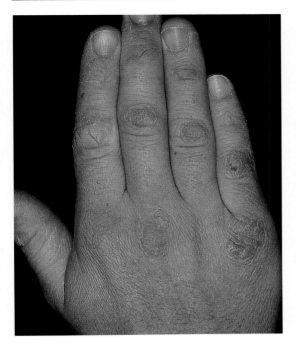

Figure 3-13
Nummular eczema. Eczematous plaques are round (coin-shaped).

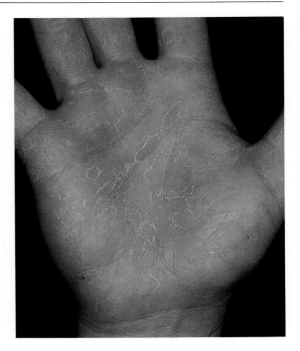

Figure 3-14
Keratolysis exfoliativa. Noninflammatory peeling of the palms that is often associated with sweating. The eruption must be differentiated from tinea of the palms.

Figure 3-15
Fingertip eczema may have a variety of causes. The skin is extremely dry and peels continuously, revealing a red, cracked, smooth surface.

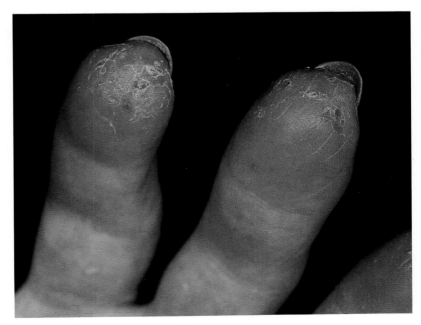

Fingertip eczema

An extremely dry chronic form of eczema of the palmar surface of the fingertips may be the result of an allergic reaction (e.g., plant bulbs, resins)[7] or may occur in children and adults as an isolated phenomenon of unknown cause (Figure 3-15). One finger or several may be involved. The skin peels from the tips distally, exposing a very dry, red, cracked, fissured, tender, or painful surface without skin lines. The process usually stops shortly before the distal interphalangeal joint is reached. Fingertip eczema may last for months or years and is resistant to treatment. Topical steroids with or without occlusion give only temporary relief. Once allergy and psoriasis have been ruled out, fingertip eczema should be managed as subacute and chronic eczema, by avoiding irritants and lubricating frequently. Tar (T-Derm, Fototar) applied twice daily has, at times, provided relief.

Hyperkeratotic eczema

An extremely thick, chronic form of eczema that occurs on the palms and occasionally the soles is seen almost exclusively in men. One or several plaques of yellow-brown dense scale increase in thickness and form deep interconnecting cracks over the surface, similar to mud drying in a river bed (Figure 3-16). The dense scale, unlike callus, is moist below the surface and is not easily pared with a blade. Patients discover that the scale is firmly adherent to the epidermis when they attempt to peel off the thick scale and expose tender bleeding areas of dermis. Hyperkeratotic eczema may result from allergy or excoriation and irritation, but in most cases the cause is not apparent. The disease is chronic and may last for years. Psoriasis and lichen simplex chronicus must be considered in the differential diagnosis. The disease is treated like chronic eczema; although the plaques respond to Group II steroid cream and occlusion, recurrences are frequent. Patch testing is indicated for recurrent disease.

Dyshidrosis

Dyshidrosis (pompholyx) is a distinctive reaction pattern confined to the palms and soles. Moderate to severe itching precedes the appearance of vesicles on the palms and sides of the fingers. The palms may be red and wet with perspiration—therefore the name dyshidrosis, which implies, incorrectly, an abnormality of sweating (Figure 3-17). The vesicles slowly disappear in 3 to 4 weeks and are replaced by 1- to 3-mm rings of scale (Figure 3-18). Waves of vesiculation may appear for an indefinite period. Irritation or attempts at treatment may induce subacute or chronic eczematous inflammation. Pustular psoriasis of the palms and soles may resemble dyshidrosis, but the vesicles of psoriasis

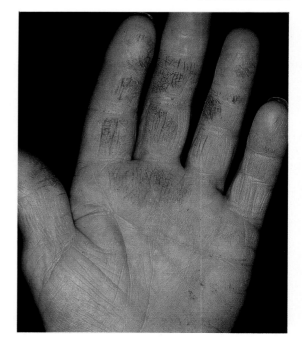

Figure 3-16
Hyperkeratotic eczema. Patches of dense yellow-brown scale occur on the palms. This patient was allergic to a steering wheel.

rapidly become cloudy with purulent fluid, and pain, rather than itching, is the chief complaint. Pustular psoriasis is chronic and the pustules do not evolve and disappear as rapidly as those of dyshidrosis. The cause of dyshidrosis is unknown, but there does seem to be some relationship to stress. There is no abnormality of eccrine sweating. Patients with atopic dermatitis are affected as frequently as others. The eruption is treated as is acute eczematous inflammation. Speculation that dyshidrosis is an allergic response to nickle ingestion has prompted attempts at control with elimination diets, but the results have been disappointing.

Id reaction

Intense inflammatory processes such as active stasis dermatitis or acute fungal infections of the feet can be accompanied by an itchy dyshidrotic-like vesicular eruption ("id reaction") (Figure 3-19). They are most common on the sides of the fingers, but may be generalized. The eruption resolves as the inflammation that initiated it resolves. The id reaction may be an allergic reaction to fungi or some antigen created during the inflammatory process. Incorrectly, almost all dyshidrotic eruptions are

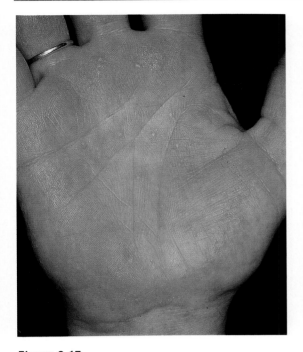

Figure 3-17
Dyshidrosis (pompholyx). The palms are red and wet with perspiration, and numerous vesicles are present.

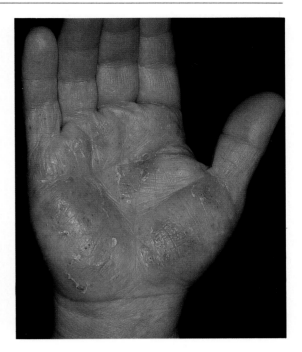

Figure 3-18
Dyshidrosis. The acute process ends as the skin peels, revealing a red, cracked base with brown spots. The brown spots are sites of previous vesiculation.

Figure 3-19
Id reaction. An acute vesicular eruption most often seen on the lateral aspects of the fingers.

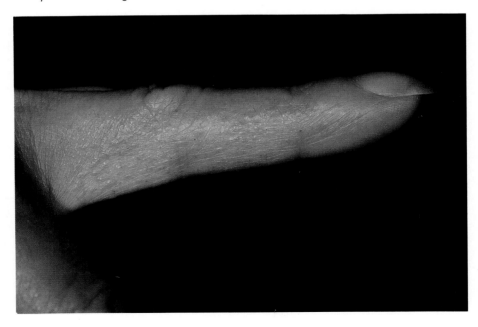

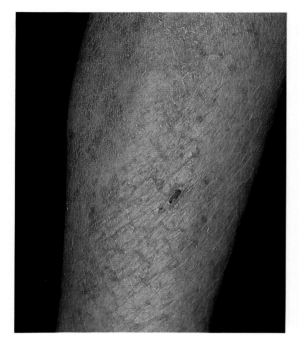

Figure 3-20
Asteatotic eczema (xerosis). The skin is extremely dry, cracked, and scaly.

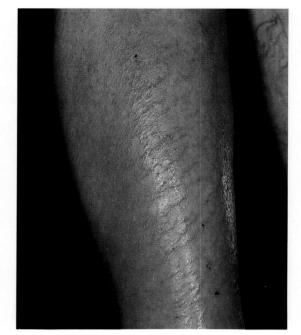

Figure 3-21
Asteatotic eczema. The cracked porcelain or "crazy paving" pattern.

called id reactions. The diagnosis of an id reaction should not be made unless there is an inflammatory process at a distant site and the id reaction disappears shortly after the inflammation is controlled.

Asteatotic Eczema

Asteatotic eczema (eczema craquelé) occurs after excess drying, especially during the winter months and among the elderly. Patients with the atopic diathesis are more likely to develop this distinctive pattern. The eruption can occur on any skin area, but it is most commonly seen on the anterolateral aspects of the lower legs. The lower legs become dry and scaly and show accentuation of the skin lines (xerosis) (Figure 3-20). Red plaques with thin, long, horizontal superficial fissures appear with further drying and scratching. Similar patterns of inflammation may appear on the trunk and upper extremities as the winter progresses. A cracked porcelain or "crazy paving" pattern of fissuring develops when short vertical fissures connect with the horizontal fissures (Figure 3-21). The term eczema craquelé is appropriately used to describe this pattern. The most severe form of this type of eczema shows an accentuation of the above pattern with deep wide horizontal fissures that ooze and are often purulent. Here pain, rather than itching, is the chief complaint.

Scratching or treatment with drying lotions such as calamine aggravates the eczematous inflammation and leads to infection with accumulation of crusts and purulent material (Figure 3-22).

Treatment. The initial stages are treated as subacute eczematous inflammation, although the most severe form may have to be treated as acute eczema. The treatment involves wet compresses and antibiotics to remove crust and suppress infection before topical steroids and lubricants are applied. Lubricating the dry skin during and after topical steroid use is essential. Avoid the use of oral steroids, because the disease will flare within a day or two once they are discontinued.

Nummular Eczema

Nummular eczema is a common disease of unknown cause occurring primarily in the middle-aged and elderly. The typical lesion is a round, coin-shaped red plaque that averages 1 to 5 cm in diameter (Figure 3-23). The lesions itch and scratching often becomes habitual. In these cases, the term nummular neurodermatitis has been used. With infection, the plaque becomes thicker and vesicles appear on the surface; in ringworm the vesicles, if present, are at the border (Figure 3-24). Unlike the thick silvery scale of psoriasis, this scale

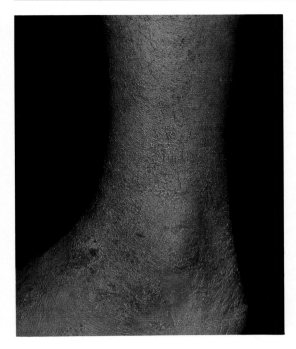

Figure 3-22
Severe asteatotic eczema with secondary infection.

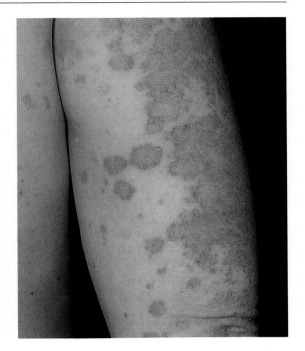

Figure 3-23
Nummular eczema. Round, eczematous plaques are of undetermined etiology.

Figure 3-24
Nummular eczema. Round, eczematous plaques are in a more acute stage than illustrated in Fig. 3-23.

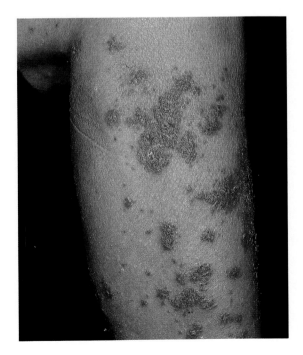

is thin and sparse, and the erythema of psoriasis is darker. Once nummular eczema is established, lesions may become more numerous, but individual ones tend to remain in the same area and do not increase in size. The disease is worse in the winter. The back of the hand is the most commonly involved site; usually only one lesion or a few lesions are present (see Figure 3-13). Other frequently involved areas are the extensor aspects of the forearms and lower legs and the flanks and hips. Lesions at these other sites tend to be more numerous. An extensive form of the disease can occur suddenly in patients with dry skin who are exposed to an irritating medicine or chemicals or those who have an active eczematous process at another site, such as stasis dermatitis on the lower legs. The lesions in these cases are round, faintly erythematous, dry, cracked, superficial, and usually confluent.

The course is variable, but it is usually chronic, with some cases resisting all attempts at treatment. Many cases become inactive after several months. Lesions may reappear at previously involved sites in recurrent cases.

Treatment. Treatment depends on the stage of activity; all stages of eczematous inflammation may be present simultaneously. The red vesicular lesions are treated as acute, the red scaling plaques as subacute, and the habitually scratched thick plaques as chronic eczematous inflammation.

Stasis Dermatitis and Ulceration

Stasis dermatitis is an eczematous eruption that occurs on the lower legs in some patients with venous insufficiency. The dermatitis may be acute, subacute, or chronic and recurrent, and it may be accompanied by ulceration. Most patients with venous insufficiency do not develop dermatitis, suggesting that genetic or environmental factors may play a role. The reason for its occurrence is unknown. Some have speculated that it represents an allergic response to an epidermal protein antigen created through increased hydrostatic pressure, whereas others feel that the skin has been compromised and is more susceptible to irritation and trauma.[8] Patients with stasis dermatitis have significantly more positive reactions when patch-tested with components of previously used topical agents.[9] Topical medications that contain potential sensitizers such as lanolin, benzocaine, parabens, and neomycin should be avoided by patients with stasis disease.

Venous insufficiency followed by edema is the fundamental change that predisposes to dermatitis and ulceration. Venous insufficiency occurs when venous return in the deep, perforating, or superficial veins is impaired by vein dilatation and valve dysfunction. Deep vein thrombophlebitis, which may have been asymptomatic at an earlier time, is the most frequent precursor of lower leg venous insufficiency. Perforating veins that carry venous blood from the superficial to the deep system dilate and become incompetent as blood pools in the deep system. The largest are posterior and superior to the lateral and medial malleoli. This is the same area where dermatitis and ulceration are most prevalent. Superficial varicosities alone are unlikely to produce venous insufficiency. Impairment of venous return leads to increased hydrostatic pressure, interstitial fluid accumulation, and edema. The edema is pitting and disappears at night with elevation. Chronic edema, trauma, infection, and inflammation lead to subcutaneous tissue fibrosis, giving the skin a firm, non-pitting, "woody" quality. Fat necrosis may follow thrombosis of small veins, which may be the most important underlying change that predisposes to ulceration. Recurrent ulceration and fat necrosis are associated with loss of subcutaneous tissue and a decrease in lower leg circumference. Advanced disease is represented by an "inverted bottle leg," in which the proximal leg swells from chronic venous obstruction and the lower leg shrinks from chronic ulceration and fat necrosis. Venous hydrostatic pressure and edema must be decreased by surgery or external compression to prevent recurrent dermatitis and ulceration. The stages in the evolution of the disease are discussed below.

Subacute inflammation. Subacute inflammation usually begins in the winter months when the legs become dry and scaly. Brown staining on the skin (hemosiderin) may have been slowly appearing for months. The pigment is iron left after disintegration of red blood cells that leaked out of veins because of increased hydrostatic pressure. Scratching induces first subacute and then chronic eczematous inflammation (Figure 3-25). Attempts at self-treatment with drying lotions (calamine) or potential sensitizers (e.g., neomycin-containing topical medicines) exacerbate and prolong the inflammation.

Acute inflammation. A red, superficial, itchy plaque may suddenly appear on the lower leg. This acute process may be eczematous inflammation, cellulitis, or both. Weeping and crusts appear. A vesicular eruption (id reaction) on the palms, trunk, or extremities sometimes accompanies this acute inflammation. The inflammation responds to antibiotics and measures to control acute and chronic subacute eczematous inflammation. The id reaction resolves spontaneously as the primary site improves.

Figure 3-25
*Stasis dermatitis in an early stage. Erythema and
erosions produced by excoriations are shown.*

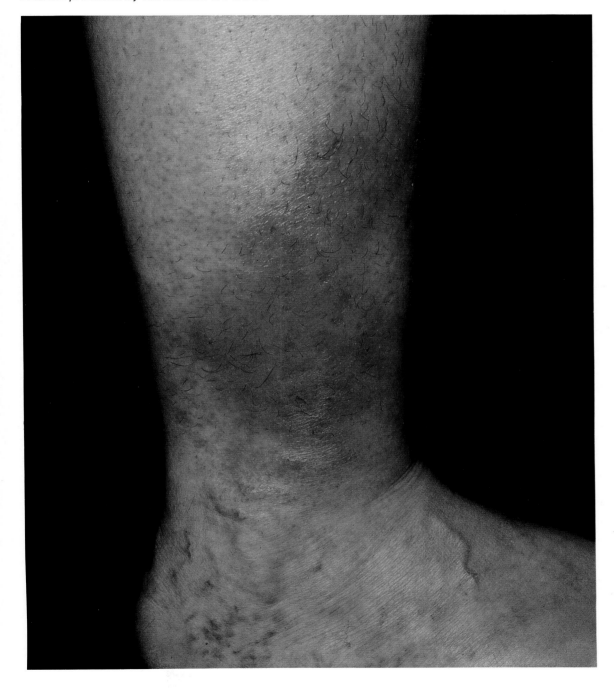

Chronic inflammation. Recurrent attacks of inflammation eventually compromise the poorly vascularized area, and the disease becomes chronic and recurrent. The typical presentation is a cyanotic red plaque over the medial malleolus. Fibrosis following chronic inflammation leads to permanent skin thickening. The skin surface in these irreversibly changed areas may have a bumpy cobblestone appearance that results from fibrosis and venous and lymph stasis. The skin remains thickened and diffusely dark brown (postinflammatory hyperpigmentation) during quiescent periods.

Ulceration and scarring. Ulceration is almost inevitable once the skin has been thickened and circulation is compromised. Ulceration may occur spontaneously or after the slightest trauma (Figure 3-26). The ulcer may remain quite small or may enlarge rapidly without any further trauma. A dull constant pain that improves with leg elevation is present in the area of the ulcer. Pain from ischemic ulcers is more intense and does not improve with elevation. The ulcers have a sharp or sloping border and may be deep or superficial. Removal of crust and debris reveals a moist base with granulation tissue. The base and surrounding skin is usually infected. Healing is slow, requiring several weeks or months. After healing, it is not uncommon to see ulcers rapidly recur. The ulcers are replaced with ivory-white sclerotic scars. Except for pain and the inconvenience of treatment, most patients tolerate this disease well and remain ambulatory.

Treatment

Topical steroids and wet dressings. The early dry superficial stage is managed as subacute eczematous inflammation. Oral antibiotics (usually those active against staphylococci) will hasten resolution if cellulitis is present. Moist exudative inflammation and moist ulcers respond to tepid wet compresses of Burow's solution or silver nitrate (0.25%) applied for 30 to 60 minutes several times a day. Wet dressings suppress bacteria and inflammation while debriding the ulcer. Adherent crust may be carefully freed with blunt-tipped scissors. Group V topical steroids are applied to eczematous skin at the periphery of the ulcer. Patients must be warned that steroid creams placed on the ulcer will stop the healing process. Elevation of the legs encourages healing.

Debrisan Wound Cleaning Beads. Debrisan beads are supplied in sterile containers of 25, 60, and 120 gm and in 4-gm packets. They are 0.1 to 0.3 mm in diameter; because of their molecular structure, they absorb low molecular weight (less than 1000) substances and possibly bacteria but not plasma proteins and fibrin. The ability of unsaturated beads to remove exudates rapidly and continuously from the ulcer results in a reduction of inflammation and edema.[10] The beads are not effective for cleaning dry ulcers and should be discontinued once healthy granulation tissue appears. The dry beads are poured directly into the ulcer at least one-quarter-inch thickness and covered with a dry dressing. A color change in the beads indicates saturation, and the beads should be washed out by irrigation or in a whirlpool and replaced with dry beads. The process is repeated until the wound is dry. Patients can be ambulatory during treatment and healing time is significantly decreased.

Benzoyl peroxide. Benzoyl peroxide, a powerful oxidizing agent commonly used for treating acne, has been shown to shorten the healing time of stasis ulcers by promoting the rapid development of healthy granulation tissue and the quick ingrowth of epithelium.[11] The slow sustained release of oxygen by benzoyl peroxide is thought to be responsible for its success. Possible complications are irritant or allergic contact dermatitis to benzoyl peroxide. A dressing is cut from sterile terrycloth to fit the ulcer exactly. It should be moistened with saline and saturated with benzoyl peroxide lotion (Benoxyl 10) or a 20% concentration prepared by the pharmacist by adding two Benzie-Paks to a 30 cc bottle of Benoxyl-10. Benzie-Paks contain benzoyl peroxide powder and are packaged with Dermik Laboratories products such as Vanoxide. A protective ointment (such as Desiten) is then applied to a wide area bordering the ulcer. Plastic film such as Saran Wrap is placed over the ulcer dressing and taped firmly in place with hypoallergenic adhesive tape such as Dermacel. The dressing is changed at 8- or 12-hour intervals. Exuberant granulation tissue is kept below the epidermal level with cauterization by a silver nitrate stick to facilitate ingrowth of epithelium.

External compression. Elimination of edema is essential during treatment and after resolution of the ulcer and dermatitis. This is accomplished by external compression by one of the following methods.

Unna boot (hard cast). A commercially available Unna paste boot (Dome paste bandage, Gelocast bandage) impregnated with zinc oxide paste may be applied soon after acute inflammation has subsided. Since the boot will not eliminate existing edema fluid, it should be applied in the morning after edema has drained.[12] At home on the morning of the day when the boot is to be applied, a gauze is placed over the ulcer and a rubberized Ace bandage is firmly wrapped in a pressure gradient fashion with greatest pressure at the ankle and the least at the knee. The patient then comes directly to the physician's office. The Ace bandage is removed, the skin is cleansed and the ulcer, if present, is debrided. A Group V topical steroid is applied to the surrounding skin if inflammation is present and lubricating creams are applied to normal skin. The Unna boot is applied, as the instructions in each

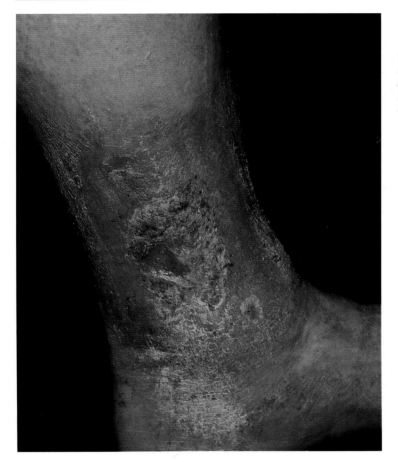

Figure 3-26
Stasis dermatitis. The skin is diffusely red, thickened, and bound down by fibrosis. Ulceration occurs with the slightest trauma.

box indicate, in layers starting behind the first metatarsal to just below the knee. Be careful not to fold or crease the bandage during application. In about 1 hour the moist bandage will dry to form a firm cast. The cast may be left exposed or wrapped with an Ace bandage to protect the other leg from abrasion with the hard cast. The boot is changed every 7 to 10 days or more frequently, if drainage from the ulcer penetrates through the boot. After healing, elastic Ace bandages are applied each morning indefinitely to prevent dependent edema.

Ace bandage and foam rubber compression. This technique is valuable for older patients who may not tolerate wearing a boot for a week; it may be applied by the patient or by a visiting nurse. Sponge rubber of the type used in furniture is more absorbent than commercially available closed cell foam rubber. The one-quarter to one-half inch thick foam rubber must be clean, but sterilization is not necessary. The rubber is shaped with scissors to extend about 3 inches beyond the ulcer margin and is beveled at the edge to avoid pressure at the margin. It is then placed over the ulcer and the ace bandage is applied in the usual pressure-gradient fashion. The rubber absorbs exudate and should be changed every 24 to 72 hours.

Custom-made support stockings (Jobst). Once ulcers have healed, lower leg compression in a pressure-gradient fashion can be maintained by a custom-fitted compression stocking. Measurements of the circumference at several points on the leg are made and are preserved on paper tape in the measuring kit provided by the Jobst Company. The measurements are taken after edema has drained following leg elevation. The amount of compression can be specified by the physician. Patients with chronic venous insufficiency who have had stasis dermatitis or ulceration require a compression of between 35-40 mm Hg. Various lengths can be purchased, but an above-the-knee length stocking may give the best results. The stockings are very difficult to apply and must be replaced periodically since they stretch. Firmly applied Ace bandages provide the same function and are inexpensive. Stockings that are not custom fitted are of little use.

Figure 3-27
Lichen simplex chronicus. This localized plaque of chronic eczematous inflammation was created by rubbing with the opposite heel.

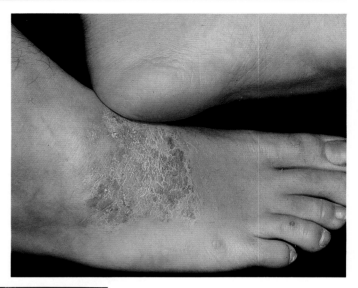

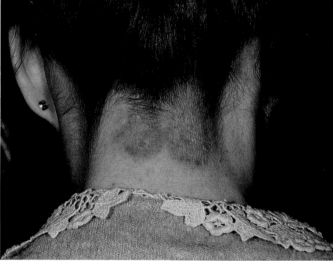

Figure 3-28
Lichen simplex nuchae occurs almost exclusively in women who scratch the back of their neck in stressful situations.

Figure 3-29
Lichen simplex chronicus of the scrotum. The skin is thickened and skin lines are accentuated, unlike the adjacent scrotal skin.

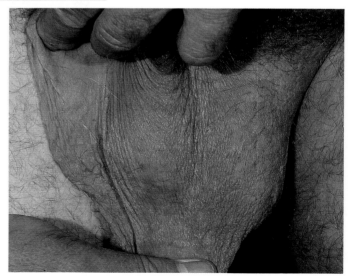

Lichen Simplex Chronicus

Lichen simplex chronicus (Figures 3-27 through 3-30) or circumscribed neurodermatitis is an eczematous eruption that is created by habitual scratching of a single localized area. The disease is more common in adults but may be seen in children. The areas most commonly affected, which are those conveniently reached, are listed in Table 3-5 in approximate order of frequency. Patients derive great pleasure in the relief that comes with frantically scratching the inflamed site. Loss of this pleasurable sensation or continued subconscious habitual scratching may explain why this eruption frequently recurs.

A typical plaque stays localized and shows little tendency to enlarge with time. Red papules coalesce to form a red, scaly, thick plaque with accentuation of skin lines (lichenification). Lichen simplex chronicus is a chronic eczematous disease, but acute changes may result from sensitization with topical medication. Moist scale, serum, crust, and pustules are signs of infection.

Lichen simplex nuchae occurs almost exclusively in women who reach for the back of the neck during stressful situations (Figure 3-28). Here the disease may spread beyond the initial well-defined plaque. Diffuse dry or moist scale, crust, and erosions extend into the posterior scalp beyond the neck. Secondary infection is common. In constant pickers, nodules are usually less than 1 cm and scattered randomly in the scalp; few nodules or many may be present.

Treatment. The patient must first understand that the rash will not clear until even minor scratching and rubbing is stopped. Scratching frequently takes place during sleep and the affected area may have to be covered. Lichen simplex chronicus is chronic eczema and is treated as outlined in the section on eczematous inflammation. Treatment of the anal area or the fold behind the ear does not require potent topical steroids as do other forms of

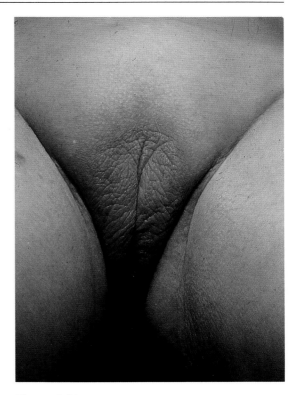

Figure 3-30
Lichen simplex chronicus of the vulva. The skin lines are markedly accentuated.

lichen simplex; rather, these intertriginous areas will respond to Group V or VI topical steroids. Lichen simplex nuchae, because of its location, is difficult to treat. Dry inflammation that extends into the scalp may be treated with a Group II steroid gel such as Topsyn applied twice daily. Moist secondarily infected areas respond to oral antibiotics and topical steroid lotions. A 2- to 3-week course of prednisone

---

TABLE 3-5

LICHEN SIMPLEX CHRONICUS: AREAS MOST COMMONLY AFFECTED LISTED IN APPROXIMATE ORDER OF FREQUENCY

Outer lower portion of lower leg	Scrotum (Figure 3-29), vulva (Figure 3-30),
Wrists and ankles (Figure 3-27)	anal area, pubis
Back (lichen simplex nuchae) and	Upper eyelids
side of neck (Figure 3-28)	Orifice of the ear
Extensor forearms near elbow	Fold behind the ear
Scalp-picker's nodules	

(20 mg twice daily) should be considered when an extensively inflamed scalp does not respond rapidly to topical treatment. Picker's nodules may be resistant to treatment, requiring monthly intralesional injections with triamcinolone acetonide (10 mg/ml, Kenalog 10 injection).

Prurigo Nodularis

Prurigo nodularis is a rare disease of unknown cause that may be considered a nodular form of lichen simplex chronicus. It resembles picker's nodules of the scalp except that the few to 20 or more nodules are randomly distributed on the extensor aspects of the arms and legs (Figure 3-31). They are created by repeated scratching. The nodules are red or brown, hard, and dome-shaped with a smooth, crusted, or warty surface; they measure 1 to 2 cm in diameter. Complaints of pruritis vary; some patients claim there is no itching and that scratching is only habitual, whereas others complain pruritis is intense.

Treatment. Prurigo nodularis is resistant to treatment and lasts indefinitely. As with picker's nodules of the scalp, repeated intralesional steroid injections may be necessary for control. Excision of individual nodules is sometimes helpful. Cryosurgery is sometimes successful.

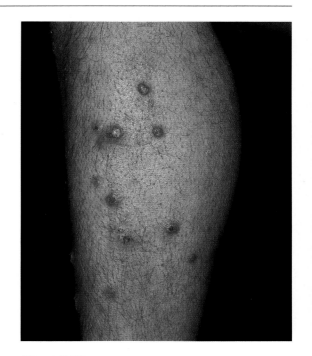

Figure 3-31
Prurigo nodularis. Thick, hard nodules usually present on the extensor surfaces of the forearms and legs result from chronic picking.

Chapped Fissured Feet

Chapped fissured feet (sweaty sock dermatitis,[13] peridigital dermatitis[14] in children) are seen only in children and may begin at about age 2. The tendency to severe chapping declines with age and is gone around the age of puberty. Onset is in early fall when the weather becomes cold, and heavy socks and impermeable shoes or boots are worn. An artificial intertrigo, as in diaper dermatitis, is created when moist socks are kept in contact with the soles. The skin in pressure areas, toes, and metatarsal regions becomes dry, brittle, and scaly and then fissured (Figure 3-32). The chapping extends onto the sides of the toes. Eventually, the entire sole may be involved; sometimes the hands are also affected (Figure 3-33). The eruption lasts throughout the winter, clears without treatment in the late spring, and predictably recurs the next fall.[15] Earlier descriptions referred to this entity as atopic winter feet in children, but the name has been changed to include patients who are not atopic. Atopic dermatitis of the feet in children occurs on the dorsal toes and usually not on the plantar surface, and it is itchy. Children with chapped fissured feet complain of soreness and pain. The affected individuals must be predisposed to chapping, because their wearing of moist socks and impermeable boots does not differ from that of unaffected children.

The differential diagnosis includes psoriasis, tinea pedis, and allergic contact dermatitis. The erythema in psoriasis is darker, and the scales shed; the scales in chapped fissured feet are adherent, and removal causes bleeding. Tinea of the feet in children is rare. Feet with the rare case of familial *Trichophyton rubrum* are pale brown and have a fine scale; fissuring is minimal, and there is little seasonal variation. Allergic contact dermatitis to shoes usually affects the dorsal aspect and spares the soles, webs, and sides of the feet. The eruption is bright red and scaly, rather than pale red and chapped.

Treatment. Group II or III topical steroids are applied twice daily, preferably with Saran Wrap occlusion at bedtime. Lubricating creams, such as Nutraplus, are applied several times each day, especially immeidately after removing moist socks to seal in moisture. The feet should not be allowed to remain moist inside shoes. Preventive measures include changing into light leather shoes after removing boots at school and changing socks one or two times every day.

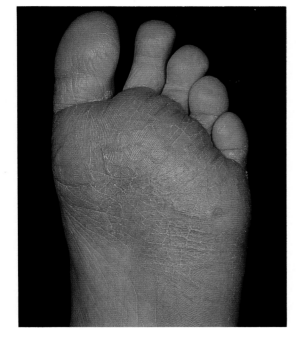

Figure 3-32
Chapped fissured feet. An early stage with erythema and cracking on pressure areas.

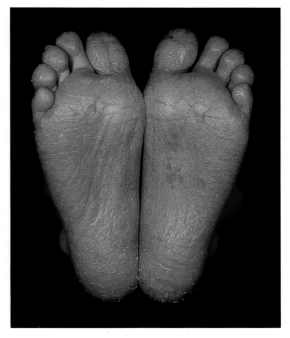

Figure 3-33
Chapped fissured feet in an advanced case in which the entire plantar surface is severely dried and fissured.

REFERENCES

1. Fisher AA: In Contact dermatitis, second edition, Philadelphia, 1973, Lea & Febiger, pp 1-11, 13-24.
2. Fisher AA: In Contact dermatitis, second edition, Philadelphia, 1973, Lea & Febiger, p 77.
3. Jordan WP Jr: Allergic contact dermatitis in hand eczema. Arch Dermatol **110:**567, 1974.
4. Adams RM: Patch testing—a recapitulation. J Am Acad Deramtol **5:**629, 1981.
5. Fisher AA: Contact dermatitis of the hands. I. Differential diagnosis. Dermatology p 62, June, 1978.
6. MacKee GM, Lewis GM: Keratolysis exfoliativa, Arch Dermatol Syph **23:**445, 1931.
7. Verspyck Mijnssen G: Pathogenesis and causative agent of "tulip finger." Br J Dermatol **81:**737, 1969.
8. Epstein S: The antigen-antibody reaction in contact dermatitis: a hypothesis and review. Ann Allergy **10:** 633, 1952.
9. Fisher AA: Prevention of contact dermatitis. NY State J Med **78:**1739, 1978.
10. Sawyer PN, Dowbak G, Sophie Z, et al: Preliminary report of efficacy of Debrisan (dextranomer) in debridement of cutaneous ulcers. Surgery **85:**201, 1979.
11. Alvarez, OM, Mertz PM, Eaglstein WH: Benzoyl peroxide and epidermal wound healing. Arch Dermatol **119:**222, 1983.
12. Nabatoff RA: Ambulatory management of lower extremity venous disease in the aged. Mt Sinai Med **47:**218, 1980.
13. Gibson WB: Sweaty sock dermatitis. Clin Pediatr **2:** 175, 1963.
14. Etna T: Peridigital dermatitis in children. Cutis **10:**325, 1972.
15. Moller H: Atopic winter feet in children. Acta Dermato-Venereologia **52:**401, 1972.

REVIEW ARTICLE

Epstein E: Hand dermatitis: practical management and current concepts. J Am Acad Dermatol **10:**395, 1984.

Chapter Four

Contact Dermatitis and Patch Testing

Contact dermatitis is an eczematous dermatitis caused by exposure to substances in the environment. Those substances act as irritants or allergens and may cause acute, subacute, or chronic eczematous inflammation. To diagnose contact dermatitis, one must first recognize that an eruption is eczematous. Contact allergies often have characteristic distribution patterns indicating that the observed eczematous eruption is caused by external rather than internal stimuli. Elimination of the suspected offending agent and appropriate treatment for eczematous inflammation are usually sufficient for managing patients with contact dermatitis effectively. However, there are many cases in which this direct approach fails; then patch testing is useful.

It is important to differentiate contact dermatitis resulting from irritation from that caused by allergy. An outline of these differences is listed in Table 4-1.

Irritant Contact Dermatitis

Irritation of the skin is the most common cause of contact dermatitis. The epidermis is a thin cellular barrier, of which the outer layer is composed of dead cells in a water-protein-lipid matrix.[1] Any process that damages any component of the barrier will compromise its function, and a nonimmunologic eczematous response may result. Repeated use of strong alkaline soap or industrial exposure to organic solvents will extract lipid from the skin. Acids may combine with water in the skin and cause dehydration. When the skin is compromised, exposure to even a weak irritant will sustain the inflammation. The intensity of the inflammation is related to the concentration of the irritant and the exposure time. Mild irritants cause dryness, fissuring, and erythema; a mild eczematous reaction may occur with continuous exposure. Continuous exposure to moisture in areas such as the hand, the diaper area,

or the skin around a colostomy may eventually cause eczematous inflammation. Strong chemicals may produce an immediate reaction. Figures 4-1 through 4-4 show examples of irritant dermatitis.

Patients vary in their ability to withstand exposure to irritants. Some people cannot tolerate frequent hand-washing, whereas others may work daily with harsh cleaning solutions without any difficulty.

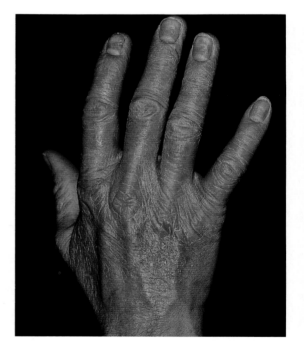

Figure 4-1
Irritant dermatitis. Chronic exposure to soap and water has caused subacute eczematous inflammation over the backs of the hands and fingers.

TABLE 4-1

CONTACT DERMATITIS: IRRITANT VERSUS ALLERGIC

	Irritant	Allergic
People at risk	Everyone	Genetically predisposed
Mechanism of response	Nonimmunologic; a physical and chemical alteration of epidermis	Delayed hypersensitivity reaction
Number of exposures required	Few to many; depends on individual's ability to maintain an effective epidermal barrier	One or several to cause sensitization
Nature of contactant	Organic solvent, soaps	Low molecular weight hapten (e.g., metals, formalin, epoxy)
Concentration of contactant required	Usually high	May be very low
Mode of onset	Usually gradual as epidermal barrier becomes compromised	Once sensitized, usually rapid; 12 to 48 hours after exposure
Distribution	Borders usually indistinct	May correspond exactly to contactant (e.g., watch band, elastic waistband)
Investigative procedure	Trial of avoidance	Trial of avoidance, patch testing, or both
Management	Protection and reduced incidence of exposure	Complete avoidance

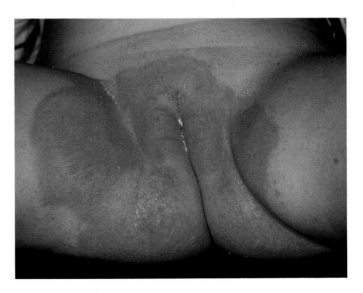

Figure 4-2
Irritant dermatitis. Long exposure to wet diapers followed by frequent washing has resulted in diffuse erythema and dry, cracked, fissured skin.

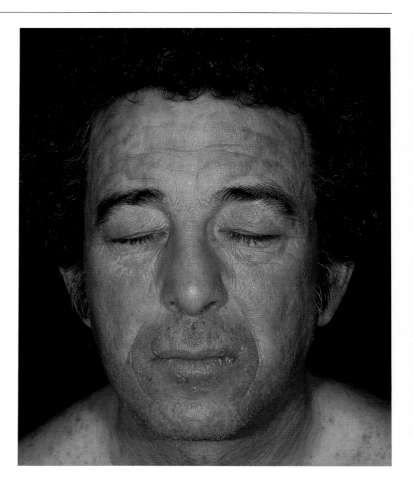

Figure 4-3
Irritant dermatitis. Exposure to industrial solvents has resulted in diffuse erythema with dryness and fissuring about the mouth.

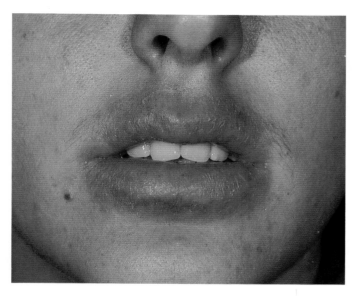

Figure 4-4
Irritant dermatitis. Repeated cycles of wetting and drying by lip licking resulted in irritant dermatitis.

Allergic Contact Dermatitis

Allergic contact dermatitis is a delayed hypersensitivity reaction that affects a limited number of individuals after one or a few exposures to an antigenic substance.

Phases

Sensitization phase. A hapten, a low molecular weight substance (e.g., nickel), penetrates the epidermis and combines with epidermal protein to form an antigen. This hapten-protein binding takes place either on or in the vicinity of Langerhans' cells, which act as an epidermal reticuloendothelial trap for antigens.[2] The Langerhans' cell is met by macrophages and T cells in the epidermis, and initial processing takes place. A message is directed to T cell precursors in the lymph nodes and sensitized T cells are formed. The sensitization phase lasts from 3 to 12 days.

Elicitation phase. On reexposure to the antigen-protein complex the sensitized T cells release lymphokines, which recruit inflammatory cells that cause eczematous inflammation. The time required for a previously sensitized individual to develop clinically apparent inflammation is generally 12 to 48 hours but may vary from 8 to 120 hours.[3]

Cross-sensitization

A hapten, the chemical structure of which is similar to the original sensitizing hapten, may cause inflammation because the immune system is unable to differentiate between the original and the chemically related antigen. Patients allergic to balsam of Peru, which is present in numerous topical preparations, may become inflamed when exposed to the chemically related benzoin in tincture of benzoin.

Systemically induced dermatitis

Patients who have been sensitized to topical medications may develop generalized eczematous inflammation if those medications or chemically related substances are ingested. Patients sensitized to ethylenediamine from contact with that chemical in topical medicines such as Mycolog cream may develop generalized inflammation following treatment with aminophylline, which contains ethylenediamine. Patients allergic to poison ivy will develop diffuse inflammation following ingestion of raw cashew nuts (Figure 4-5). Cashew nut oil is chemically related to the oleoresin of the poison ivy plant.

Clinical presentation

The intensity of inflammation depends on the degree of sensitivity and the concentration of the antigen. Strong sensitizers such as the oleoresin of poison ivy may produce intense inflammation in low concentrations, whereas weak sensitizers may cause only erythema.

The pattern of inflammation is an important consideration when attempting to differentiate allergic contact dermatitis from other causes of eczematous inflammation. The pattern of inflammation may correspond exactly to the offending substance. The diagnosis is obvious when inflammation is confined specifically to the area under a watch band, shoe, or elastic waist band.

The location of inflammation may provide a clue to the source of the antigen. Table 4-2 lists substances that are common causes of inflammation in specific body regions. Table 4-3 lists substances commonly encountered in specific professions.

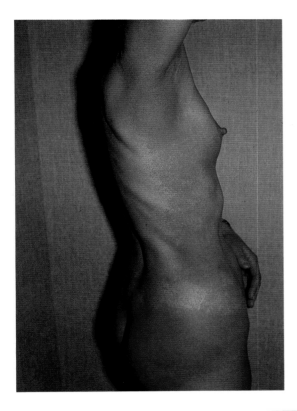

Figure 4-5
Diffuse allergic reaction occurring in a patient allergic to poison ivy who has ingested raw cashew nuts, the oil of which cross-reacts with the oleoresin of poison ivy.

TABLE 4-2

CONTACT DERMATITIS: DISTRIBUTION DIAGNOSIS

Location	Material
Scalp and ears	Shampoo, hair dyes, topical medicines, metal earrings, eye glasses
Eyelid	Nail polish (transferred by rubbing), cosmetics, contact lens solution, metal eyelash curlers
Face	Airborne allergens (poison ivy from burning leaves, ragweed), cosmetics, sunscreens, acne medications (e.g., benzoyl peroxide), after-shave lotion
Neck	Necklaces, airborne allergens (ragweed), perfumes, after-shave lotion
Trunk	Topical medication, sunscreens, poison ivy, plants (phototoxic reactions), clothing, undergarments (e.g., spandex bra, elastic waistband), metal belt buckles
Axillae	Deodorant (axillary vault), clothing (axillary folds)
Arms	Same as hand; watch and watchband
Hands	Soaps and detergents, foods, poison ivy, industrial solvents and oils, cement, metal (pots, rings), topical medications
Genitals	Poison ivy (transferred by hand), rubber condoms
Anal region	Hemorrhoid preparations (benzocaine, nupercaine), Mycolog cream
Lower legs	Topical medication (benzocaine, lanolin, neomycin, parabens), dye in socks
Feet	Shoes (rubber or leather), cement spilling into boots

TABLE 4-3

CONTACT DERMATITIS: OCCUPATIONAL EXPOSURE

Occupation	Irritants	Allergens
Beauticians	Wet work (shampoos)	Hair tints, permanent solution, shampoos (formaldehyde)
Construction workers	Fuels, lubricants, cement	Cement (chromium, cobalt), epoxy, glues, paints, solvents, rubber, chrome-tanned leather gloves
Chefs, bartenders, bakers	Moist foods, juices, corn, pineapple juice	Orange and lemon peel (oil of limonene), mango, carrot, parsnips, parsley, celery; spices (e.g., capsicum, cinnamon, cloves, nutmeg, vanilla cloves)
Farmers	Milker's eczema (detergents), tractor lubricants and fuels	Malathion, pyrethrum insecticides, fungicides, rubber, ragweed, marsh elder
Forest products industry	Wet work (wood processing)	Poison ivy and oak, plants growing on bark (e.g., lichens, liverworts)
Medical and surgical personnel	Surgical scrubbing	Rubber gloves, glutaraldehyde (germicides), acrylic monomer in cement (orthopedic surgeons), penicillin, chlorpromazine, benzalkonium chloride, neomycin
Printing industry	Alcohols, alkalis, grease	Polyfunctional acrylic monomers, epoxy acrylate oligomers, isocyanate compounds (all used in a new ink-drying method)

Rhus dermatitis

In the United States, poison ivy, poison oak, and poison sumac produce more cases of allergic contact dermatitis than all other contactants combined. These plants belong to the Anacardiaceae family and the genus *Rhus*. All parts of the plant contain a potent sensitizing oleoresin called urushiol. Other plants in that family, such as the cashew nut,[4] contain similar sensitizing chemicals that may cross-react with Rhus.

Poison ivy and poison oak are neither ivy nor oak species. Poison ivy plants vary greatly throughout the United States. They grow in the form of woody vines attached to trees or objects for support, trailing shrubs predominantly found on the ground, or erect woody shrubs. Frequently, they grow with other shrubs or vines and are unnoticed. Leaves of common poison ivy are extremely variable, but the three leaflets are a constant characteristic (Figure 4-6). The most common type of leaf has smooth margins. The old saying "Leaflets three, let it be" is a reminder of this consistent leaf characteristic but may lead to undue suspicion of some harmless plants. One leaf leads off each node on the twig,

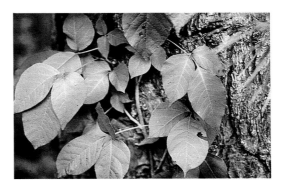

Figure 4-6
Poison ivy. Three leaflets; only one leaf leads off from each node on the twig.

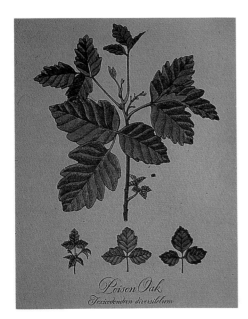

Figure 4-7
Poison oak. Leaflets occur in threes but are lobed. (Courtesy of Syntex Laboratories, Inc.)

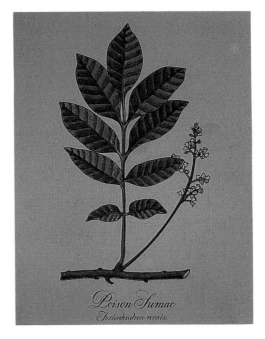

Figure 4-8
Poison sumac. Pairs of leaflets with a single leaflet at the end of the twig. (Courtesy of Syntex Laboratories, Inc.)

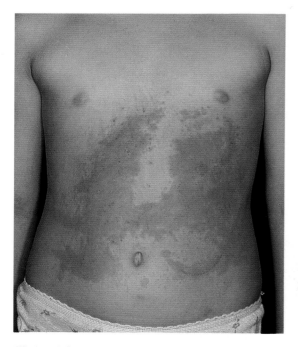

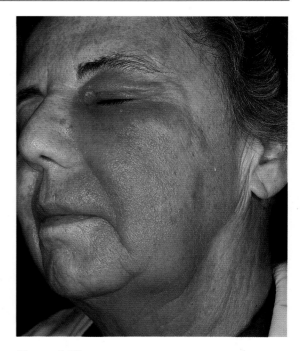

Figure 4-9
Poison ivy dermatitis. Diffuse erythema with linear lesions.

Figure 4-10
Poison ivy dermatitis. Diffuse erythema with vesicles over the entire surface.

and leaves never occur in pairs along the stem. Some plants bear clusters of white berry-like fruits that originate from the stems. The leaves turn a brilliant color in the fall.

Poison oak or oak-leaf ivy occurs as a low-growing shrub. Stems generally grow upright. Leaflets occur in threes but are lobed, similar to the leaves of some kinds of oak (Figure 4-7). Poison oak is found in the southeastern United States and along the West Coast.

Poison sumac grows as a coarse woody shrub or small tree, rather than as a vine. Mature plants range in height from 5 feet to small trees that may reach 25 feet. Poison sumac occurs chiefly in the eastern half of the United States and grows in swamps and bogs. Leaves of poison sumac consist of 7 to 13 leaflets, arranged in pairs, with a single leaflet at the end of the mid-rib (Figure 4-8). The leaflets are oval, elongated, and have smooth margins. They are 3 to 4 inches long and 1 to 2 inches wide. In early spring their color is bright orange. Later, they become dark green, turning a brilliant red-orange in the fall. Poison sumac has clusters of white fruit, whereas all other forms of sumac have red fruits that together form a distinctive terminal seed head.

Clinical presentation. Rhus dermatitis occurs from contact with the leaf or internal parts of the stem or root and can be acquired from roots and stems in the fall and winter. The clinical presentation varies with the quantity of oleoresin contacting the skin, the pattern in which contact was made, individual susceptibilty, and regional variation in cutaneous reactivity. Small quantities of oleoresin produce only erythema, whereas large quantities cause intense vesiculation (Figures 4-9 to 4-11). The highly characteristic linear lesions are created when part of the plant is drawn across the skin or from streaking the oleoresin while scratching. Diffuse or unusual patterns of inflammation occur when the oleoresin is acquired from contaminated animal hair or clothing or from smoke while burning the plant. The eruption may appear as quickly as 8 hours after contact or be delayed for a week or more. Appearance of new lesions a week after contact is confusing to the patient, who attributes these new lesions to the spread of the disease by touching active lesions or from contamination with blister fluid. Blister fluid does not contain the oleoresin and, contrary to popular belief, cannot spread the inflammation. Washing the skin with any type of soap inactivates and removes all surface oleoresin, there-

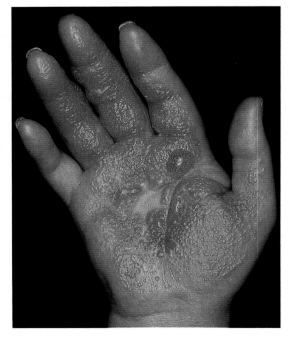

Figure 4-11
Poison ivy dermatitis. Vesicles and bullae appeared within 24 hours of pulling up poison ivy plants.

by preventing further contamination. Clothing must also be washed.

Treatment of inflammation. See the section on treatment of acute and subacute eczematous inflammation in Chapter 3.

Prophylactic treatment. Complete desensitization cannot be accomplished. A trial of hyposensitization may be considered for patients who have continuous disease during the summer months. Hollister-Stier Laboratories has poison ivy oleoresin available in capsule form for oral hyposensitization. The program is started 4 months before anticipated exposure and consists of daily ingestion of increasing quantities of oleoresin. Pruritus ani is a complication of oral hyposensitization.

Shoe dermatitis and rubber allergy

Fungal infections, psoriasis, and atopic dermatitis are common causes of inflammation of the feet. Shoe allergy, while less common, should always be considered in the differential diagnosis, particularly in children. Shoe allergy typically appears as subacute eczematous inflammation over the dorsa of the feet, particularly the toes (Figures 4-12 and 4-13). The interdigital spaces are spared, in contrast to tinea pedis. The inflammation is usually bi-

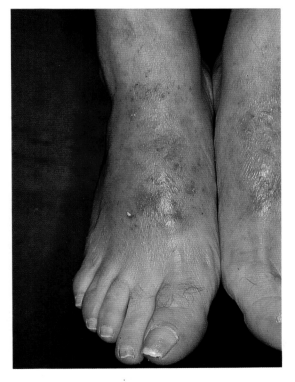

Figure 4-13
Shoe contact dermatitis. Sharply defined plaques formed under a shoe lining impregnated with rubber cement.

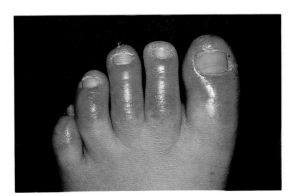

Figure 4-12
Shoe contact dermatitis. The toe webs are spared, in contrast to tinea pedis.

lateral, but unilateral involvement does not preclude the diagnosis of allergy. The thick skin of the soles is more resistant to allergens. Sweaty sock dermatitis, an irritant reaction in children caused by excessive perspiration, is seen as diffuse dryness with fissuring on the toes, webs, and soles. These irritated areas may become eczematous and appear as shoe contact dermatitis.[5]

Mercaptobenzothiazole, a rubber component of adhesives used to cement shoe uppers, and potassium bichromate, a leather tanning agent, are common causes of shoe allergy.[6] These chemicals are leached out by sweat.

Allergy to rubber compounds is also seen with adhesive bandages and surgical gloves. Hypoallergic dressings are available at most pharmacies. Surgeons with rubber sensitivity may use Elastyren hypoallergenic surgical gloves. Unlike latex rubber, Elastyren is not vulcanized and therefore contains no metal oxides, sulfur, accelerators, or mercaptobenzothiazole, sensitizers commonly found in rubber products. Elastyren gloves are imported from Denmark and marketed by Hermal Pharmaceutical Laboratories, Oak Hill, NY.

Diagnosis. Patch testing is required to confirm the diagnosis of allergy. First patch test with pieces of the shoe that cover the inflamed site (Figure 4-14). Cut a 1-inch square piece of material from the shoe and round off the corners to prevent irritation. Separate glued surfaces and patch test with all layers. Moisten each layer with water and apply the samples to the upper outer arm, cover with tape, and proceed as described in the section on patch testing. In some cases, patch testing with the standard patch test series may be required to establish the diagnosis.

Management. Patients with shoe allergy must control perspiration. Socks should be changed at least once every day. An absorbent powder such as Z-Sorb applied to the feet may be helpful. Aluminum chloride hexahydrate in a 20% solution (Drysol) applied at bedtime is a highly effective antiperspirant. Most vinyl shoes are acceptable substitutes for rubber- and chrome-sensitive patients. Inflammation of the soles may be prevented by inserting a barrier such as Dr. Scholl's Air Foam Pads or Johnson's Odor-Eaters. Once perspiration is controlled, it may be possible for sensitized patients to wear both leather shoes and shoes with rubber cement.

Metal dermatitis
Nickel

In the United States, nickel is one of the most common causes of allergic contact dermatitis. Women are affected much more frequently than men. Ear piercing and wearing clip-on earrings brings metal into direct contact with skin, an ideal setting for sensitization to occur (Figure 4-15). Ears should be pierced with stainless steel instruments, and stainless steel studs should be worn until com-

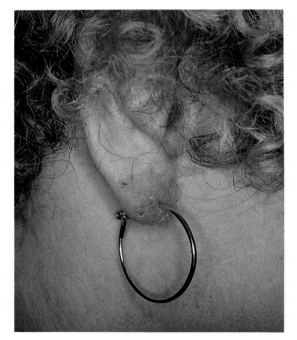

Figure 4-15
Nickel allergy. A classic presentation.

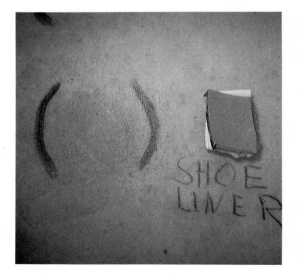

Figure 4-14
Patient in Fig. 4-13 was patch tested with a piece of shoe lining. A 2+ positive allergic reaction occurred within 48 hours.

plete epithelialization takes place. Some so-called hypoallergenic earrings may sensitize individuals.

Men are usually sensitized in an industrial setting.[7] Avoidance is the only means of preventing inflammation. However, nickel can be found everywhere. Sources of contact are necklaces, scissors, door handles, watch bands, bracelets, belt buckles (Figure 4-16), and screws in orthopedic implants.

The dimethylglyoxime (DMG) spot test for nickel involves adding two solutions to a metal surface. If the solution turns pink, the test is positive.[8]

Chromates

The trivalent and hexavalent dichromate compounds are sensitizers. Chromate is possibly the most common sensitizer for men in industrialized countries.[9] Sources are cement, photographic processes, metal, and dyes. Cement is the most common cause of chromate allergy.[10] Cement acts both as an irritant and as a sensitizer. Most cement workers experience dryness of the skin when first exposed, but most seem to adapt. Severe alkali burns occur on the lower legs of men whose skin is in direct contact with wet cement.[11] The most severe burns occur when cement spills over the boot top and is held next to the skin (Figure 4-17). Industrial workers sensitized to chromates in cement develop eczematous inflammation on the backs of the hands and forearms. The source of contact is frequently not appreciated until these patients fail to respond to both topical and systemic steroids. Once the patient is removed from contact with cement, response to treatment is rapid.

Further examples of allergic contact dermatitis are illustrated in Figures 4-18 to 4-22.

Figure 4-16
Nickel allergy. Belt buckle rubbed against abdomen when the patient bent over.

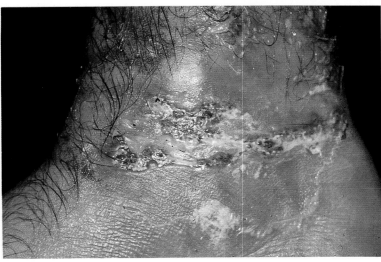

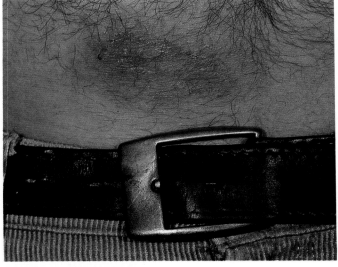

Figure 4-17
Severe irritant dermatitis from contact with wet cement.

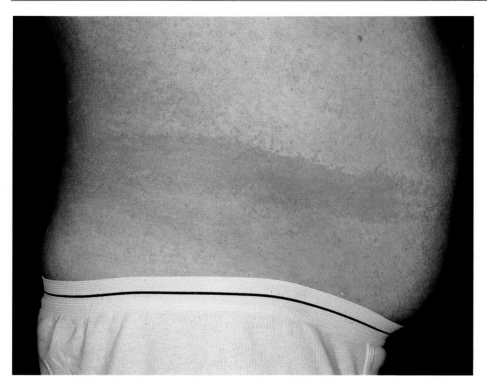

Figure 4-18
Allergic contact dermatitis to rubber band of underwear. Washing clothes with bleach may make the rubber allergenic.

Figure 4-19
Allergic contact dermatitis to dye in a body suit.

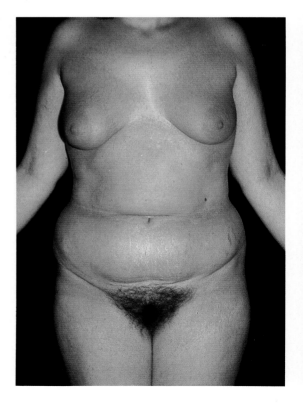

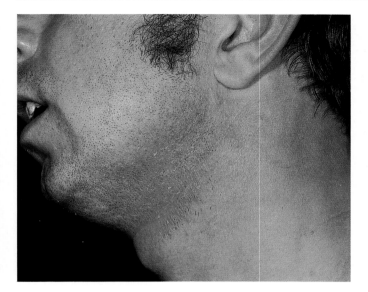

Figure 4-20
Allergic contact dermatitis to benzoyl peroxide in a topical acne preparation.

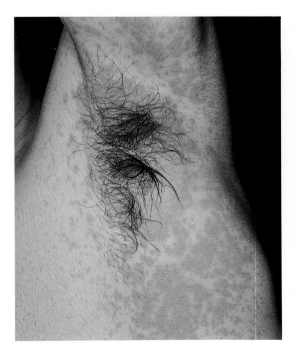

Figure 4-21
Allergic contact dermatitis to a spray deodorant.

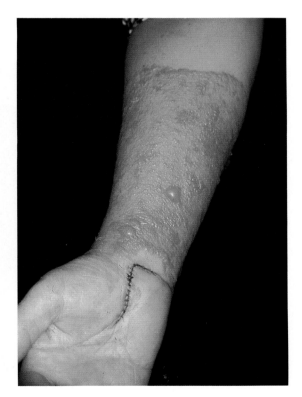

Figure 4-22
Allergic contact dermatitis to benzoin under a cast.

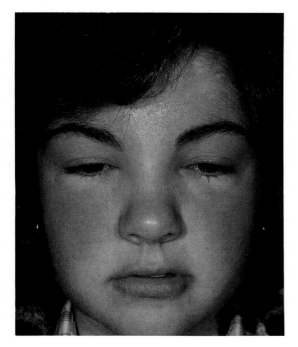

Figure 4-23
A beautician with diffuse erythema of the face.

Figure 4-24
The patient in Fig. 4-23 was patch tested with several of the preparations used at work. Many positive reactions of varying intensity appeared.

Diagnosis of Contact Dermatitis

Determining the allergens responsible for allergic contact dermatitis requires a medical history, physical examination, and in some instances patch testing. Historical points of interest are date of onset, relationship to work (improves during weekends or vacation), and types of products used in skin care. The number of different creams, lotions, cosmetics, and topical medications that patients can accumulate is amazing. Persistent questioning may eventually uncover the responsible antigen. Patch testing should not be attempted until the patient has had time to ponder the questions raised by the physician. In many cases all that is required is to avoid the suspected offending material. Patch testing is indicated for cases in which inflammation persists despite avoidance and appropriate topical therapy. Patch testing is not useful as a diagnostic test for irritant contact dermatitis, since this is a non-immunologically mediated inflammatory reaction.

Patch testing

Open patch test. The suspected allergen is applied to the skin of the upper outer arm and left uncovered. Application is repeated twice daily for 2 days and read as described below.

Use test. The suspected cream or cosmetic is used on a site distant from the original eruption. Suitable areas for testing are the outer arm or the

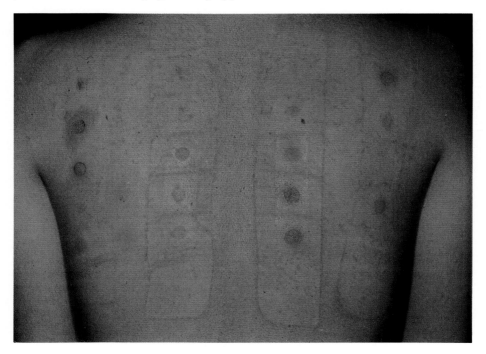

skin of the anticubital fossa. The material is applied for at least one week.

Closed patch test. The material is applied to the skin and covered with an adhesive bandage. The bandage is removed in 48 hours for initial interpretation (Figures 4-23 and 4-24). Solid objects such as shoe leather, wood, or rubber materials or nonirritating material such as skin moisturizers, topical medicines, or cosmetics are well suited to this technique.

Only bland material should be applied directly to the skin surface. Caustic industrial solvents must be diluted. Patch testing with a high concentration of caustic material may lead to skin necrosis. Petrolatum is generally the most suitable vehicle for dispersion of test materials. The concentration required to elicit a response varies with each chemical and appropriate concentrations for testing can be found in standard text books dealing with contact dermatitis. If intense itching occurs, patches should be removed from test sites. A negative patch test with this direct technique does not rule out the diagnosis of allergy. The concentration of material tested may be too weak to elicit a response, or one component of a topical medication (e.g., topical steroids) may suppress the allergic reaction induced by another component of the same cream.

If this technique fails or if the clinical presentation is that of allergic contact dermatitis but a source cannot be uncovered by the history and physical examination, then patch testing with the Standard Patch Test Series should be considered.

Standard patch test series

Testing with groups of allergens is generally performed by physicians who frequently see contact dermatitis and have experience with the problems involved in accurately determining the significance of test results. A group of chemicals that have proved to be frequent or important causes of allergic contact dermatitis have been assembled into a standard patch test series by the North American Contact Dermatitis Group (Table 4-4).[12]

The American Academy of Dermatology (AAD) Patch Test Kit for 1984-85 contains 20 allergens and a manual entitled "Patch Testing in Allergic Contact Dermatitis." An exposure list of the products that contain the 20 allergens is also available The kit may be ordered from Dermatology Services, Inc., P. O. Box 192, Evanston, IL, 60204, at a cost of $80 for AAD members and $100 for nonmembers. A perfume screening series with 14 allergens and a vehicle-and-preservative screening series with eight allergens is also available.

TABLE 4-4

1984-1985 PATCH TEST KIT ALLERGENS AND EXAMPLES OF COMMON SOURCES

Allergen	Example of source
Benzocaine, 5%	Topical anesthetics
Imidazolidinyl urea, 2% aqueous	Preservative in creams and cosmetics
Thiuram mixture, 1%	Rubber products
Wool (lanolin) alcohols, 30%	Cosmetics, medicated creams
Neomycin sulfate, 20%	Topical medications
p-Phenylenediamine, 1%	Hair dyes, inks
Mercaptobenzothiazole, 1%	Rubber products
p-Tertiary-butylphenol formaldehyde resin, 1%	Adhesive and rubber systems
Thimerosal (Merthiolate), 0.1%	Eye, ear, nose preparations
Formaldehyde, 2% aqueous	Glues, paper, clothing, cosmetics
Carba mix, 3%	Rubber cements and sealants
Rosin (colophony), 20%	Adhesives, cements, cleaners
PPD mixture, 0.6% (black rubber mixture)	Rubber products
Ethylenediamine dihydrochloride, 1%	Mycolog cream
Quaternium-15, 2%	Cosmetics
Mercapto mixture, 1%	Shoes, rubber products
Epoxy resin, 1%	Glue, pastes
Balsam of Peru, 25%	Cosmetics
Potassium dichromate, 0.5%	Cement
Nickel sulfate, 2.5%	Earrings, metal tools

Figure 4-25
Patch testing with the allergens of the standard series of the North American Contact Dermatitis Group. Allergens are applied to an aluminum patch test tape.

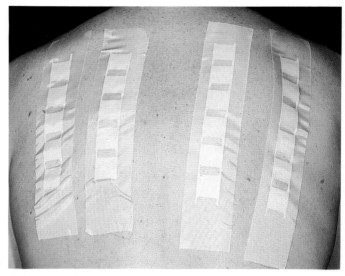

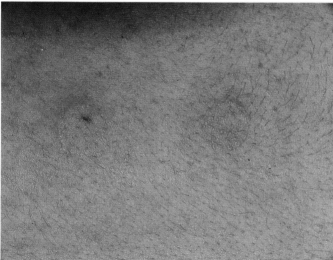

Figure 4-26
A 2+ positive patch test reaction with erythema and vesicles.

Figure 4-27
A 3+ positive patch test reaction with vesicles and bullae.

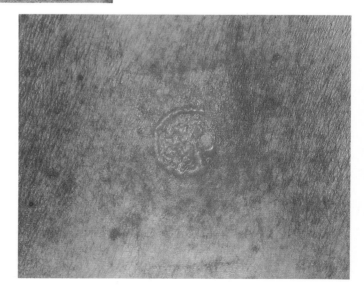

The AAD makes revisions and additions to ensure that the standard series best reflects the sensitivities currently prevalent in the population. The test battery is only a screening procedure and does not test for all of the possible environmental allergens. Corticosteroids such as prednisone in doses of 15 mg/day or the equivalent may inhibit patch test reactions.[13]

Technique. The material to be tested is applied to a holding device (Finn chamber or patch) (Figure 4-25) and is then applied to the skin with tape (e.g., Blenderm). The back is the preferred site. The test strips remain on the site for 48 hours and are read 20 minutes after removal. The area around the test site is marked with paint (e.g., 0.5% gentian violet) at the time of initial testing and again at 48 hours. Patients return 2 to 3 days after patch removal to check for delayed reactions.

Patch test reading and interpretation. The test reactions are graded at each reading as follows:

Doubtful reaction. Faint macular erythema only
+ = Weak (nonvesicular) positive reaction; erythema, infiltration, possibly papules
++ = Strong (vesicular) positive reaction; erythema, infiltration, papules, vesicles (Figure 4-26)
+++ = Extreme positive reaction; bullous reaction (Figure 4-27)
− = Negative reaction
IR = Irritant reaction of different types
NT = Not tested

Allergic versus irritant test reactions

It is important to determine whether the test response is caused by allergy or a nonspecific irritant reaction. Strong allergic reactions are vesicular and may spread beyond the test site. Strong irritant reactions exhibit a deep erythema resembling a burn. There is no morphologic method of distinguishing a weak irritant patch test from a weak allergic test. Commercially prepared antigens are formulated to minimize irritant reactions. Irritant test responses result from either hyperirritability of the skin or the application of an irritating concentration of a test substance. Irritation is avoided by applying tests only on normal skin that has not been washed or cleaned with alcohol.

The excited skin syndrome (angry back). A strongly positive reaction may produce a state of skin hyperreactivity in which other patch test sites, particularly those with minimal irritation, become reactive.[14] Patients who have multiple strong test reactions should be retested at a later date with one antigen at a time (Figure 4-28).

Relevance of test results. There are a number of possible conclusions that may be drawn from the test results:

• The allergen eliciting the positive test is directly responsible for the patient's dermatitis.
• A chemically related or cross-reacting material is responsible for the dermatitis.
• The patient has not recently been in contact with the indicated allergen and, although allergic to that specific chemical, it is not relevant to the present condition.
• The test is negative but would be positive if a sufficient concentration of test chemical were used.
• The positive test is an irritant reaction and is irrelevant.

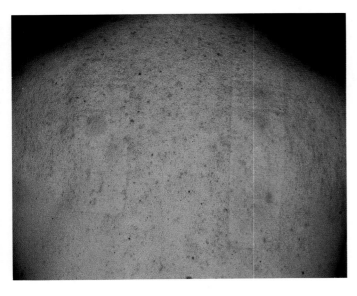

Figure 4-28
The excited skin syndrome. Several tests have become positive, and the severe reactions have stimulated inflammation over the entire back.

REFERENCES

1. Blank IH: Factors which influence the water content of the stratum corneum. J Invest Dermatol **18:**433, 1952.
2. Stingl G, Katz SI, Green I, et al: The functional role of Langerhans cells. J Invest Dermatol **74:**315, 1980.
3. Silberberg I, Baer RL, Rosenthal SA: The role of Langerhans cells in allergic contact hypersensitivity: a review of findings in man and guinea pigs. J Invest Dermatol **66:**210, 1976.
4. Marks JG Jr, Demelfi T, McCarthy MA, et al: Dermatitis from cashew nuts. J Am Acad Dermatol **10:**627, 1984.
5. Jillson OF: You name it. Cutis **27:**461, 1981.
6. Dahl MV: Allergic contact dermatitis from foot wear. Minn Med **58:**871, 1975.
7. Cronin E: Metals in contact dermatitis. Edinburgh, 1980, Churchill Livingstone.
8. Fisher AA: Metal dermatitis: some questions and answers. Cutis **19:**156, 1977.
9. North American Contact Dermatitis Group: Epidemiology of contact dermatitis in North America. Arch Dermatol **108:**537, 1972.
10. Burrows D, Calnan CD: Cement dermatitis. II. Clinical aspects. Trans St. John's Hosp Dermatol Soc **51:**27, 1965.
11. Flowers MW: Burn hazard with cement. Br Med J **i:** 1250, 1978.
12. Adams RM: Patch testing—a recapitulation. J Am Acad Dermatol **5:**629, 1981.
13. Feverman E, Levy A: A study of the effect of prednisone and an antihistamine on patch test reactions. Br J Dermatol **86:**68, 1972.
14. Bruynzeel DP, van Ketal WG, von Blomberg-van der Flier M, et al: Angry back or the excited skin syndrome: a prospective study. J Am Acad Dermatol **8:** 392, 1983.

Chapter Five

Atopic Dermatitis

Atopic dermatitis is a characteristic, easily recognizable disease that generally begins early in life and follows an unpredictable course. The term "atopy" was introduced years ago to describe patients who had a personal or family history of one or more of the following diseases: hayfever, asthma, extremely dry skin, and eczema. Recent data show that between 7 and 24 individuals per 1000 have atopic dermatitis.[1] The highest incidence is among children. Fifty percent of those patients who have atopic dermatitis will develop asthma or hayfever. Seventy percent of atopic patients have a family history of one or more of the principal atopic features of asthma, hayfever, or eczematous dermatitis.[2] Patients with the most severe disease are twice as likely to have persistant disease.[3] Those without a family history have a better prognosis. The pattern of inheritance is unknown, but available data suggest that it is polygenic.

There are two common misconceptions about atopic dermatitis. The first is that it is a stress-related or emotional disorder. It is true that patients with inflammation lasting for months or years seem to be more irritable, but this is a normal response to a frustrating disease. The second misconception is that atopic skin disease is precipitated by an allergic reaction. Atopic individuals frequently have respiratory allergies and, when skin-tested, are informed that they are allergic to "everything." Although patients with atopic dermatitis may react with a wheal when challenged with a needle during skin testing, this is a characteristic of atopic skin and is not necessarily a manifestation of allergy. All evidence to date shows that in most cases atopic dermatitis is precipitated by environmental stress on genetically compromised skin and not by interaction with allergens.

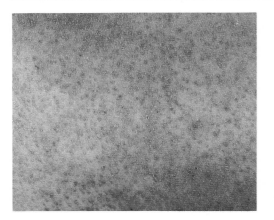

Figure 5-1
Atopic dermatitis. Papular lesions are common in the antecubital and popliteal fossae: Papules become confluent and form plaques.

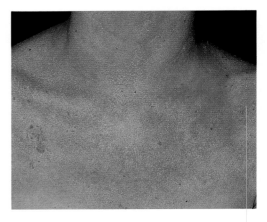

Figure 5-2
Atopic dermatitis. Eczematous dermatitis with diffuse erythema and scaling on the neck and chest.

Immunology

A number of abnormalities of the immune system have been documented. These facts have not, however, provided an explanation for the pathogenesis of atopic dermatitis. Atopic patients frequently show positive scratch and intradermal reactions to a number of antigens. Avoiding those antigens rarely improves the dermatitis. Serum IgE levels are elevated above 200 IU/ml in 80% to 90% of patients with atopic dermatitis, whereas levels are less than 200 IU/ml in 70% of normal adults.[4] Patients with extremely active disease may have IgE levels greater than 1000 IU. However, 20% of patients with atopic dermatitis have normal or below normal levels of IgE. The levels of IgE do not necessarily correlate with the activity of the disease; therefore, elevated serum IgE levels can only be considered supporting evidence for the disease.[5]

Several facts suggest disordered cell-mediated immunity in atopic dermatitis. Patients both with and without active disease may develop severe diffuse cutaneous infection with the herpes simplex virus (eczema herpeticum). Mothers with active herpes labialis should avoid direct contact of the active lesion with their child's skin, as in kissing, especially if the child has dermatitis.

Atopic patients have an increased susceptibility to viral infections, such as warts and molluscum contagiosum, and to cutaneous fungal infections.[6] The incidence of contact allergy is lower than normal in atopic patients, and they do not develop poison ivy after exposure as often as do nonatopic individuals. However, humoral immunity seems to be normal.

Clinical Aspects

Abnormally dry skin and a lowered threshold for itching are important features of atopic dermatitis. Scratching creates most of the characteristic patterns of the disease. Most atopic patients make a determined effort to control their scratching, but during sleep, conscious control is lost; under warm covers they scratch and a rash appears. The itch-scratch cycle is established and conscious effort is no longer sufficient to control scratching. The act of scratching becomes habitual and the disease progresses.

There is no single primary lesion in atopic dermatitis. Rather, several patterns and types of lesions may be produced by exposure to external stimuli or may be precipitated by scratching. These types of lesions are papules (Figure 5-1), eczematous dermatitis with redness and scaling (Figure 5-2), and lichenification (Figure 5-3). Lichenification represents a thickening of the epidermis. It is a highly characteristic lesion, with normal skin lines accentuated to resemble a washboard. These so-called primary responses are altered by excoriation and infection. Although the cutaneous manifestations of the atopic diathesis are varied, they have characteristic age-determined patterns. Knowledge of these patterns is useful; many patients, however, will have a nonclassic picture. Atopic dermatitis may stop after an indefinite time or may progress from infancy to adulthood with little or no relief. Fifty-eight percent of infants with atopic dermatitis were found to have persistent inflammation 15 to 17 years later.[7] Atopic dermatitis is arbitrarily divided into three phases.

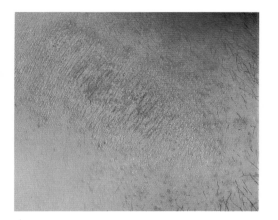

Figure 5-3
Atopic dermatitis. Lichenification with accentuation of normal skin lines. This lichenified plaque is surrounded by papules.

Infant phase

The infant phase is from birth to 2 years. Infants are rarely born with atopic eczema, but typically they develop the first signs of inflammation during the third month of life. Most common is a baby who during the winter months develops dry, red scaling areas confined to the cheeks, but the perioral and perinasal areas are spared (Figure 5-4). The chin is often involved and initially may be more inflamed than are the cheeks. This results from the irritation of drooling and subsequent repeated washing. Inflammation may spread to involve the perinasal and perioral area as the winter progresses (Figure 5-5). Habitual lip licking in an atopic child results in oozing, crusting, and scaling on the lips and perioral skin (Figure 5-6). Many infants do not excoriate during these early stages, and the rash remains localized and chronic. Repeated scratching or washing creates red, scaling, oozing plaques on the cheeks (Figure 5-7), a classic appearance for infantile eczema. At this stage the infant is uncomfortable and becomes restless and agitated during sleep.

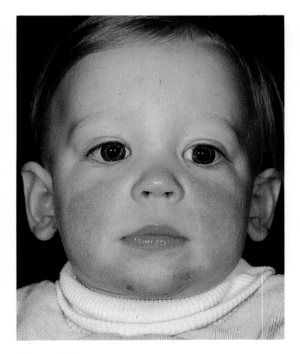

Figure 5-4
Atopic dermatitis. A common appearance in children with erythema and scaling confined to the cheeks and sparing the perioral and perinasal area.

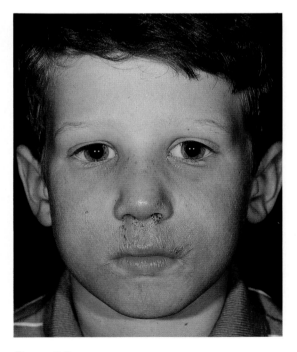

Figure 5-5
Atopic dermatitis. Progression of inflammation to involve the perioral and perinasal areas.

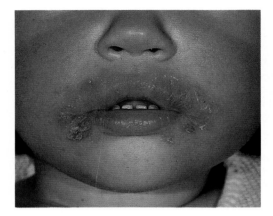

Figure 5-6
Habitual lip licking in an atopic child produces
erythema and scaling that eventually may lead to
secondary infection.

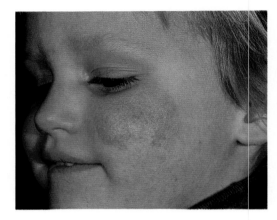

Figure 5-7
Atopic dermatitis. Typical appearance of infantile
atopic dermatitis with inflammation on the cheeks.

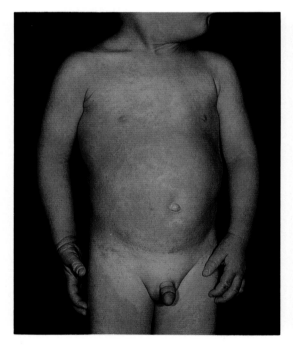

Figure 5-8
Generalized infantile atopic dermatitis sparing the
diaper area, which is protected from scratching.

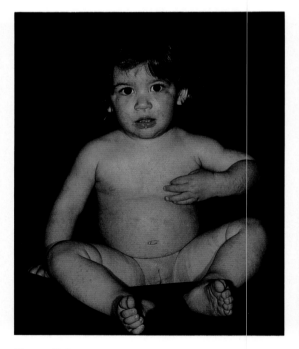

Figure 5-9
Generalized infantile atopic dermatitis. All areas
are inflamed, including the diaper area that has
been irritated by moisture. The thick papules and
plaques on the extensor surface of the arms were
created by scratching.

A small but significant number of infants have a generalized eruption consisting of papules, redness, scaling, and areas of lichenification. The diaper area is often spared (Figure 5-8). Lichenification may be in the fossa and crease areas, or it may be confined to a favorite easily reached spot, such as directly below the diaper, the back of the hand, or the extensor forearm (Figure 5-9). Prolonged atopic dermatitis with increasing discomfort disturbs sleep, and both the parents and child may be distraught.

For years, foods such as milk, wheat, eggs, juices, and beef have been suspected as etiologic factors, but their role in producing or exacerbating inflammation had not been proved. Some physicians believe that atopic disease may be delayed or prevented by breast feeding and withholding those foods in early infancy. A recent study in children with atopic dermatitis showed that certain foods could elicit a number of symptoms within 10 to 90 minutes of challenge. These patients had a significant mean rise in plasma histamine concentration. Positive prick skin tests of the foods inducing allergic symptoms were found in most patients.[8] It seems likely that ingestion of specific food allergens in sensitized patients, which leads to release of histamine, could result in cutaneous pruritus, itching, and subsequently typical eczematous inflammation. Food restriction, such as omitting cows' milk or wheat cereal, might be considered for infants and children when more conventional forms of management have failed. The course of the disease may be influenced by events such as teething, respiratory infection, and adverse emotional stimulus. The dis-ease is chronic, with periods of exacerbation and remission. Atopic dermatitis resolves in about 50% of infants by 18 months, but the others progress to the childhood phase, and a different pattern evolves.

Childhood phase

In the childhood phase (2 to 12 years) the most common appearance of atopic dermatitis is inflammation in flexural areas (i.e., the antecubital fossa, neck, wrists, and ankles [Figures 5-10 and 5-11]). These areas of extension and flexion perspire with exertion. Perspiring stimulates burning and intense itching and initiates the itch-scratch cycle. Tight clothing that contains heat around the neck or extremities further aggravates the problem. Inflammation typically begins in one of the fossa or about the neck. The rash may remain localized to one or two areas or progress to involve the neck, antecubital and popliteal fossae, wrists, and ankles. The eruption begins with papules that rapidly coalesce into plaques; these become lichenified when scratched. The plaques may be pale and mildly inflamed with little tendency to change (Figure 5-12); if intensely scratched, they may be bright red and scaling with erosions. The border may be sharp and well defined as in psoriasis (Figure 5-13) or poorly defined with papules extraneous to the lichenified areas. Even with repeated scratching a few patients never develop lichenification. The exudative lesions typical of the infant phase are not as common, but can occur. Most patients with chronic lesions tolerate their disease and sleep well.

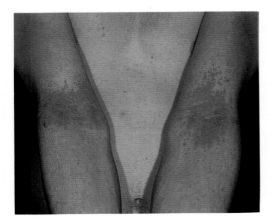

Figure 5-10
Atopic dermatitis. Classic appearance of confluent papules forming plaques in the antecubital fossa.

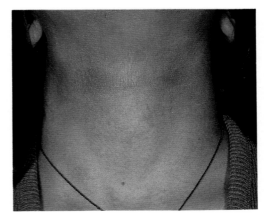

Figure 5-11
Atopic dermatitis. Classic appearance of erythema and diffuse scaling about the neck.

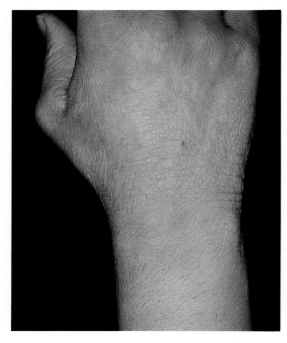

Figure 5-12
Atopic dermatitis. A chronically inflamed lichenified plaque on the wrist.

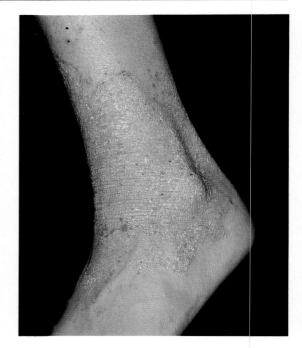

Figure 5-13
Sharply defined lichenified plaque with a silvery scale showing some of the features of psoriasis. Erosions are present.

Figure 5-14
Hypopigmentation in the antecubital fossa caused by destruction of melanocytes by chronic scratching.

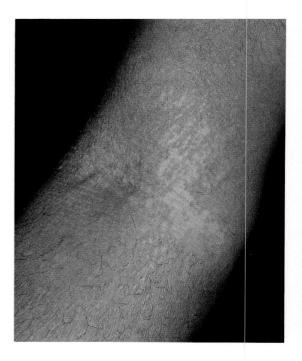

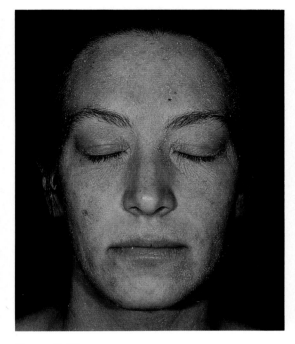

Figure 5-15
Generalized atopic dermatitis. Diffuse erythema and scaling are present.

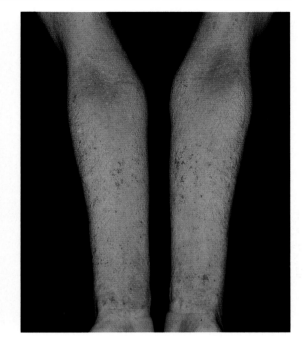

Figure 5-16
Generalized atopic dermatitis. Extension of inflammation beyond the classic areas of involvement. Numerous infected erosions are present.

Constant scratching may lead to destruction of melanocytes, resulting in areas of hypopigmentation that become more obvious when the inflammation subsides. These hypopigmented areas fade with time (Figure 5-14). Additional exacerbating factors such as heat, cold dry air, emotional stress, or any other factor that stimulates scratching may cause the inflammation to extend beyond the confines of the crease areas (Figures 5-15 and 5-16). Inflammation to this extent is incapacitating. Normal duration of sleep cannot be maintained, and schoolwork or job performance deteriorates; these people are miserable. They discover that standing in a hot shower gives considerable temporary relief, but further progression is inevitable with the drying effect produced by repeated wetting and drying. In the more advanced cases, hospitalization is required. Most patients with this pattern of inflammation will be in remission by age 30,[9] but in a few patients the disease becomes chronic, or improves only to relapse during a change of season or at some other period of transition. Their dermatitis becomes a lifelong ordeal.

Adult phase

The adult phase of atopic dermatitis begins near the onset of puberty. The reason for the resurgence of inflammation at this time is not understood, but it may be related to hormonal changes or to the stress of early adolescence. Adults may have no history of dermatitis in earlier years, but this is unusual. As in the childhood phase, localized inflammation with lichenification is the most common pattern. One area or several areas may be involved. There are several characteristic appearances.

Inflammation in flexural areas. Inflammation in flexural areas is common and is identical to childhood flexural inflammation.

Hand dermatitis. Hand dermatitis may be the most common expression of the atopic diathesis in the adult (see Chapter 3). Adults are exposed to a variety of irritating chemicals in the home and at work, and most wash more frequently than do children. Irritation causes redness and scaling on the dorsal aspect of the hand or about the fingers. Itching develops, and the inevitable scratching results in lichenification or oozing and crusting. A few or all

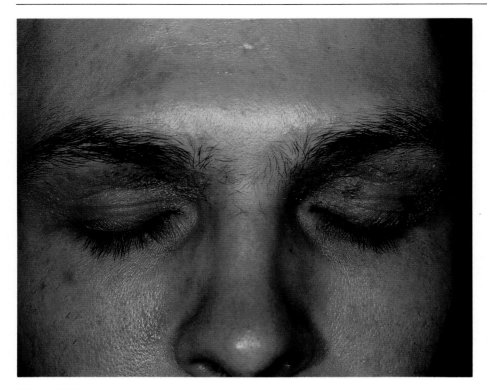

Figure 5-17
Atopic dermatitis of the upper eyelids, an area that is often rubbed with the back of the hand.

of the fingertip pads may be involved. They may be dry and chronically peeling or red and fissured. The eruption may be painful, chronic, and resistant to treatment. Psoriasis may have an identical appearance.

Inflammation around eyes. The eyelids are thin, frequently exposed to irritants, and easily traumatized by scratching. Many adults with atopic dermatitis have inflammation localized to the upper lids (Figure 5-17). They may claim to be allergic to something, but elimination of suspected allergens may not solve the problem. Habitual rubbing with the back of the hand is typical. If an attempt at controlling inflammation fails, then patch testing should be considered to eliminate allergic contact dermatitis.

Lichenification of anogenital area. Lichenification of the anogenital area is probably more common in atopic patients. Intertriginous areas that are warm and moist can become irritated and itch. Lichenification of the vulva, scrotum, and rectum may develop with habitual scratching. These areas are resistant to treatment, and inflammation may last for years. Modesty often delays the visit to the physi-

cian, and the untreated lichenified plaques become very thick. Emotional factors should also be considered with this isolated phenomenon.

Associated Features

Dry skin and xerosis

Dry skin is an important feature of the atopic state (see also Chapter 3). Drier than normal skin may appear at any age, and it is not unusual for infants to have dry scaling skin on the lower legs. Dry skin is sensitive, easily irritated, and itchy. It is the itching that provides the basis for the development of various forms of atopic dermatitis. In other words, it is the itch that rashes. Dry skin is most often located on the extensor surfaces of the legs and arms, but in susceptible individuals it may involve the entire cutaneous surface. Individual variation is great, and some atopic patients never develop anything more than dry skin in the winter. As winter approaches, humidity falls and water is lost from the outermost layer of the skin. The skin becomes drier as winter continues, and scaling skin becomes cracked and

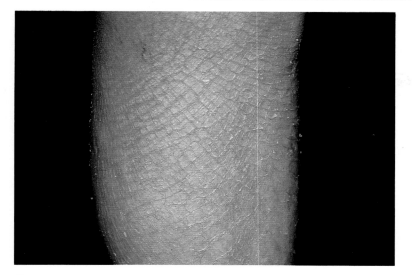

Figure 5-18
Dominant ichthyosis vulgaris. White translucent quadrangular scales on the extensor aspects of the arms and legs. This form is significantly associated with atopy.

fissured. Dry areas are washed repeatedly, and eventually the epidermal barrier can no longer maintain its integrity; erythema may appear. Overwashing and drying may produce redness with horizontal linear splits, particularly on the lower legs of the elderly, giving a cracked or crazed porcelain appearance (see Chapter 3, Figures 3-20 through 3-22).

Ichthyosis vulgaris

Ichthyosis is a disorder of keratinization characterized by the development of dry rectangular scales. There are many forms of ichthyosis. Dominant ichthyosis vulgaris may occur as a distinct entity, or it may be found in the atopic patient. These patients with ichthyosis vulgaris often have keratosis pilaris and hyperlinear exaggerated palm creases. The infant may show only dry scaling skin during the winter. With age, however, the changes become more extensive, and small, fine white translucent scales appear on the extensor aspects of the arms and legs (Figure 5-18). These scales are smaller and lighter in color than the large brown polygonal scales of sex-linked ichthyosis vulgaris that occurs exclusively in males (Figure 5-19). The scaling of the dominant form does not encroach on the axillae and fossae, as is seen in the sex-linked type. Scaling rarely involves the entire cutaneous surface. The condition tends to improve with age.

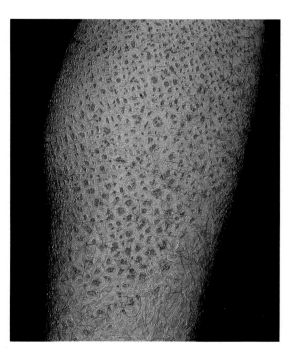

Figure 5-19
Sex-linked ichthyosis vulgaris. Large brown quadrangular scales that may encroach on the antecubital and popliteal fossae. Compare this presentation with Figure 5-18. There is no association with atopy.

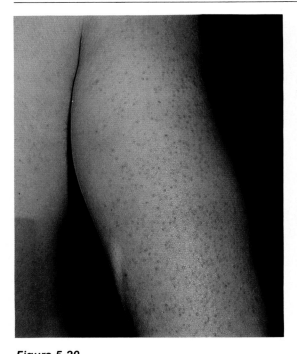

Figure 5-20
Keratosis pilaris. Small follicular papules are most commonly found on the posterolateral aspects of the upper arms.

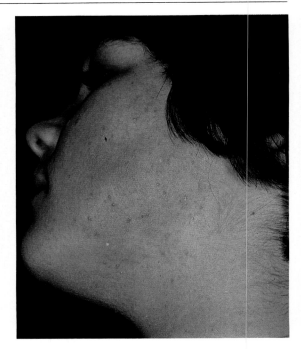

Figure 5-21
Keratosis pilaris. This is common on the face of children and is frequently confused with acne.

Keratosis pilaris

Keratosis pilaris is so common that it is probably physiologic. It does, however, seem to be more common and more extensive in the atopic patient. Small (1 to 2 mm) rough follicular papules or pustules may appear at any age and are common in young children. The peak incidence occurs during adolescence, and the problem tends to improve thereafter. The posterolateral aspects of the upper arms (Figure 5-20) and anterior thighs are frequently involved, but any area, with the exception of the palms and soles, may be involved. Lesions on the face may be confused with acne, but the uniform small size and association with dry skin and chapping differentiate keratosis pilaris from pustular acne (Figure 5-21). The eruption may be generalized, resembling heat rash or miliaria. Most cases are asymptomatic, but the lesions may be red, inflammatory, and pustular and resemble bacterial folliculitis, particularly on the thighs (Figure 5-22). In the adult generalized form, a red halo appears at the periphery of the keratotic papule (Figure 5-23). This unusual diffuse pattern in adults persists indefinitely. Systemic steroid therapy may greatly accentuate both the lesion and the distribution, result-

ing in numerous follicular pustules. No treatment other than lubrication is required for localized asymptomatic lesions.

Patients with widespread atypical or psychologically troubling keratosis pilaris may be treated with the following program devised by Novick.[10] The patient should first be advised about measures to prevent excessive skin dryness (see Exacerbating Factors below).

Patients with a prominent inflammatory component to the lesions should apply a Group V, emollient-based, topical steroid preparation twice daily until overall inflammation is markedly reduced. This is usually achieved in 7 days. At this point the topical steroid should be discontinued.

Following a daily shower the patient should gently pat-dry the skin, leaving it moist. A pharmacist-compounded preparation consisting of salicylic acid 2% to 3% in urea cream (Carmol 20) should then be gently massaged into the moist skin with a polyester cleaning sponge (e.g., Buf-Puf). During the first week, affected areas should be lightly massaged for about 5 seconds. After the sponge massage the residual cream should be gently rubbed into the skin with the fingertips. If

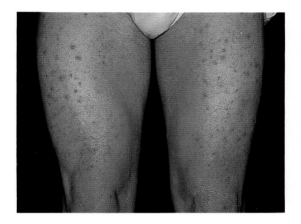

Figure 5-22
Keratosis pilaris. Infected lesions in a uniform distribution. Typical bacterial folliculitis has a haphazard distribution.

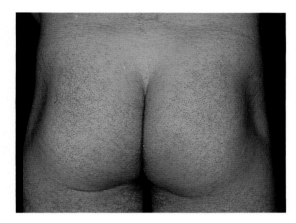

Figure 5-23
Keratosis pilaris. Diffuse lesions are occasionally seen in adults. This type lasts indefinitely.

no irritation has resulted after the first week, the patient may increase the pressure of the massage or the duration of massage by 5 seconds or both every 2 or 3 days; skin tolerance to the abrasion must be built up gradually. Patients will seldom require more than 20 seconds on each area daily to establish satisfactory control.

Once satisfactory control is obtained, the frequency of treatment may be reduced to once or twice weekly and straight 20% urea cream (Carmol 20), an over-the-counter item, substituted.

Hyperlinear palmar creases

Atopic patients frequently reveal an accentuation of the major skin creases of the palms (Figure 5-24), which may be present in infancy and become more prominent as age and severity of skin inflammation increase. The changes might be initiated by rubbing or scratching and may be a form of lichenification or thickening without eczematous inflammation, peculiar to the area. Patients with accentuated skin creases seem to have more extensive inflammation on the body and a longer disease course. Occasionally patients without atopic dermatitis have accentuated palm creases.

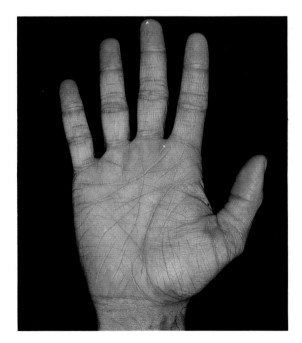

Figure 5-24
Hyperlinear palmar creases. Seen frequently in patients with severe atopic dermatitis.

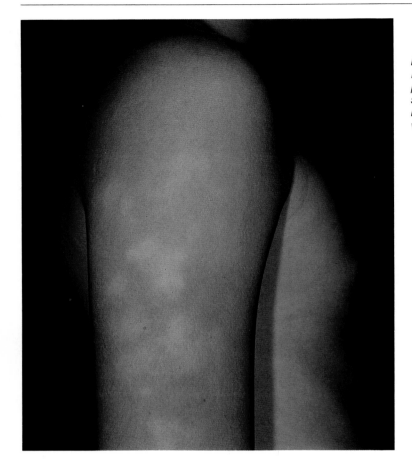

Figure 5-25
Pityriasis alba. Irregular hypo-pigmented areas are frequently seen in atopic patients and are not to be confused with tinea versicolor or vitiligo.

Pityriasis alba

Pityriasis alba is a common disorder that is characterized by asymptomatic, hypopigmented, slightly elevated fine scaling plaque with indistinct borders. The condition, which involves the face and lateral upper arms, appears in young children and usually disappears by early adulthood. The white round-to-oval areas vary in size but generally average 2 to 4 cm in diameter (Figure 5-25). Lesions become obvious in the summer months when the areas fail to tan. Parents are concerned about its appearance but should be assured that the loss of pigment is not permanent, as in vitiligo. Vitiligo and the fungal infection tinea versicolor both appear to be white, but the margin between normal and hypopigmented skin in vitiligo is distinct. Tinea versicolor is rarely located on the face, and the hypopigmented areas are more numerous and often confluent. Examination of a potassium hydroxide slide preparation of the scale will quickly settle the question. No treatment other than lubrication should be attempted unless the patches become eczematous.

Atopic pleats

The appearance of an extra line on the lower eyelid (Dennie-Morgan infraorbital fold) has been considered a distinguishing feature of the atopic patient. Since this extra line may also appear in the nonatopic patient, it is an unreliable sign of the atopic state.

Cataracts and keratoconus

Analysis of a large group of atopic patients showed about a 10% incidence of cataracts.[11] The reason for their development is not understood. Most are asymptomatic and can be detected only by slit-lamp examination. Two types have been reported: the "complicated type," which begins at the posterior pole in the immediate subcapsular region, and the anterior plaque or shield-like opacity, which lies subcapsularly and in the pupillary zone.[12] The anterior plaque type is the most frequently described. Posterior subcapsular cataracts are a well established complication of systemic steroid therapy. Recent data suggest that there is no safe dose of corticosteroids and that individual susceptibility may determine the threshold for development of cataracts.[13] It may be that atopic patients have a lower threshold or a greater tendency to develop cataracts, particularly when challenged with systemic steroids. This fact must be considered for the unusual atopic patient who requires systemic steroids for short-term control. Malpractice suits have been filed against physicians who prescribed systemic steroids for patients who subsequently developed cataracts.

Keratoconus (elongation and protrusion of the corneal surface) has been considered as being more common in the atopic state. However, the incidence is low, and it does not appear to be associated with cataracts.

Exacerbating Factors

Factors that promote dryness or increase the desire to scratch worsen atopic dermatitis. Understanding and controlling these aggravating factors are essential to the successful management of atopic dermatitis.

Temperature change

Atopic patients do not tolerate sudden changes in temperature. Sweating induces itching, particularly in the antecubital and popliteal fossae, to a greater extent than in the normal individual. Lying under warm blankets, entering a warm room, and physical stress all intensify the desire to scratch. A sudden lowering of temperature, such as leaving a warm shower, promotes itching. Wearing clothing that tends to contain heat should be discouraged.

Decreased humidity

The beginning of fall heralds the onset of a difficult period for atopic patients. Cold air cannot support much humidity. The moisture-containing outer first layer of the skin reaches equilibrium with the atmosphere and consequently holds less moisture. Dry skin is less supple, more fragile, and more easily irritated. Pruritus is established, the rash appears, and the long winter months in the northern states may be a difficult period to endure. Commercially available humidifiers can offer some relief by increasing the humidity in the house above 50%. Discourage patients from lathering their extremities while they are bathing.

Excessive washing

Repeated washing and drying remove water-binding lipids from the first layer of the skin. Daily baths may be tolerated in the summer months but will lead to excessive dryness in the fall and winter.

Contact with irritating substances

Wool, household and industrial chemicals, cosmetics, and some soaps and detergents promote irritation and inflammation in the atopic patient. The inflammation is frequently interpreted as an allergic reaction by patients who claim they are allergic to almost everything they touch. These complaints reflect an intolerance to irritation. Although some atopic patients do develop allergic contact dermatitis, the incidence is lower than in the general population.

Emotional stress

Stressful situations can have a profound effect on the course of atopic dermatitis. A stable course can quickly degenerate, and localized inflammation may almost overnight become extensive. Patients are well aware of this phenomenon and regretfully believe that they are responsible for their disease. This notion is reinforced by relatives and friends who assure them that their disease "is caused by your nerves." Explaining that atopic dermatitis is an inherited disease that is made worse, rather than caused, by emotional stress is reassuring.

Treatment

Treatment goals consist of attempting to eliminate inflammation and infection, hydrating the skin, and controlling exacerbating factors. Most patients can be brought under adequate control in less than 3 weeks. Possible reasons for failure to respond include poor patient compliance, allergic contact dermatitis to a topical medicine, the simultaneous occurrence of asthma or hayfever, inadequate sedation, continued emotional stress, and ingestion of specific food allergens in sensitized patients.

Topical steroids or tar ointments are used to control inflammation. Oral antibiotics are more effective for eradicating infection than topical antibiotics.

Infants

Infants with dry, red, scaling plaques on the cheeks will respond to Group V, VI, or VII topical steroids applied twice daily for 6 to 10 days. Parents are instructed to decrease the frequency of washing, start lubrication with a bland lubricant during the initial phase of the treatment period, and continue lubrication long after topical steroids have been discontinued. Antistaphylococcal antibiotics are required only if there is moderate serum and crusting. Cracking around the lips is controlled in a similar manner, but heavier lubricants (such as Chapstick) are used after the inflammation is clear. Infants with more generalized inflammation require 10 to 21 days of a Group V, VI, or VII topical steroid applied 3 times a day. Secondary infection often accompanies generalized inflammation, and an appropriate antistaphylococcal antibiotic such as cephalexin suspension (Keflex) twice daily is required.

Children and adults

Lichenified plaques in older children and adults respond to Groups II through V topical steroids under occlusion dressing (Figure 5-26). Occlusive therapy for 10 to 14 days is preferred if the plaques are resistant to treatment, or occlusion may be used from the onset after infection has been controlled if the plaque is very thick. Diffuse inflammation involving the face, trunk, and extremities is treated with Group V topical steroids applied 3 times a day. Systemic antibiotics are almost invariably required. Exudative areas with serum and crust should be treated with a Burow's solution compress for 20 minutes 3 times a day for 2 to 3 days. Dryness and cracking with fissures occur if compressing is prolonged. Resistant cases may be treated with Group V topical steroids applied before and after vinyl suit occlusion. The suit may be worn to bed or used 2 hours twice a day. All signs of infection such as serum and crust should be clear before initiating occlusive therapy. A 10-day course of 20 mg of prednisone twice daily is needed only rarely to control difficult cases.

Oral and intramuscular steroid therapy has a number of disadvantages. The relapse rate is high, with inflammation returning shortly after the medication is discontinued. Enthusiasm for topical therapy diminishes once the patient has experienced the rapid clearing produced by systemic therapy, prompting patient requests to try systemic therapy again. The answer should be no. Hospitalization with topical medication and sedation is indicated for the atopic patient with generalized inflammation who does not respond to routine measures. The association of atopic cataracts with systemic steroid therapy has been discussed. Tar ointments were the mainstay of therapy before topical steroids were introduced. They were effective and had few side effects but did not work quickly. Tar in a lubricating

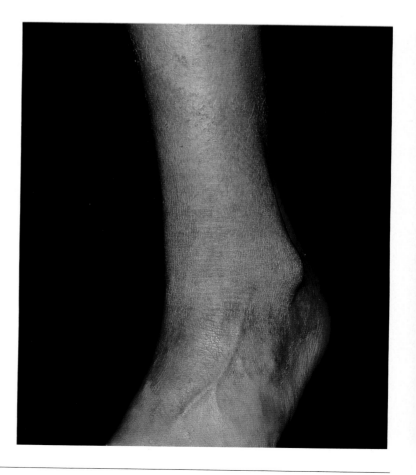

Figure 5-26
Response to treatment. Lichenified plaque shown in Figure 5-13 after 7 days of a Group IV topical steroid under occlusion dressing.

base such as T-Derm or Fototar applied twice a day is an effective alternative to topical steroids. Intensely inflamed areas should first be controlled with topical steroids. Tar ointments can then be used to complete therapy. Tar can be used as an initial therapy for chronic superficial plaques.

Lubrication

Restoring moisture to the skin increases the rate of healing and establishes a durable barrier against further drying and irritation. A variety of lotions and creams is available, and most are adequate for rehydration (see Table 2-1). Their use should be encouraged, particularly during the winter months. Patients should be cautioned that lotions may sting shortly after application. This may be a property of the base or a specific ingredient such as lactic acid. If itching or stinging continue with each application, another product should be selected. If inflammation occurs after use of a lubricant, then allergic contact dermatitis to a preservative or a perfume should be considered. Bath oils are an effective method of lubrication, but they can make the tub slippery and dangerous for older patients. In order to be effective, a sufficient amount of oil must be used to create an oily feeling on the skin when leaving the tub. Septic systems may be adversely affected by prolonged use of bath oils. A mild soap should be used infrequently (see Table 2-1); Dove, Keri, Purpose, Oilatum, and Basis are adequate. Ivory is drying and should be avoided.

Sedation

Antihistamines relieve itching, have a calming effect, and aid more comfortable sleep. They should be considered for both infants and adults. Antihistamines may be prescribed on a continuous basis or only before bedtime, depending on the needs of the individual. Continuing antihistamines for a short period after inflammation has subsided assists a smooth course of recovery. Hydroxyzine (Atarax, Durrax, Vistaril) is well tolerated by most patients, and the dosage can be varied over a wide range with little risk of side effects.

REFERENCES

1. Johnson ML: Prevalence of dermatologic disease among persons 1-74 years of age: United States. In Advance data from vital and health statistics of the national center for health statistics, No. 4, Jan. 26, 1977.
2. Cormane RH: B and T cells in dermatitis. Mayo Clin Proc **49**:531, 1974.
3. Roth HL, Kierland RR: The natural history of atopic dermatitis. Arch Dermatol **89**:209, 1964.
4. Dahl MV: Atopic dermatitis. In Clinical immunodermatology. Chicago, 1981, Year Book Medical Publishers, Inc.
5. Stone SP, Muller SA, Glech GJ: IgE levels in atopic dermatitis. Arch Dermatol **108**:806, 1973.
6. Hanifin JM, Ray LF, Lobitz WC Jr: Immunologic reactivity in dermatophytosis. Br J Dermatol **90**:1, 1974.
7. Musgrove K, Morgan JK: Infantile eczema. Br J Dermatol **95**:365, 1976.
8. Sampson HH, Jolie PL: Increased plasma histamine concentrations after food challenges in children with atopic dermatitis. N Engl J Med **311**:372, 1984.
9. Soloman LM: Atopic dermatitis in dermatology. Philadelphia, 1975, W.B. Saunders Co.
10. Novick NE: Practical management of widespread, atypical keratosis pilaris. J Am Acad Dermatol **11**: 305, 1984.
11. Roth HL, Kierland RR: The natural history of atopic dermatitis. Arch Dermatol **89**:209, 1964.
12. Rosen E: Atopic cataract. Springfield, Ill, 1959, Charles C Thomas, Publisher.
13. Skalka HW, Prachal JT: Effects of corticosteroids on cataract formation. Arch Ophthalmol **98**:1773, 1980.

Urticaria

Urticaria, also referred to as hives or wheals, is a common and distinctive reaction pattern. Hives may occur at any age; up to 20% of the population will have at least one episode during a lifetime. Hives may be more common in atopic patients. Urticaria is classified as acute or chronic. The majority of cases are acute, lasting from hours to a few weeks. Because most individuals can diagnose urticaria and realize that it is a self-limited condition, they do not seek medical attention. The etiology of acute urticaria has been determined in many cases, but the cause of chronic urticaria (arbitrarily defined as hives lasting longer than 6 weeks) has been determined in only 5% to 20% of cases.[1] Patients with chronic urticaria present a major problem in diagnosis and management. These patients are often subjected to detailed and expensive medical evaluations that usually prove unrewarding. Recent studies have demonstrated the value of a complete history and physical examination followed by the judicious use of laboratory studies in evaluating the results of the examination.

Clinical Aspects

A hive or wheal is an erythematous or white non-pitting edematous plaque that changes in size and shape by peripheral extension or regression during the few hours or days that the individual lesion exists. The hive results from localized capillary vasodilatation, followed by transudation of protein-rich fluid into the surrounding tissue, and resolves when the fluid is slowly reabsorbed.

The evolution of urticaria is a dynamic process. New lesions are evolving as older ones resolve. Lesions vary in size from the 1 to 3 mm edematous papules of cholinergic urticaria to giant hives, a single lesion of which may cover an extremity. They may be round or oval; when confluent, they become polycyclic (Figure 6-1). A portion of the border either may not form or may be reabsorbed, giving the appearance of incomplete rings (Figure 6-2). Hives may be uniformly red or white, or the edematous border may be red and the remainder of the surface white. This variation in color is usually present in hives that are superficial. Thicker plaques have a uniform color (Figures 6-1 and 6-3).

Hives may be surrounded by a clear or red halo. Thicker plaques that result from massive transudation of fluid into the dermis and subcutaneous tissue are referred to as angioedema. These thick firm plaques, like typical hives, may occur on any skin surface, but they usually involve the lips, larynx (causing hoarseness or sore throat), and mucosa of the gastrointestinal tract (causing abdominal pain) (Figures 6-4 and 6-5). Bullae or purpura may appear in areas of intense swelling. Purpura and scaling may result as the lesions or urticarial vasculitis clear. Hives usually have a haphazard distribution, but those elicited by physical stimuli have characteristic features and distribution.

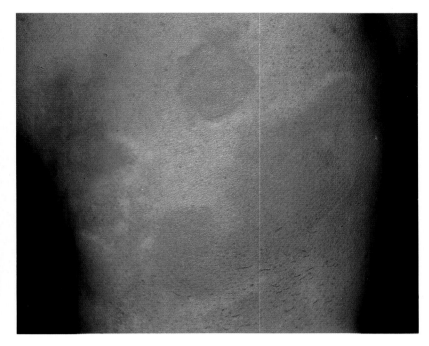

Figure 6-1
Hives. The most characteristic presentation is
uniformly red edematous plaques surrounded by
a faint white halo.

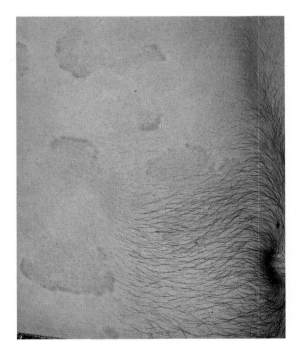

Figure 6-2
Hives. Polycyclic pattern.

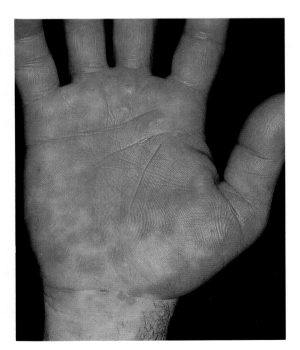

Figure 6-3
Hives. The entire palm is affected and is greatly
swollen. The lesions resemble those of erythema
multiforme.

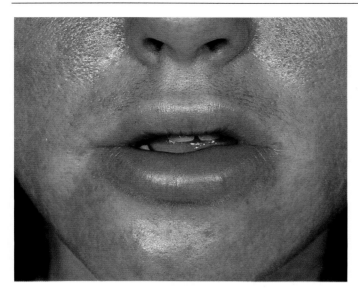

Figure 6-4
Angioedema. Urticarial swelling of the lower lip.

Figure 6-5
Angioedema. Massive swelling of the entire central area of the back.

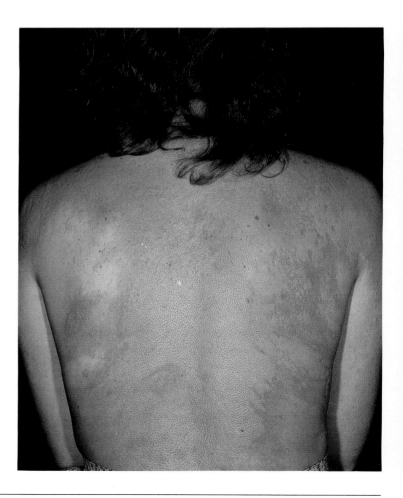

Pathophysiology

Histamine is the most important chemical mediator of urticaria. When injected into skin, histamine produces the triple response of Lewis, the features of which are local erythema (vasodilatation), the flare characterized by erythema beyond the border of the local erythema, and a wheal produced from leakage of fluid from the postcapillary venule.

Histamine induces vascular changes by a number of mechanisms (Figure 6-6). Blood vessels contain two (and possibly more) receptors for histamine. The two most studied are designated H_1 and H_2. When stimulated by histamine, H_1 receptors cause an axon reflex, vasodilatation, and pruritus. They are blocked by the vast majority of clinically available antihistamines called H_1 antagonists (e.g., chlorpheniramine), which occupy the receptor site and prevent attachment of histamine.[2] H_2 receptor stimulation results in vasodilatation. H_2 receptors are also present on the mast cell membrane surface and, when stimulated, inhibit further production of histamine. Cimetidine and ranitidine are clinically available H_2 blocking agent (antihistamine). H_2 receptors are present at other sites and mediate gastric acid secretion, atrial contraction, and uterine contraction.

Histamine causes endothelial cell contraction, which allows vascular fluid to leak between the cells through the vessel wall, contributing to tissue edema and wheal formation. Histamine is contained in the granules of mast cells. A variety of immunologic, nonimmunologic, physical, and chemical stimuli may be responsible for the degranulation of mast cell granules and the release of histamine into the surrounding tissue and circulation (Figure 6-7). All such stimuli appear to initiate the release of histamine by first reacting with different cell membrane receptors. Activation of one group of receptors stimulates the conversion of adenosine triphosphate (ATP) to cyclic adenosine monophosphate (AMP), and activation of another group stimulates conversion of guanosine triphosphate (GTP) to cyclic guanosine monophosphate (GMP).[3] Increasing intracellular concentrations of cyclic GMP lead to histamine release, whereas increasing concentrations of cyclic AMP inhibit histamine release.

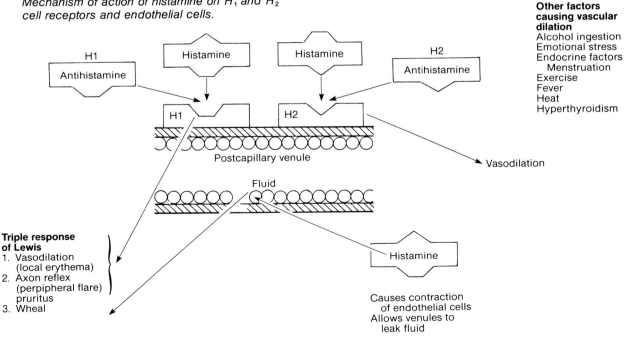

Figure 6-6

Mechanism of action of histamine on H_1 and H_2 cell receptors and endothelial cells.

Other factors causing vascular dilation
Alcohol ingestion
Emotional stress
Endocrine factors
  Menstruation
Exercise
Fever
Heat
Hyperthyroidism

Triple response of Lewis
1. Vasodilation (local erythema)
2. Axon reflex (perpipheral flare) pruritus
3. Wheal

Postcapillary venule

Vasodilation

Fluid

Histamine

Causes contraction of endothelial cells
Allows venules to leak fluid

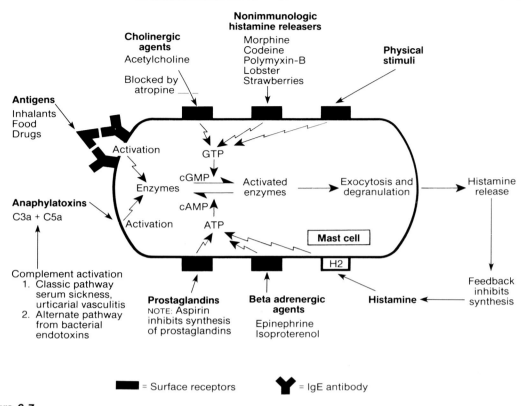

Figure 6-7
Pathophysiology of histamine release.

Histamine regulation
Factors increasing histamine release

Cell membrane–bound IgE plus antigen. Circulating antigens to foods, drugs, or inhalants interact with cell membrane–bound IgE.[4] This type I hypersensitivity reaction is probably responsible for most cases of acute urticaria.

Anaphylotoxins C3a and C5a. Complement may be activated to produce the anaphylotoxins C3a and C5a by either the classic or alternate pathway.[5] Complement activation via the classic pathway is initiated by the combination of circulating IgG or IgM with an antigen such as a drug. Type III hypersensitivity reactions (Arthus-type reaction) occur with deposition of insoluble immune complexes of IgG or IgM in vessel walls. Release of anaphylotoxins may take place during an Arthus-type reaction and accounts for the urticaria in serum sickness, hepatitis, and urticarial vasculitis.

Nonimmunologic release of histamine. Pharmacologic mediators such as acetylcholine, morphine, or strawberries react directly with cell membrane–bound mediators to release histamine.[6] The physical urticarias may be induced by both direct stimulation of cell membrane receptors and immunologic mechanisms.

Factors decreasing histamine release

Histamine. Histamine interacts with an H_2 mast cell surface receptor to inhibit further release of histamine. Therefore, histamine acts by feedback inhibition as an antihistamine in this case.

Beta-adrenergic agents. Beta-adrenergic agents such as epinephrine are powerful suppressors of histamine release. Their function may be influenced by steroid hormones, which may help explain why prednisone is sometimes useful for treating urticaria.

Prostaglandins. Prostaglandins may act as cell surface receptors to inhibit release of histamine. Aspirin inhibits the synthesis of certain prostaglandins.[7] This may explain why salicylates induce hives in a nonimmunologic way in many patients with chronic urticaria.

Evaluation

General evaluation of urticaria is outlined in Table 6-1, and the known causes are listed in Table 6-2. Knowledge of the etiologic factors will help direct the history and physical examination.

Determine that the patient actually has urticaria by skin examination. Urticaria induced by physical stimuli should be considered first in order to avoid an unnecessarily lengthy evaluation.

Determine whether hives are acute or chronic. There are no routine laboratory studies for the evaluation of acute urticaria. If acute (i.e., present for less than 6 weeks), perform a history and physical examination, with selected laboratory studies to investigate any abnormalities in the examination.[8] Drugs, foods, pollens, and physical stimuli are common causes of acute urticaria, and particular attention should be paid to these factors during the initial

---

TABLE 6-1

EVALUATION OF URTICARIA

Skin examination for the characteristics of hives
  Size
    Papular—cholinergic urticaria, bites
    Plaque—most cases
  Thickness
    Superficial—most cases
    Deep—angioedema
  Distribution
    Generalized—ingestants, inhalents, internal disease
    Localized—physical urticarias, contact urticaria
  Duration of individual lesion
    Less than 1 hour—physical urticarias, typical hives
    Less than 24 hours—typical hives
    More than 24 hours—urticarial vasculitis; scaling and purpura appear as hive resolves
Complete medical history
  Duration
    Acute—days to few weeks
    Chronic—more than 6 weeks
  Time of appearance
    Time of day
    Time of year
      Constant—food, internal disease
      Seasonal—inhalent allergy
  Environment
    Home—clear while at work or on vacation
    Work—contact or inhalant of chemicals
  Appearance after physical stimuli (physical urticaria)
    Scratching, pressure, exercise, sun exposure, cold
  Associated with arthralgia and fever
    Juvenile rheumatoid arthritis, rheumatic fever, serum sickness, systemic lupus erythematosus, urticarial vasculitis, viral hepatitis
Complete physical examination
  Sources of infection (e.g., sinus and gum infections)
  Internal disease, thyroid examination, etc.
Laboratory evaluation
  Acute and chronic urticaria—studies to confirm findings of history and physical examination
  Chronic urticaria—studies to consider, if cause not found:
    Sinus and dental films
    Change of environment
    Salicylate-free diet
    Skin biopsy of urticarial plaque (rule out urticarial vasculitis)

TABLE 6-2

ETIOLOGIC CLASSIFICATION OF URTICARIA

Foods
    Fish, shellfish, nuts, eggs, chocolate, strawberries, tomatoes, pork, cow's milk, cheese, wheat, yeast
Food additives
    Salicylates, benzoates, penicillin, dyes such as tartrazine
Drugs
    Penicillin, aspirin, sulfonamides; also drugs that cause a nonimmunologic release of histamine, e.g., morphine, codeine, polymyxin, dextran, curare, quinine
Infections
    Chronic bacterial infections (e.g., sinus, dental, chest, gallbladder, urinary tract), fungal infections (dermatophytosis, candidiasis), viral infections (viral hepatitis, infectious mononucleosis, coxsackie), protozoal and helminth infections (intestinal worms, malaria)
Inhalants
    Pollens, mold spores, animal danders, house dust, aerosols, volatile chemicals
Internal disease
    Serum sickness, systemic lupus erythematosus, hyperthyroidism, carcinomas, lymphomas, juvenile rheumatoid arthritis (Still's disease), leukocytoclastic vasculitis, polycythemia vera (acne urticata—urticarial papule surmounted by a vesicle), rheumatic fever
Physical stimuli (the physical urticarias)
    Dermographism, pressure urticaria, cholinergic urticaria, solar urticaria, cold urticaria, urticarias induced by heat, vibration, water (aquagenic)
Nonimmunologic contact urticaria
    Plants (nettles), animals (caterpillars, jellyfish), medications (cinnamic aldehyde, compound 48/80, dimethyl sulfoxide)
Immunologic or uncertain mechanism contact urticaria
    Ammonium persulfate used in hair bleaches, chemicals, foods, textiles, wood, saliva, cosmetics, perfumes
Skin diseases
    Urticaria pigmentosa (mastocytosis), dermatitis herpetiformis, pemphigoid, amyloidosis
Pregnancy
Genetic, autosomal dominant (all rare)
    Hereditary angioedema, cholinergic urticaria with progressive nerve deafness and amyloidosis of the kidney, familial cold urticaria, vibratory urticaria

evaluation.[9] Once all possible causes are eliminated, the patient is treated with antihistamines to suppress the hives and stop the itching. The approach in the early stages is conservative, because most of the cases end spontaneously in a short time and do not recur.

Chronic urticaria

Patients who have a history of hives lasting for 6 or more weeks are classified as having chronic urticaria. The patient must understand that the course of this disease is unpredictable; it may last for months or years. During the evaluation the patient should be assured that antihistamines will decrease discomfort. The patient should also be told that although the evaluation may be lengthy and is often unrewarding, in most cases the disease ends spontaneously. Patients who understand the nature of this disease will not become discouraged so easily, nor will they be as apt to go from physician to physician seeking a cure.

There are many studies in the literature on chronic urticaria.[10-12] Most demonstrate that if the cause is not found after investigation of abnormalities elicited during the history and physical examination, there is little chance that the cause will be determined. It is tempting to order laboratory tests such as antinuclear antibody levels (ANA) and stool examination for ova and parasites in an effort to be

TABLE 6-3

THE SALICYLATE, AZO DYE, AND BENZOIC ACID–FREE DIET: THE FOLLOWING FOODS MAY BE EATEN

Bread	Cereals (not flavored)	Rice
Sugar	Salad oils (not flavored)	Butter
Eggs	Milk	Cream
Beef	Chicken	Turkey
Fish	Lettuce	Parsley
Mushrooms	Potatoes	Plain rolls
Crackers	Veal	Lamb
Pork	Peanuts	Cottage cheese
Beans	Lima beans	Parsnips
Corn	Olives	Artichokes
Asparagus	Bean sprouts	Green beans
Wax beans	Beets	Beet greens
Broccoli	Brussels sprouts	Cabbage
Carrots	Cauliflower	Celery
Swiss chard	Chives	Eggplant
Lettuce	Onions	Pineapples
Pumpkin	Radishes	Spinach
Squash	Turnip greens	Turnips
Dates	Figs	Loganberries
Mango	Pears	
Tangerines		

thorough, but results of studies do not support this approach.[8] However, there are certain tests and procedures that might be considered when the initial evaluation has proved unrewarding.

Sinus films. In one study,[8] sinus films were found to be abnormal in 17% of patients with chronic urticaria. The presence of sinus disease was not suspected in any of the patients before the radiologic studies. In all patients with sinus involvement who were also treated for acute sinusitis, the urticaria cleared and subsequent x-ray films showed no sinus disorders. Since the pathologic disorder was not evident on history or physical examination, the authors recommended that sinus films should be considered for all patients with chronic urticaria, especially of recent onset.

Change of environment. Since the environment consists of numerous antigens, patients should consider a trial period of 1 or 2 weeks of separation from home and work, preferably with a geographic change.

Salicylate-free diet. Salicylate-free diets[13] may be beneficial (Tables 6-3 and 6-4). Several studies revealed that a significant number of patients with chronic urticaria developed hives when challenged with food coloring azo dyes (e.g., tartrazine), salicylates, and benzoic acid food preservatives.[14,15]

While these substances may not be the primary cause of the urticaria in such patients, they may be an aggravating factor. The salicylate, azo dye, and benzoic acid–free diet is not extremely restrictive and may be worth the effort for difficult cases.

Other procedures. Other procedures such as the prick test to *Candida albicans,* challenge test to live food yeasts, antifungal therapy, and low yeast diet may be useful. One study revealed that *C albicans* sensitivity is an important factor in about 26% of patients with chronic urticaria.[16] Prick tests to standard yeast allergens were performed by depositing a drop of the allergens on the skin and introducing a hypodermic needle into the epidermis parallel to the skin surface to the length of the bevel. Prick test sites were examined after 15 minutes; any wheal of 4 mm diameter or more was interpreted as a positive reading. Whealing, induration, or both occurring 4 to 8 hours after the test was considered positive. Patients with a positive prick test who respond with hives when challenged with commercially available bakers' yeast are treated according to the protocol for elimination of yeast, outlined in Table 6-5.

Skin biopsy. Patients with hives characteristic of urticarial vasculitis should have a biopsy taken of the urticarial plaque.

TABLE 6-4

SOURCES OF SALICYLATES, AZO DYES, AND BENZOIC ACID

Foods containing natural salicylate

Almonds	Currants	Nectarines
Apples	Dewberries	Oranges
Apricots	Gooseberries	Peaches
Bananas	Grapefruit	Pickles
Blackberries	Grapes or raisins	Plums or prunes
Blueberries	Green peas	Raspberries
Boysenberries	Green peppers	Strawberries
Cherries	Lemons	Tabasco peppers
Cucumbers	Melons	Tomatoes

Foods containing salicylates, azo dyes, or benzoic acid

Most foods containing artificial color or flavors, such as breakfast cereals (Cheerios, Sugar Jets, Bran Flakes, Product 19, Raisin Bran, Sugar Pops), bakery goods (dinner rolls, cinnamon rolls, cake mixes, frosting mixes, cookie mixes, tarts, turnovers, brownie mixes), puddings, mints, flavored candies, flavored chips (Whistles, taco chips), ice cream, jellies, jams, macaroni and spaghetti (certain brands), some packaged and canned soups, mayonnaise, salad dressings, luncheon meats (salami, bologna), frank-furters, oleomargarine, ketchup (certain brands), mustard, cider and wine vinegars, canned fish (anchovies, herring, sardines, caviar, cleaned shellfish), fruit gelatins, some cheeses, flavored sauces, surface-treated fish (can be washed away)

Beverages containing salicylates, azo dyes, or benzoic acid

Root beer	Flavored colas
Cider	Fruit juices
Wine	Kool-aids
Gin	Beer
Distilled liquor (except vodka)	

Drugs and other products

Aspirin and aspirin-containing compounds (hundreds of preparations), toothpaste and toothpowder, mint flavors, mouthwashes, lozenges, gum, some antihistamines

TABLE 6-5

PROTOCOL FOR ELIMINATION OF YEAST

Anti-*Candida* treatment
1. Nystatin tablet, 1,000,000 units 3 times a day for 2 weeks, followed by nystatin tablet 500,000 units 3 times a day for 2 weeks
2. Nystatin tablet 1,000,000 units, dissolve in mouth twice daily for 1 week
3. Miconazole vaginal cream, insert in vaginal tract before bedtime for 2 weeks

Low yeast diet

The following foods must not be eaten: breads, buns, sausage, wines, beer, cider, grapes, sultana raisins, cheese, vinegar, tomato ketchup, pickles

If the patient improves, the low yeast diet is continued and nystatin is gradually tapered and then discontinued

The Physical Urticarias

During the initial examination, whether the hives are elicited by physical stimuli should be determined. Patients with these distinctive hives may be spared a detailed evaluation; they simply require an explanation of their condition and its treatment. A major distinguishing feature of the physical urticarias is that attacks are brief, lasting only 30 to 60 minutes.[17] In typical urticaria, individual lesions last from hours to a few days. The one exception in physical urticarias is a type of pressure urticaria that may last for several hours.

Dermographism

Also known as "skin writing," dermographism is the most common of the physical urticarias and is produced by rubbing or stroking the skin. A tongue blade drawn firmly across the patient's arm or back will elicit an exaggerated triple response of Lewis (Figure 6-8). Erythema is followed by edema and a surrounding red flare. As a control the examining physician should perform this test on his or her own arm at the same time. The exaggerated edema and red flare appear within minutes. The tendency to be dermographic appears at any age and may last for months or years. It may be preceded by infection, antibiotic therapy, or emotional upset, but in most cases the cause is unknown.

The degree of urticarial response varies. A patient will be highly reactive for months and then appear to be in remission, only to have symptoms recur (Figure 6-9). Patients complain of linear itchy wheals from scratching or wheals at the site of friction from clothing. Delayed dermographism, in

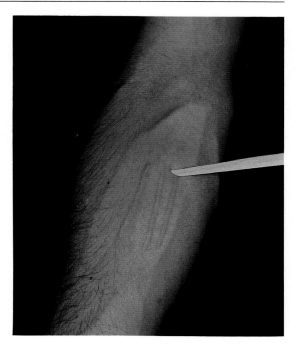

Figure 6-8
Dermographism. A tongue blade drawn firmly across the arm will elicit urticaria in susceptible individuals.

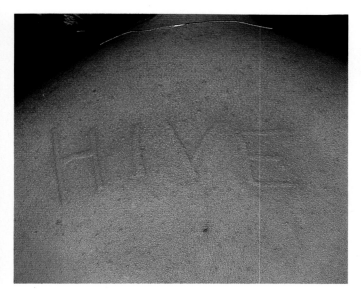

Figure 6-9
Dermographism. A highly sensitive patient.

which the immediate urticarial response is followed in 1 to 6 hours by a wheal that persists for 24 to 48 hours, is rare. Treatment is not necessary unless the patient is highly sensitive and reacts continually to the slightest trauma. Short courses of antihistamines (e.g., hydroxyzine in relatively low doses, 10 to 25 mg every 4 hours) provide adequate relief.

Pressure urticaria

A deep, itchy, painful swelling occurring 4 to 6 hours after pressure has been applied to an area and lasting 8 to 48 hours is characteristic of this uncommon form of physical urticaria. The feet and buttocks are the most common sites. Since the swelling occurs hours after the application of pressure, the cause may not be immediately apparent. Repeated deep swelling in the same area is the clue to the diagnosis. Patients with dermographism may have whealing from pressure that occurs immediately, rather than hours later.

Cholinergic urticaria

Round papular wheals 1 to 3 mm in diameter that are surrounded by a slight to extensive red flare occurring after exercise, exposure to heat, or emotional stress are diagnostic of this most distinctive type of hives (Figure 6-10). Typically, the hives occur during or shortly after exercise. However, their onset may be delayed for about an hour after stimulation. Cholinergic urticaria may become confluent and resemble typical hives, appear simultaneously with typical hives and angioedema, or be accompanied by wheezing. The condition is most common in young adults and resolves spontaneously after months or years.

The diagnosis is suspected from a history of developing small itchy bumps following strenuous activity and is confirmed by experimentally reproducing the lesions. Challenge with an intradermal injection of cholinergic drugs such as methacholine chloride (Mecholyl) is diagnostic in some patients. A more reliable method is to ask the patient to run in place for 10 to 15 minutes and then to observe him or her for 1 hour to detect the typical micropapular hives. Symptoms are avoided by limiting strenuous exercise and showering with warm water. Antihistamines taken 1 hour before exercise attenuates the eruption, but the side effect of drowsiness is often unacceptable.

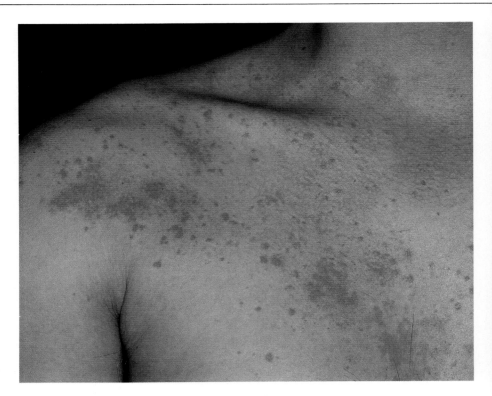

Figure 6-10
Cholinergic urticaria. Round red papular wheels that occur in response to exercise, heat, or emotional stress.

Solar urticaria

Hives occurring minutes after exposure of the skin to sun and disappearing in less than 1 hour are called solar urticaria. Previously exposed tanned skin may not react when exposed to ultraviolet light. Hives induced by exposure to ultraviolet light must be distinguished from the much more common sun-related condition of polymorphic light eruption. Lesions of polymorphic light eruption are rarely urticarial. They occur hours after exposure and persist for several days.

There are several different wavelengths that can cause solar urticaria.[18] An individual will react to a specific wavelength or a narrow band of the light spectrum, usually within the range of 290 to 500 nm. Those reacting to light above 400 nm (visible light) will develop hives even when exposed through glass. Solar urticaria has been described in patients with connective tissue diseases and porphyria. The wavelength responsible for solar urticaria is identified by phototesting. Antihistamines, sunscreens, and graded exposure to increasing amounts of light are effective treatments.

Cold urticaria

Cold urticaria occurs in both familial and acquired forms. The familial form is a dominantly transmitted autosomal disorder that is rare. Acquired cold urticaria begins in adolescence and resolves spontaneously. Hives occur with a sudden drop in air temperature or during exposure to cold water. Swimming in cold water may result in massive transudation of fluid into the skin, leading to hypotension and possibly death. Like dermographism, cold urticaria often begins after infection, drug therapy, or emotional stress. The diagnosis is made by inducing a hive with an ice cube held against the skin for 1 to 5 minutes (Figure 6-11). Patients are informed of the nature of the illness and must learn to protect themselves from a sudden increase or decrease in temperature. Antihistamines provide some relief.

Heat, water, and vibration urticarias

Other physical stimuli such as heat, water of any temperature, or vibration are rare causes of urticaria.

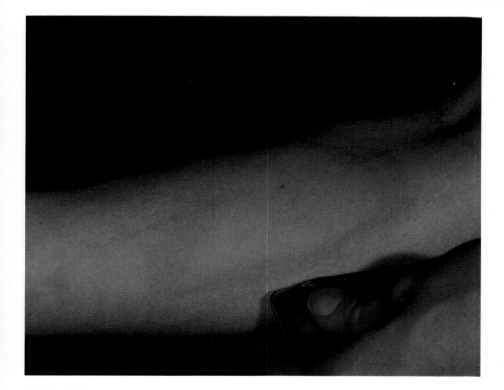

Figure 6-11
Cold urticaria. The hive occurred within minutes of holding an ice cube against the skin.

The Contact Urticaria Syndrome

Contact urticaria is characterized by a wheal and flare occurring within 30 to 60 minutes after cutaneous exposure to certain agents. Direct contact of the skin with these agents may cause wheal-and-flare response restricted to the area of contact, generalized urticaria, urticaria and asthma, or urticaria combined with an anaphylactoid reaction. In addition, some patients experience rhinitis, laryngeal edema, and abdominal disturbances. Urticaria occurs after the absorption of material through the skin and is elicited by nonimmunologic and immunologic mechanisms. Nonimmunologic, histamine-releasing substances are produced by certain plants (nettles), animals (caterpillars, jellyfish), and medications (dimethyl sulfoxide [DMSO]).[19,20] The mechanism by which woods, plants, foods, cosmetics, animal hair, and dander cause contact urticaria has not been defined. The term "protein contact dermatitis" is used when an immediate reaction occurs after eczematous skin is exposed to certain types of food (fish, garlic, onion, cives, cucumber, parsley, tomato), animal (cow hair and dander), or plant substances. Cooks who complain of burning or stinging when handling certain foods may have the contact urticaria syndrome.

Most patients give a history of relapsing deramtitis or generalized urticarial attacks rather than a localized hive, whereas others complain only of localized sensations of itching, burning, and tingling. Since there is no standard test battery for routine evaluation of contact urticaria, a careful history concerning the occurrence of immediate reactions, whether localized or generalized, is essential. An open patch test may be performed by applying a drop of the suspected substance to the ventral forearm and observing the site for a wheal 30 to 60 minutes later. Closed or intradermal tests may be associated with more intense or generalized reactions.

Urticarial Vasculitis

A group of patients has been identified with chronic urticaria and distinctive clinical and laboratory findings.[21,22] The urticarial plaques in most patients with chronic urticaria evolve completely in less than 24 hours and disappear while new plaques are appearing. A few patients with chronic urticaria have hives that persist for 24 to 72 hours; with resolution of lesions, they may have residual changes of purpura, scaling, and hyperpigmentation (Figure 6-12). Some of these patients complain of burning or painful lesions rather than pruritus. Erythema multiforme–like lesions may also be present. All of these patients have systemic com-

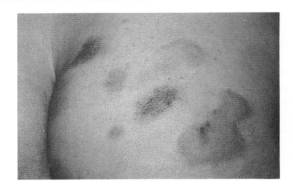

Figure 6-12
Urticarial vasculitis. Purpura occurs as the hive resolves.

plaints, with arthralgia being the most common. Other less common complaints in order of frequency are arthritis, gastrointestinal pain or distress, fever, and generalized adenopathy. As with typical cutaneous vasculitis, most patients have an elevated erythrocyte sedimentation rate and hypocomplementemia (depressed CH50, C4, or C2).

Biopsy in most cases shows a histologic picture indistinguishable from that seen in cutaneous necrotizing vasculitis (palpable purpura). In this case, fragmentation of leukocytes and fibrinoid deposition occur in the walls of postcapillary venules, a pattern called "leukocytoclastic vasculitis."

This disease, which has clinical features of urticaria and histologic features of vasculitis, may represent a midpoint in the spectrum of hypersensitivity diseases between urticaria and cutaneous necrotizing vasculitis. Unfortunately, as with most of the other related diseases, the etiology is not clear.

Treatment of Urticaria

For the majority of patients, acute and chronic urticaria may be controlled with antihistamines. In a simplified form, Figure 6-6 shows that histamine and antihistamines have similar chemical structures and that both fit into and compete for the same receptor site. Antihistamines do not block the release of histamine. If histamine has been released before an antihistamine is taken, the receptor sites will be occupied and the antihistamine will have no effect. The majority of antihistamines that are available are H_1 antagonists (i.e., compete for the H_1 receptor sites). Cimetidine and ranitidine are the only H_2 antagonists available at this time. Antihistamines control urticaria by inhibiting vasodilatation and vessel fluid loss. Antihistamines also have anticholinergic

TABLE 6-6

ANTIHISTAMINES*

Generic Name	Trade Name	Dosage (mg)	Dosing Intervals (hrs)	Degree of Drowsiness
Alkylamines				
Brompheniramine maleate	Dimetane	4	4-6	+
Chlorpheniramine maleate	Chlor-Trimeton	4 Liquid 2 mg/ 5 ml	6-8	+ +
Dexchlorpheniramine maleate	Polaramine	2 Liquid 2 mg/ 5 ml	4-6	+
Triprolidine HCl	Actidil	2.5	6-8	+ +
Ethanolamines				
Carbinoxamine maleate	Clistin	4	6-8	+ +
Clemastine fumarate	Tavist-1	1.34	8-12	+ +
	Tavist	2.68	8-12	+ +
Diphenhydramine HCl	Benadryl	25, 50 Liquid 12.5 mg/ 5 ml	4-8	+ + +
Ethylenediamines				
Tripelennamine HCl	PBZ	25, 50 Liquid 25 mg/ 5 ml	4-6	+ + + +
Hydroxyzines				
Hydroxyzine HCl	Atarax	10, 25, 50, 100 Syrup 10 mg/ 5 ml	4-8	+
Hydroxyzine HCl	Durrax	10, 25		
Hydroxyzine pamoate	Vistaril	25, 50, 100 Syrup 25 mg/ 5 ml		
Piperidine				
Azatadine maleate	Optimine	1	12	+
Cyproheptadine HCl	Periactin	4	8	+ + +
Phenothiazines				
Methdilazine HCl	Tacaryl	4 (chewable), 8	6-12	+
Promethazine HCl	Phenergan	12.5, 25, 50 Liquid 6.25 mg/ 5 ml	4-6	+ + + +
Trimeprazine	Temaril	2.5	6-12	+ + + +

*Several are available as timed release capsules.

(dry mouth, blurred vision, constipation, dizziness), sedative, antipruritic, and antiemetic effects.

The antihistamines are grouped according to chemical structure (Table 6-6). Those drugs in each group have similar actions and side effects. If a patient does not respond to an agent in one group, it may be assumed that other drugs in that group will also be ineffective, and an agent from a different group should be selected.

Acute and chronic urticaria

Treatment for acute and chronic urticaria should begin with hydroxyzine, a drug with powerful antihistamine, sedative, and antipruritic properties. The dosage may be regulated over a wide range to fit the needs of the individual patient. For adults, begin with 10 mg every 4 hours and increase the dose as required to 25 to 100 mg every 4 hours. Some patients will not respond to hydroxyzine, and antihistamines from other groups, such as diphenhydramine, chlorpheniramine, clemastine, or azatadine, may be selected.

Patients who are sensitive to salicylates or tartrazine must avoid antihistamines containing tartrazine dyes. The tablet forms of Atarax, Durrax, Optimine, and Periactin are examples of dye-free antihistamines.

It would seem that the combination of an H_1 and H_2 antihistamine would provide optimum effects. The results of studies are conflicting but generally show that the combination is no more effective than an H_1 blocking agent used alone, except for dermographism, in which the combination of chlorpheniramine (H_1) and cimetidine (H_2) is clearly more effective.[23] Oral corticosteroids should be considered only in refractory cases. Their effect, although sometimes useful, is unpredictable.

Severe urticaria or angioedema requires epinephrine. Epinephrine solutions have a rapid onset of effect but a short duration of action. The dosage for adults is a 1:1000 solution (0.2 to 1 ml) given either subcutaneously or intramuscularly. The epinephrine suspensions provide both prompt and prolonged effect up to 8 hours. For adults 0.1 to 0.3 ml of the 1:200 suspension is given subcutaneously.

Urticarial vasculitis responds in some cases to indomethacin.[24] Dosage required for control ranges from 25 mg 3 times a day to 50 mg 4 times a day. Many patients on this schedule will be free of lesions within 3 weeks. Signs and symptoms recur within 48 hours of terminating the medication.

Physical urticaria

For physical urticaria measures should be taken to avoid the physical stimulus, and symptoms may be treated as outlined for treatment of acute and chronic urticaria. As mentioned in that section, the combination of an H_1 and H_2 antihistamine may be more effective than an H_1 antihistamine alone for severe dermographism.

REFERENCES

1. Champion RH, Roberts SOB, Carpenter RE, et al: Urticaria and angioedema: a review of 554 patients. Br J Dermatol **81**:588, 1969.
2. Beaven MA: Histamine and its participation in dermatological disorders. Part 1. Prog Dermatol **11**(4):16, 1977.
3. Beaven MA: Histamine and its participation in dermatological disorders. Part II. Its role in pathological reactions and diseases. Prog Dermatol **11**(5):24, 1977.
4. Ishizaka T, Ishizaka K: Triggering of histamine release from rat mast cells by divalent antibodies against IgE receptors. J Immunol **120**:800, 1978.
5. Grant JA, Dupree E, Goldman AS: Complement mediated release of histamine from human basophils. Clin Res **23**:292, 1975.
6. Lorenz W, Doenicke A: Histamine release in clinical conditions. Mt Sinai J Med **45**:357, 1978.
7. Collier HOJ; Prostaglandins and aspirin. Nature **232**:17, 1971.
8. Jacobson KW, Branch LB, Nelson HS: Laboratory tests in chronic urticaria. JAMA **243**:1644, 1980.
9. Monroe EW, Jones HE: Urticaria—an updated review. Arch Dermatol **113**:80, 1977.
10. Miller DA, Geraldine FL, Akers WA: Chronic urticaria. Am J Med **44**:68, 1968.
11. Fisherman EW, Cohen GN: Recurring and chronic urticaria: identification of etiologies. Ann Allergy **36**:401, 1976.
12. Juhlin L: Recurrent urticaria: clinical investigation of 330 patients. Br J Dermatol **104**:369, 1981.
13. Noid HE, Schulze TW, Winkelmann RK: Diet plan for patients with salicylate-induced urticaria. Arch Dermatol **109**:866, 1974.
14. Rudzki E, Czubalski K, Grzywa Z: Detection of urticaria with food additives intolerance by means of diet. Dermatologica **161**:57, 1980.
15. Michaelsson G, Juhlin L: Urticaria induced by preservatives and dye additives in food and drugs. Br J Dermatol **88**:525, 1973.
16. James J, Warin RP: An assessment of the role of Candida albicans and food yeasts in chronic urticaria. Br J Dermatol **84**:227, 1971.
17. Jorizzo JL, Smith EB: The physical urticarias: an update and review. Arch Dermatol **118**:194, 1982.
18. Rauits M, Armstrong RB, Harber LC: Solar urticaria: clinical features and wavelength dependence. Arch Dermatol **118**:228, 1982.
19. Von Krogh, Maibach HI: The contact urticaria syndrome—an updated review. J Am Acad Dermatol **5**:328, 1981.
20. Fisher AA: Contact urticaria due to medicants, chemicals, and foods. Cutis **30**:168, 1982.
21. Soter NA: Chronic urticaria as a manifestation of necrotizing venulitis. N Engl J Med **296**:1440, 1977.
22. Monroe EF: Urticarial vasculitis: an updated review. J Am Acad Dermatol **5**:88, 1981.
23. Kaur S, Greaves M, Eftekhari N: Factitious urticaria (dermographism) treatment by cimetidine and chlorpheniramine in a randomized double-blind study. Br J Dermatol **104**:185, 1981.
24. Millns JL: The therapeutic response of urticarial vasculitis to indomethacin. J Am Acad Dermatol **3**:349, 1980.

Chapter Seven

Acne, Rosacea, and Related Diseases

Acne

Acne, a disease of the pilosebaceous unit, appears in males and females near puberty and in most cases becomes less active as adolescence ends. The intensity and duration of activity vary for each individual.

The disease may be minor, with only a few comedones or papules, or it may occur as the highly inflammatory and diffusely scarring acne conglobata. The severest forms of acne occur more frequently in males, but the disease tends to be more persistent in females, who may have flares before menstrual periods, which continue until menopause.

Acne is too often dismissed as a minor affliction not worthy of treatment. Believing that the affliction is a phase of the growing process which will soon disappear, parents put off seeking medical advice. Permanent scarring of the skin and the psyche can result from such inaction. The disease, however, has implications far beyond the few marks that may appear on the face. The lesions cannot be hidden under clothing; each is prominently displayed and detracts significantly from one's personal appearance and self-esteem. Taunting and ridicule from peers are demoralizing. Having to appear publicly with the lesions such as those depicted on the following pages creates embarrassment and frustration.

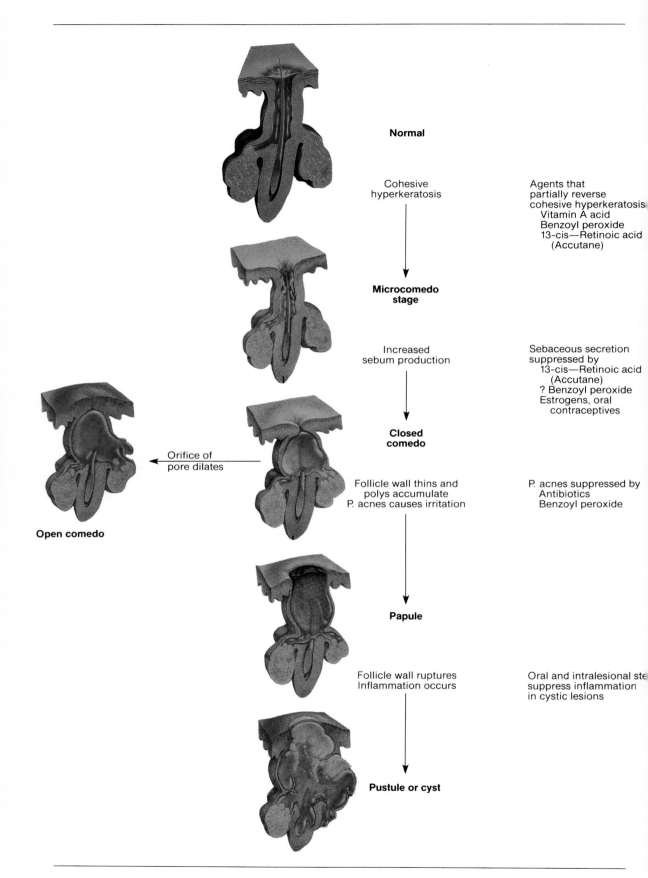

Normal

Cohesive
hyperkeratosis

Agents that
partially reverse
cohesive hyperkeratosis
Vitamin A acid
Benzoyl peroxide
13-cis—Retinoic acid
(Accutane)

Microcomedo
stage

Increased
sebum production

Sebaceous secretion
suppressed by
13-cis—Retinoic acid
(Accutane)
? Benzoyl peroxide
Estrogens, oral
contraceptives

Closed
comedo

Orifice of
pore dilates

Open comedo

Follicle wall thins and
polys accumulate
P. acnes causes irritation

P. acnes suppressed by
Antibiotics
Benzoyl peroxide

Papule

Follicle wall ruptures
Inflammation occurs

Oral and intralesional ste
suppress inflammation
in cystic lesions

Pustule or cyst

Figure 7-1 (opposite)

Figure 7-1 (opposite)
Pathogenesis of acne and effects of therapeutic agents. (Photographs courtesy Ortho Pharmaceutical Corporation.)

Etiology and pathogenesis

Much has been learned about the pathophysiology of acne.[1,2] Figure 7-1 illustrates the evolution of the different acne lesions and the mechanism of action of several therapeutic agents. Acne is a disease involving the pilosebaceous unit and is most frequent and intense in areas where sebaceous glands are largest and most numerous.

Sebaceous glands are located throughout the entire body except the palms, soles, dorsa of the feet, and lower lip. They are largest and most numerous on the face, chest, back, and upper outer arms. Clusters of glands appear as relatively large visible white globules on the buccal mucosa (Fordyce's spots), the vermilion border of the upper lip (Figure 7-2), the female areolae (Montgomery's tubercles), the labia minora, the prepuce, and around the anus.

Sebaceous glands are large in newborn infants, but regress shortly after birth. They remain relatively small in infancy and most of childhood, but enlarge once again in prepuberty. Sebaceous glands contain cells that produce a complex mixture of oily material. Sebaceous cells mature, die, and fragment and are then extruded into the sebaceous duct. Here they combine with the desquamating cells of the lower hair follicle and finally arrive at the skin surface as sebum.

Acne begins at the microscopic level when an increased number of cornified cells remain adherent to the follicular canal (cohesive hyperkeratosis) directly above the opening of the sebaceous gland duct. The resulting plug is called a microcomedo. Factors causing increased sebaceous secretion influence the eventual size of the follicular plug. The plug enlarges behind a very small follicular orifice at the skin surface and becomes visible as a closed comedo (firm white papule). An open comedo (blackhead) occurs if the follicular orifice dilates. Melanin accumulation rather than dirt accounts for the black color.[3] Further increase in the size of a blackhead will dilate the pore, but will not result in inflammation. Continuing sebaceous secretion behind the small follicular orifice of a closed comedo may, in combination with other factors, result in the formation of a red inflamed papule or pustule.

Hormones influence sebaceous gland secretion. Testosterone is converted to dihydrotestosterone in the skin and acts directly on the sebaceous gland to increase its size and metabolic rate. Estrogens, through a less well-defined mechanism, decrease sebaceous gland secretion.[4] The normal skin resident, *Propionibacterium acnes* (formerly termed *Corynebacterium acnes*), which is usually sensitive to several antibiotics such as tetracycline, appears to play a role in creating an inflammatory lesion. *P acnes* synthesizes lipases that convert the triglycerides in sebum to free fatty acids, which may be irritating and comedogenic.[5] They may secrete substances that are chemotactic for polymorphonuclear leukocytes and possibly mediate inflammation by stimulation of immune mechanisms.[6] Whatever the cause, the follicular wall thins, becomes inflamed (red papule), and then ruptures, releasing part of the comedo into the dermis. An intense inflammatory reaction results in the formation of the acne pustule or cyst.

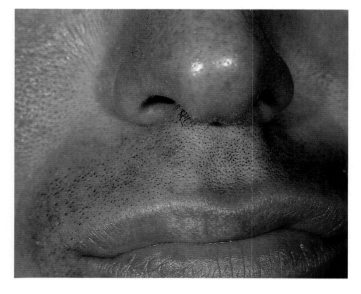

Figure 7-2
Clusters of sebaceous glands (tiny white-yellow spots) are normally present on the vermilion border of the upper lip.

Therapeutic agents for treatment of acne

Topical and oral agents act at various stages (Figure 7-1) in the evolution of an acne lesion and may be used alone or in combination to enhance efficacy. Most cases are controlled with combinations of vitamin A acid, benzoyl peroxide, and antibiotics. Topical agents should be applied to the entire affected area to treat existing lesions and to prevent the development of new ones.

Vitamin A acid

Vitamin A acid (VAA), also known as retinoic acid (Retin-A) or tretinoin, is available in various preparations: Retin-A solution (0.05%) is the strongest and most irritating. Retin-A gel (0.025% or 0.01%) is drying and indicated for oily skin, whereas Retin-A cream (0.1% or 0.05%) is lubricating and indicated for dry skin.

Vitamin A acid, an oxidation product of vitamin A, initiates increased cell turnover in both normal follicles and comedones and reduces the cohesion between keratinized cells. It acts specifically on microcomedones (the precursor lesion of all forms of acne), causing fragmentation and expulsion of the microplug, expulsion of comedones, and conversion of closed comedones to open comedones.[7] Inflammation may occur during this process. Continuous topical application leads to thinning of the stratum corneum. Removing the protective stratum corneum causes the skin to become more susceptible to sunburn and sun damage and to irritation from wind, cold, or dryness. Irritants such as astringents, alcohol, and acne soaps will not be as well tolerated as previously. The incidence of contact allergy is very low. Because of the direct action of tretinoin on the microcomedo, many clinicians believe this agent is appropriate for all forms of acne.

Principles of treatment. Wash skin gently with a mild soap (Purpose, Basis, etc.) no more than 2 to 3 times each day, using the hands rather than a wash cloth. Avoid special acne or abrasive soaps. To minimize possible irritation, wait 20 to 30 minutes for the skin to dry completely. Apply tretinoin in a thin layer once daily, using only enough to cover the skin. Avoid the corners of the nose, the mouth, and the eyes; these areas are the most sensitive and the most easily irritated. Apply tretinoin to the chin less frequently during the initial stages of therapy since the chin is sensitive and is usually the first area to be inflamed. Patients with sensitive skin or those who live in cold dry climates should apply tretinoin less frequently during the initial weeks of treatment. Sunscreens should be worn during the summer months if exposure is anticipated.

Response to treatment

One to four weeks. During the first few weeks, patients may experience redness, burning, or peeling. Those with excessive irritation should use less frequent applications (i.e., every other day or every third day or apply medication after supper and wash it off 2 to 3 hours later). Most patients adapt to treatment within 4 weeks and return to daily applications. Those tolerating daily applications may be advanced to a higher dosage or to the more potent solution.

Three to six weeks. New papules and pustules may appear as comedones, which become irritated during the process of being dislodged. Patients unaware of this phenomenon may discontinue treatment. Some patients never get any worse and sometimes begin to improve dramatically by the fifth or sixth week.

After six weeks. Most patients improve by the ninth to twelfth week and exhibit continuous improvement thereafter. Some patients never adapt to tretinoin and experience constant irritation or continue to worsen. An alternate treatment should be chosen if adaptation has not occurred by 8 weeks.

Benzoyl peroxide

Examples of benzoyl peroxide (BP) preparations are water-based gels (Benzac W 5% and 10%; Persa-gel W, 5% and 10%), alcohol-based gel (Benzagel, 5% and 10%), acetone-based gel (Persa-gel, 5% and 10%), Neutrogena Acne Mask (5%), and the new combination product Benzamycin (3% erythromycin, 5% benzoyl peroxide).

Benzoyl peroxide is available over the counter and by prescription. Gels may be alcohol-, water-, or acetone-based. Water-based gels are less irritating, but alcohol-based gels, if tolerated, may be more effective. Strengths available are 2.5%, 5%, and 10%. Benzoyl peroxide is also available in a soap base in strengths varying from 4% to 10%.

Benzoyl peroxide is keratolytic and in low concentrations produces mild desquamation, whereas higher concentrations or frequent applications result in scaliness and peeling. BP penetrates into the hair follicle and disrupts the microcomedo; it is therefore considered a comedolytic agent like vitamin A acid.[8] BP causes a significant reduction in the concentration of free fatty acids via its antibacterial effect on *P acnes*,[9] presumably by release of free radical oxygen capable of oxidizing bacterial proteins. BP seems to reduce the size of the sebaceous gland, but whether sebum secretion is suppressed is still unknown. Approximately 2% of patients develop allergic contact dermatitis to benzoyl peroxide.

Principles of treatment. Benzoyl peroxide should be applied in a thin layer to the entire affected area. Most patients experience mild erythema and scaling during the first few days of treatment with even the lowest concentrations, but most will adapt in a week or two. It was previously held that vigorous peeling was necessary for maximum therapeutic effect; although many patients improved with this technique, others became worse. Recent studies show that an adequate therapeutic result can be obtained by starting with daily applications of the 2.5% or 5% gel and gradually increasing or decreasing frequency of application and strength until mild dryness and peeling occur.[10] The sudden appearance of diffuse erythema and vesiculation suggests contact allergy to BP.

Oral antibiotics

Antibiotics have been used for approximately 3 decades for the treatment of papular, pustular, and cystic acne. Their major effect is believed to ensue from their ability to decrease follicular populations of *Propionibacterium acnes*.[11] The role of *P acnes* in the pathogenesis of acne is not completely understood. Conversion of triglycerides in sebum by bacterial lipases to irritating free fatty acids is one possible mechanism of action. Antibiotic-resistant strains of *P acne* have recently been discovered.[12]

Tetracycline. Tetracycline hydrochloride (TCN) is the most widely prescribed oral antibiotic for acne. It is safe, effective, and inexpensive. One major disadvantage is the requirement that this drug not be taken with food (particularly dairy products), certain antacids, and iron, all of which interfere with the intestinal absorption of TCN. Failure to adhere to these restrictions accounts for many of the reported therapeutic failures. Efficacy and compliance are obtained by starting TCN at 500 mg twice daily and continuing this dosage until a significant decrease in the number of inflamed lesions occurs, usually in 3 to 6 weeks. Thereafter the dosage may be decreased to 250 mg twice daily, or oral therapy can be discontinued in favor of topical antibiotics. Patients with severe pustular and cystic acne or those not responding to 1 gm per day may require high dose TCN (1.5 to 3.0 gm per day) for control.[13] These higher dosages are generally well tolerated even for extended periods. Patients failing to respond after 6 weeks of adequate dosage of oral TCN should be introduced to an alternate treatment. For unknown reasons a significant number of patients who take TCN exactly as directed will not respond to high doses, whereas others respond favorably to 250 mg daily or every other day and flare when attempts are made to discontinue treatment.

The incidence of photosensitivity to TCN is very low. All women should be warned about the increased incidence of *Candida albicans* vaginitis that results from taking antibiotics. The package labeling of oral contraceptives warns that reduced efficacy and increased incidence of breakthrough bleeding may occur with tetracyclines and other antibiotics. Although this association has not been proved, it is prudent to inform patients of this risk until more data are available.

Erythromycin. Erythromycin (e.g., E-Mycin 250 or 333 mg; ERYC 250 mg; EES 400) is possibly slightly less effective than tetracycline at the same dosage levels and is more expensive. The advantages include better patient compliance with the newer enteric coated forms, which are absorbed adequately when taken with food, and a lower incidence of *C. albicans* vaginitis than that found with equivalent dosages of TCN.

Minocycline. Minocycline (Minocin 50 and 100 mg capsules and scored tablets) is a tetracycline derivative that has proved valuable in cases of pustular acne that have failed to respond to conventional oral antibiotic therapy. One study comparing minocycline (50 mg 3 times a day) with tetracycline (250 mg 4 times a day) revealed that minocycline resulted in significant improvement in patients who did not respond to tetracycline.

Patients who responded to tetracycline had significantly advanced improvement when switched to minocycline.[14] The usual initial dose is 50 to 100 mg twice daily. The dosage is tapered when a significant decrease in the number of lesions is observed, usually in 3 to 6 weeks. Minocycline is highly lipid-soluble and readily penetrates the cerebrospinal fluid, causing in some patients dose-related ataxia, vertigo, nausea, and vomiting. In susceptible individuals, central nervous system (CNS) side effects occur with the first few doses of medication. If these reactions persist after decreasing the dosage or taking capsules with food, alternative therapy is indicated. A blue-gray pigmentation of the skin, oral mucosa, nails, and thyroid gland has been found in some patients, usually those taking high dose minocycline for extended periods.[15,16] Skin pigmentation has been most frequently reported in acne scars and has also been observed as blue-black 1- to 2-cm macules on the anterior aspect of the lower legs.[17] Lower leg pigmentation may be mistaken for bruises. Pigmentation may persist for long periods after minocycline has been discontinued. The consequences of these deposits are unknown.

Clindamycin. Clindamycin (75- and 150-gm capsules) is a highly effective oral antibiotic for the control of acne. Its use has been curtailed in recent years because of its association with severe pseudomembranous colitis caused by *Clostridium difficile*,[18] which fortunately responds in most cases to oral or intravenous vancomycin hydrochloride. Clindamycin is effective in dosages ranging from 75 to 300 mg twice daily.

Ampicillin. Long-term use of oral antibiotics for treatment of acne may result in the appearance of cysts and pustules that yield Gram-negative organisms when cultured.[19] Ampicillin (250- and 500-mg capsules) is effective for this so-called Gram-negative acne. Ampicillin is often effective for treatment of conventional mild to moderately inflammatory acne and is a safe alternative for patients who fail to respond to tetracycline.[20] Ampicillin may be prescribed for acne in pregnancy or during lactation. A dosage of 500 mg twice each day is maintained until satisfactory control is achieved; the dosage is then decreased. Some patients will experience a flare of activity at lower dosages and must resume taking 500 mg twice each day.

Trimethoprim and sulfamethoxazole. Trimethoprim and sulfamethoxazole (Bactrim, Septra), like ampicillin, is useful for treating Gram-negative acne. The adult dose is 160 mg of trimethoprim/800 mg of sulfamethoxazole once or twice daily.

Topical antibiotics

Commercially available topical antibiotics include tetracycline (Topicycline lotion), erythromycin (A/T/S, EryDerm, Staticin, and T-Stat lotions), clindamycin (Cleocin-T lotion), meclocycline (Meclan cream), and Benzamycin (3% erythromycin, 5% benzoyl peroxide). Clinical trials have demonstrated that twice daily application of topical antibiotics is at least as effective as oral tetracycline at 250 mg twice daily.[21] Extemporaneous formulation of topical antibiotics is no longer necessary; commercial preparations with predictable stability are available. All lotions are alcohol-based and may produce some irritation. Topicycline and EryDerm do not contain propylene glycol and may be less irritating to some patients. Meclan cream is the least irritating of the commercially available topical antibiotics.

Drying and peeling agents

The oldest technique for treating acne is to use agents that induce a continuous mild drying and peeling of the skin. Over-the-counter products used for this purpose contain sulfur, salicyclic acid, resorcinol, and benzoyl peroxide. Before the use of tretinoin and antibiotics, this approach secured very acceptable results for some patients. A paperback book intended for the general public entitled *Clear Skin*[22] presents a comprehensive, easily understood explanation of the drying and peeling method and is recommended for patients who elect this method of treatment. The goal is to establish a mild continuous peel by varying the frequency of application and strength of the agent. The drying and peeling technique can be recommended for patients who are reluctant to visit the physician or to parents inquiring about children who are beginning to develop acne. If improvement is negligible after an 8-week trial, the patient should consider evaluation by a physician.

Lime sulfur solution (calcium polysulfide and calcium thiosulfate). Commercially available preparations that contain lime sulfur solution are Vlem-Dome (lime sulfur solution in 4-ml packets) and Vlemasque (sulfurated lime in a paste).

Sulfurated lime solution applied in a hot compress is very effective and is indicated for patients with severe active inflammatory nodulocystic acne. The mechanism of action is unknown. Cysts may evolve and rapidly become inactive as drying and peeling occur. Patients should be cautioned about the unpleasant odor of sulfur produced in mixing and applying the solution.

The solution is made by adding a 4-ml packet of Vlem-Dome to 1 pint of hot water. A cotton compress (e.g., several folds of bed sheet) is dipped into the hot solution, squeezed gently to retain a maximum amount of fluid, and applied to the entire affected area for 20 to 30 minutes once or twice a day until moderate erythema and peeling occurs. The frequency of application is modified to produce the desired result and treatment can be continued for days or weeks until control is obtained. No other topical treatment should be used during this time.

Vlemasque paste, applied as a mask and washed off one-half hour later, is useful for milder forms of pustular and cystic acne.

Estrogens

Estrogens in the form of anovulatory agents are effective in the treatment of acne for some women. For years, women had reported clearing of treatment-resistant acne after using oral contraceptives. Unfortunately, in many instances the acne flared and became worse after oral contraception was discontinued. Fear of disease exacerbation prompted many women to continue treatment even after contraception was no longer desired. Some women had noticed the opposite effect. While they were using oral contraceptives, their acne worsened and became resistant to conventional therapy. These women had usually taken agents such as Ovral,[23] which has a relative androgenic effect.

Most oral contraceptives contain combinations of estrogens and progestational agents. The estrogen component (either mestranol or ethinyl estradiol) has a sebum-inhibiting effect. The progestational agent may modify the effect of the estrogen; these effects depend upon the type and amount of progestin present. Some progestins, such as norgestrel in Ovral, have both androgen activity and marked antiestrogen activity, which counteracts the effectiveness of the estrogen. The progestins norethynodrel and ethynodiol diacetate have very little antiestrogen or androgen activity; therefore, products such as Enovid-E, Ovulen, and Demulen would be expected to be effective. Products containing 100 μg of mestranol are the most effective, but have a greater risk of side effects than the lower dose pills. Oral contraceptives may be considered if all forms of conventional acne treatment have failed. Selection of an appropriate agent may provide the additional benefit of effective acne therapy

TABLE 7-1

COMPOSITION AND RELATIVE ANDROGENICITY OF SELECTED ORAL CONTRACEPTIVES

Brand name	Estrogen	mg	Progestin	mg	Relative androgenicity of progestin*
Enovid, 5 mg	Mestranol	75	Norethynodrel	5	0
Enovid, 10 mg	Mestranol	150	Norethynodrel	9.85	0
Enovid-E	Mestranol	100	Norethynodrel	2.5	0
Norinyl, 2 mg	Mestranol	100	Norethindrone	2	2
Ortho-Novum, 2 mg	Mestranol	100	Norethindrone	2	2
Ovulen	Mestranol	100	Ethynodiol diacetate	1	1
Norinyl 1 + 80	Mestranol	80	Norethindrone	1	2
Ortho-Novum 1 80	Mestranol	80	Norethindrone	1	2
Demulen	Ethinyl estradiol	50	Ethynodiol diacetate	1	1
Norinyl 1 + 50	Mestranol	50	Norethindrone	1	2
Ortho-Novum 1/50	Mestranol	50	Norethindrone	1	2
Ovral	Ethinyl estradiol	50	Norgestrel	0.5	4

From Shalita, A.R. Sibulkin, D.: Acne vulgaris: pathogenesis and treatment—systemic treatment. Dermatol. Allergy Nov 1979, p 45.
*Scale of 0 to 4.

TABLE 7-2

PHARMACOLOGIC EFFECTS OF PROGESTINS USED IN ORAL CONTRACEPTIVES

	Progestin	Estrogen	Antiestrogen	Androgen
Norgestrel	+++*	0	+++	+++
Ethynodiol diacetate	++	+*	+*	++
Norethindrone acetate	+	+	+++	++
Norethindrone	+	+*	+++	++
Norethynodrel	+	+++	0	0

From Facts and Comparisons. Section on Oral Contraceptives 1981.
Key: +++, pronounced effect; ++, moderate effect; +, slight effect; 0, no effect.
*Has estrogenic effect at low doses; may have antiestrogenic effect at higher doses.

for those women who have chosen anovulatory agents for birth control.

The characteristics of most commonly used oral contraceptives are outlined in Table 7-1. Table 7-2 summarizes the effects of the various progestins.

Patients should be cautioned that taking antibiotics such as tetracycline with oral contraceptives may increase their risk of developing candida vaginitis. As mentioned in the discussion of tetracycline, some oral antibiotics may render oral contraceptives less effective.

Isotretinoin (Accutane 10, 20, 40 mg capsules)

Isotretinoin (13-cis retinoic acid), an oral retinoid related to vitamin A, is an effective agent for control of cystic acne. It is indicated for patients with severe cystic acne who have failed to respond to conventional therapy and patients with severe noncystic inflammatory acne which is treatment-resistant and demonstrates a potential for scarring. Age is not a limiting factor in patient selection. At dosages of 1 mg/kg/day, sebum production decreases

TABLE 7-3

INCIDENCE OF CLINICAL SIDE EFFECTS OF ISOTRETINOIN

Cheilitis, dry lips	90%
Dry skin, desquamation of central face, pruritus, nonspecific symptoms related to dryness of nose and mouth, epistaxis	80%
Conjunctivitis	38%
Musculoskeletal symptoms	16%
Rash, thinning of hair, peeling of palms and soles, skin infections, nonspecific gastrointestinal symptoms, headache, and increased susceptibility to sunburn	5%

to about 10% of pretreatment values and the sebaceous glands decrease in size.[24] These effects persist for an indefinite period when therapy is discontinued. Maximum inhibition is reached by the third or fourth week. Within a week patients normally notice drying and chapping of facial skin and skin oiliness disappears quickly.

During the first month there is usually a reduction in superficial lesions such as papules and pustules. A significant reduction in the number of cysts normally takes at least 8 weeks. Facial lesions respond faster than trunk lesions.[25]

Side effects. Side effects occur frequently (Table 7-3). They may appear before visible therapeutic effects, are dose-related, and generally disappear shortly after discontinuing treatment. Cheilitis is the most common side effect, occurring in virtually all patients. Application of emollients should be started with the initiation of therapy to minimize drying. Exuberant granulation tissue may occur at the sites of healing acne lesions and is more likely to develop in patients who have preexisting crusted, draining, or ulcerated lesions. Granulation tissue can be controlled with intralesional steroid injections or silver nitrate sticks. Isotretinoin therapy induces an elevation of plasma triglycerides in approximately 25% of patients. Abnormalities of serum triglycerides are usually reversible upon cessation of isotretinoin therapy. Approximately 40% of patients develop an elevated sedimentation rate during treatment. Since teratogenicity occurs in humans, women entering therapy must not be pregnant and must take effective measures to avoid pregnancy through therapy. Accutane contains the preservative parabens; those patients with a proven allergy to parabens can not receive Accutane.

Laboratory studies. Before starting treatment, confirm that female patients are not pregnant. Initial laboratory studies should include a determination of triglycerides and cholesterol. Triglyceride determination should be repeated after 2 to 3 weeks of treatment and again tested at 4 to 6 weeks. If the triglyceride level at 4 to 6 weeks of treatment exceeds 350 to 400 mg/dl, the blood lipids should be repeated at no less than 2- to 3-week intervals to determine whether the triglyceride concentration increases further or levels off. If the value becomes greater than 700 to 800 mg/dl, the drug should be stopped to reduce the risk of the development of pancreatitis. Perform a complete blood count and liver function tests before treatment, after 4 to 6 weeks of treatment, and at the end of treatment.

Isotretinoin therapy. The isotretinoin therapy program is as follows. Isotretinoin is given in 2 divided doses daily preferably with meals. The basic dosage schedule is 1.0 mg/kg/day maintained for 20 weeks. Although patients demonstrate significant improvement with lower dosages, studies have shown that the longest remissions are realized when isotretinoin is maintained at 1.0 mg/kg/day or higher for 20 weeks.[26] Those patients who have severe cystic acne of the chest and back often require 2 mg/kg/day. See Table 7-4 for correct dosages. Many patients will experience a moderate to severe flare of acne during the initial weeks of treatment. This adverse reaction can be minimized by starting isotretinoin at 10 mg twice daily and gradually increasing the dosage during the first 4 to 6 weeks until the therapeutic levels are reached. Discontinue treatment at the end of 20 weeks and observe for 2 to 5 months. Those with persistent severe acne may receive a second course of treatment.

Prednisone

Prednisone has a limited but definite place in the management of acne.[27] Nodulocystic acne can be resistant to all forms of conventional topical and antibiotic therapy. Lime sulfur solution compresses (Vlem-Dome) may offer no relief. Nodulocystic acne can be destructive, producing widespread disfigurement through scarring. Intervention with powerful antiinflammatory agents should not be postponed in the case of rapidly advancing disease. Deep cysts improve only slowly with isotretinoin, and much permanent damage can occur while one is waiting for an effect.

Prednisone therapy. The procedure for the use of prednisone is as follows. For rapidly advancing or

TABLE 7-4

ISOTRETINOIN DOSING BY BODY WEIGHT*

Body weight		Total mg/day	
KILOGRAMS	POUNDS	1 MG/KG	2 MG/KG
40	88	40	80
50	110	50	100
60	132	60	120
70	154	70	140
80	176	80	160
90	198	90	180
100	220	100	200

*1 to 2 mg/kg/day given in two divided doses for 15 to 20 weeks. Patients with disease primarily on the chest and back or those weighing over 70 kg may require doses at the higher end of this range.

painful cystic acne, prednisone should be started at 40 to 60 mg/day given in divided doses twice daily. Maintain this dose until a majority of lesions are significantly improved and then begin to taper. Lower the dosage to 30 mg given as a single dose in the morning. The dose can be tapered by 5 mg each week until 20 mg is reached, at which point prednisone can be further tapered to 30 mg every other day and withdrawn in 5 mg increments every 4 days. Some patients respond well to this program and therefore do not require isotretinoin treatment. It is not necessary to subject patients to extensive courses of prednisone. Patients who are flaring after a short course of prednisone therapy may be started on isotretinoin.

Intralesional corticosteroids

Individual nodulocystic lesions can be effectively treated with a single injection of triamcinolone acetonide (Kenalog) delivered with a 27- or 30-gauge needle. Triamcinolone is available in 10 mg/ml suspension and can be diluted with 1% lidocaine or physiologic saline. Saline is preferred because injections of lidocaine mixtures are painful. A 2.5 to 5.0 mg/ml concentration is usually an adequate injection for suppressing inflammation.

Intralesional corticosteroid therapy. The procedure for the use of intralesional corticosteroids is as follows. Shake the bottle of steroid solution very thoroughly to disperse the white suspension. Shake the syringe immediately before injection. Insert the needle through the thinnest portion of the cyst roof and deposit 0.1 to 0.3 ml of solution into the cyst cavity. This quantity will momentarily blanch most cysts. Atrophy may occur if steroids are injected into the base of the cyst. Patients can be assured that if skin depression occurs, it is temporary in most cases and gradually resolves in 4 to 6 months. Multiple cysts can be injected in the course of one session. Intralesional injection is used specifically to supplement other programs.

It is comforting for patients to know that if a large painful cyst appears fast relief is available with this relatively painless procedure. Occasionally, intralesional steroid injections may be given for small papules and pustules when rapid resolution is desired. However, prolonged continuous use of intralesional steroids has resulted in adrenal suppression.

Acne surgery

Acne surgery is the manual removal of comedones and the drainage of pustules and cysts. When performed correctly, acne surgery speeds resolution and rapidly enhances cosmetic appearance.

The procedure for acne surgery is as follows. Three instruments are used: the round loop comedo extractor, the oval loop acne extractor or Schamberg, and the #11 pointed-tip scalpel blade. Removal of open comedones enhances the patient's appearance. By use of either type of extractor, most comedones can easily be expressed with uniform smooth pressure. Lesions that offer resistance are loosened and sometimes disengaged by inserting the point of a #11 blade into the blackhead and elevating. The orifice of the closed comedo must be enlarged before pressure can be applied. Following the angle of the follicle, insert the scalpel point with the sharp edge up about 1 mm into the tiny orifice. Draw the blade slightly forward and up; then apply pressure with the extractor to remove the sometimes surprisingly large quantity of soft white material. After the head of the white pustule is nicked with the #11 blade, pustules are easily drained by pressing the material with the acne extractor. Cysts are preferably managed by intralesional injection because incision and drainage may cause scarring. Pustules and cysts that have a thin effaced roof in which fluid contents are easily ballotted are drained through a small incision by manual pressure. Make a short incision (about 3 mm) to prevent scarring. After drainage, a #1 curette may be inserted through the incision on the cyst to dislodge chunks of necrotic tissue.

Scar revision. Many patients are self-conscious about the pitted and crater-like scars that remain as a permanent record of previous inflammation. Some people will endure any procedure and spare no expense to rid themselves of the minutest scar. A variety of procedures is available to remove or revise scars. A dermatologic or plastic surgeon is best equipped to perform such procedures. The subspecialty of dermatologic surgery is expanding, but at the present time most dermatologic surgeons are located at university centers.

Generally, it is advisable to wait until disease activity has been low or absent for several months. Scars improve with time as they atrophy. The color contrast is often the most troublesome aspect of postinflammatory acne. Inflamed lesions may leave a flat or depressed red scar that is so obvious patients mistake the mark for an active lesion. The color will fade and approach skin tones in 4 to 12 months. The following techniques are those most commonly used for scar revision.

Dermabrasion. Dermabrasion (see also Chapter 26) has been practiced for years and when performed correctly is a valuable technique for decreasing the depth of pitted scars. The epidermis and part of the dermis are planed away with a high-speed motor-driven finely abrasive brush or wheel. A major portion of the face may be treated during a single session. Reepithelialization takes 3 to 4 weeks. The procedure may have to be repeated once or twice to obtain optimal results. Adverse affects include additional scarring and permanent loss of pigment. The creation of hypopigmented areas is a common side effect and for this reason many surgeons advise against using this technique for patients with dark skin.

Scar excision. Many pitted scars are too deep to be planed by dermabrasion. These deep or "ice pick" scars may be excised and closed carefully with gratifying results. Some dermatologic surgeons remove the scars with a punch biopsy. The plug is removed and the scar is separated from the subcutaneous tissue. The remaining round core of fat and dermis is replaced in the round hole and held at the surface with a Steri-strip. The autograft is rapidly fibrosed into place and the epidermis subsequently regenerates. There are several modifications of this technique.

Bovine dermal collagen implants (Zyderm). A new processing technique has been developed to render bovine collagen nonantigenic and suitable for augmenting scars in humans (see Chapter 26). Lidocaine-dispersed collagen is supplied in preloaded syringes for intradermal injection. It is indicated in the dermal augmentation of a variety of deficiencies including acne scars. Soft, distensible lesions with smooth margins are the most amenable to correction, whereas ice pick acne and tiny punched lesions do not respond as well.

Approach to acne therapy

Many patients are embarrassed to ask for help. Any feeling of apathy or indifference on the part of the physician will be sensed by the patient and treatment will fail. It should be emphatically stated that both the treatment and positive results are most important to all concerned. A brief discussion of the pathogenesis should be included to explain that acne is inherited and that the disease may be active for years.

TABLE 7-5

CHART FOR DOCUMENTING PROGRESS OF ACNE TREATMENT
(NUMBER OF PAPULES, PUSTULES, CYSTS AT EACH VISIT)

	Date of office visit				
	1	2	3	4	5
Forehead					
(R) cheek					
(L) cheek					
Chest					
Back					

Several myths about acne should be discussed. For example, it should be stated that greasy foods cause obesity, not acne, but that moderate dietary restriction is appropriate if the patient desires it. In the same context, since acne is not caused by dirt (the pigment in blackheads is melanin), excessive washing is unnecessary and interferes with most treatment programs.

Female patients should be informed that moderate use of nongreasy lubricants and water-based cosmetics is usually well tolerated, but that a gradual decrease in the use of cosmetics is encouraged as the acne improves. If female patients are taking oral contraceptives, a change in estrogen and progestin combinations may be all that is necessary. The patient should be informed that gentle manipulation of pustules is tolerated, but excoriation produces permanent scarring. Erythema and pigmentation after resolution of pustules and cysts takes many months to fade.

Patients should not have inappropriate expectations. Acne can in most cases be controlled but not cured. The patient should be encouraged to ask questions about the disease, the course of treatment, and results.

Initial evaluation

Determine the types of lesions present (i.e., comedones, pustules, or cysts). Make a chart as illustrated in Table 7-5 and record the number of pustules on the forehead, right and left cheeks, chest, and back during each visit. Indicate the approximate number of comedones.

Determine the degree of skin sensitivity by inquiring about experiences with topical medicines and soaps. Degree of pigmentation and hair color are not the sole determinants of skin sensitivity. Patients with the atopic diathesis generally do not tolerate aggressive drying therapy.

Select therapy appropriate to the type of acne; refer to the previous section on therapeutic agents for specific details. A program can generally be established for most patients after 3 visits, but some difficult cases require continuous supervision. Emphasize that for maximum effect treatment must be continuous and prolonged. Patients who had only a few lesions that quickly cleared may be given a trial period without treatment 6 to 8 weeks after clearing. In an attempt to suppress further activity, those patients who have numerous lesions should remain on continuous topical treatment for several months. The patient's propensity to scarring must be ascertained. Patients vary in their tendency to develop scars. Some demonstrate little scarring even after significant inflammation, whereas others develop a scar from nearly every inflammatory papular or pustular lesion. This latter group requires aggressive therapy to prevent further damage.

The following treatment programs are offered only as a guide. Modifications will have to be made for each individual.

Comedo or closed comedo acne

Closed comedo acne (Figures 7-3 and 7-4) responds slowly. A large mass of sebaceous material is impacted behind a very small follicular orifice. The

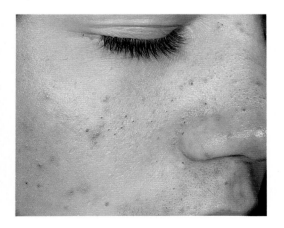

Figure 7-3
Comedones (blackheads) are occasionally inflamed.

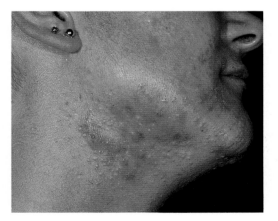

Figure 7-4
Closed comedones (whiteheads). Tiny white dome-shaped papules with a tiny follicular orifice. Several lesions depicted here are inflamed.

orifice may enlarge during treatment, making extraction by acne surgery possible.

First visit. Tretinoin is the most effective agent for this type of acne. In treating with this drug select the base and strength according to skin sensitivity. Apply once each evening or less frequently if irritation develops. Express large open comedones; many will be difficult to remove. Several weeks of tretinoin treatment will facilitate easier extraction.

Second visit (week 5). Adjust the strength of tretinoin. Start benzoyl peroxide gel, either 2.5% or 5%. Apply once each day or less frequently if irritation develops. Comedones may become inflamed during treatment. No alteration of therapy will be necessary if a few papules appear, but topical or oral antibiotics should be considered for significant inflammation. Either substitute a topical antibiotic for benzoyl peroxide, use Benzamycin (3% erythromycin, 5% benzoyl peroxide), or begin oral antibiotics.

Third visit (week 10). The patient should have adapted to using combination treatment. Some patients experience no irritation while using tretinoin and may begin to apply it more than once daily.

Pustular acne

Mild to moderate inflammation. Pustular acne with mild to moderate inflammation is defined here as fewer than 20 pustules (Figure 7-5).

First visit. Initially apply tretinoin and benzoyl peroxide gel on alternate evenings. Start with the lowest concentration of tretinoin gel or cream and 2.5% or 5% benzoyl peroxide gel. After the initial adjustment period, attempt to use tretinoin each night and benzoyl peroxide each morning. Tetracycline should be prescribed for patients with 10 to 20 pustules. Express pustules and open comedones.

Second visit (week 5). Increase strength of tretinoin or benzoyl peroxide or both if the patient has adapted to initial concentrations. Introduce tetracycline or another antibiotic if the number of pustules has not decreased. Express pustules and open comedones.

Third visit (week 10). By the tenth week a program of topical therapy should have been established that results in some dryness and mild erythema without irritation; there should be a significant decrease in the number of pustules. A few closed comedones will have disappeared, but they usually require much longer continuous therapy. If the number of pustules has not changed significantly, establish that tetracycline is being taken correctly. If directions have been followed, either increase the dose of tetracycline or start minocycline at full dosage. If there are any signs of irritation, decrease the frequency and strength of topical medicines. Irritation, particularly around the mandibular areas and neck, will worsen pustular acne. Inject resistant inflamed pustules with triamcinolone acetonide (Kenalog).

Those who have responded well may begin to taper and eventually discontinue tetracycline. A topical antibiotic or Benzamycin may be substituted for benzoyl peroxide. Continue topical therapy for extended periods.

Moderate to severe inflammation. Patients who have moderate to severe acne (more than 20 pustules) are temporarily disfigured (Figures 7-6 to 7-8). Their disease may have been gradually worsening or be virulent at onset. The exposive onset of pustules can sometimes be precipitated by stress. There may be few to negligible visible comedones. Affected areas should not be irritated during the initial stages of therapy.

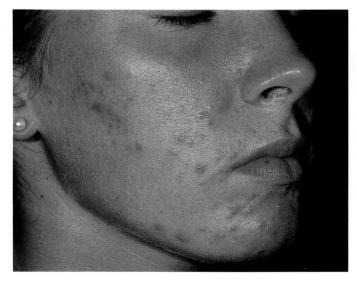

Figure 7-5
Pustular acne. Lesions are discrete and moderately inflamed.

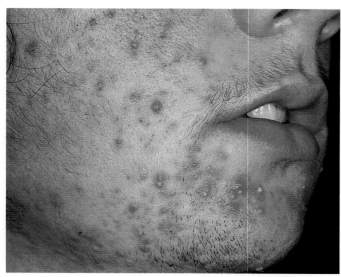

Figure 7-6
Pustular acne. Many pustules are present and several have become confluent on the chin area.

Figure 7-7
Pustular acne. Numerous lesions were present for months. The round red macules are areas of previous activity.

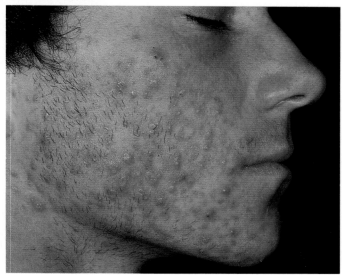

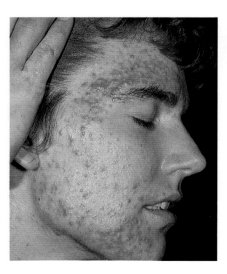

Figure 7-8
Severe pustular acne with masses of confluent pustules on the forehead and in the chin area.

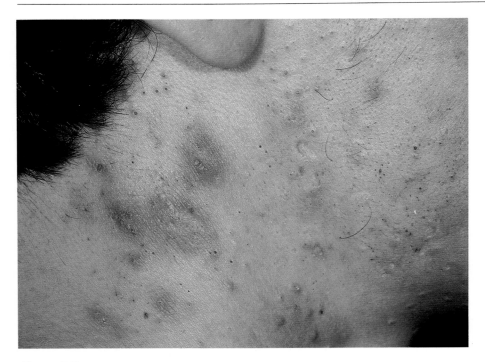

Figure 7-9
Localized cystic acne. Cystic lesions appeared in this patient, who has chronic comedo and pustular acne.

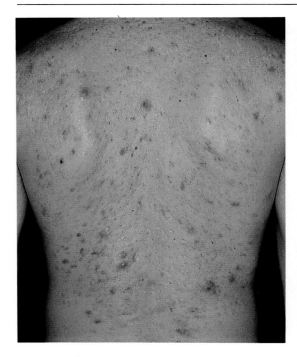

Figure 7-10
Cystic acne. Years of activity have left numerous scars over the entire back. Several active cysts are present.

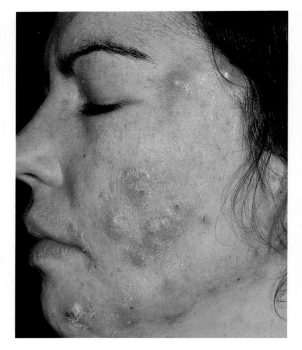

Figure 7-11
Cystic acne. The lesions in this patient are primarily cystic. Only a few pustules and comedones are present.

First visit. Begin tetracycline or erythromycin in full doses for moderately inflamed cases. Consider using minocycline for the more extensive and acutely inflamed cases. Begin either 2.5% or 5% benzoyl peroxide and apply once or twice daily during the initial weeks of therapy; avoid irritation. Vlemasque may be applied for one-half hour every other night. Frequency of use should be adjusted to avoid irritation. Gently express pustules.

Second visit (week 5). A significant response will occur in many patients and the antibiotic dosage may be slowly tapered, but not discontinued. Patients on tetracycline or erythromycin who display little improvement should switch to minocycline. Those on minocycline may have the dosage maintained or increased. Begin combination topical therapy on alternate days (tretinoin gel 0.01% one day, benzoyl peroxide 2.5% or 5% the next). Increase frequency of use until slight dryness and erythema occurs. Introduce or continue Vlemasque as tolerated.

Third visit (week 10). Many patients will have improved; therefore, plans should be made for tapering and discontinuing oral antibiotics. Some pa-

tients respond very well to lower doses of oral antibiotics and require tetracycline, 250 mg daily or every other day for control. Those patients may be safely maintained on low-dose oral antibiotics for extended periods. Patients not responding to conventional therapy may be colonized by Gram-negative organisms. Culture the pustules and cysts and start an appropriate antibiotic such as ampicillin. The response may be dramatic.

Combinations of tretinoin, benzoyl peroxide, topical antibiotics, and Vlemasque should be continued for months in an attempt to suppress recurrent activity. Consider isotretinoin, a short course of prednisone, or intralesional triamcinolone injections for antibiotic-resistant acne in patients who demonstrate a potential for scarring.

Nodulocystic acne

Nodulocystic acne includes localized cystic acne (few cysts on face, chest, or back) (Figure 7-9), diffuse cystic acne (wide areas of face, chest, and back) (Figures 7-10 and 7-11), pyoderma faciale (inflamed cysts localized to the face in females) (Figure 7-12), and acne conglobata (highly inflam-

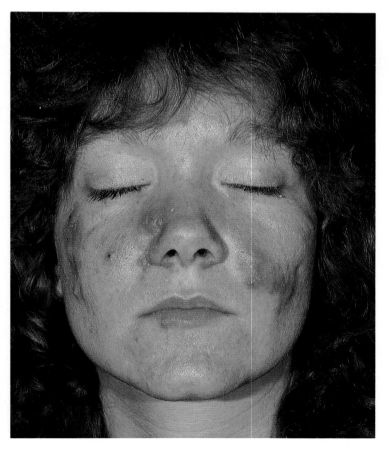

Figure 7-12
Pyoderma faciale. Confluent cysts remain localized to the face. This disease occurs almost exclusively in females.

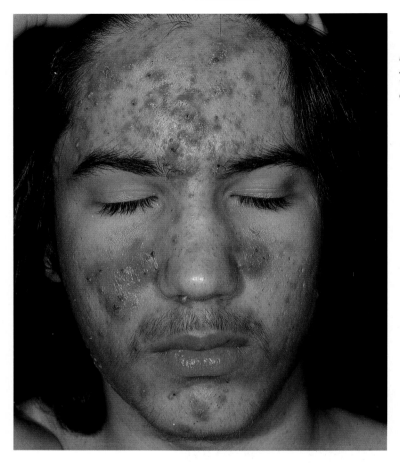

Figure 7-13
*Acne conglobata. Large cysts
with multiple deep
communicating tracts.*

matory, with cysts that communicate under the skin, abscesses, and burrowing sinus tracts) (Figures 7-13 and 7-14).

Cystic acne is a serious and sometimes devastating disease that requires vigorous treatment. The face, chest, back, and upper arms may be permanently mutilated by numerous atrophic or hypertrophic scars. The physical appearance may be so unattractive that teenagers refuse to attend school and adults fear going to work. Patients sometimes delay seeking help, hoping that improvement will occur spontaneously; consequently, the disease may be quite advanced when first viewed by the physician.

Patients with a few inflamed cysts can be managed with a program similar to that outlined for inflammatory acne. Oral antibiotics, conventional topical therapy, and periodic intralesional triamcinolone injections may keep this problem under adequate control.

Extensive cystic acne requires a different approach. There are two less common variants of cystic acne. Pyoderma faciale is a distinct variant of cystic acne, which remains confined to the face. Women, generally over the age of 20, experience the rapid onset of large sore erythematous-to-purple cysts, predominantly on the central portion of the cheeks. Purulent drainage from cysts occurs spontaneously or with minor trauma. A traumatic emotional experience has been associated with some cases. Comedones are absent, and scarring occurs in most cases.[28]

Cultures will help differentiate this condition from Gram-negative acne. A recent review demonstrated that the disease could be effectively managed by omitting prednisone and using sulfur lime compresses and oral antibiotics.[29]

Acne conglobata is a chronic highly inflammatory form of acne in which involved areas contain a mixture of double comedones (two blackheads that communicate under the skin), papules, pustules, communicating cysts, abscesses, and draining sinus tracts. The disease may linger for years, ending with deep atrophic or keloidal scarring.

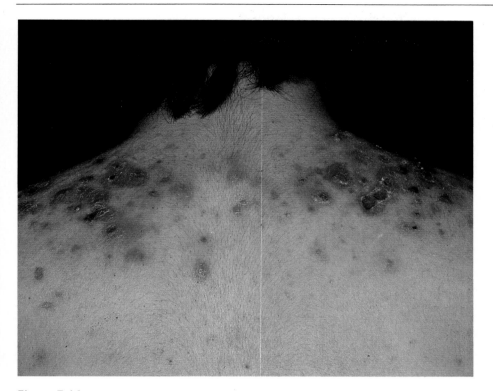

Figure 7-14
Acne conglobata. Abscesses and ulcerated cysts are found over most of the upper shoulder area.

First visit. Be optimistic; assure the patient that effective treatment is available. Tell patients that they will be followed closely and, if the disease becomes very active, will be seen at least weekly until the condition is adequately controlled. Patients with multiple draining cysts may be better managed in the hospital. A primary therapeutic goal is to avoid scarring by terminating the intense inflammation quickly; prednisone is sometimes required. Incise and drain cysts with thin roofs. Inject deeper cysts with triamcinolone 2.5 to 5.0 mg/ml. Hot sulfur lime (Vlem-Dome) compresses are the mainstay of initial therapy for extensive inflammatory cystic acne. They are applied for 20 to 30 minutes 1 to 4 times a day as tolerated to produce erythema and peeling. Cysts will evolve and should be drained, sometimes on a daily basis. Start tetracycline or minocycline in full doses. Consider initiating isotretinoin therapy for patients with extensive involvement or those who have a propensity to scar. For highly active cases, start prednisone (adult dose 20 mg 2 or 3 times a day). Prednisone should not be withheld while wait-

ing for weeks for antibiotics or isotretinoin to take effect.

Two to three weeks after initial visit. For patients who improve, if the acute phase ends during this period, sulfur lime compresses may be tapered and discontinued. Continue antibiotics and begin topical therapy as described in the sections on advanced pustular acne. Minor flares are controlled with intralesional injections. Patients taking isotretinoin should taper other forms of therapy as improvement is noted.

Patients initially treated with conventional topical therapy and antibiotics who do not improve should discontinue sulfur lime compresses and minocycline if the disease remains active. Start prednisone, 40 to 60 mg/day. Benzoyl peroxide gel (5%) is applied with enough frequency to create dryness without irritation. Isotretinoin may be started simultaneously and continued for a full course while prednisone and topical therapy are tapered. An alternative program is to begin with isotretinoin as the only oral medication while using benzoyl peroxide and

Vlemasque until isotretinoin starts to cause skin dryness.

Gram-negative acne

Patients with a long history of treatment with oral antibiotics for acne may suddenly develop superficial pustules around the nose or nodules and cysts on the cheeks. Cultures of these lesions reveal species of *Enterobacter, Klebsiella,* or *Proteus.*[30] Selection of the appropriate antibiotic is made after antibiotic sensitivities. Ampicillin or trimethoprim-sulfamethoxazole (Bactrim, Septra) are generally the appropriate drugs. Gram-negative acne responds quickly to the proper antibiotic; once the gram-negative organisms have been eradicated, conventional antibiotics may again be useful. Isotretinoin has been successful for resistant cases of gram-negative acne.[31]

Steroid acne

In predisposed individuals, sudden onset of follicular pustules and papules may occur shortly after starting oral corticosteroids.[32] The pustules of steroid acne (Figure 7-15) differ from acne vulgaris by being of uniform size and symmetric distribution, usually on the neck, chest, and back. Steroid-induced acne is rare before puberty. This drug eruption is not a contraindication to continued or future use of oral corticosteroids. Combination therapy with tretinoin and benzoyl peroxide is effective.

Neonatal acne

Acneiform lesions (Figure 7-16) confined to the nose and cheeks may be present at birth or may develop in early infancy.[33] The lesions clear without treatment as the large sebaceous glands of the infant become smaller and less active.

Occupational acne

An extensive diffuse eruption of large comedones and pustules (Figure 7-17) may occur in some individuals exposed to certain industrial chemicals,[34] including chlorinated hydrocarbons and other industrial solvents, coal tar derivatives, and oils. Lesions occur on the extremities and trunk where clothing saturated with chemicals has been in prolonged close contact with the skin. Patients predisposed to this form of acne must avoid exposure by wearing protective clothing or finding other work. Treatment is the same as for inflammatory acne.

Acne mechanica

Mechanical pressure may induce an acneiform eruption (Figure 7-18). Common causes include forehead guards of sports helmets, chin straps, and orthopedic braces.[35]

Acne cosmetica

Postadolescent women who regularly apply layers of cosmetics may develop closed and open comedones, papules, and pustules.[36] This may be the patient's first experience with acne. Traditionally, the comedogenicity of a given cosmetic foundation has been tested by its ability to produce comedones in the ear of a rabbit. More recently, trials with specific cosmetics on women have revealed that some formulations cause acne, some have no effect, and some may result in decreasing the number of comedones. Until specific formulations are tested in humans and their comedogenic potential is known, patients should be advised to use light water-based cosmetics and to avoid cosmetic programs that advocate applying multiple layers of cream-based cleansers and coverups.

One alternative to cosmetics is the use of tinted acne preparations (Table 7-6). These are drying but generally well received by patients.

Acne excoriée des jeune filles

Most acne patients will attempt to drain comedones and pustules with moderate finger pressure. Occasionally, a young woman with little or no acne will develop several deep linear erosions on the face (Figure 7-19).[37] This inappropriate attempt to eradicate lesions causes scarring. Women may deny or be oblivious to their manipulation. It should

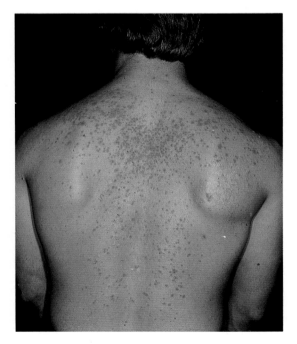

Figure 7-15
Steroid acne. Numerous papules and pustules are of uniform size and symmetrically distributed.

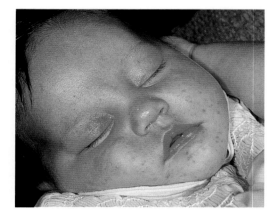

Figure 7-16
Neonatal acne. Small papules and pustules commonly occur on the cheeks and nose of infants.

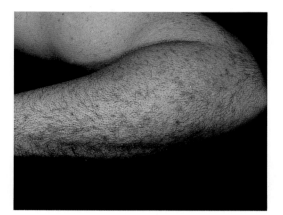

Figure 7-17
Occupational acne. Comedones, papules, and pustules occur in areas exposed to oils and industrial solvents.

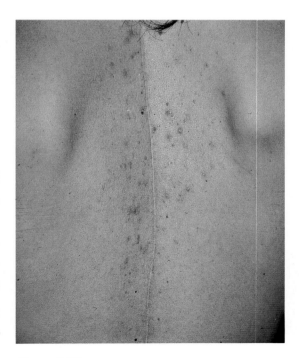

Figure 7-18
Acne mechanica. Comedones, papules, and pustules occurred after a few weeks of wearing a back brace.

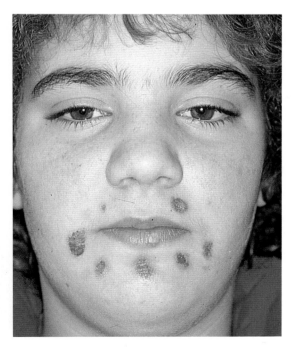

Figure 7-19
Acne excoriée des jeunes filles. Erosions and ulcers are created by inappropriate attempts to drain acne lesions.

TABLE 7-6

COSMETIC SUBSTITUTIONS (TINTED ACNE LOTIONS)

Brand names	Active ingredients	Availability
Sulfacet-R*	Sodium sulfacetamide 10%, sulfur 5%	Rx
Loroxide*	Benzoyl peroxide 5.5%, chlorhydroxyquinoline 0.25%	OTC
Rezamid*	5% sulfur, 2% resorcinol, 0.5% parachlorometaxylenol	OTC
Acnomel	8% sulfur, 2% resorcinol	OTC

*"Color blend" is provided that enables the patient to alter the basic shade of the lotion to match the skin color.

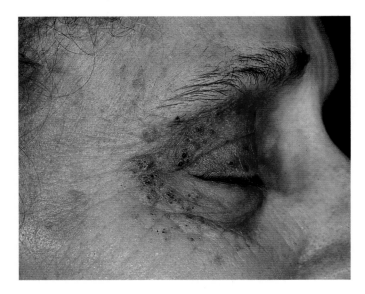

Figure 7-20
Senile comedones. Large comedones may appear around the eyes and temples in the middle-aged and older individuals. Sunlight is a predisposing factor.

Figure 7-21
Milia. Tiny white dome-shaped cysts that occur about the eyes and cheeks. There is no obvious follicular opening like that seen with closed comedones.

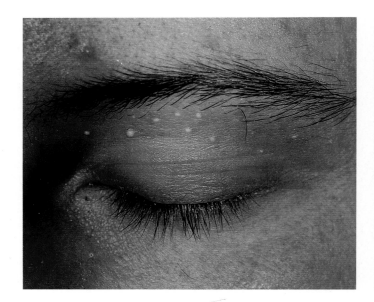

be explained that such lesions can occur only with manipulation and that the lesions may be unconsciously created during sleep. Once this is explained, many women are capable of exercising adequate restraint. Those unable to refrain from excoriation may benefit from psychiaric care.

Senile comedones

Excessive exposure to sunlight in predisposed individuals causes large open and closed comedones around the eyes and on the temples (Figure 7-20). Inflammation very rarely occurs, and comedones can be easily expressed with acne surgery techniques. Tretinoin may be used to loosen impacted comedones. Once cleared, the comedones may not return for years, and tretinoin may be discontinued.

Milia

Milia are tiny white pea-shaped cysts that commonly occur on the face and especially around the eyes (Figure 7-21). They also occur in scars and during the healing process in lesions of porphyria cutanea tarda. Milia may occur spontaneously or after habitual rubbing of the eyelids. They have no opening on the surface and cannot be expressed like blackheads. They are easily drained by the same procedure used to drain closed comedones.

Perioral dermatitis

Perioral dermatitis (PD) (Figure 7-22) is a distinct eruption resembling acne occurring in young women. Papules and pustules on an erythematous and sometimes scaling base are confined to the chin and nasolabial folds while sparing a clear zone around the vermilion border. Prolonged use of fluorinated steroid creams were thought to be the primary cause when this entity was described over 25 years ago. However, in recent years most women have denied use of such creams. PD occurs in an area where drying agents are poorly tolerated; topical preparations such as benzoyl peroxide, tretinoin, and alcohol-based antibiotic lotions aggravate the eruption.

Treatment. Perioral dermatitis uniformly responds in 2 to 3 weeks to 1 gm per day of tetracycline or erythromycin.[38] Once the eruption is cleared, the dose may be tapered gradually and then discontinued in 4 to 5 weeks. Patients with renewed activity should have an additional course of antibiotics and start meclocycline (Meclan) cream once or twice daily as tolerated. Continue oral antibiotics at maintenance levels if this cream does not provide adequate control. Nonfluorinated steroids (Group VII) such as hydrocortisone may at times be required to suppress erythema and scaling. Fluorinated steroids must be avoided.

Figure 7-22
Perioral dermatitis. Tiny papules and pustules are located around the mouth. The eruption occurs almost exclusively in females.

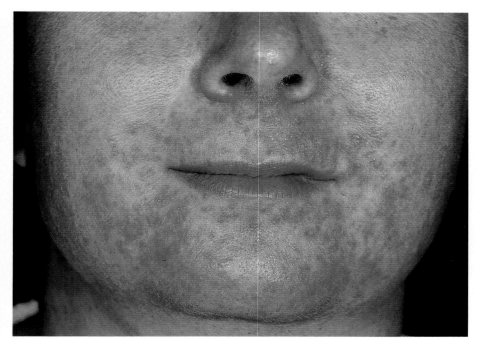

Rosacea (Acne Rosacea)

W.C. Fields drank excessively and had clusters of papules and pustules on red swollen telangiectatic skin of his cheeks and forehead. The red bulbous nose completed the full-blown syndrome of active rosacea. Patients with rosacea are defensive about their appearance and must explain to unbelieving friends that they do not imbibe. The etiology is in fact unknown. Alcohol may accentuate erythema but does not cause the disease. Sunlight precipitates acute episodes. Coffee and caffeine-containing products once topped the list of forbidden foods in the arbitrarily conceived elimination diets recommended as a major part of the management of rosacea. It is the heat of coffee, not its caffeine content, that leads to flushing.[39] Hot drinks of any type should be avoided by patients with rosacea.

Rosacea occurs after the age of 30 and is most common in people of Celtic origin. The resemblance to acne is at times striking. The cardinal features are erythema, edema, papules and pustules, and telangiectasia. One or all of these features may be present. The disease is chronic, lasting for years, with episodes of activity followed by quiescent periods of variable length. The eruption appears on the forehead, cheeks, and nose (Figure 7-23). Most patients have some erythema, with less than 10 papules and pustules at any one time. At the other end of the spectrum are those with numerous pustules, telangiectasia, diffuse erythema, oily skin, and edema, particularly of the cheeks and nose. Chronic deep inflammation of the nose leads to an irreversible hypertrophy called rhinophyma (Figure 7-24). A mild conjunctivitis with soreness, grittiness, and lacrimation occurs in about 50% of cases. Conjunctival injection is sometimes prominent.

Treatment. Both the skin and eye manifestations of rosacea respond uniformly to either tetracycline or erythromycin. Start with 1 gm per day in divided doses as for acne and taper to the minimum dosage that provides adequate control. Topical antibiotics may be attempted, but most cases will require long-term low-dose oral antibiotics. Patients who remain clear for months should periodically be given a trial period without medication. However, many patients promptly revert to the low-dose oral regimen. Patients with rhinophyma may benefit from specialized surgical procedures performed by plastic or dermatologic surgeons.[40] Isotretinoin has controlled severe rosacea.[31,41]

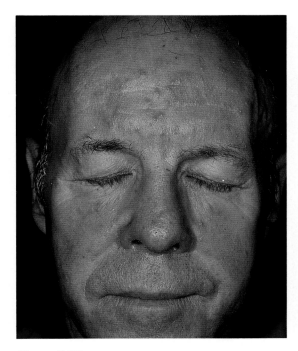

Figure 7-23
Rosacea. Pustules and erythema occur on the forehead, cheeks, and nose.

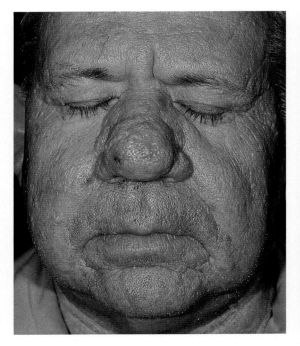

Figure 7-24
Rosacea and rhinophyma. Chronic rosacea of the nose has caused irreversible hypertrophy (rhinophyma).

Hidradenitis Suppurativa

Hidradentitis suppurativa is a chronic suppurative and scarring disease occurring in the axillae, the anogenital regions, and under the female breast (Figures 7-25 and 7-26). The disease is more common in obese females. A hallmark of hidradenitis is the double comedo, a blackhead with 2 surface openings that communicate under the skin. This distinctive lesion may be present for years before other symptoms appear. Unlike acne, once this disease begins it becomes progressive and self-perpetuating. The pathogenesis is disputed. Some claim that, like acne, the initial event is the formation of a keratinous follicular plug, whereas others believe that apocrine duct occlusion is the primary event. Extensive deep dermal inflammation results in large painful abscesses. The healing process permanently alters the dermis. Cord-like bands of scar tissue criss-cross the axillae. Reepithelialization leads to meandering epithelial-lined sinus tracts in which foreign material and bacteria become trapped. As with acne, the role of bacteria in the pathogenesis is unclear. The course varies among individuals from an occasional cyst in the axilla to diffuse abscess formation in the inguinal region.

Treatment. Antiperspirants should probably be avoided. Tretinoin cream (0.05) may prevent duct occlusion, but it is irritating and must be used cautiously. As with acne vulgaris, long-term oral antibiotics may prevent inflammation. Large cysts should be drained and obesity must be controlled. Surgical excision of chronically draining and inflamed skin with application of a split thickness graft is at times the only solution. Isotretinoin may be a useful adjunctive therapy.[41]

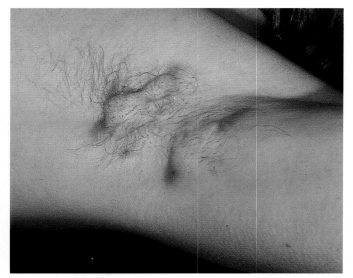

Figure 7-25
Hidradenitis suppurativa. A chronic suppurative and scarring disease.

Figure 7-26
Hidradenitis suppurativa. The disease may remain localized or involve large areas of the groin or anal area.

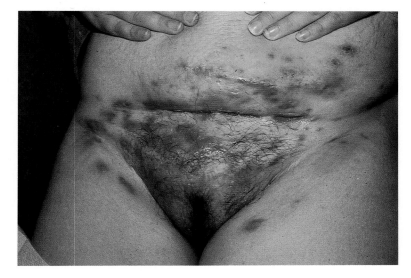

Miliaria

Miliaria or heat rash is a common phenomenon occurring in predisposed individuals during periods of exertion or heat exposure. Eccrine sweat duct occlusion is the initial event. The duct ruptures, leaks sweat into the surrounding tissues, and induces an inflammatory response. Occlusion occurs at 3 different levels to produce 3 distinct forms of miliaria. The papular and vesicular lesions that resemble pustules of folliculitis have one major distinguishing feature. They are not follicular and therefore do not have a penetrating hair shaft. Follicular pustules are likely to be infectious, whereas nonfollicular papules, vesicles, and pustules like those seen in miliaria are usually noninfectious.

Miliaria crystallina

In miliaria crystallina (Figure 7-27), occlusion of the eccrine duct at the skin surface results in accumulation of sweat under the stratum corneum. The sweat-filled vesicle is so near the skin surface that it appears as a clear dew drop. There is little or no erythema and the lesions are asymptomatic. The vesicles appear individually or in clusters and are most frequently seen in infants or bedridden overheated patients. Rupture of a vesicle produces a drop of clear fluid. A cool water compress and proper ventilation is all that is necessary to treat this self-limited process.

Miliaria rubra

Miliaria rubra (prickly heat, heat rash) (Figure 7-28), the most common of the sweat-retention diseases, results from occlusion of the intraepidermal section of the eccrine sweat duct. Papules and vesicles surrounded by a red halo or diffuse erythema develop as the inflammatory response develops. Instead of itching, the eruption is accompanied by a stinging or prickling sensation. The eruption occurs underneath clothing or in areas prone to sweating after exertion or overheating; the palms and soles are spared. The disease is usually self-limited, but some patients never adapt to hot climates and must therefore make a geographic change to aid their condition.

Treatment consists of removing the patient to a cool air-conditioned area. Frequent application of a mild antiinflammatory lotion will relieve symptoms and shorten the duration of inflammation. The patient can prepare this lotion by adding the contents of a 15-gm tube of a Group V steroid cream (e.g., betamethasone cream, 0.1) to 2 ounces of water.

Miliaria profunda

Miliaria profunda is observed in the tropics after the patient has had several bouts of miliaria rubra. Occlusion of the dermal section of the eccrine duct is followed by a white papular eruption.

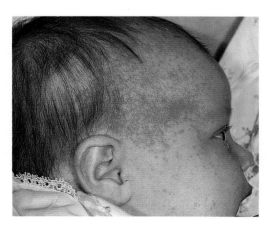

Figure 7-27
Miliaria crystallina. Eccrine sweat duct occlusion at the skin surface results in a cluster of vesicles filled with clear fluid.

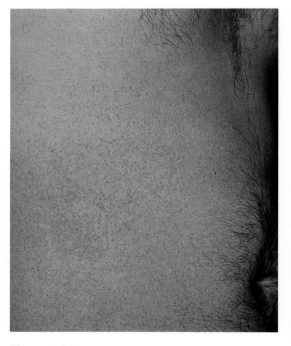

Figure 7-28
Miliaria (prickly heat). A diffuse eruption of tiny papules and vesicles occurs after exertion or overheating.

REFERENCES

1. Kligman AM: An overview of acne. J Invest Dermatol **62:**268, 1974.
2. Strauss JS, Pouchi PE, Downing DT: Acne: perspectives. J Invest Dermatol **62:**321, 1974.
3. Blair C, Lewis CA: The pigment of comedones. Br J Dermatol **82:**572, 1970.
4. Forstrom L: The influence of sex hormones on acne. Acta Derm Venereol Suppl (Stockh) **89:**27, 1980.
5. Marples RR, McGinley KJ, Mills OH: Microbiology of comedones in acne vulgaris. J Invest Dermatol **60:**80, 1973.
6. Puhvel SM, Sakamoto MA: Cytotaxin production by comedonal bacteria (Propionibacterim acnes, propionibacterium granulosum, and staphylococcus epidermis). J Invest Dermatol **74:**36, 1980.
7. Thomas JR, Doyle JA: The therapeutic uses of topical vitamin A acid. J Am Acad Dermatol **4:**505, 1981.
8. Cotterill JA: Benzoyl peroxide. Acta Derm Venereol Suppl **89:**57, 1980.
9. Cunliffe WJ, Holland KT: The effect of benzoyl peroxide on acne. Acta Derm Venereol **61**(3):267, 1981.
10. Lassus A: Local treatment of acne. A clinical study and evaluation of the effect of different concentrations of benzoyl peroxide gel. Curr Med Res Opin **7**(6):370, 1981.
11. Pochi PE, Straus JS: Antibiotic sensitivity of corynebacterium acne (propionibacterium acne). J Invest Dermatol **36:**423, 1961.
12. Leyden JJ, McGinley KJ, Cavalieri S, et al: Propionibacterium acnes resistance to antibiotics in acne patients. J Am Acad Dermatol **8:**41, 1983.
13. Baer RL, Leshaw SM, Shalita AR: High dose tetracycline therapy in severe acne. Arch Dermatol **110:**83, 1974.
14. Rossman RE: Minocycline treatment of tetracycline-resistant and tetracycline-responsive acne vulgaris. Cutis **27:**196, 1981.
15. Fenske NA, Millns JL, Greer KE: Minocycline-induced pigmentation at sites of cutaneous inflammation. JAMA **244:**1103, 1980.
16. Simons JJ, Morales A: Minocycline and generalized cutaneous pigmentation. J Am Acad Dermatol **3:**244, 1980.
17. Fitzpatrick TB: Comment on blue-gray dermal pigmentation associated with high-dose prolonged minocycline ingestion. Dermatologic Capsule and Comment Nov-Dec, 1980, p 10.
18. Bartlett JG, Moon N, Change TW, et al: Role of *Clostridium difficile* in antibiotic-associated pseudomembranous solitis. Gastroenterology **75:**778, 1978.
19. Leyden JJ, Marples RR, Mills OH Jr, et al: Gram-negative folliculitis: a complication of antibiotic therapy in acne vulgaris. Br J Dermatol **88:**583, 1973.
20. Shore RN: Usefulness of ampicillin in treatment of acne vulgaris. J Am Acad Dermatol **9:**604, 1983.
21. Gratton D, Raymond GP, Guertin-Larochelle S, et al: Topical clindamycin versus systemic tetracycline in the treatment of acne: results of a multiclinic trial. J Am Acad Dermatol **7:**50, 1982.
22. Flandermeyer KL: Clear skin: a step-by-step program to stop pimples, blackheads, acne. Boston, 1979, Little, Brown & Company.
23. Shalita AR, Sibulkin D: Acne vulgaris: Pathogenesis and treatment: systemic treatment. Dermatology Nov. 1979, pp 45-51.
24. Strauss JS, Stranier AM: Changes in long-term sebum production from isotretinoin therapy. J Am Acad Dermatol **6:**751, 1982.
25. Peck GL, Olsen TG, Butkus D, et al: Isotretinoin versus placebo in the treatment of cystic acne: a randomized double-blind study. J Am Acad Dermatol **6:**735, 1982.
26. Strauss JS, Rapini RP, Shalita AR, et al: Isotretinoin therapy for acne: results of a multicenter dose-response study. J Am Acad Dermatol **10:**490, 1984.
27. Shalita AR, Berstein JE: Acne Vulgaris: current concepts in pathogenesis and treatment. Curr Concepts Skin Disorders, Fall 1982, pp 3-6.
28. Plewig G, Kligman AM: Acne: morphogenesis and treatment. Berlin, 1975, Springer-Verlag.
29. Massa MC, Daniel WP: Pyoderma faciale: a clinical study of twenty-nine patients. J Am Acad Dermatol **6:**85, 1982.
30. Feibleman CE, Rasmussen JE: Gram-negative acne. Cutis **25:**194, 1980.
31. Plewig G, Nikolowski J, Wolff HH: Action of isotretinoin in acne rosacea and gram-negative folliculitis. J Am Acad Dermatol **6:**766, 1982.
32. Hitch JM: Acneiform eruptions induced by drugs and chemicals. JAMA **200:**879, 1967.
33. Tromovitch TT, Abrams AA, Jacobs PH: Acne in infancy. Am J Dis Child **106:**230, 1963.
34. Crow KD: Chloracne: a critical review including a comparison of two series of cases of acne from chlornaphthalene and pitch fumes. Trans St Johns Hosp Dermatol Soc **65:**79, 1970.
35. Mills OH, Kligman AM: Acne mechanica. Arch Dermatol **111:**481, 1975.
36. Kligman AM, Mills OH: "Acne cosmetica." Arch Dermatol **106:**843, 1972.
37. Albrecht H, Schonfelder T: Acne excoriee des jeunes filles: psychiatrically considered. Arch Klin Exp Dermatol **223:**506, 1965.
38. Sneddon IB: Treatment of steroid-induced rosacea and perioral dermatitis. Dermatologica **152**(suppl 1): 231, 1976.
39. Wilkin JK: Oral thermal-induced flushing in erythematotelangiectatic rosacea. J Invest Dermatol **76:**15, 1981.
40. Verde SF, Oliveira ADS, Picoto ADS, et al: How we treat rhinophyma. J Dermatol Surg Oncol **6:**560, 1980.
41. Shalita AR, Cunningham WJ, Leyden JJ, et al: Isotretinoin treatment of acne and related disorders: an update. J Am Acad Dermatol **9:**629, 1983.

Chapter Eight

Psoriasis and Related Diseases

Psoriasis

Psoriasis is a national health problem afflicting millions of people.[1] The disease is transmitted genetically, most likely with a dominant mode of variable penetrance; the etiology is unknown.[2] Men and women are equally affected. Environmental influences may modify the course, severity, and age of onset. Extent and severity vary widely. Psoriasis frequently begins in childhood when the first episode may be stimulated by infection as in guttate psoriasis. Many millions of people may have the potential to develop psoriasis, with only the correct combination of environmental factors needed to precipitate the disease. Stress, for example, may precipitate an episode.

Clinical manifestations

The lesions of psoriasis are distinctive. They begin as red scaling papules that coalesce to form round to oval plaques that are well defined from the surrounding normal skin (Figure 8-1). The scale is adherent, silvery white, and reveals bleeding points when removed (Auspitz's sign). Scale may become extremely dense, especially on the scalp. Scale forms but is macerated and dispersed in intertriginous areas; therefore, the psoriatic plaques of skin folds appear only as smooth red plaques with a macerated surface. The most common site for an intertriginous plaque is the intergluteal fold; this is referred to as gluteal pinking (Figure 8-2). The deep rich red color is another characteristic feature and remains constant in all areas. Psoriasis can be precipitated by trauma (scratching, sunburn, or surgery), the so-called isomorphic or Koebner's phenomenon (Figures 8-3, 8-9, and 8-12). Pruritus is highly variable. Although psoriasis can affect any cutaneous surface, certain areas are favored and should be examined in all patients in whom the diagnosis of psoriasis is suspected. Those areas are the elbows and knees, the scalp, the gluteal cleft, and the finger and toenails.

Figure 8-1
Psoriasis. Typical oval plaque with well-defined borders and silvery scale.

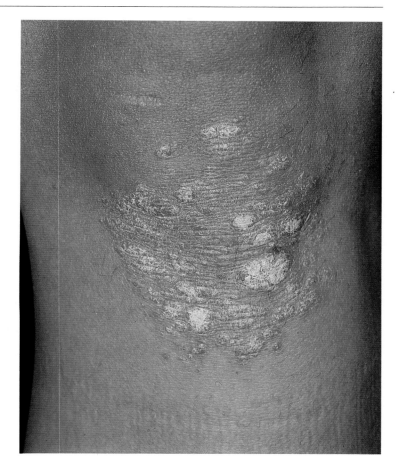

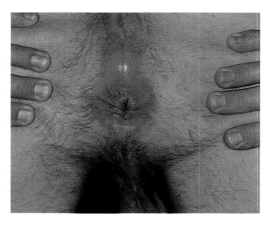

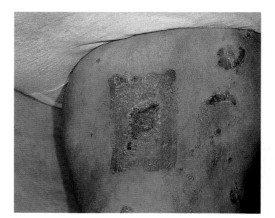

Figure 8-2
Psoriasis. Gluteal pinking, a common lesion in patients with psoriasis. Intertriginous psoriatic plaques retain the rich red color typical of skin lesions but do not retain scale.

Figure 8-3
Psoriasis. The Koebner phenomenon. Psoriasis has appeared on the donor site of the skin graft.

The disease affects the extensor more than the flexor surfaces and usually spares the palms, soles, and face. Most patients have chronic localized disease, but there are several other presentations. Localized plaques may be confused with eczema or seborrheic dermatitis and the guttate form with many small lesions can resemble secondary syphilis or pityriasis rosea.

Histology

The psoriatic epidermis contains a large number of mitoses. There is epidermal hyperplasia and scale, the final product of the abnormally functioning epidermis. The dermis contains enlarged and tortuous capillaries that are very close to the skin surface and impart a characteristic erythematous hue to the lesions. Bleeding occurs (Auspitz's sign) when the capillaries are ruptured as scale is removed.

Clinical presentations

There are variations in morphology, including chronic plaque psoriasis, guttate psoriasis (acute eruptive psoriasis), generalized pustular psoriasis, localized pustular psoriasis, psoriasis of the palms and soles, psoriatic erythroderma, and light-sensitive psoriasis. There is psoriasis of specific areas, such as scalp psoriasis, localized pustular psoriasis, psoriasis of the palms and soles, psoriasis of flexural sites (psoriasis inversus), psoriasis of the nails, and psoriatic arthritis.

Chronic plaque psoriasis. Chronic noninflammatory well defined plaques are the most common presentation of psoriasis. Lesions can appear anywhere on the cutaneous surface. They enlarge to a certain size and then tend to remain stable for months or years (Figure 8-4). A temporary brown or red macule remains when the plaque subsides after treatment or spontaneously clearing.

Guttate psoriasis. Over 30% of psoriatic patients have their first episode before age 20; in many instances, an episode of guttate psoriasis is the first indication of the patient's propensity for the disease. Streptococcal pharyngitis or viral upper respiratory infection may precede the eruption by 1 or 2 weeks.[3,4] A few to many pinpoint to 1-cm red scaling papules suddenly appear on the trunk and extremities, sparing the palms and soles (Figures 8-5 and 8-6). Lesions increase in diameter with time. The scalp and face may also be involved. Pruritus is variable. Guttate psoriasis may resolve spontaneously in weeks or months; it responds more readily to treatment than does chronic plaque psoriasis. Throat cultures should be taken to rule out streptococcal infection. There is a high incidence of positive antistreptolysin O titers in this group.

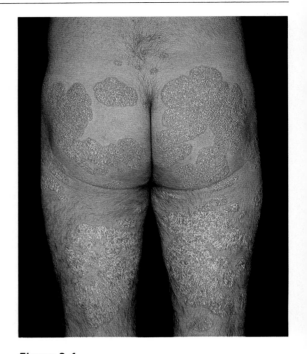

Figure 8-4
Chronic plaque psoriasis. Noninflamed plaques tend to remain fixed in position for months.

Generalized pustular psoriasis. This rare form of psoriasis (also called von Zumbusch's psoriasis) is a serious and sometimes fatal disease. Erythema suddenly appears in the flexural areas and migrates to other body surfaces. Numerous tiny sterile pustules evolve from an erythematous base and coalesce into lakes of pus (Figure 8-7). The superficial upper epidermal pustules are easily ruptured. The patient is febrile and has leukocytosis. Topical medications such as tar and anthralin may precipitate episodes in patients with unstable or labile psoriasis.[5] Withdrawal of both topical and systemic steroids has precipitated flares. Relapses are common.[6]

Psoriatic erythroderma. Generalized erythrodermic psoriasis, like generalized pustular psoriasis, is a severe, unstable, highly labile disease that may appear as the initial manifestation of psoriasis but usually occurs in patients with previous chronic disease (Figure 8-8). Infections or overzealous irritating therapy may precipitate an episode. Methotraxate is used if rapid control is not obtained with topical steroids. Tar, anthralin, and light should be avoided.

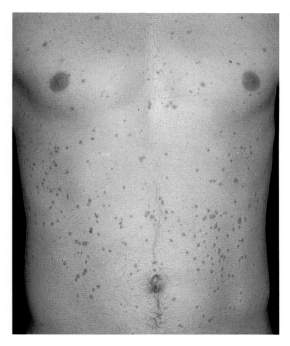

Figure 8-5
Guttate psoriasis. Numerous uniformly small lesions may abruptly occur following streptococcal pharyngitis.

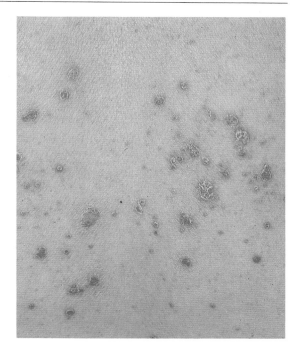

Figure 8-6
Guttate psoriasis. Numerous pinpoint to 1-cm lesions develop typical psoriatic scale soon after appearance.

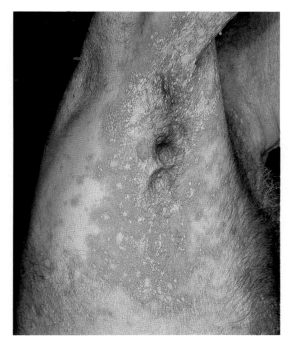

Figure 8-7
Generalized pustular psoriasis. An erythematous plaque has evolved numerous sterile pustules, which in many areas have coalesced.

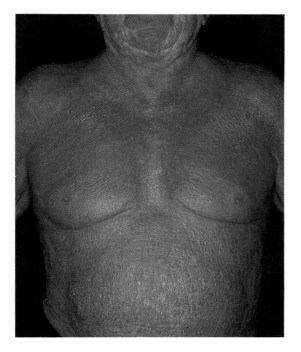

Figure 8-8
Psoriatic erythroderma. Generalized erythema occurred shortly after this patient discontinued use of methotrexate.

Figure 8-9
Light-induced psoriasis.
Overexposure to sunlight
precipitated this diffuse flare
of psoriasis. The midback was
protected by a wide halter strap.

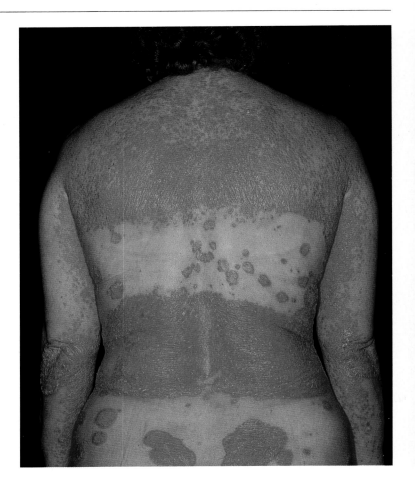

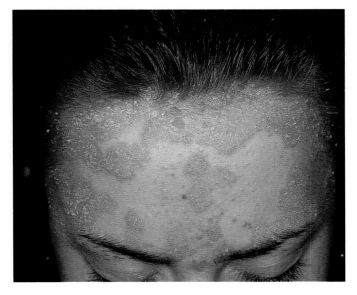

Figure 8-10
Psoriasis of the scalp. Plaques typically
form in the scalp and along the hair
margin. Occasionally plaques will
occur on the face.

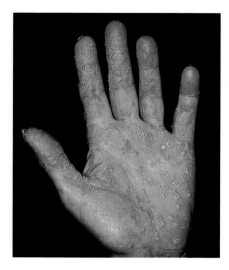

Figure 8-11
Psoriasis of the palms. In this instance plaques are similar to those that appear on the body.

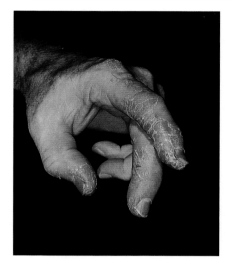

Figure 8-12
Psoriasis of the fingertips. The eruption appears eczematous, but the rich red hue is typical of psoriasis. This eruption occurred as a Koebner phenomenon in a surgeon.

Light-sensitive psoriasis. Psoriatic patients wait for sunny summer months when in most cases the disease responds predictably to ultraviolet light. However, too much of a good thing can be dangerous, especially for the patient who gets sunburned in an anxious attempt to clear the disease rapidly. As a result of the Koebner phenomenon, guttate lesions or a painful diffusely inflamed plaque forms in the burned areas (Figure 8-9). Plaques subsequently converge onto the clear previously protected sites. Some psoriatic patients do not tolerate ultraviolet light of any intensity.

Psoriasis of the scalp. The scalp is a favored site for psoriasis and may be the only site affected. Plaques are similar to those of the skin except that the scale is more readily retained; it is possibly anchored by hair. Extension of the plaques onto the forehead is relatively common (Figure 8-10). A dense, tight-feeling scale can cover the entire scalp. Even in the most severe cases, the hair is not permanently lost. Tinea amiantacea, a distinct scaling eruption of the scalp observed in children, is described in the section concerning seborrheic dermatitis.

Psoriasis of the palms and soles. The palms and soles may be involved as part of a generalized eruption (Figure 8-11) or they may be the only manifestation of disease.[7] There are several presentations. Superficial red plaques with thick brown scale may be indistinguishable from chronic eczema (Figure 8-12). Smooth deep red plaques are similar to those found in the flexural area (Figure 8-13).

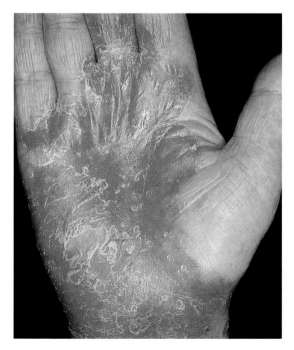

Figure 8-13
Psoriasis of the hand. Deep red smooth plaque in a patient with typical lesions on the body.

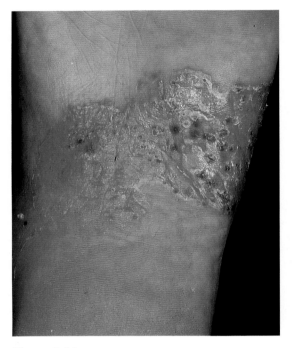

Figure 8-14
Pustular psoriasis of the soles. An early case in a typical location.

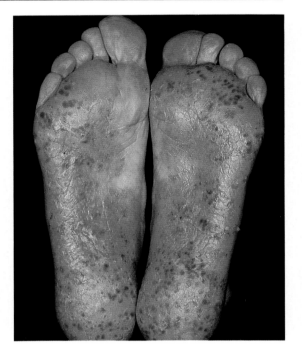

Figure 8-15
Pustular psoriasis of the soles. This is a chronic disease in which the soles may remain inflamed for years.

Figure 8-16
Pustular psoriasis of the digits. The eruption has remained localized in this one finger for years.

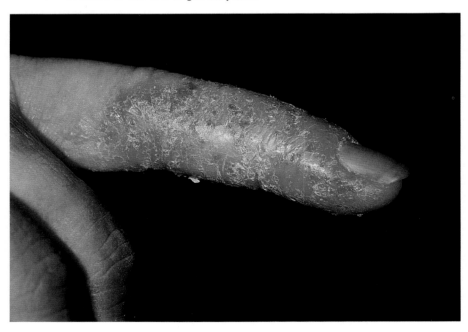

Pustular psoriasis of the palms and soles.
Pustules first appear on the middle portion of the palms and insteps of the soles; they may either remain localized or spread (Figures 8-14 and 8-15). The pustules do not rupture but turn dark brown and scaly as they reach the surface. The surrounding skin becomes pink, smooth, and tender. A thick crust may later cover the affected area. The course is chronic, lasting for years while the patient endures periods of partial remission followed by exacerbations so painful as to affect mobility. Treatment is less than adequate, but most patients remain active and reasonably comfortable.

Pustular psoriasis of the digits. This severe localized variant of psoriasis, also known as acrodermatitis continua, may remain localized to one finger for years. Vesicles rupture, resulting in a tender, diffusely eroded and fissured surface which continually exudes serum. The loosely adherent moist crust is easily shed, but continually recurs (Figure 8-16). Localized pustular psoriasis is highly resistant to therapy.

Psoriasis of the flexural or intertriginous areas. In psoriasis of the flexural or intertriginous areas the gluteal fold, axillae, groin, submammary folds, retroauricular fold, and the glans of the uncircumcised penis may be affected. The deep red, smooth, glistening plaques may extend to and stop at the junction of the skin folds, as with intertrigo or candida infections. The surface is moist and contains macerated white debris. Infection, friction, and heat may induce flexural psoriasis, a Koebner phenomenon. Cracking and fissures are common at the base of the crease, particularly in the groin, gluteal cleft, and superior and posterior auricular fold (Figure 8-17). As with typical psoriatic plaques, the margin is distinct. Pustules beyond the plaque border suggest secondary yeast infection. Infants and young children may develop flexural psoriasis of the groin, which extends onto the diaper area.

Psoriasis of the nails. Nail changes are characteristic of psoriasis and the nails of patients should be examined. (See chapter on nail disease). These changes offer supporting evidence for the diagnosis of psoriasis when skin changes are equivocal or absent.

Pitting. Nail pitting is the best known and possibly the most frequent psoriatic nail abnormality (Figure 8-18). Nail plate cells are shed in much the same way as psoriatic scale is shed, leaving a variable number of tiny punched-out depressions on the nail plate surface. They emerge from under the cuticle and grow out with the nail. Many other cutaneous diseases (e.g., eczema, fungal infections, and alopecia areata) may cause pitting, or it may occur as an isolated finding as a normal variation.

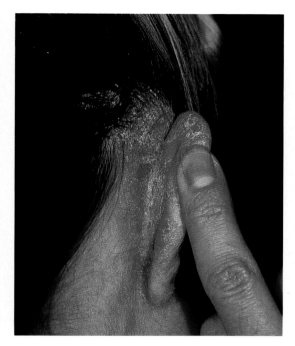

Figure 8-17
Psoriasis of the posterior auricular fold.

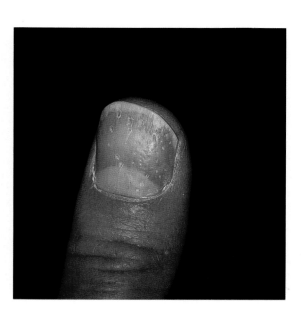

Figure 8-18
Psoriasis of the nails. Pitting is the best known psoriatic nail abnormality.

TABLE 8-1

PSORIATIC ARTHRITIS

Type	Percentage of all psoriatic arthritis	Features
Asymmetric arthritis (one or more joints)	60-70%	Joints of fingers and toes ("sausage finger")
Symmetric polyarthritis	15%	Clinically resembles rheumatoid arthritis, rheumatoid factor negative
Distal interphalangeal joint disease	5%	Mild, chronic, associated with nail disease
Destructive polyarthritis (arthritis mutilans)	5%	Osteolysis of small bones of hands and feet; gross deformity; joint subluxation
Ankylosing spondylitis	5%	With or without peripheral joint disease

Adapted from Moll JMH: The clinical spectrum of psoriatic arthritis. Clin Orthop **143**:66, 1979.

Onycholysis. Psoriasis of the nail bed causes separation of the nail from the nail bed. Unlike the uniform separation caused by pressure on long nails, the nail detaches in an irregular manner. The nail plate turns yellow, simulating a fungal infection.

Subungual debris. This is analogous to fungal infection; the nail bed scale is retained, forcing the distal nail to separate from the nail bed.

Nail deformity. Extensive involvement of the nail matrix results in a nail losing its structural integrity, resulting in fragmentation and crumbling (Figure 8-19).

Psoriatic arthritis. Psoriatic arthritis is a distinct form of arthritis in which the rheumatoid factor is usually negative. The incidence in the psoriatic population is between 5% and 7%. Onset may occur any time, but peak occurrence is between ages 30 and 50; women are more frequently affected than men.[8] Cases of arthritis have been reported to develop after trauma. There are five recognized presentations (Table 8-1).[9]

Asymmetric arthritis. The most common pattern is an asymmetric arthritis involving one or more joints of the fingers and toes (Figure 8-20). Usually one or more proximal interphalangeal (PIP), distal interphalangeal (DIP), metatarsophalangeal, or metacarpophalangeal joints are involved. During the acute phase the joint is red, warm, and painful. Continued inflammation promotes soft tissue swelling on either side of the joint ("sausage finger") and restrict mobility.

Symmetric arthritis. A symmetric polyarthritis resembling rheumatoid arthritis occurs, but the rheumatoid factor is negative.

DIP joint disease. Perhaps the most characteristic presentation of arthritis with psoriasis is involvement of the distal interphalangeal joints of the hands and feet with associated psoriatic nail disease. The disease is chronic but mild, is not disabling, and accounts for approximately 5% of patients with psoriatic arthritis.

Arthritis mutilans. The most severe form of psoriatic arthritis involves osteolysis of any of the small bones of the hands and feet. Gross deformity and subluxation are attributed to this condition. Severe osteolysis leads to digital telescoping, producing the "opera glass" deformity. This deformity may also be seen in rheumatoid arthritis.

Ankylosing spondylitis. This occurs as an isolated phenomenon or in association with peripheral joint disease. HLA–B27 is present in over 90% of patients with psoriatic arthritis and peripheral arthritis.[10]

Seventy percent of patients with rheumatoid arthritis have a positive rheumatoid factor, whereas those with psoriatic arthritis have an incidence equivalent to the normal population, about 5%.[11]

Nail involvement occurs in over 80% of patients with psoriatic arthritis, compared with 30% of patients with uncomplicated psoriasis.[12]

Treatment of psoriatic arthritis. Early psoriatic arthritis is treated with salicylates or nonsteroidal antiinflammatory agents. Antimalarials are contraindicated because of the risk of exfoliative dermatitis in patients with psoriasis. Systemic corticosteroids are avoided because of rebound of the skin disease upon withdrawal. For advanced disease, methotrexate controls both the joint and skin diseases.[13]

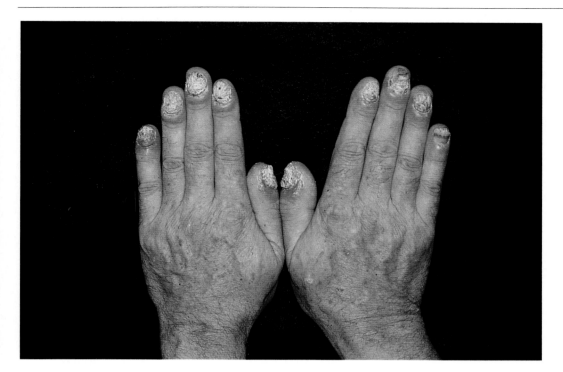

Figure 8-19
Psoriasis of the nails. Extensive involvement of
each nail matrix has caused all nails to be poorly
formed.

Figure 8-20
Psoriatic arthritis. Asymmetric arthritis pattern.

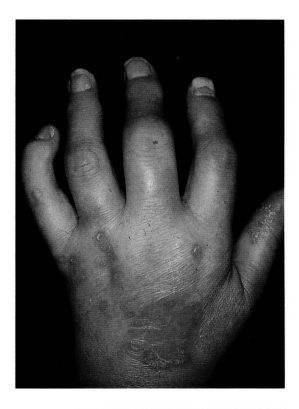

Treatment

Many topical and systemic agents are available for the treatment of psoriasis. With the exception of methotrexate, all require lengthy treatment to give relief, which is frequently only temporary. The most effective topical programs use ultraviolet light in combination with topical steroids, tar, or anthralin. Ultraviolet light in intensities high enough to be effective can be obtained from natural sunlight or commercially available light cabinets. Inexpensive single-bulb tanning lights are less effective. Some dermatologists have light cabinets; patients with extensive psoriasis are best treated in that setting. Effective programs can be designed for patients who do not have access to a therapeutic light source or for patients who have limited disease. Without light, tar is moderately effective, but persistent use of anthralin can clear the disease and offers the patient substantial remission periods.

The most common form of psoriasis seen by the practitioner is the localized chronic plaque disease involving the skin and scalp (Figures 8-1 and 8-4). Before instituting therapy, one must determine whether the plaque is inflamed (Figure 8-21). Some topical medications are irritating and can precipitate further activity, an example of the Koebner phenomenon. Inflammation should be suppressed with

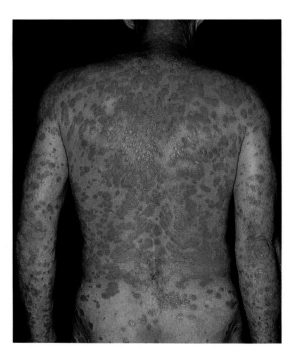

Figure 8-21
Inflammatory plaque psoriasis. A patient with such highly inflamed disease must not be treated initially with irritating medicines such as anthralin.

topical steroid and/or antibiotics before initiating other treatment programs.

A plaque is effectively treated when induration has disappeared. Residual erythema or brown hyperpigmentation is common when the plaque clears; patients frequently mistake the residual color for disease and continue treatment. If the plaque can not be felt by drawing the finger over the skin surface, treatment can be terminated.

Topical therapy

Topical steroids. Topical steroids (see Chapter 2) give fast but temporary relief. They are most useful for reducing inflammation and controlling itching. Initially, when the patient is introduced to topical steroids, the results are most gratifying. However, tachyphylaxis, or tolerance, occurs and the medication becomes less effective with continued use. Patients remember the initial response and continue topical steroids in anticipation of continued effectiveness. Long-term use of topical steroids results in atrophy and telangiectasia. Once the inflammation is suppressed and the plaque becomes chronic, tar or anthralin can be started.

Topical steroids are useful for relieving itching and treating inflamed and intertriginous plaques. A Group I to V topical steroid applied 2 or 4 times a day in a cream or ointment base is required for best results; however, Group V topical steroids applied twice daily should be used on the intertriginous areas and the face. Some plaques will resolve completely, but most will remain only partially reduced with continued application. Continuous application for more than 3 weeks should be discouraged. Remissions are very brief and the plaques may return shortly after treatment is terminated. Topical steroid creams applied under an occlusive plastic dressing promote more rapid clearing, but remissions are not extended. Topical steroid solutions are useful for scalp psoriasis. Intralesional injections of small plaques with triamcinolone acetonide (Kenalog, 5 to 10 mg/ml) almost invariably clear the lesion and accord long-term remission. Atrophy may occur with the 10-mg/ml concentration.

Anthralin. For years anthralin has been used effectively in conjunction with ultraviolet light to treat psoriasis. The principal objection was the mess and staining involved in its use. Anthralin is now practical for home therapy because of the new schedules that involve short treatment times (short contact method).[14]

Anthralin paste in high concentration (0.5% to 4%) is applied to the plaque. Care must be taken to protect normal skin and anthralin should not be applied to intertriginous areas or to the face. The medicine is washed off 10 to 30 minutes later and lubricants are applied to avoid dryness. A 2-hour contact period is more effective than short-contact therapy

TABLE 8-2

ANTHRALIN (DITHRANOL)*

Anthra-Derm (ointment)	0.1%, 0.25%, 0.5%, 1.0%
	In 45-gm tubes
Drithocreme (cream)	0.1%, 0.25%, 0.5%, 1.0%
	In 50-gm tubes
Dritho-scalp (cream)	0.25%, 0.5%
	In 50-gm tubes
Lasan (cream)	0.1%, 0.2%, 0.4%, 1.0%
	In 60-gm tubes

*Higher concentrations must be compounded by the pharmacist. (See Table 8-3.)

TABLE 8-3

ANTHRALIN PASTE (INSTRUCTIONS FOR THE PHARMACIST)

Anthralin	X%
Salicylic acid	4%
Paraffin	5%
Zinc oxide paste (qs)	100%

1. Heat the zinc oxide in the mixing bowl of the variable speed mixer and the paraffin in a water bath.
2. Levigate the powders in a small amount of mineral oil.
3. When the zinc oxide is soft and the paraffin melted, add all ingredients and mix until the product is somewhat congealed.
4. Package into 2 oz ointment jars.

and should be used in patients who fail to respond to the short-contact regimen.[15] A mild erythema may occur. This treatment is continued daily unless irritation occurs. If inflammation occurs, discontinue anthralin and treat with Group II to V topical steroid until improvement is noted. Reintroduce anthralin at a lower concentration and continue daily treatment. The goal is to maintain a daily schedule using the highest concentration of anthralin tolerated without inducing inflammation. Anthralin is commercially available in concentrations ranging from 0.1% to 1.0% (Table 8-2). Higher concentrations must be compounded by the pharmacist; a formula is found in Table 8-3. Patients must be cautioned about irritation and staining. Hands should be washed carefully after application, taking care to avoid eye contact. In a matter of weeks skin stain fades, but purple clothing stains are permanent (Figure 8-22).

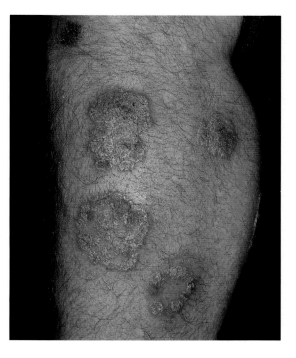

Figure 8-22
Psoriatic plaques under treatment with anthralin. As with all forms of treatment, plaques first clear in the center.

TABLE 8-4

COAL TAR PREPARATIONS

Estar Gel	5% in 13.8% alcohol 90 gm
Fototar Cream	1.6% 85 gm
Fototar Stik	5% 15 gm
PsoriGel	7.5% in 1% alcohol 120 gm
T-Derm	5% lotion

TABLE 8-5

ANTISEBORRHEIC SHAMPOOS

Selenium sulfide*	Pyrithione zinc
2.5% Selsun, Exsel	2% Head and Shoulders, Sebulon
1% Selsun Blue	1% Danex, Zincon
Coal tar†	Sulfur and sal acid
10% Xseb T	Sebulex
5% Vanseb T, Tegrin, Ionil T	Vanseb
4.3% Pentrax	Meted
0.5% Sebutone	

*Higher concentration more effective.
†Higher concentration slightly more effective but unpleasant.

Tar and ultraviolet light. Tar enhances the effectiveness of ultraviolet light.[16] For the most effective therapeutic response, a tar preparation may be applied 2 or more hours before anticipated ultraviolet light exposure. There are several commercially available tar preparations (Table 8-4). Some are drying, whereas others with a lubricating base (e.g., T-Derm and Fototar) are well tolerated. Therapeutic light sources that emit ultraviolet light in the range of 290 to 320 nm are the most effective;[17] long-wave ultraviolet light (UVA) in the 320- to 400-nm range is less effective for combined use with tar. An intensive program called the Goeckerman regimen combines the daily application of tar with short-wave ultraviolet light (UVB) exposure; it is safe, highly effective and possibly produces the longest remission periods.[18] However, a major commitment of time and money is required. Many larger hospitals provide inpatient facilities for this 3-week program. Patients with diffuse or poorly responsive psoriasis may leave the hospital with gratifying results. The Goeckerman regimen can also be used on an outpatient basis.[19]

Recent studies suggest that application of lubricants before UVB exposure provides results similar to tar and UVB.[20] A tar concentrate such as Balnetar can be added to the bath water as a substitute for tar ointments and lotions. Tar solution soaks are useful for psoriasis of the palms and soles. The feet can be soaked for 1 hour each day in a basin of warm water and Balnetar.

Treating the scalp. The scalp is a difficult area to treat because hair interferes with the application of medicine. Symptoms of tenderness and itching vary considerably. The goal is to provide symptomatic and cosmetic relief. It is unnecessary and impractical to attempt to have the scalp remain constantly clear.

Moderate scalp involvement. When used at least every other day, tar shampoos (Table 8-5) may be effective in controlling moderate scaling. Corticosteroid solutions are very expensive, but a minute amount can cover a wide area. Steroid gels (e.g., Lidex gel, Topicort gel) thoroughly penetrate hair and are effective. Small plaques are effectively treated with intralesional steroid injections of triamcinolone acetonide (e.g., Kenalog) 5 to 10 mg/ml. Remissions after use of intralesional steroids are much longer than those after topical steroids.

Diffuse scalp involvement. Diffuse disease or plaques with dense scale require more intensive therapy. Baker's P & S liquid (phenol, sodium chloride, and liquid paraffin) applied to the scalp at bedtime and washed out in the morning is moderately effective in reducing scale. Baker's liquid is pleasant and well tolerated for extended periods. Large plaques with thick scale require more intensive treatment; once control is achieved, tar shampoos should be used for maintenance.

Treatment of diffuse and thick scalp psoriasis. Three different programs can be used. All use oil- or ointment base preparations for scale penetration. They are applied at bedtime and washed out each morning with strong detergents such as Dawn dishwashing liquid. Topical steroid solutions can be applied during the day.

Liquor carbonis detergens (LCD), an extract of crude oil tar, 10% to 15%, is mixed with Nivea oil by the pharmacist. At bedtime the unpleasant mixture is liberally massaged into the scalp plaques. The mixture may be warmed before application to enhance scale penetration. A shower cap will protect pillows. An impressive amount of scale is removed in the first few days. Nightly applications are continued for at least 3 weeks or until the scalp is acceptably clear.

A mixture of 20% cade oil, 10% sulfur, and 5% salicylic acid in unibase to make 3 oz is very effective for stubborn plaques. Warming the mixture before application enhances penetration. It is applied each night and washed out in morning.

Anthralin ointment applied each evening and removed in the morning is another method for treating resistant scalp psoriasis. A short-contact method similar to that previously described for anthralin is used; apply 0.25% to 2% anthralin ointment and wash completely 10 to 20 minutes after application.

Systemic therapy

Methotrexate. Psoriatic skin has more cells in replication at any one time than normal skin. Methotrexate (MTX) by its inhibitory effect on DNA synthesis, apparently functions as a direct suppressor of psoriatic epidermal cell reproduction.[21] This drug has been successfully used for years in treating psoriasis. In general, a patient should not be started on MTX until all other forms of control have been attempted, including hospitalization. The major disadvantage of methotrexate is its potential for causing liver damage. Strict guidelines have been established for its use; they[22] are discussed below.

Indications. Methotrexate is indicated in the control of recalcitrant psoriasis not responsive to topical therapy when the psoriasis is physically, emotionally, or economically life-ruining. Candidates for MTX therapy are patients with the following: psoriatic erythroderma, psoriatic arthritis, acute pustular psoriasis, localized pustular psoriasis, psoriasis in body areas preventing employment, and extensive psoriasis.

Contraindications. Methotrexate can cause liver damage. Relative contraindications include significant renal or liver abnormalities, pregnancy, hepatitis, cirrhosis, severe anemia, leukopenia, thrombocytopenia, excessive alcohol consumption, or active infectious disease. Unreliable patients and men and women of reproductive age not using contraceptive measures should also be excluded.

Laboratory studies. If feasible, a liver biopsy should be performed prior to treatment. Liver scans have no place in the evaluation of methotrexate-induced liver toxicity. After therapy is instituted, liver biopsies are obtained at intervals of 1 to 1.5 gm cumulative dose of MTX.[23] The factors governing the decision to obtain a repeat liver biopsy are the value of liver function tests and the presence or absence of risk factors such as alcohol, arsenic, lowered renal function, obesity, or diabetes. The decision to proceed with additional MTX is also governed by the findings of the liver biopsy. A leukocyte and platelet count is obtained at 1- to 4-week intervals.

Dosage schedules. Two dosage schedules are used for the average 70-kg adult. The first is a single weekly dose of 7.5 to 25 mg per week orally or 7.5 to 100 mg per week intravenously or intramuscularly.[24] The second is a divided oral dose schedule of 2.5 to 5 mg at 12-hour intervals, with three doses each week.[25] The dosage is gradually increased by 2.5 mg per week; generally the total dose should not exceed 25 mg per week.

Photochemotherapy. The FDA approved photochemotherapy treatment for psoriasis in early 1982. The treatment, known as PUVA,[26] is so designated because of the use of a class of drugs called psoralens (the P) along with exposure to UVA. The specific psoralen drug approved for use in PUVA therapy is methoxsalen. Patients ingest a prescribed dose of methoxsalen approximately 2 hours before being exposed to a carefully measured amount of UVA light in a uniquely designed enclosure. The drug apparently couples with and inhibits DNA synthesis after activation with ultraviolet light in the UVA region (320 to 400 nm), thereby decreasing cellular proliferation. The drug dosage is based on body weight, and the amount of initial energy delivered is based on the degree of skin pigmentation and ability to sunburn. Patients are treated 2 to 3 times each week during the clearing phase; this requires approximately 20 treatments. Over 80% of patients clear and can be maintained with periodic treatments; the maintenance schedule varies with each individual.[27] Light does not penetrate hair; scalp psoriasis must be treated with conventional therapy.

The advantages of PUVA are that it controls severe psoriasis with relatively few maintenance treatments and that it can be done on an outpatient basis. The short-term side effects include dark tanning, pruritus, nausea, and severe sunburn. Patients must protect their eyes with special glasses for the remainder of the treatment day and the following day to prevent potential psoralen-induced cataracts. The known long-term side effects include accelerated skin aging and an increased incidence of skin cancers.[28]

Photochemotherapy is an ideal treatment modality for some patients. Patients should be selected only by physicians experienced in the treatment of all forms of psoriasis.

Systemic corticosteroids. Systemic steroids rapidly clear psoriasis; unfortunately in many instances the disease worsens, occasionally evolving into pustular psoriasis when corticosteroids are withdrawn.[29] For this reason systemic corticosteroids have been abandoned as a routine treatment for psoriasis.

Seborrheic Dermatitis

Seborrheic dermatitis is a common chronic inflammatory disease with a characteristic pattern for different age groups. The etiology is unknown, but heredity is almost certainly an integral factor. In adults seborrheic dermatitis tends to persist, but it does undergo periods of remission and exacerbation. The extent of involvement among patients varies widely. Most cases can be adequately controlled.

Infants (cradle cap)

Infants commonly develop a greasy adherent scale on the vertex of the scalp. Minor amounts of scale are easily removed by frequent shampooing with products containing sulfur and salicylic acid (e.g., Sebulex shampoo). Scale may accumulate and become thick and adherent over much of the scalp and may be accompanied by inflammation (Figure 8-23). Secondary infection can occur. Patients with serum and crust are treated with oral

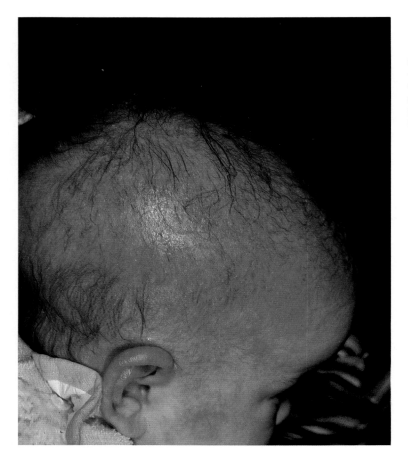

Figure 8-23
Seborrheic dermatitis (cradle cap). Diffuse inflammation with secondary infection. Much of the scale from this child's scalp was removed with shampoos.

antistaphylococcal antibiotics. Once infection is controlled, erythema and scaling can be suppressed with Group VI or VII topical steroid creams or lotions. Dense thick adherent scale is removed by applying warm mineral or olive oil to the scalp and washing several hours later with detergents such as Dawn dishwashing liquid. Attempt to prolong remissions with frequent use of salicyclic acid or tar shampoos (Table 8-5).

Young children (tinea amiantacea and blepharitis)

Tinea amiantacea is a characteristic eruption of unknown etiology. Mothers of afflicted children often recall episodes of cradle cap during infancy. Some authors believe that tinea amiantacea is a form of eczema or psoriasis. One patch or several patches of dense scale appear anywhere on the scalp and may persist for months before the parent notices temporary hair loss or the distinctive large, oval, yellow-white plates of scale firmly adherent to the scalp and hair (Figure 8-24). The scale binds to the hair and is drawn up with the growing hair, a characteristic sign. Patches of dense scale range from 2 to 10 cm. The scale suggests fungal scalp disease, therefore the designation tinea. Amiantacea, meaning asbestos, refers to the plate-like quality of the scale, which resembles genuine asbestos.

Warm 10% LCD in Nivea oil (prescribe 8 oz; it must be prepared by the pharmacist) is applied to the scalp at bedtime and removed by shampooing each morning with Dawn dishwashing liquid. The scale is completely removed in 1 to 3 weeks and tar shampoos are used for maintenance. Periodic recurrences are similarly treated.

White scale adherent to the eyelashes and lid margins with variable amounts of erythema is characteristic of seborrheic blepharitis (Figure 8-25).

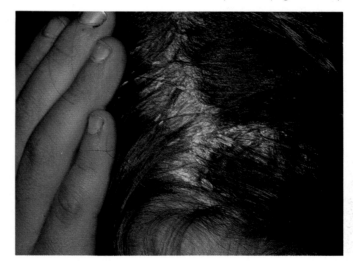

Figure 8-24
Seborrheic dermatitis (tinea amiantacea). The scalp contains dense patches of scale. Large plates of yellow-white scale firmly adhere to the hair shafts.

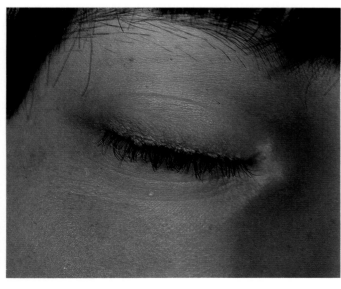

Figure 8-25
Seborrheic dermatitis (blepharitis).

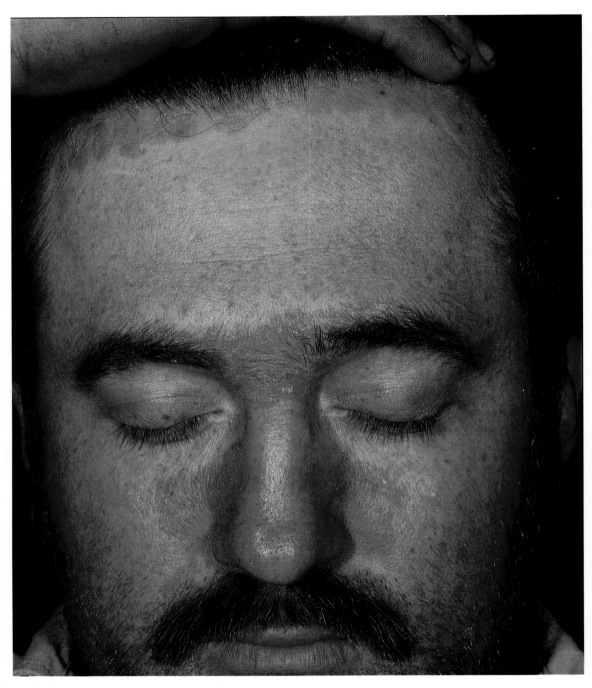

Figure 8-26
Seborrheic dermatitis in an adult with extensive
involvement in all of the characteristic sites.

The disease produces some discomfort and is unbecoming. It persists for years and is resistant to treatment. Scale may be suppressed by frequent washing with zinc- or tar-containing antidandruff shampoos (Table 8-5). Although topical steroid creams and lotions suppress this disease, prolonged use of such preparations around the eyes may cause glaucoma and therefore should be avoided.[30]

Adolescents and adults (classic seborrheic dermatitis)

Most individuals periodically experience fine, dry, white scalp scaling with minor itching; this is dandruff. They tend to attribute this condition to a dry scalp and consequently avoid hair washing. However, avoidance of washing allows scale to accumulate and inflammation may occur. Patients with minor amounts of dandruff should be encouraged to wash every day or every other day with antidandruff shampoos (Table 8-5). Fine, dry, white or yellow scale may occur on an inflamed base. The distribution of scaling and inflammation may be more diffuse and occur in the seborrheic areas: scalp and scalp margins, eyebrows, base of eyelashes, nasolabial folds, external ear canals, posterior auricular fold, and presternal area (Figure 8-26). The axillae, inframammary folds, groin, and umbilicus are less frequently affected. Scaling of the ears may be misjudged as eczema or fungus infection. Its presence in association with characteristic scaling in other typical areas assists in supporting the diagnosis. Once established, the disease tends to persist to a variable degree. Older patients, particularly the bedridden or those with neurologic problems such as Parkinson's disease, tend to have a more chronic and extensive form of classic seborrheic dermatitis. Occasionally the scalp scale may be diffuse, thick, and adherent. Differentiation from psoriasis may be impossible. Patients should be reassured that seborrheic dermatitis does not cause permanent hair loss.

Treatment consists of frequent washing of all affected areas including the face and chest with anti-seborrheic shampoo. Remaining inflamed areas respond quickly to Group V topical steroid creams. Steroid lotions may be applied to the scalp twice daily. Patients must be cautioned that topical steroids should not be used as maintenance therapy. Dense diffuse scalp scaling is treated with 10% LCD in Nivea oil as previously described for cradle cap. Adults may apply the oil preparation at bedtime and cover with a shower cap. Treatment is repeated each night until the scalp is clear, about 1 to 3 weeks.

Pityriasis Rosea

Pityriasis rosea (PR) is a common, benign, usually asymptomatic, distinctive self-limiting skin eruption of unknown etiology. There is some evidence that it is viral in origin. It is predominant among women by a margin of 1.5 to 1. More than 75% of patients are between the ages of 10 and 35 years, with a mean age of 23 years and a range of 4 months to 78 years. Two percent of patients have a recurrence.[31] The incidence of the disease is higher during the colder months. Twenty percent of patients have a recent history of acute infection with fatigue, headache, sore throat, lymphadenitis, and fever; the disease may be more common in atopic individuals. Pityriasis rosea has several unique features, but variant patterns do exist, which may create confusion between this disease and secondary syphilis, guttate psoriasis, viral exanthems, tinea, nummular eczema, and drug eruptions.

Typically, a single 2- to 10-cm round-to-oval lesion, the herald patch, abruptly appears. It may occur anywhere on the body but is most frequently located on the trunk or proximal extremities. The herald patch retains the same features as the subsequent oval lesions. At this stage many patients are convinced that they have ringworm. Within a few days to several weeks, smaller lesions appear and reach their maximum number in 1 to 2 weeks (Figure 8-27). They are typically limited to the trunk

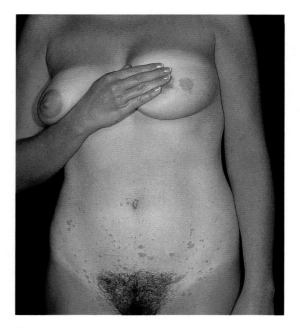

Figure 8-27
Pityriasis rosea. A herald patch is present on the breast. Subsequent lesions commonly begin in the lower abdominal region.

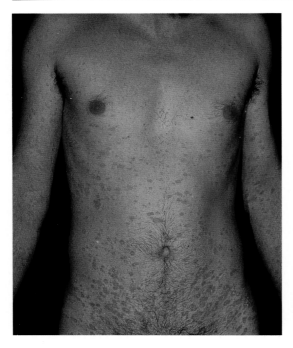

Figure 8-28
Pityriasis rosea. The fully evolved eruption 2 weeks after onset.

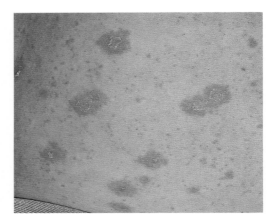

Figure 8-29
Pityriasis rosea. Both small oval plaques and multiple small papules are present. Occasionally, the eruption will consist only of small papules.

Figure 8-30
Pityriasis rosea. A ring of tissue-like scale (collarette scale) remains attached within the border of the plaque.

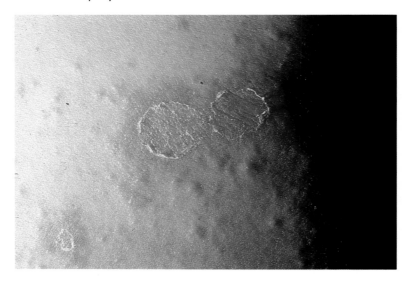

and proximal extremities, but in extensive cases they develop on the arms, legs, and face (Figure 8-28). Individual lesions are salmon pink in whites and hyperpigmented in blacks. Many of the earliest lesions are papular, but in most cases the typical 1- to 2-cm oval plaques appear (Figure 8-29). A fine wrinkled tissue-like scale remains attached within the border of the plaque giving the characteristic ring of scale, called collarette scale (Figure 8-30). The long axis of the oval plaques is oriented along skin lines. Numerous lesions on the back, oriented along skin lines, give the appearance of drooping pine-tree branches, therefore the designation Christmas tree distribution. The number of lesions varies from a few to hundreds, which in rare instances seem to cover the entire skin surface. Some cases are asymptomatic, but many patients complain of mild transient itching. Severe itching may accompany extensive inflammatory eruptions. The disease clears spontaneously in 1 to 3 months. Postinflammatory hyperpigmentation may occur, especially in blacks.

Diagnosis. Diagnosis is made by clinical appearance. Tinea can be ruled out with a potassium hydroxide examination. Secondary syphilis may be indistinguishable from pityriasis rosea, especially if the herald patch is absent. A VDRL for syphilis should be ordered, especially if the herald patch is absent. A biopsy reveals nonspecific features and is of little aid. Pityriasis rosea may also be mimicked by psoriasis and nummular eczema.

Management. Whether pityriasis rosea is contagious in unknown. The disease is benign and self-limited and does not appear to affect the fetus of the pregnant woman; therefore, isolation is unnecessary. Group V topical steroids and oral antihistamines may be used as needed for itching. The rare extensive case with intense itching will respond to a 1- to 2-week course of prednisone, 10 mg 3 times a day. Direct sun exposure will hasten the resolution of individual lesions, while those in protected areas such as under bathing suits will remain[32] (Figure 8-27).

Lichen Planus

Lichen planus (LP) is a unique inflammatory cutaneous and mucous membrane reaction pattern. The customary age of onset is between 30 and 70 years. Although the disease may occur at any age, it is rare in children younger than 5. There are a number of clinical forms and the number of lesions varies from a few chronic papules to acute generalized disease (Table 8-6). The etiology is unknown, but some patients with LP have a deficiency of glucose-6-phosphate dehydrogenase in their epidermis.[33] Eruptions from drugs (gold, chloroquine, methyl-dopa, penicillamine, etc.), chemical exposure (film processing), bacterial infections (secondary syphilis), and post-bone marrow transplants (graft-versus-host reaction) that have a similar appearance are referred to as lichenoid.

TABLE 8-6

VARIOUS PATTERNS OF LICHEN PLANUS

Various patterns of lichen planus	Most common site
Actinic	Sun exposed areas
Annular	Trunk, external genitalia
Atrophic	Any area
Erosioulcerative	Soles of feet, mouth
Follicular (lichen plano pilaris)	Scalp
Guttate (numerous small papules)	Trunk
Hypertrophic	Lower limbs (especially ankles)
Linear	Zosteriform (leg), scratched area
Nail disease	Finger nails
Papular (localized)	Flexor surface (wrists and forearms)
Vesiculobullous	Lower limbs, mouth

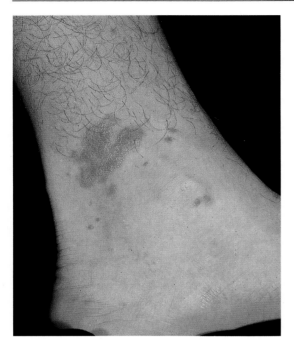

Figure 8-31
Lichen planus. A characteristic lesion of planar, polyangular purple papules with lacey reticular criss-crossed whitish lines (Wickham's stria) on the surface.

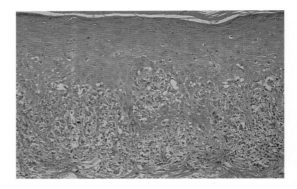

Figure 8-32
Lichen planus. The epidermis is thickened. The epidermodermal junction is indistinct. There is a band of chronic inflammatory cells in the upper dermis. Melanin pigment is dispersed throughout the inflammatory infiltrate.

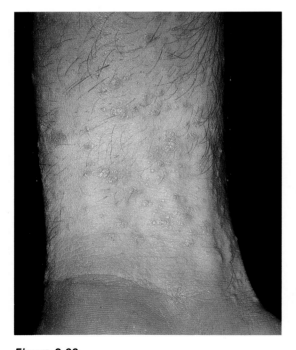

Figure 8-33
Localized lichen planus. Early lesions are present on the flexor surface of the wrists, a common site for localized lichen planus.

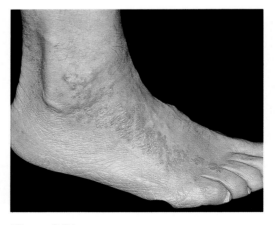

Figure 8-34
Localized lichen planus. Papules become thicker and confluent with time.

The morphology and distribution of the lesions are characteristic (Figure 8-31). The primary lesion is a 2- to 10-mm flat-topped papule with an irregular angulated border (polygonal papules). Close inspection of the surface shows a lacy, reticular pattern of criss-crossed whitish lines (Wickham's stria) that can be accentuated by a drop of immersion oil. Histologically, Wickham's stria are areas of focal epidermal thickening (Figure 8-32). Newly evolving lesions are pink-white, but over time they assume a distinctive violaceous hue with a peculiar waxy luster. Lesions that persist for months may become thicker and dark red (hypertrophic lichen planus). Papules aggregate into different patterns. Patterns are usually haphazard clusters, but they may be annular, diffusely papular (guttate), or linear, appearing in response to a scratch (Koebner phenomenon). Rarely, a line of papules may extend the length of an extremity. Vesicles or bullae may appear on preexisting lesions or on normal skin. The clinical features of lichen planus can be remembered by learning the five P's: pruritic, planar (flat-topped), polyangular, purple papules.

Localized papules

Papules are most commonly located on the flexor surfaces of the wrists and forearms (Figure 8-33), the legs immediately above the ankles (Figure 8-34), and the lumbar region (Figures 8-38 and 8-39). Itching is variable; 20% of patients with LP do not itch. Some patients with generalized involvement have minimal symptoms, whereas others display intolerable pruritus. The course is unpredictable. Some patients experience spontaneous remission in a few months, but the most common localized papular form tends toward chronicity and endures on the average for approximately 4 years. Twenty percent of patients have a recurrence of LP.

Hypertrophic lichen planus

This second most common cutaneous pattern may occur on any body region, but is typically found on the pretibial areas of the legs and ankles (Figure 8-35). After a long time, papules lose their characteristic features and become confluent as reddish-brown or purplish thickened round-to-elongated (band-like) plaques with a rough or verrucous surface; itching may be severe. Lesions continue for months or years, averaging about 8 years, and may be perpetuated by scratching. After the lesions clear, a dark brown pigmentation remains.

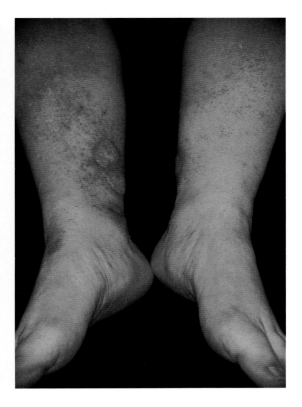

Figure 8-35
Hypertrophic lichen planus. Thick reddish-brown plaques are most often present on the lower legs.

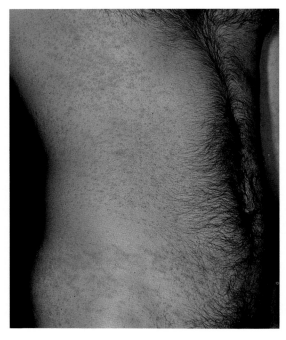

Figure 8-36
Generalized lichen planus.

Figure 8-37
Generalized lichen planus. Numerous pinpoint whitish-purple papules.

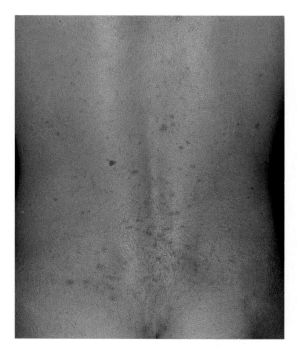

Figure 8-38
Generalized lichen planus. Papules are larger and are confluent in the lower back region.

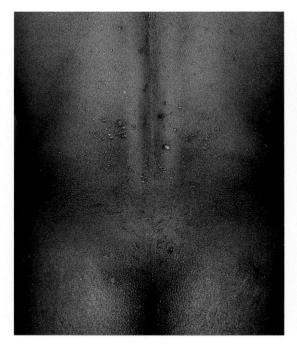

Figure 8-39
Generalized lichen planus. Lesions are usually darkly pigmented in blacks.

Generalized lichen planus and lichenoid drug eruptions

LP may occur abruptly as a generalized intensely pruritic eruption (Figure 8-36). Initially, the papules are pinpoint, numerous, and isolated (Figure 8-37). The papules may remain discrete or become confluent as large red eczematous-like thin plaques. A highly characteristic diffuse dark brown postinflammatory pigmentation remains as the disease clears. Before resolving spontaneously, untreated generalized LP continues for approximately 8 months. Lichenoid drug eruptions are frequently of this diffuse type.[34,35] Low-grade fever may be present in the first few days and lesions appear on the trunk, extremities, and lower back (Figures 8-38 and 8-39). The disease is seldom seen on the face or scalp and is rare on the palms and soles.

Lichen planus of the palms and soles

LP of the palms and soles generally occurs as an isolated phenomenon, but may appear simultaneously with disease in other areas. The lesions differ from classic lesions of LP in that the papules are larger and aggregate into semitranslucent plaques with a globular waxy surface (Figure 8-40). Itching may be intolerable. Ulceration may occur and lesions of the feet may be so resistant to treatment that surgical excision and grafting are required.[36] The disease may last indefinitely.

Follicular lichen planus

Follicular LP is also known as lichen planopilaris. Lesions localized to the hair follicles may occur alone or with papular LP. Follicular LP presenting as pinpoint, hyperkeratotic, follicular projections is the most common form of LP found in the scalp, where papular lesions are rarely observed. Hair loss occurs and may be permanent if the disease is sufficiently active to cause scarring. Lichen planus of the scalp is a disease that causes scarring alopecia.

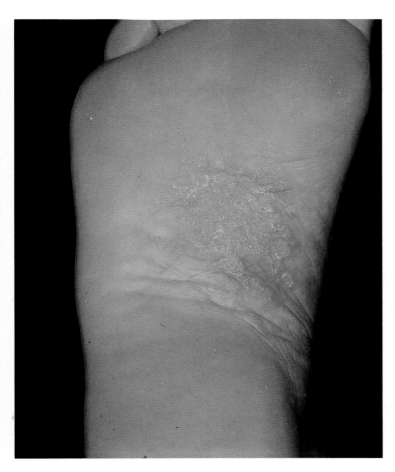

Figure 8-40
Lichen planus of the soles.
Thick semitranslucent plaques.

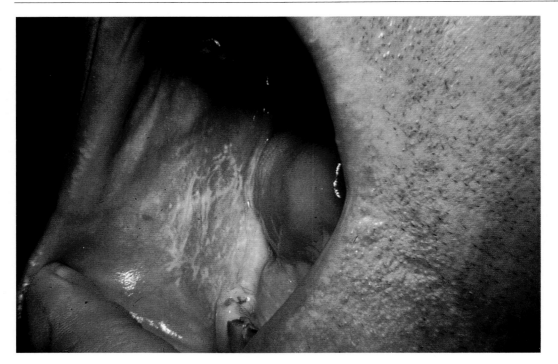

Figure 8-41
Mucous membrane lichen planus. A lacey white
pattern is present on the buccal mucosa.
(Courtesy of Gerald Shklar, B.Sc., D.D.S., M.S.,
Harvard School of Dental Medicine.)

Figure 8-42
Lichen planus on the penis. A lacey white pattern
identical to that seen on the buccal mucosa.

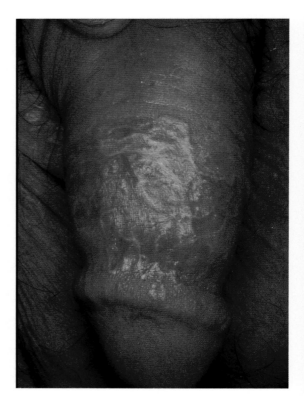

Mucous membrane lichen planus

Mucous membrane involvement is observed in over 50% of patients with LP. Lesions may be located on the tongue and lips, but the most common site is the buccal mucosa (Figure 8-41). There are two stages of severity. The most common form is the nonerosive, generally asymptomatic, dendritic branching or lacy white network pattern seen on the buccal mucosa. White papules and plaques may appear with time. The oral cavity should always be examined if the diagnosis of cutaneous LP is suspected. The presence of this dendritic pattern is solid supporting evidence for the diagnosis of cutaneous LP.

A more difficult form is erosive mucosal LP. Localized or extensive ulcerations may involve any area of the oral cavity. Chronic ulcerative lesions rarely undergo malignant degeneration. Superficial and erosive lesions are less commonly found on the glans penis (Figure 8-42), vulvovaginal region, and anus.

Nails

Nail changes most frequently accompany generalized LP, but rarely occur as the only manifestation of disease. They include proximal to distal linear depressions or grooves and partial or complete destruction of the nail plate. See the chapter on nail disease.

Diagnosis

The diagnosis of LP can be made clinically, but a skin biopsy will eliminate any doubt.[37] Direct immunofluorescence of skin is not routinely performed for the diagnosis of LP. The skin shows numerous ovoid globular deposits of IgE, IgM, IgA, and complement and a thick, linear band of fibrinogen at the dermoepidermal junction.[38] LP is not considered an immunologically mediated disease. The deposition of all types of immunoglobulin is considered to be a nonspecific response to inflammation. Circulating antibodies have not been found; therefore, indirect immunofluorescence is negative.

Treatment

Therapy for cutaneous lichen planus

Topical steroids. Group I or II topical steroids in a cream or cintment base applied 3 times per day are used as initial treatment for localized disease. They relieve itching, but the lesions are slow to clear. Plastic occlusion will enhance the effectiveness of topical steroids.

Intralesional steroids. Triamcinolone acetonide (Kenalog), 5 to 10 mg/ml, may reduce the hypertrophic lesions located on the wrists and lower legs. Injections may be repeated every 3 or 4 weeks.

Systemic steroids. Generalized severely pruritic lichen planus responds to oral corticosteroids. For adults, a 2- to 4-week course of prednisone, 20 mg twice daily, is usually sufficient to clear the disease. To prevent recurrence, gradually decrease the dosage over a 3-week period.

Antihistamines. Antihistamines such as hydroxyzine (Atarax, Durrax), 10 to 25 mg every 4 hours, may provide satisfactory relief from itching.

Oral griseofulvin (500 mg daily for 4 to 6 weeks) has been reported to reduce itching and flatten lesions in 70% of patients,[39] but most reports have shown this treatment to be ineffective.

PUVA. A bilateral comparison study demonstrated that PUVA is an effective therapy for generalized, symptomatic lichen planus and suggested that maintenance therapy might not be required once complete clearance is attained.[40]

Therapy for mucous membrane lichen planus

Triamcinolone in Orabase twice daily is the initial treatment for oral LP. The medication is placed on the lesions, but not rubbed in. Massaging the special cream base will result in loss of adhesiveness.

Intralesional steroids in a single submucosal injection, 0.5 to 1 ml, of methylprednisolone acetate (Depo-Medrol) 40 mg/ml may be sufficient to heal erosive oral LP within 1 week.[41]

Topical tretinoin incorporated into Orabase at a 0.1% strength was reported effective after 2 months of continuous treatment for all forms of oral LP.[42] Presently this preparation is not commecially available. Tretinoin must be ordered from the manufacturer for compounding.

Figure 8-43
Lichen sclerosus et atrophicus. Early
lesions are ivory-colored flat-topped
slightly raised papules with follicular
plugs.

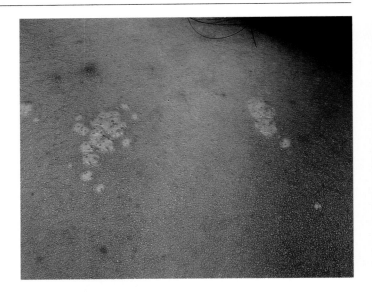

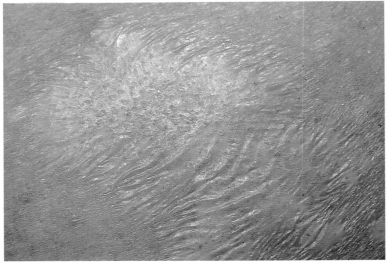

Figure 8-44
Lichen sclerosus et atrophicus.
Papular lesions as illustrated in
Figure 8-43 coalesce to form
atrophic plaques with a
wrinkled surface. White to brown
horny follicular plugs appear
on the surface, a feature
referred to as "delling."

Figure 8-45
Lichen sclerosus et atrophicus.
There is epidermal atrophy and
a keratotic plug. A zone of edema
and collagen homogenization is
present in the upper dermis.

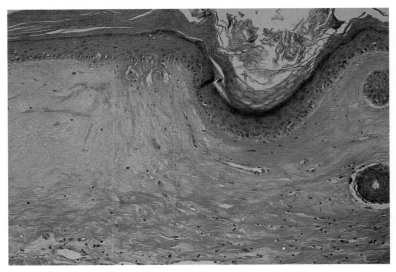

Lichen Sclerosus et Atrophicus

Lichen sclerosus et atrophicus (LSA) is an uncommon but distinctive chronic cutaneous disease of unknown origin. Cases in females outnumber males by 10:1. Although the trunk and extremities may be affected, the disease has a predilection for the vulva, perianal area, and groin. Most lesions appear spontaneously, but some may be induced by trauma (Koebner phenomenon). At a glance LSA may be confused with guttate morphea, lichen planus, or discoid lupus erythematosus. The difference becomes evident upon closer inspection of the surface features. Early lesions are small, smooth, pink or ivory, flat-topped, slightly raised papules. White-to-brown horny follicular plugs appear on the surface; this feature is referred to as "delling" (Figure 8-43). Delling is not observed in lichen planus or morphea. In time, clusters of papules may coalesce to form small oval plaques with a dull or glistening, smooth, white, atrophic, wrinkled surface (Figure 8-44). Histologically, the interface area between the dermis and epidermis appears to have dissolved (Figure 8-45). The overlying unsupported thin atrophic epidermis contracts, giving the appearance of wrinkled tissue paper.

Anogenital lesions in females

In most cases, anogenital lesions are distinctive. All of the following patterns may be present in the same individual. The first is a white atrophic plaque in the shape of an hourglass or inverted keyhole encircling the vagina and rectum (Figure 8-46). This most distinctive pattern is seen in prepubertal females as well as adults. Prepubertal LSA may occur in infants and resolves without sequelae in about two-thirds of cases at or just before menarche. The disease persists in about one-third of the patient.[43] Typically, the adult form appears after menopause and has a lengthy duration. Lesions itch and may show evidence of excoriation.

Intertriginous (skin crease) lesions involve the groin and anal area and are subject to friction and maceration. The delicate thin white wrinkled compromised skin breaks down to become hemorrhagic and eroded, simulating irritant or candidal intertrigo (Figure 8-47). Bullae may precede erosions.

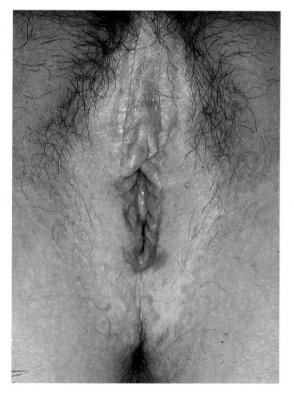

Figure 8-46
Lichen sclerosus et atrophicus. A white atrophic plaque encircles the vagina and rectum (inverted keyhole pattern).

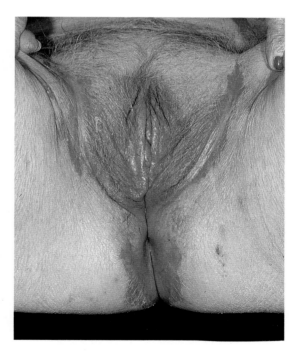

Figure 8-47
Lichen sclerosus et atrophicus. Atrophic hemorrhagic intertriginous lesions that simulate candida intertrigo.

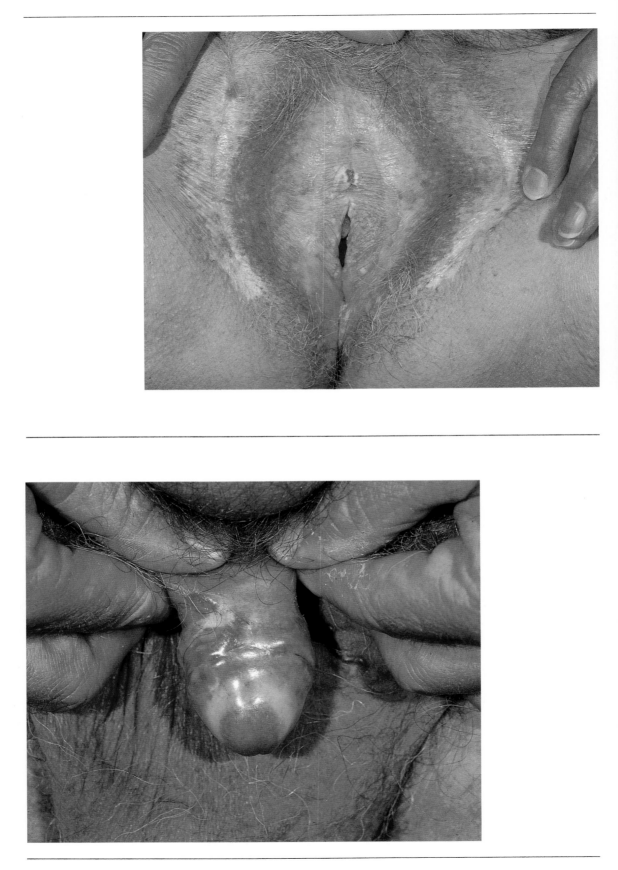

Figure 8-48 (opposite, top)
Lichen sclerosus et atrophicus of the vulva (kraurosis vulvae). The crease areas are atrophic and wrinkled, the labia is hyperpigmented, and the introitus is contracted and ulcerated.

Figure 8-49 (opposite, bottom)
Lichen sclerosus et atrophicus of the penis (balanitis xerotica obliterans). The glans is smooth, white, and atrophic. Erosions are present on the prepuce.

LSA of the vulva (kraurosis vulvae) is a distressing problem. The disease is chronic and painful and interferes with sexual activity. Atrophic fragile tissue erodes, becomes macerated, and heals slowly. Repeated cycles of erosion and healing induce contraction of the vaginal introitus and atrophy of the clitoris and labia minora (Figure 8-48). A watery discharge may be present. Squamous cell carcinoma, particularly of the clitoris or labia minora, has been reported in about 3% of patients with chronic LSA.[44] Therefore, biopsy should be considered in lesions that are white and raised (leukoplakia), fissured or ulcerated, and unresponsive to medical therapy.

One report showed that women with untreated, vulvar lichen sclerosus had significantly decreased serum levels of dihydrotestosterone and androstenedione and significantly higher than normal serum levels of free testosterone. Total testosterone levels were normal. Estrogen and sex hormone–binding globulin levels were normal.[45]

LSA of the penis

In LSA of the penis (balanitis xerotica obliterans), the patient complains initially of recurrent balanitis which may be intensified by intercourse; the shaft may be involved. The white atrophic plaques occur on the glans and prepuce and erode and heal with contraction. Encroachment into the urinary meatus may lead to stricture. As with vaginal LSA, degeneration into squamous cell carcinoma is rare.

Management

In general, the diagnosis of LSA can be made by clinical observation, but a biopsy may be necessary for confirmation. As previously stated, chronically fissured, ulcerated, or hyperplastic lesions should be biopsied to rule out the possibility of squamous cell carcinoma.

Topical steroid creams should be the first program of treatment for uncomplicated lesions. The creams suppress itching and may correct some of the pathologic changes. Group V topical steroid creams are applied twice daily for 2 weeks. If there is no improvement, a short trial period of Group II or III topical steroids is worth the effort. Vaginal and vulvar candidiasis may occur. Atrophy of the vulva may result from continuous application of topical steroids. Use should be discontinued and replaced with bland lubricants such as Nutraplus cream when a favorable response is obtained.

Intralesional steroids such as trimacinolone acetonide (Kenalog), 2.5 to 5 mg/ml, may be useful for areas not responding to topical therapy.

Testosterone propionate in a bland ointment has been reported to be partially effective for vulvar[45] and penile LSA. A 2% testosterone ointment is prescribed. The pharmacist is instructed to add 5 ml of testosterone propionate in oil (100 mg/ml) to 25 gm of white petrolatum. The ointment is applied at bedtime and in the morning each day until lesions improve. Two or three months may be required before improvement is noted. One report demonstrated that during the period of testosterone application, both total testosterone and dihydrotestosterone levels increased significantly, resulting in values higher than those in untreated, normal women. The increase in levels of free testosterone were not significant.[45] Side effects such as increased libido and clitoral hypertrophy may occur with long-term use.

REFERENCES

1. Johnson MT: Skin conditions and related need for medical care among persons 1-74, United States, 1971-1974. Data from the National Health Survey. Washington DC, 1978, DHEW Publication No. (PHS) 79-1660.
2. Watson W, Cann HM, Farber EM, et al: Genetics of psoriasis. Arch Dermatol **105**:197, 1972.
3. Watson W, Farber EM: Psoriasis in childhood. Pediatr Clin North Am **18**:875, 1971.
4. Whyte HJ, Baughman RD: Acute guttate psoriasis and streptococcal infection. Arch Dermatol **89**:350, 1964.
5. Ogawa M, Baughman RD, Clendenning WE: Generalized pustular psoriasis: induction by topical use of coal tar. Arch Dermatol **99**:671, 1969.
6. Baker H, Ryan TJ: Generalized pustular psoriasis: a clinical and epidemiological study of 104 cases. Br J Dermatol **80**:771, 1968.
7. Ashurst PJC: Relapsing pustular eruptions of the hands and feet. Br J Dermatol **776**:169, 1964.
8. Cohen GL: Psoriatic arthritis. Prog Dermatol **10**:2, 5, 1976.
9. Moll JMH: The clinical spectrum of psoriatic arthritis. Clin Orthop **143**:66, 1979.
10. Brewerton DA: HLA-B27 and the inheritance of susceptiblity to rheumatic diseases. Arthritis Rheum **19**:656, 1976.
11. Wright V: Psoriatic arthritis. Ann Rheum Dis **20**:123, 1961.

12. Wright V: Rheumatism and psoriasis: a reevaluation. Am J Med **27**:454, 1959.

13. Willkens RF, Williams HJ, Ward JR: Randomized double-blind placebo-controlled trial of low-dose pulse methotrexate in psoriatic lesions. Arthritis Rheum **27**:376, 1984.

14. Lowe NJ, Ashton RE, Koudsi H, et al: Anthralin for psoriasis: short-contact anthralin therapy compared with topical steroid and conventional anthralin. J Am Acad Dermatol **10**:69, 1984.

15. Statham BN, Ryatt KS, Rowell NR: Anthralin therapy for psoriasis. J Am Acad Dermatol **11**:303, 1984.

16. Levine MJ, White HAD, Parrish JA: Components of the Goeckerman regimen. J Invest Dermatol **73**:170, 1979.

17. Parrish, JA, Jaenicke KF: Action spectrum for phototherapy of psoriasis. J Invest Dermatol **76**:359, 1981.

18. Perry HO, Soderstrom CW, Schultze RW: The Goeckerman treatment of psoriasis. Arch Dermatol **98**:178, 1968.

19. DesGroseilliers J-P, Cullen AE, Rouleau GA: Ambulatory Goeckerman treatment of psoriasis: experience with 200 patients. Can Med Associ J **124**:1018, 1981.

20. Adrain RM, Parrish JA, Momtaz-T K, et al: Outpatient phototherapy of psoriasis. Arch Dermatol **117**:623, 1981.

21. Bleyer WA: The clinical pharmacology of methotrexate. Cancer **41**:36, 1978.

22. Roenigk, HH Jr, Auerbach R, Maibach HI, et al: Methotrexate guidelines—revised. J Am Acad Dermatol **6**:145, 1982.

23. Weinstein GD: Chemotherapy for psoraisis. Dermatol Clin **2**(3):431, 1984.

24. Roenigk H, Fowler-Bergfeld W, Curtis G: Methotrexate for psoriasis in weekly oral doses. Arch Dermatol **99**:86, 1969.

25. Weinstein G, Frost P: Methotrexate for psoriasis: a new therapeutic schedule. Arch Dermatol **103**:33, 1971.

26. Parrish JA, Fitzpatrick TB, Tannenbaum L, et al: Photochemotherapy of psoriasis with oral methoxsalen and long wave ultraviolet light. N Engl J Med **291**:1207, 1974.

27. Roenigk HH Jr, Farber EM, Storrs F, et al: Photochemotherapy for psoriasis: a clinical cooperative study of PUVA-48 and PUVA-64. Arch Dermatol **115**:576, 1979.

28. Stern RS, Laird N, Melski J, et al: Cutaneous squamous cell carcinoma in patients treated with PUVA. N Engl J Med **310**:1156, 1984.

29. Baker H, Ryan TJ: Generalized pustular psoriasis: a clinical and epidemiological study of 104 cases. Br J Dermatol **80**:771, 1968.

30. Brubaker RF, Halpin JA: Open angle glaucoma associated with topical administration of flurandrenolide to the eye. Mayo Clin Proc **50**:320, 1975.

31. Chuang T-Y, Ilstrup DM, Perry HO, et al: Pityriasis rosea in Rochester, Minnesota, 1969 to 1978: a 10-year epidemiologic study. J Am Acad Dermatol **7**:80, 1982.

32. Baden HP, Provan J: Sunlight and pityriasis rosea. Arch Dermatol (letter) **113**:377, 1977.

33. Black MM: What is going on in lichen planus? Clin Exp Dermatol **2**:303, 1977.

34. Almeyda J, Levantine A: Lichenoid drug eruptions. Br J Dermatol **85**:604, 1971.

35. DeGraciansky P, Boulle S: Skin disease from color developers. Br J Dermatol **78**:297, 1966.

36. Grotty CP, Daniel SU WP, Winkelmann RK: Ulcerative lichen planus: follow-up of surgical excision and grafting. Arch Dermatol **116**:1252, 1980.

37. Ragas A, Ackerman AB: Evolution, maturation, and regression of lesions of lichen planus: new Observations and correlations of clinical and histologic findings. Am J Dermatopathol **3**:5, 1981.

38. Varelzidis A, Tosca A, Perissios A, et al: Immunohistochemistry in lichen planus. Dermatologica **159**:137, 1979.

39. Sehgal VH, Bikhchandani R, Koranne RV, et al: Histopathological evaluation of griseofulvin therapy in lichen planus: a double-blind controlled study. Dermatologica **161**:22, 1980.

40. Gonzalez E, Momtaz-T K, Freedman S: Bilateral comparison of generalized lichen planus treated with psoralens and ultraviolet A. J Am Acad Dermatol **10**:958, 1984.

41. Ferguson MM: Treatment of erosive lichen planus of the oral mucosa with depot steroids. Lancet **2**:771, 1977.

42. Sloberg K, Hersle K, Mobacken H, et al: Topical tretinoin therapy and oral lichen planus. Arch Dermatol **115**:716, 1979.

43. Sanchez NP, Mihm MC: Reactive and neoplastic epithelial alterations of the vulva: a classification of the vulvar dystrophies from the dermatopathologist's viewpoint. J Am Acad Dermatol **6**:378, 1982.

44. Wallace HJ: Lichen sclerosis et atrophicus. Trans St Johns Hosp Dermatol Soc **57**:9, 1971.

45. Friedrich EG Jr, Kalra PS: Serum levels of sex hormones in vulvar lichen sclerosus, and the effect of topical testosterone. N Engl J Med **310**:488, 1984.

Chapter Nine

Bacterial Infections

Impetigo

Impetigo is a common, contagious, superficial skin infection produced by streptococci, staphylococci, or a combination of both bacteria. It has a specific clinical presentation that differs from other cutaneous streptococcal or staphylococcal infections such as folliculitis and erysipelas. Children in close physical contact with each other have a higher rate of infection than do adults. Most cases appear in the late summer and early fall. Symptoms of itching and soreness are mild, and systemic symptoms are infrequent. Impetigo may occur after a minor skin injury such as an insect bite, but it most frequently develops on apparently unimpaired skin. The disease is self-limiting, but when untreated it may last for weeks or months. Poststreptococcal glomerulonephritis may follow impetigo. Rheumatic fever has not been reported as a complication.

Two patterns of infection, bullous and vesicular impetigo, have been described in the literature. Both begin as vesicles with a thin, fragile roof consisting only of stratum corneum.

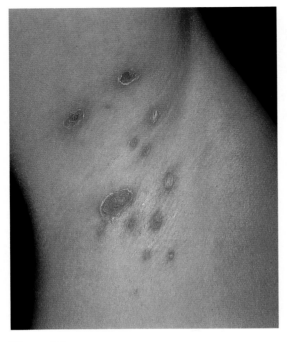

Figure 9-1
Bullous impetigo. Lesions are present in all
stages of development. Bullae rupture, exposing
a lesion with an eroded surface and peripheral
scale.

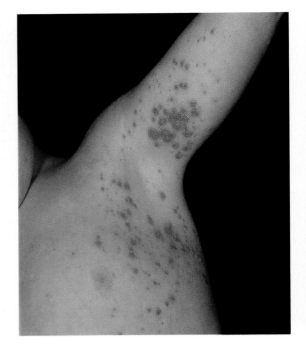

Figure 9-2
Bullous impetigo. The lesions initially were
present on the arm and autoinoculated the chest.

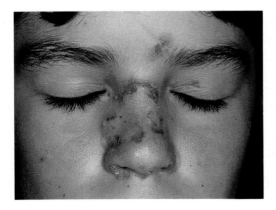

Figure 9-3
Bullous impetigo. Bullae have collapsed and
disappeared. The lesion is in the process of
peripheral extension. Note involvement of both
nares.

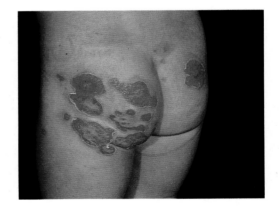

Figure 9-4
Bullous impetigo. Huge lesions with a glistening
eroded base and a collarette of moist scale.

Bullous impetigo

Bullous impetigo *(Staphylococcus aureus)* is most common in infants and children and typically occurs on the face, but it may infect any surface on the body. There may be a few lesions localized in one area, or the lesions may be so numerous and widely scattered that they resemble poison ivy. One vesicle or more enlarges rapidly to form bullae in which the contents turn from clear to cloudy. The center of the thin-roofed bullae collapses, but the peripheral area may retain fluid for many days in an innertube-shaped rim. A thin, flat, honey-colored crust appears in the center of the bulla and, if removed, discloses a bright red, inflamed, moist base that oozes serum. In most cases, a tinea-like scaling border replaces the fluid-filled rim as the round lesions enlarge and become contiguous with the others (Figures 9-1 to 9-5). In some untreated cases, lesions may extend radially and retain a narrow, bullous innertube-rim. These individual lesions may reach 2 to 8 cm and then cease to enlarge, but they may remain chronic for months (Figures 9-6 and 9-7). Thick crust accumulates in these longer-lasting lesions. Lesions heal with hyperpigmentation in black patients. Regional lymphadenitis is uncommon with pure staphylococcal impetigo. There is some evidence that the responsible staphylococci colonize in the nose and then spread to normal skin before infection.[1]

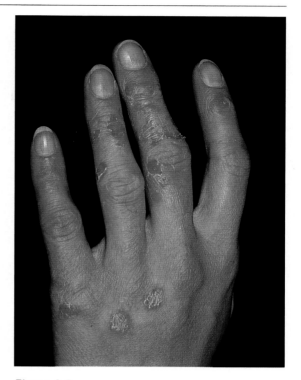

Figure 9-5
Bullous impetigo is occasionally seen on the hand and is often mistaken for eczema.

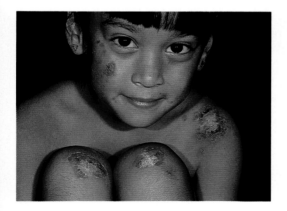

Figure 9-6
Impetigo. A bullous rim extended slowly for weeks. No topical or oral treatment had been attempted.

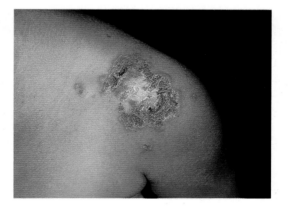

Figure 9-7
Bullous impetigo. The right shoulder of the patient in Figure 9-6. There is a bullous rim; a thick crust covers eroded and ulcerated surfaces. These lesions have features of both impetigo and ecthyma.

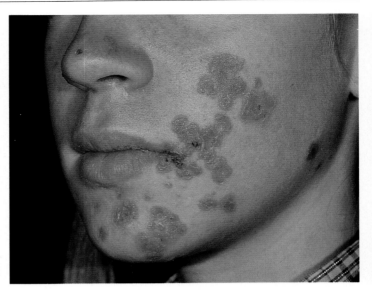

Figure 9-8
Vesicular impetigo. A thick, honey-yellow, adherent crust covers the entire eroded surface.

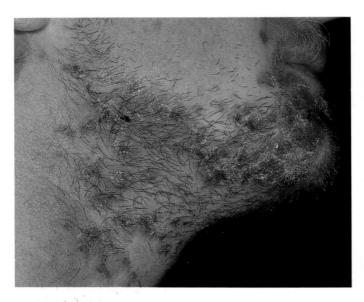

Figure 9-9
Impetigo. Shaving caused rapid dissemination of the infection throughout the beard area.

Vesicular impetigo

Vesicular impetigo (streptococci) originates as a small vesicle that ruptures to expose a red, moist base. A honey-yellow to white-brown firmly adherent crust accumulates as the lesion extends radially (Figures 9-8 and 9-9). Satellite lesions appear beyond the periphery. Untreated streptococcal impetigo lasts for weeks and may extend in a continuous manner to involve a wide area (Figure 9-10). Most cases heal without scarring. A pure culture of

streptococci may sometimes be isolated from beginning lesions, but most lesions promptly become contaminated with staphylococci. Regional lymphadenitis is common. The reservoirs for streptococcal infection include the unimpaired normal skin or the lesions of other individuals, rather than the respiratory tract.[2] The antistreptolysin O (ASO) titer does not rise to a significant level after impetigo,[3] although anti-DNase B rises to high levels after streptococcal impetigo.[4]

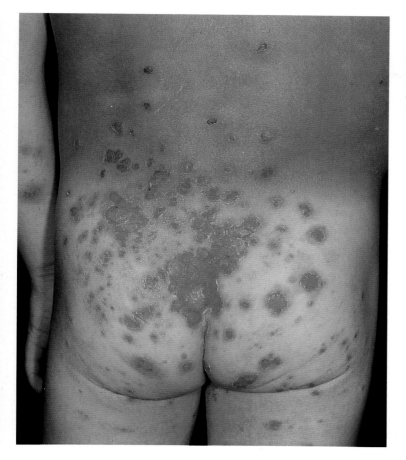

Figure 9-10
Impetigo. Widespread dissemination followed 3 weeks of treatment with a Group IV topical steroid.

Acute nephritis

Acute nephritis tends to occur when many individuals in a family have impetigo. Most cases occur in the southern part of the United States. Infants under 1½ years of age are rarely affected by nephritis following impetigo. The highest incidence of nephritis following impetigo is in children between 2 and 4 years of age.[5] Skin infection with a known strain of nephritogenic streptococci seldom results in acute nephritis in children over 6 years of age. This is in contrast to throat infection with nephritogenic strains, which cause acute nephritis in young adults as well as in children. The latent period between the acquisition of a nephritogenic streptococcus in skin lesions and the onset of acute nephritis varies between 1 and 5 weeks and averages 10 days.[6] The overall incidence of acute nephritis with impetigo varies between 2% and 5%, but, in the presence of a nephritogenic strain of streptococcus, the rate varies between 10% to 15%. During the initial streptococcal infection, hematuria and proteinuria may be found in approximately one-third of the patients. The urinary findings disappear for several days before development of poststreptococcal acute glomerulonephritis. The overall incidence and clinical features of acute nephritis[6] are as follows.

Hematuria occurs in 90%. Gross hematuria occurs in 25% followed by microscopic hematuria with erythrocyte casts and proteinuria that lasts for a variable time. Edema occurs in a majority of patients; the degree varies with the amount of dietary sodium. In the early morning, periorbital edema and lower extremity swelling are present. Hypertension occurs in 60%; adults have moderate elevation of blood pressure, in the range of 160/100 mm Hg; children are close to normal. Again, the degree of hypertension varies with dietary sodium. Cerebral symptoms (headache and disturbance of consciousness), congestive heart failure, and acute renal failure are less common.

Laboratory findings

After impetigo, ASO titer elevations are low or absent, but anti-DNase B and antihyaluronidase increase significantly. Total serum complement activity is low during initial stages of acute nephritis. The C3 level parallels the total serum complement. Sedimentation rate parallels the activity of the disease. C-reactive protein is usually normal. Cultures of the pharynx and any skin lesion should be made. The serotype of group A streptococcus responsible is determined by typing with M-group antisera. M serotypes associated with acute nephritis are 2, 49, 55, 57, and 60.[7]

Acute nephritis heals without therapeutic intervention. Symptoms and signs such as hypertension should be managed as they occur.

Treatment of impetigo

Impetigo may resolve spontaneously or become chronic and widespread. Some physicians use only local therapy such as mechanical debridement of crusts, washing with antibacterial soaps, and applying antibacterial creams. Local treatment does not treat noncontiguous evolving lesions. The oral or parenteral administration of antibiotics results in a higher and more predictable cure rate. Although the efficacy of systemic antibiotics in preventing acute nephritis has not been conclusively demonstrated, the possibility exists; this is additional justification for recommending systemic therapy.

Previously, penicillin had been recommended as the drug of choice; however, most laboratories report a high incidence of penicillin-resistant staphylococci. Since most cases of impetigo have a mixed infection of staphylococci and streptococci, penicillin is no longer the drug of choice. Unreliable patients in whom intramuscular benzathine penicillin may be used to eradicate the streptococci are an exception. A 10-day course of the appropriate oral dose of erythromycin, cloxacillin, dicloxacillin, or cephalexin will induce rapid healing.

If oral treatment must be avoided, then the following local measures are useful. Wash the involved area twice each day with an antibacterial soap such as Hibiclens or Betadine. Washing the entire body with these soaps may prevent recurrence at distant sites. Crusts should be removed inasmuch as they block the penetration of antibacterial creams. To facilitate removal, crusts are softened by soaking with a wet cloth compress. Then apply antibacterial topical preparations such as iodine ointment (Betadine) or combination ointments such as Neosporin (neomycin, bacitracin, and polymyxin B) directly on the lesions. Infected children should be briefly isolated until treatment is under way.

Ecthyma

Ecthyma has many features similar to impetigo. The lesions begin as vesicles and bullae. They then rupture to form an adherent crust which, when removed, exposes an ulcer rather than the erosion of impetigo (Figures 9-6 and 9-7). The lesion may remain fixed in size and resolve without treatment or it may extend slowly, forming indolent ulcers with very thick oyster shell–like crusts. This type of lesion occurs most commonly on the legs, where there are usually less than 10 lesions. Another more diffuse form occurs on the buttocks and legs of children who excoriate. Except for the thick crusts and underlying ulcers, the picture is almost identical to diffuse streptococcal impetigo. Lesions heal with scarring. Ecthyma is initiated by group A beta-hemolytic streptococci, but the lesions quickly become contaminated with staphylococci. Treat with a 10-day course of oral antibiotics such as dicloxacillin, erythromycin, or one of the cephalosporins such as cephalexin.

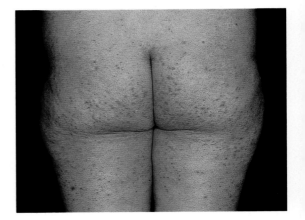

Figure 9-11
Superficial folliculitis after long periods of sitting in a tight garment.

TABLE 9-1

DISEASES PRESENTING AS FOLLICULITIS

Superficial folliculitis	Deep folliculitis
Staphylococcal folliculitis (Bockhart's impetigo)	Furuncle and carbuncle
Pseudofolliculitis barbae (from shaving)	Sycosis (inflammation of the entire depth of the follicle)
Superficial fungal infections (dermatophytes)	Sycosis (beard area): Sycosis barbae, bacterial or fungal
Cutaneous candidiasis (pustules also occur outside the hair follicle)	Sycosis (scalp): folliculitis decalvans, bacterial
Acne vulgaris	Acne vulgaris, cystic
Acne, mechanically or chemically induced	Gram-negative acne
Steroid acne after withdrawal of topical steroids	Pseudomonas folliculitis
Keratosis pilaris	Dermatophyte fungal infections

Folliculitis

Folliculitis is inflammation of the hair follicle caused by infection, chemical irritation, or physical injury. Inflammation may be superficial or deep in the hair follicle. Folliculitis is common and is seen as a component of a variety of inflammatory skin diseases (Table 9-1). In superficial folliculitis, the inflammation is confined to the upper part of the hair follicle, and is characterized by a painless or tender pustule that eventually heals without scarring (Figures 9-11 and 9-12). In many instances, the hair shaft in the center of the pustule cannot be appreciated. Inflammation of the entire follicle or the deeper portion of the hair follicle begins as a swollen red mass, which eventually may point at the surface as a somewhat larger pustule than that seen in superficial folliculitis (Figure 9-13). Deeper lesions are painful and may heal with scarring.

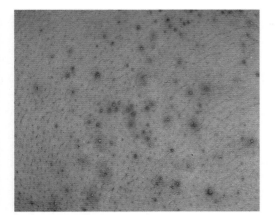

Figure 9-12
A closer view of the patient in Figure 9-11 showing tiny follicular pustules.

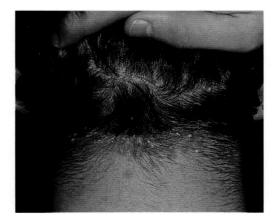

Figure 9-13
Deep folliculitis. Follicular pustules are surrounded by erythema and swelling. The entire follicular structure is inflamed. Staphylococci were isolated by culture.

Staphylococcal folliculitis

Staphylococcal folliculitis is the most common form of infectious folliculitis. One pustule or a group of pustules may appear, usually without fever or other systemic symptoms on any body surface. Infectious folliculitis that appears spontaneously is called Bockhart's impetigo (Figures 9-14 and 9-15). In this type, follicular pustules appear in crops on the face and limbs and resolve in 1 or 2 weeks. Bockhart's impetigo is not as infectious as vesicular or bullous impetigo. Staphylococcal folliculitis may be caused by injury, abrasion, or nearby surgical wounds or draining abscesses. It may also be a complication of occlusive topical steroid therapy (Figures 9-16 and 9-17), particularly if moist lesions are occluded for many hours. Follicular pustules are cultured, not by touching the pustule with a cotton swab, but by scraping off the entire pustule with a #15 blade and depositing the material on the cotton swab of a transport medium kit. Most cases can be treated with a Burow's tepid wet compress. Appropriate oral antibiotics are used for resistant cases.

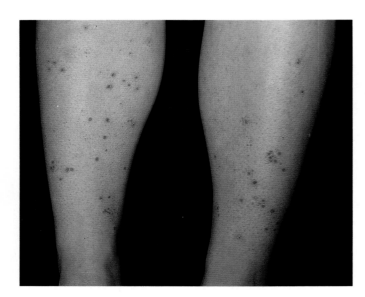

Figure 9-14
Bockhart's impetigo. Tiny follicular pustules evolve to round, superficially eroded lesions with the same appearance as vesicular impetigo.

Figure 9-15
Bockhart's impetigo. A closer view of the patient in Figure 9-14 illustrating the follicular location of the lesions.

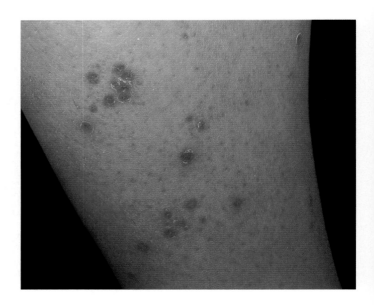

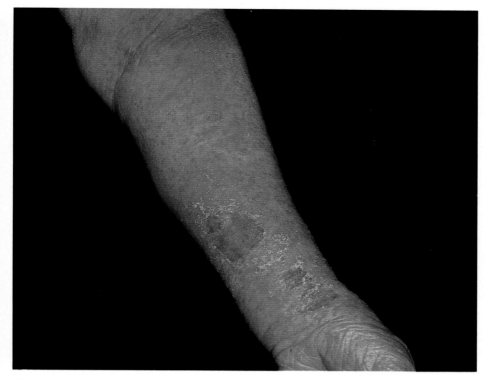

Figure 9-16
Staphylococcal folliculitis. Numerous pustules occurred hours after occlusion of a moist eczematous process with a Group V topical steroid and plastic dressing.

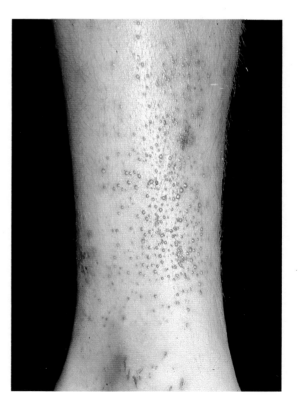

Figure 9-17
Staphylococcal folliculitis. Follicular pustules appeared after the patient's lower extremity had been occluded with a topical steroid and a plastic dressing for 24 hours. Gram-negative organisms may also flourish after long periods of plastic occlusion.

Pseudofolliculitis

Pseudofolliculitis is a foreign body reaction to hair; clinically, there is less inflammation than with staphylococcal folliculitis. The condition is most commonly seen on the neck of blacks with spiral hair. If cut below the surface by shaving, the sharp-tipped whisker may curve into the follicular wall or emerge and curve back to penetrate the skin. A tender red papule or pustule occurs at the point of entry and remains until the hair is removed. Normal bacterial flora may eventually be replaced by pathogenic organisms if the process becomes chronic. Pseudofolliculitis of the beard is a significant problem in the armed services (Figure 9-18).

This is a mechanical problem and must be treated as such. Each imbedded hair shaft must be dislodged by inserting a firm, pointed instrument such as a Hagedorn needle or the needle of a syringe under the hair loop and firmly elevating it. Shaving should be discontinued until all of the red papules have resolved. Shaving may then be resumed with a double-edge razor (Trac II), shaving only with the grain. Shaving closely with multiple razor strokes should be avoided. A foil-guarded shaver (brand name PFB)* is reported to result in a reduction in the number of lesions and minimizes trauma to existing lesions.[8] The best results are obtained when the PFB razor is used with Edge gel shaving cream. Specially designed electric razors (Remington's Black Man's Razor, Norelco's Black Man's Razor) may also be used. If these measures fail, shaving must be discontinued indefinitely.

Keratosis pilaris

Keratosis pilaris is a common finding on the posterolateral aspects of the upper arms and anterior thighs. The eruption is probably more common in patients with atopic dermatitis (see Chapter 5). Clinically, a group of small, pinpoint, follicular pustules remains in the same area for years. Histologic studies show that the inflammation actually occurs outside of the hair follicle. Scratching, tight-fitting clothing, or treating with abrasives may infect these sterile pustules. It is important to recognize this entity in order to avoid unnecessary treatment. Many patients object to these small sometimes unsightly bumps. The treatment of keratosis pilaris is described in Chapter 5.

*Disposable PFB razors ($19.80 per 2 dozen) may be ordered from Shenandoah Supply Co., PO Box 2097, Staunton, VA 24401. Telephone 703 885-1118.

Sycosis barbae

Sycosis implies follicular inflammation of the entire depth of the hair follicle and may be caused by infection with *Staphylococcus aureus* or dermatophyte fungi (see Chapter 11 for a discussion of fungal sycosis). This disease occurs only in men who shave, beginning with the appearance of small follicular papules or pustules and rapidly becoming more diffuse as shaving continues (Figure 9-19). Reaction to the disease varies greatly with the individual. Infiltration about the follicle may be slight or extensive. The more infiltrated cases heal with scarring. In chronic cases the pustules may remain confined to one area such as the upper lip or neck. The hairs are epilated with difficulty in staphylococcal sycosis and with relative ease in fungal sycosis. Hairs should be removed and examined for fungi, and the purulent material should be cultured. The now rare folliculitis decalvans is a more destructive and chronic form of sycosis found in the scalp and other hairy areas. This begins with pustules, becomes granulomatous, and heals with scarring alopecia.

Treatment consists of using appropriate oral antibiotics (e.g., erythromycin, dicloxacillin, cephalexin) for at least 2 weeks or until all signs of inflammation have cleared. Recurrences are not uncommon and require an additional course of oral antibiotics. Shaving should be performed with a thoroughly cleaned razor head until the eruption has cleared.

Figure 9-18 (opposite, top)
Pseudofolliculitis. Staphylococcal folliculitis is simulated when hair curves into and penetrates the skin, causing a foreign body–type reaction.

Figure 9-19 (opposite, bottom)
Sycosis barbae. Deep follicular pustules.

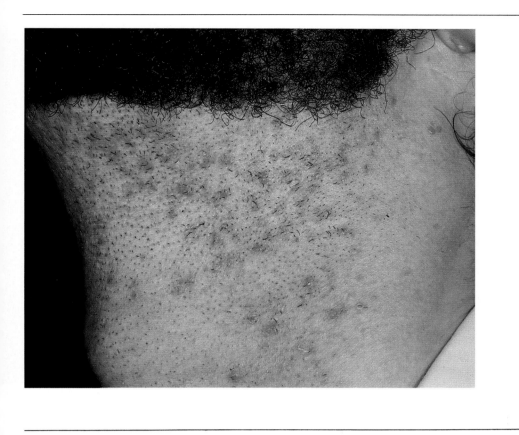

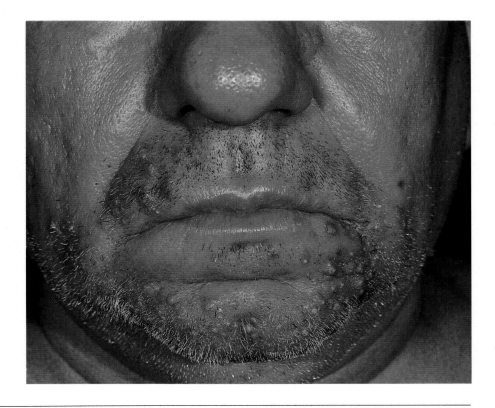

Cellulitis

Cellulitis is an infection of the dermis and subcutaneous tissue caused by a group A streptococcus and *Staphylococcus aureus;* it is rarely caused by other organisms, such as non-group A streptococcus, *Haemophilus influenzae* type B, or *Pseudomonas aeruginosa.* Cellulitis typically occurs near surgical wounds or a cutaneous ulcer or, like erysipelas, may develop in apparently normal skin.

Clinical manifestations

Streptococcal cellulitis. Streptococcal cellulitis is characterized by an expanding red, swollen, tender-to-painful plaque with an indefinite border that may cover a wide area (Figure 9-20). Chills and fever occur as acute cellulitis spreads rapidly, becomes edematous, and sometimes develops bullae or suppurates. Less acute forms detected around a stasis leg ulcer spread slowly and may appear as an area of erythema with no swelling or fever.

Red, sometimes painful streaks of lymphangitis may extend toward regional lymph nodes. As with erysipelas, repeated attacks of cellulitis can cause impairment of lymphatic drainage, which predisposes to more infection and permanent swelling. This series of events takes place most commonly in the lower legs of patients with venous stasis and ulceration. The end stage with dermal fibrosis, lymphedema, and epidermal thickening on the lower leg is called elephantiasis nostras.

Material for Gram stain and culture may be obtained from needle aspiration of the border region. Treatment should be started immediately and, if appropriate, altered according to laboratory results.

***Haemophilus influenzae* type B cellulitis.** *Haemophilus influenzae* type B (HIb) cellulitis should be suspected when an infant develops high fever and a mildly painful, salmon pink to purplish blue indurated plaque on one cheek that, unlike erysipelas, is poorly demarcated. One extensive study[9] provides the following information: Fever is present in 92% of patients, and unilateral or bilateral otitis media is present in 68%. The organism may be cultured from blood (86%), cerebrospinal fluid (7.5%), middle ear fluid (96%), and lesion aspirate fluid (51%). Meningitis was present in 7.6% of the infants, which in some was asymptomatic and required lumbar puncture for demonstration. Therefore lumbar puncture should be obtained in all patients. *H influenzae* cellulitis occurring about the umbilicus was diagnosed in an adult whose son was being treated for an ear infection.[10] A blood culture was positive for HIb.

Pseudomonas cellulitis. Pseudomonas cellulitis is described in the section on pseudomonas infection.

Treatment. A penicillinase-resistant penicillin, erythromycin, or cephalosporin is effective for staphylococcal or streptococcal cellulitis. Patients with recurrent disease may be treated with prophylactic doses of antibiotics (e.g., penicillin, 250 to 500 mg of phenoxymethyl penicillin) for months or years. Pain can be relieved with cool, wet Burow's compresses. To provide coverage against beta lactamase–producing strains of HIb, initial antimicrobial therapy should be with ampicillin and chloramphenicol. One of the drugs may be discontinued after the susceptibility of the offending organism is known. Cephamandole should not be used unless meningitis has been excluded.

Tinea pedis and recurrent cellulitis after saphenous venectomy

Recurrent cellulitis of the leg has been reported to occur after saphenous venectomy for coronary artery bypass grafting.[11,12] The patients develop acute onset of fever, erythema, and swelling of the leg. The disease resembles streptococcal cellulitis. Tinea pedis has been observed on the foot of the infected leg. The fungal infection may be an important factor in the pathogenesis of the cellulitis. Breaks in the dermal barrier due to fungal infection may permit entry of bacteria through the skin. The cellulitis responded initially to intravenous antibiotics followed by additional oral therapy. The fungal infection is treated topically or systemically as outlined in Chapter 11.

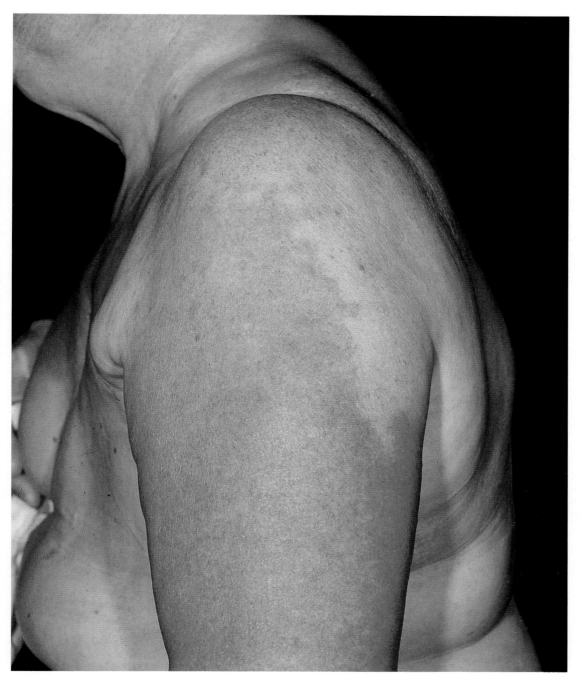

Figure 9-20
Cellulitis. Infected area is tender, deep red, and swollen.

Erysipelas

The archaic term "St. Anthony's Fire" accurately describes the intensity of this eruption. Erysipelas is an acute, inflammatory, superficial skin infection caused most frequently by group A streptococci. Erysipelas may originate in a traumatic or surgical wound, but no portal of entry can be found in most cases. The lower legs, face, and ears are most frequently involved. In the pre-antibiotic era, erysipelas was a feared disease with a significant mortality rate, particularly in infants. Most contemporary cases are of moderate intensity and have a benign course.

Clinical manifestations. After prodromal symptoms ranging from 4 to 48 hours and consisting of malaise, chills, and fever (101° to 104° F) and occasionally anorexia and vomiting, there appears at the site of infection one or more red, tender, firm spots. These spots rapidly increase in size, forming a tense, red, hot, uniformly elevated shining patch with an irregular outline and a sharply defined, raised border (Figure 9-21). As the process develops, the color becomes a dark firey red, and vesicles may appear at the advancing border and over the surface. Symptoms of itching, burning, tenderness, and pain may be moderate to severe. Without treatment, the rash reaches its height in approximately 1 week and subsides slowly over the next 1 to 2 weeks.

In some particularly susceptible people, erysipelas may recur frequently for a long period of time and, by obstruction of the lymphatics, cause permanent thickening of the skin (lymphedema).[13] Subsequent attacks may be initiated by the slightest trauma or occur spontaneously to cause further irreversible skin thickening. The pinna and lower legs are particularly susceptible to this recurrent pattern (Figure 9-22). Erysipelas is more superficial and demarcated from normal skin than cellulitis.

Treatment. Treatment is the same as for streptococcal cellulitis. Recurrent cases may require long-term prophylactic treatment with low-dose penicillin.

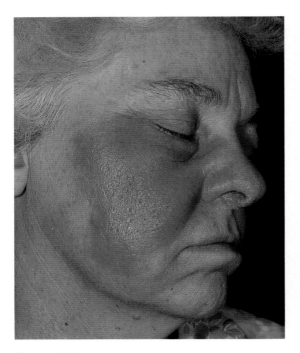

Figure 9-21
Erysipelas. Streptococcal cellulitis. The acute phase with intense erythema.

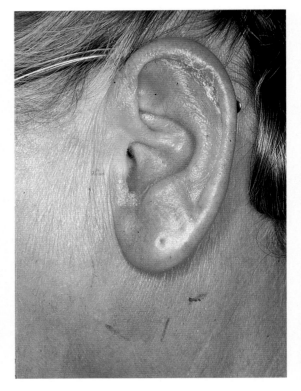

Figure 9-22
Erysipelas. Recurrent episodes of infection have resulted in lymphatic obstruction and caused permanent thickening of the skin.

Furuncles and Carbuncles

A furuncle, or boil, is an acute infection of a hair follicle; therefore, it does not occur on hairless areas such as the palms and soles. They may occur at any other site, particularly in areas prone to friction or minor trauma, such as underneath a belt or on the anterior thighs. Furuncles are uncommon in children but increase in frequency after puberty. *Staphylococcus aureus* is the most common pathogen. The infecting strain may be found during quiescent periods in the nares and perineum. There is evidence that the anterior nares is the primary site from which the staphylococcus is disseminated to the skin. Substituting a nonpathogenic strain of staphylococcus in the anterior nares has proven successful for treatment of recurrent staphylococcal furunculosis.

Furunculosis occurs as a self-limited infection in which one or several lesions are present or as a chronic, recurrent disease lasting for months or years and affecting one or several family members. Most patients with sporadic or recurrent furunculosis appear to be otherwise normal and have an intact immune system.

One disease in which an immune defect has been found to predispose to recurrent furunculosis is the hyperimmunoglobulinemia E–staphylococcal abscess syndrome, in which large abscesses with little erythema or inflammation ("cold abscess") appear in young girls with an atopic-like dermatitis, eosinophilia, elevated IgE, and a profound defect in neutrophil granulocyte chemotaxis. Diabetic patients probably do not have a predisposition to furunculosis or other cutaneous infections.

Clinical manifestations. The lesion begins as a deep, tender, firm, red, 1- to 5-cm nodule that becomes fluctuant in a few days (Figure 9-23). The temperature is normal and no systemic symptoms are present. Pain becomes moderate to severe as purulent material accumulates and is most intense in areas where expansion is restricted, such as the neck and external auditory canal. The abscess either remains deep and reabsorbs or points and ruptures through the surface. The abscess cavity contains a surprisingly large quantity of pus and white chunks of necrotic tissue. The point of rupture heals with scarring.

Carbuncles are aggregates of infected follicles. The infection originates deep in the dermis and the subcutaneous tissue and forms a broad, red, swollen, slowly evolving, deep, painful mass that points and drains through multiple openings. Malaise, chills, and fever precede or occur during the active phase. Deep extension into the subcutaneous tissue may be followed by sloughing and extensive scarring. Areas with thick dermis (i.e., the back of the neck, the back of the trunk and the lateral aspects of the thighs) are the preferred sites. In the pre-antibiotic era, some fatalities occurred.

Treatment

Warm compresses. Many furuncles are self-limited and will respond well to frequent applications of a moist, warm compress, which provides comfort and probably encourages localization and pointing of the abscess.

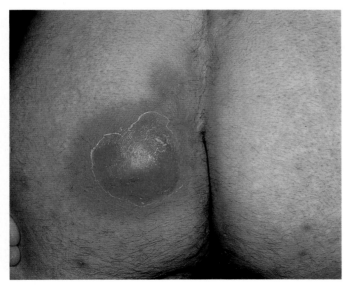

Figure 9-23
Furuncle (boil). Enlarged swollen mass with purulent material beginning to exude from several points on the surface.

Incision, drainage, and packing. The primary management of cutaneous abscesses should be incision and drainage. In general, routine culture and antibiotic therapy are not indicated for localized abscesses in patients with presumably normal host defenses.[14] The abscess is not ready for drainage until the skin has thinned and the underlying mass becomes soft and fluctuant. The skin around the central area is anesthetized with 1% Xylocaine. A #11 pointed, lance-shaped surgical blade is inserted and drawn through the thin effaced skin, following skin lines and creating an opening from which pus may easily be expressed with light pressure. Care must be taken to avoid extending the incision into firm noneffaced skin. A curette is inserted through the opening and carefully drawn back and forth to break adhesions and dislodge fragments of necrotic tissue. Continuous drainage may be promoted by packing the larger cavities with a long ribbon of iodoform gauze. The end of the ribbon is inserted through a curette loop. The curette is then turned to secure the gauze, inserted deep into the cavity, twisted in the reverse direction, and removed concurrently while supporting the gauze in place with a thin-tipped forceps. Next, the gauze is worked into the cavity with the forceps until resistance is met. The gauze quickly becomes saturated and should be removed hours later and replaced with a fresh packing.

Antibiotics. Patients with recurrent furunculosis learn that they can sometimes stop the progression of an abscess by starting antistaphylococcal antibiotics at the first sign of the typical localized swelling and erythema; they continue to use antibiotics for 5 to 10 days. Antibiotics should be started immediately in order to attenuate the evolving abscess. Antibiotics have little effect once the abscess has become fluctuant.

Management of recurrent furunculosis

A few patients have repeated episodes of furuncles that last for months and years. Several members of a family may be affected. Most of these patients are normal with an intact immune system. The problem seems to be related to chronic carriage of a particular strain of staphylococci in the nares and on the skin. Therapy goals are to decrease or eliminate the pathogenic strain. In the most difficult cases, implanting a less aggressive strain may prevent recurrence. There are two programs to be considered. The first involves suppression of staphylococci[15] on the skin and nares and the second involves suppression and replacement with a nonpathogenic strain (502A bacterial interference).[16]

Suppression of pathogenic staphylococci. Culture the organism and determine sensitivity. Begin therapeutic doses of appropriate antibiotics, initially for 21 days; if that fails, begin another course to last for 1 to 3 months.

Wash the entire body and the fingernails with a nailbrush each day for 1 to 3 weeks with Betadine, Hibiclens, or pHisoHex soap. The frequency of washing should be decreased if the skin becomes dry.

After showering, bacitracin ointment is applied to both anterior nares with a cotton swab. The following sanitary practices should be stressed: towels, washcloths, and sheets should be changed daily; wound dressings should be changed frequently; shaving instruments must be thoroughly cleaned each day; and nose picking must be avoided.

502A bacterial interference. Using the method of Russell W. Steele, MD,[17] culture the nose and any active lesion on the patient to document resistant staphylococcal strains. Culture other family members if spread of the disease in the family has been previously noted.

The patient and infected household members are given dicloxacillin, 250 mg 4 times a day. Infants and children are given proportionately smaller doses (50 mg/kg/day divided into 4 doses). The patient and family are then advised to shower twice daily with pHisoHex or Dial soap. After showering, bacitracin ointment is applied with a cotton swab to both anterior naries. Treatment is continued for 7 to 10 days. All treatment (topical and oral) is then discontinued for 48 hours.

Two days after medication is stopped, the anterior nasal mucosa is inoculated with *Staphylococcus aureus* 502A.* The stock bacteria comes freeze-dried in a glass vial and is reconstituted by adding trypticase soy broth to the vial. This material is prepared by streaking a trypticase soy agar plate with stock slant of 502A. After 48 hours of growth on the inoculated plate, a single yellow-pigmented colony is selected and inoculated into 10 to 20 ml of trypticase soy broth. This is grown overnight at 35° to 37° C and is subsequently used to colonize the anterior naries of the patient and family.

For inoculation, the patient's head is tilted back and the anterior naries are swabbed with this culture while the patient sniffs the material back into the naries and the nasopharynx. Two soaked cotton swabs of culture material are applied to each naries during a treatment session.

Follow-up clinical data is obtained 1 month later from the family and the process is repeated only if control of subcutaneous abscesses has not been achieved.

*Ordered by hospital laboratory from the American Type Culture Collection, 12301 Parklawn Dr., Rockville, MD 20852; phone 301-881-2600; cost is approximately $50 per vial.

Staphylococcal Scalded Skin Syndrome

Staphylococcal scalded skin syndrome (SSSS) is also known as Ritter's disease. Three clinical entities (SSSS, staphylococcal scarlatiniform eruption, and bullous impetigo) are caused by an epidermolytic toxin elaborated by *S aureus,* phage group II including types 55, 71, 3A, 3B, and 3C.[18] Two antigenically distinct forms of epidermolytic toxin (ET A and ET B) have been identified.[19] The toxin is antigenic and when elaborated elicits an antibody response. Epidermolytic toxin antibody is present in 75% of normal people over the age of 10 years, a fact that may explain the rarity of SSSS in adults.

SSSS is most often seen in infants and begins with a localized, often inapparent, *S aureus* infection of the conjunctivae, throat, nares, or umbilicus. The disease begins with diffuse, tender erythema; the skin has a sandpaper-like texture similar to that seen in scarlet fever. However, the rash of scarlet fever is not tender. The temperature rises and within 1 or 2 days the skin wrinkles, forms transient bullae, and peels off in large sheets leaving a moist, red, glistening surface (Figure 9-24). Minor pressure induces skin separation (Nikolsky's sign). The area of involvement may be localized but is often generalized. Evaporative fluid loss from large areas is associated with increased fluid loss and dehydration. A yellow crust forms and the denuded surface dries and cracks. Healing occurs in 7 to 10 days, accompanied by desquamation similar to that seen in scarlet fever.

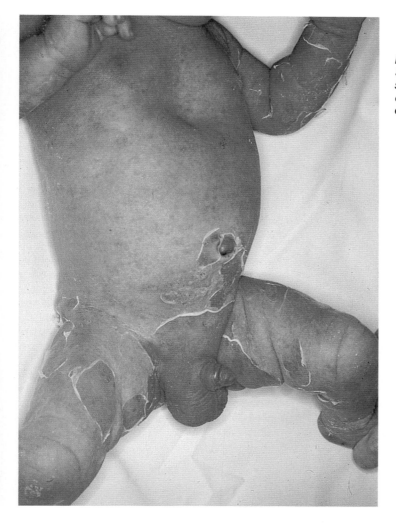

Figure 9-24
Staphylococcal scalded skin syndrome. Exfoliative phase, during which time the upper epidermis is shed.

Staphylococcal scarlatiniform eruption is similar to SSSS, except that the skin does not blister or peel.

Diagnosis. In SSSS, splitting of the epidermis occurs high in the epidermis in the stratum granulosum; inflammation is scant. Thin-roofed bullae are flaccid and rupture easily. Toxic epidermal necrolysis is a rare syndrome, usually seen in adults, which is caused by drugs or a viral infection. The clinical appearance is similar to SSSS, but biopsy shows separation at the dermo-epidermal junction and an intense inflammatory infiltrate. Cultures should be taken from the eye, nose, throat, bullae, and any obviously infected area. Cultures of the skin are often negative.

Treatment. Corticosteroids are contraindicated because they interfere with host defense mechanisms.[20] Hospitalization and intravenous antibiotic therapy is desirable for extensive cases. Patients with limited disease may be managed at home with oral antibiotics. Most of the toxin-producing S aureus produces penicillinase; therefore, drugs such as methicillin should be administered. Topical antibiotics are not necessary. The patient's skin should be lubricated with bland light lotions such as Keri and washed infrequently. Wet dressing may cause further drying and cracking.

Pseudomonas Aeruginosa Infection

Pseudomonas aeruginosa is a gram-negative aerobic bacillus found in the normal skin and intestinal flora of relatively few individuals. The bacteria may colonize warm, moist areas such as skin folds (toe webs), ear canals, burns, ulcers, and areas beneath nails. It is also found in the moist areas of sinks and drains and in poorly preserved topical creams and ointments. Certain strains of *P aeruginosa* produce the blue-green pigment pyocyanin or a yellow-green pigment pyoverdin (fluorescein) that can be demonstrated with a Wood's light. The green color may be evident both clinically and in cultures. An organic metabolite may impart a fruity odor to some cutaneous lesions. *Pseudomonas* survives poorly in an acid environment. There are many serotypes. Occasionally, other species such as *P putrefaciens* are of clinical significance.

Pseudomonas folliculitis

From 8 to 72 hours after using a contaminated whirlpool or home hot tub, 53% to 82% of those exposed will develop pseudomonas folliculitis.[21] Showering after using the contaminated facility offers no protection. The typical patient has a few to more than fifty 0.5- to 3-cm pruritic, round, urticarial plaques with a central papule or pustule located on all skin surfaces except the head, but the areas most often infected are those primarily covered by bathing suits (Figures 9-25 and 9-26). The eruption, in most cases, clears in 7 to 10 days, leaving round spots of red-brown postinflammatory hyperpigmentation.[22] Malaise and fatigue may occur during the initial few days of the eruption. Patients have been reported to have recurrent crops of lesions for as many as 3 months. *P aeruginosa* serotype 0-11 was implicated in most reports, possibly implying that this subgroup is particularly adapted for survival in hot, chlorinated water. Risk of infection increases according to time spent in the whirlpool, the number of people using the pool (increased organic carbon debris from sloughed keratin) and duration of time between chlorination. The risk of infection decreases when the water is changed frequently and the chlorine level is kept well above the recommended concentration for the facility.[23]

Treatment. The infection is self-limited, but a 2.5% acetic acid wet compress applied for 20 minutes twice daily or gentamicin cream (Garamycin) applied 3 times a day may hasten resolution. Vinegar is 5% acetic acid.

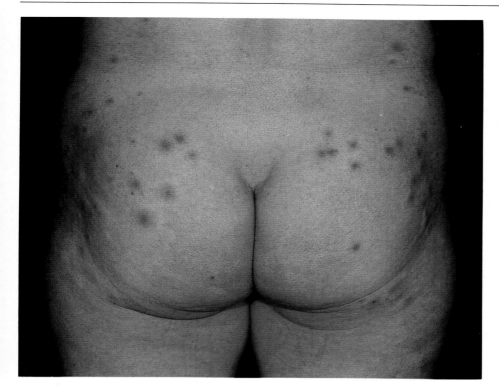

Figure 9-25
Pseudomonas folliculitis. Urticarial plaques surmounted by pustules located primarily in the areas covered by the bathing suit.

Figure 9-26
Pseudomonas folliculitis. Round, red 0.5 cm urticarial plaques surmounted by a centrally located papule or pustule. These lesions are larger than those seen with staphylococcal folliculitis.

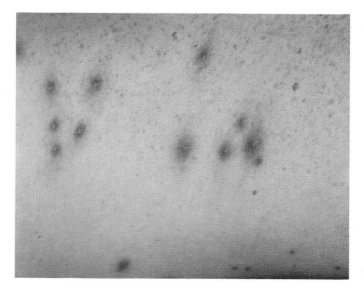

Pseudomonas cellulitis

Pseudomonas cellulitis may be a localized phenomenon or it may occur during pseudomonas septicemia. The localized form occurs as a secondary infection of tinea of the toe webs or groin (Figure 9-27), bed sores, stasis ulcers, burns, or grafted areas. Maceration or occlusion of these cutaneous lesions predisposes to secondary infection with *Pseudomonas*. Suppression of normal bacterial flora by broad-spectrum antibiotics encourage secondary infection. The skin becomes painful and turns a dusky red (Figure 9-27). Bluish-green purulent material with a grape-juice or "mousey" odor accumulates as the red indurated area becomes macerated and then eroded. Vesicles and pustules may occur as satellite lesions. The eruption may spread to cover wide areas and be accompanied by systemic symptoms. Pseudomonas septicemia may produce a deep, indurated, necrotic cellulitis that resembles other forms of infectious cellulitis.

Treatment. Treatment consists of 2.5% acetic acid (vinegar is 5%) wet compresses applied for 20 minutes 4 times a day.

External otitis

External otitis is an inflammation of the external auditory canal. It occurs in a mild self-limited form (swimmer's ear) or as an acute and chronic recurrent debilitating disease. The normally acidic cerumen inhibits Gram-negative bacterial growth and forms a protective layer that discourages maceration. Swimming or excessive manipulation while cleaning the canal may disrupt this natural barrier. Inflammatory diseases such as psoriasis, seborrheic dermatitis, and eczematous dermatitis disrupt the normal barrier and predispose to infection. *Pseudomonas* is the most common bacteria isolated from both mild and severe external otitis.[24] Most cases, however, represent a mixed infection with other gram-negative (*Proteus mirabilis, Klebsiella pneumoniae*) and gram-positive (*Staphylococcus epidermidis,* beta hemolytic streptococcus) bacteria. Fungal infection with candida or *Aspergillus niger* sometimes occurs and may be the primary pathogens.[25]

Figure 9-27
Pseudomonas cellulitis. Inflamed area has a "mousey" or grape juice-like odor.

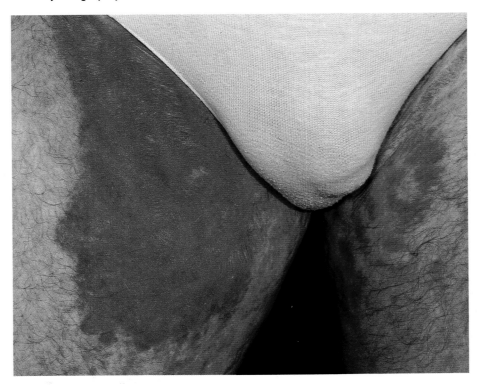

The early stages are characterized by erythema, edema, and an accumulation of moist cellular debris in the canal. Traction on the pinna or tragus may elicit pain. If the disease progresses, erythema radiates into the pinna and purulent material partly obstructs the exudes from the canal. Pain becomes constant and more intense. Cellulitis of the pinna and skin surrounding the ear accompanied by a dense mucopurulent exudate exuding from the canal may result from infection with pseudomonas (Figure 9-28). However, in most cases, this indicates secondary infection with staphylococci and streptococci. The lymphatics of the external ear may be permanently damaged during an attack of cellulitis, predisposing to recurrent episodes of streptococcal erysipelas of the pinna. Recurrent attacks are brought on by manipulation or the slightest trauma.

Eczematous inflammation and infection of the external ear and surrounding skin, referred to by some as infectious eczematoid dermatitis, may occur for a variety of reasons, such as irritation from purulent exudate, scratching and manipulation, or allergy to topical medications.

Treatment. The external auditory canal is cleansed. Squamous debris, cerumen, and pus are removed by suction or irrigation with an ear syringe.

Acidification is accomplished with 2% acetic acid (VōSol Otic Solution or Otic Domeboro Solution) or 2% acetic acid with 1% hydrocortisone (VōSol HC Otic Solution). Instill 5 drops in the canal 4 times a day. Acidification creates an environment that is inhospitable to gram-negative bacteria and fungi.

Topical antibiotics should be considered if canal inflammation does not resolve in less than 1 week. A culture of canal drainage is obtained. Antibiotic otic solutions such as Cortisporin Otic Suspension (polymyxin B-neomycin-hydrocortisone) or Coly-Mycin S Otic (colistin sulfate-neomycin-hydrocortisone) are instilled into the canal several times each day until the infection has resolved.

Ear wicks are made of strands of cotton or fine cloth and are inserted into the canal to act as a conduit for applications of otic solutions. If properly saturated, they will keep medication in contact with all surfaces of the canal. Solution must be added almost hourly to maintain saturation. New wicks are inserted daily. The use of a wick is usually unnecessary for mild inflammation, but this procedure may be considered when the canal is partially obstructed by swelling and edema.

Topical steroids, wet compresses, and oral antibiotics are used when eczematous inflammation and infection occur on the external ear and surrounding skin (see Chapter 3 for discussion of the treatment of eczematous inflammation).

Toe web infection

A thick, white, macerated scale with a green discoloration may appear in the toe webs of people who wear heavy wet boots. Wood's light examination reveals a greenish fluorescence. *Pseudomonas* or a mixed flora of *Pseudomonas* and fungi may be isolated from the soggy scale. The webs are treated with applications of Castellani Paint 3 times a day, followed by various measures to promote dryness of the feet.

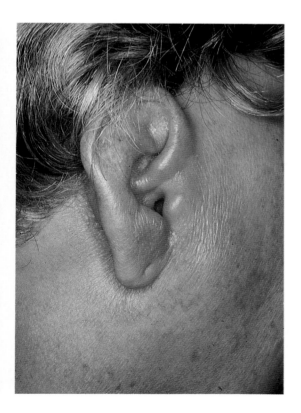

Figure 9-28
Pseudomonas cellulitis. The entire pinna and surrounding skin have become inflamed after an episode of external otitis.

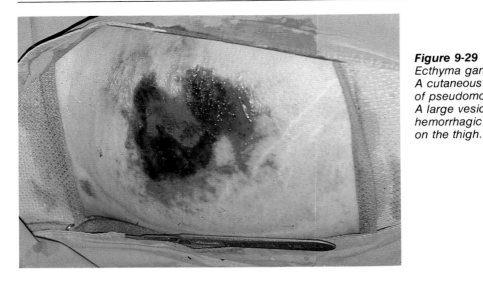

Figure 9-29
*Ecthyma gangrenosum.
A cutaneous manifestation
of pseudomonas septicemia.
A large vesicular bullous
hemorrhagic mass is located
on the thigh.*

Ecthyma gangrenosum

Ecthyma gangrenosum, not to be confused with pyoderma gangrenosum or streptococcal ecthyma, is a rare but highly characteristic entity that is pathognomonic of pseudomonas septicemia. There are usually less than 10 lesions; these occur most commonly on the legs and buttocks.[26] They begin as isolated, red, purpuric macules, vesicles, or bullae that may remain localized or, more typically, extend over several centimeters, the central area becoming hemorrhagic and necrotic (Figure 9-29). Ulcers are treated with acetic acid or silver nitrate wet compresses while appropriate measures are taken to treat the septicemia.

Pitted Keratolysis

Pitted keratolysis is an asymptomatic eruption of the weight-bearing surfaces of the soles. It is characterized by many circular or longitudinal punched-out depressions in the skin surface (Figures 9-30 and 9-31). The eruption is limited to the stratum corneum and causes little or no inflammation. Hyperhidrosis, moist socks, or immersion of the feet favors its development. There may be a few circular pits that remain unnoticed, or the entire weight-bearing surface may be covered with annular furrows. Several bacteria have been implicated, including *Dermatophilus congolensis* and species of corynebacterium and streptomyces.[27] These organisms are not easily cultured, but the filamentous and coccoid microorganisms can be demonstrated by hematoxylin and eosin staining of a formalin-fixed section of shaved stratum corneum prepared for histopathology. The clinical presentation is so characteristic that laboratory confirmation is usually not necessary.

Treatment. Treatment consists of promoting dryness. Socks should be changed frequently. Rapid clearing occurs with twice daily application of 20% aluminum chloride (hexahydrate), commercially available as Drysol. For resistant cases, apply Drysol to the feet at bedtime and cover with a plastic bag. The bag is removed each morning, and the feet, if dry, are lubricated with a light lotion such as Neutraderm. This is repeated every evening until the condition clears. Treatment can then be employed periodically when necessary. Application twice a day of alcohol-based benzoyl peroxide (PanOxyl 5), topical erythromycin (A/T/S, Staticin), or Benzamycin may also be useful.

Figure 9-30
Pitted keratolysis. Deep longitudinal furrows are located primarily on weight-bearing surfaces.

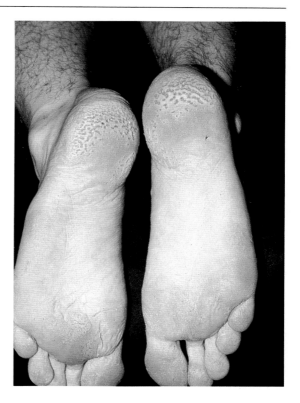

Figure 9-31
Pitted keratolysis. The skin around the deep pits is often wet and macerated.

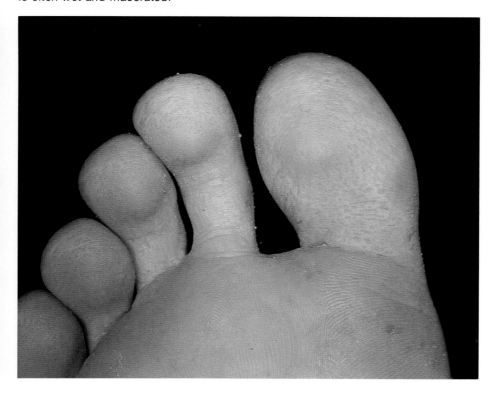

Trichomycosis Axillaris

Trichomycosis axillaris is an asymptomatic infection of axillary hairs caused by a corynebacterium. The hair shaft becomes coated with adherent yellow (occasionally red or black), firm concretions (Figure 9-32). Hyperhidrosis is often present. The hair should be shaved and hyperhidrosis controlled with antiperspirants.

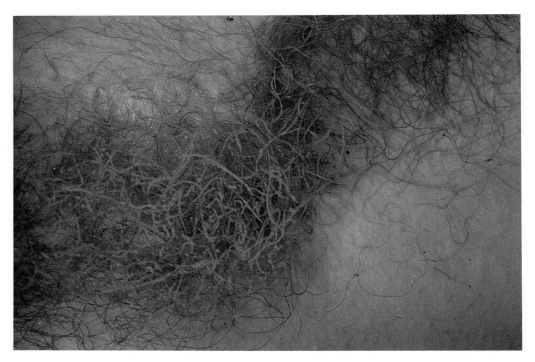

Figure 9-32
Trichomycosis axillaris. Yellow concretions are adherent to the axillary hair. These concretions are composed of a mass of diphtheroid organisms and not fungi.

REFERENCES

1. Miles AA, William REO, Clayton-Cooper B: Carriage of Staphylococcus aureus (pyogenes) in man and its relation to wound infections. J Pathol Bacteriol **56:**513, 1944.
2. Peter G, Smith AL: Group A streptococcal infections of the skin and pharynx. N Engl J Med **297:**311, 1977.
3. Bisno AL, Nelson KE, Waytz P, et al: Factors influencing serum antibody response in streptococcal pyoderma. J Lab Clin Med **81:**410, 1973.
4. Kaplan, EL, Anthony BF, Chapman SS, et al: The influence of the site of infection in the immune response to group A streptococci. J Clin Invest **49:**1405, 1970.
5. Fison TN: Acute glomerulonephritis in infancy. Arch Dis Child **31:**101, 1956.
6. Fine RN: Clinical manifestations and diagnosis of post-streptococcal acute glomerulonephritis—post streptococcal acute glomerulonephritis: fact and controversy. Ann Intern Med **91:**76, 1979.
7. Dillon HC: Streptococcal infection of the skin and their complications: impetigo and nephritis. In Streptococci and streptococcal diseases: Recognition, understanding and management. New York, 1972, Academic Press.
8. Alexander AM: Evaluation of a foil-guarded shaver in the management of pseudo folliculitis barbae. Cutis **27:** May 1981.
9. Ginsburg CM: Hemophilus influenzae type B buccal cellulitis. J Am Acad Dermatol **4:**661, 1981.
10. Shaw RA, Plouffe JF: Haemophilus influenzae cellulitis in an adult. Arch Intern Med **139:**368, 1979.
11. Greenberg J, De Sanctis RW, Mills RM: Vein-donor-leg cellulitis after coronary artery bypass surgery. Ann Intern Med **97:**565, 1982.
12. Baddour LM, Bisno AL: Recurrent cellulitis after saphenous venectomy for coronary bypass surgery. Ann Intern Med **97:**493, 1982.
13. Maibach HI, Hacker P: Bacterial infections of the skin. In Dermatology. Philadelphia, 1975, W.B. Saunders Co.
14. Meislin HW, Lerner SA, Graves MH, et al: Cutaneous abscesses: anaerobic and aerobic bacteriology and outpatient management. Ann Intern Med **87:**145, 1977.
15. Arndt KA: Manual of dermatologic therapeutics. Second edition. Boston, 1978, Little, Brown and Company.
16. Steele RW: Recurrent staphylococcal infection in families. Arch Dermatol **116:**189, 1980.
17. Steele RW: Immunology for the practicing physician. Norwalk, Conn, 1983, Appleton-Century-Crofts, pp 72-73.
18. Melish ME: Staphylococci, streptococci and the skin. Semin Dermatol **1:**101, 1982.
19. Elias PM, Fritsch P, Epstein EH: Staphylococcal scalded skin syndrome. Arch Dermatol **113:**207, 1977.
20. Rudolph RI, Schwartz W, Leyden JJ: Treatment of staphylococcal toxic epidermal necrolysis. Arch Dermatol **110:**559, 1974.
21. Sausker WF, Aeling JL, Fitzpatrick JE, et al: Pseudomonas folliculitis acquired from a health spa whirlpool. JAMA **239:**2362, 1978.
22. Zacherle BJ, Silver DS: Hot tub folliculitis. Arch Intern Med **142:**1620, 1982.
23. Khabbaz RF, McKinley TW, Goodman RA, et al: Pseudomonas aeruginosa serotype 0.9: new cause of whirlpool-associated dermatitis. Am J Med **74:**73, 1983.
24. Gardiner LJ, Sasaki CT: Acute external otitis (swimmer's ear). Dermatology July, 1981, p. 25.
25. Haley LD: Etiology of otomycology. Arch Otolaryng **52:**202, 1952.
26. Hall JH, Callaway JL, Tindall JP, et al: *Pseudomonas aeruginosa* in dermatology. Arch Dermatol **97:**312, 1968.
27. Young CN: Pitted keratolysis. Trans St. Johns Hosp Dermatol Soc **60:**77, 1974.

Chapter Ten

Sexually Transmitted Bacterial Infections

Gonorrhea

Gonorrhea is a common sexually transmitted disease. The responsible organism, *Neisseria gonorrhoeae,* can survive only in a moist environment approximating body temperature and is transmitted only by sexual contact (genital, genital-oral, or genital-rectal) with an infected person. It is not transmitted through toilet seats or the like. Purulent burning urethritis in males and asymptomatic endocervicitis in females are the most common forms of the disease, but gonorrhea is also found at other sites. All forms of the disease have the potential for evolving into a bacteremic phase, producing the arthritis-dermatitis syndrome. From an epidemiologic point of view the disease is becoming more difficult to control because of the increasing number of asymptomatic male carriers. All forms of the disease previously responded to penicillin, but resistant strains have emerged.

N gonorrhoeae is a gram-negative cocci found in pairs (diplococci) within polymorphonuclear leukocytes in purulent material. The bacterium is an obligate aerobe that grows best in an atmosphere of 5% to 10% CO_2. A modified Thayer-Martin medium (chocolate agar) incubated in a candle jar to elevate CO_2 levels provides optimal conditions for isolation.

N gonorrhoeae is differentiated from nonpathogenic strains such as *N meningitidis,* which may be normal flora in the pharynx, by colony morphology and sugar fermentation patterns. Specificity about the source of the culture is necessary so that the laboratory will perform all the tests necessary for differentiation from normal flora.

N gonorrhoeae is a fragile organism that survives only in humans and quickly dies if all of its environmental requirements are not met. The organism can survive only in blood and on simple epithelium such as that found in the urethra, endocervix, rectum, pharynx, and prepubertal vaginal tract. It does not survive on the stratified epithelium of the skin and postpubertal vaginal tract. The bacteria must be kept moist with isotonic body fluids and will die if not maintained close to body temperature. A slightly alkaline medium is required, such as that found in the endocervix and in the vagina during the immediate premenstrual and menstrual phases. The antibodies produced during the disease offer little protection from future attacks but can be measured with some newly developed tests. A fluorescent antibody test identifies the organism in tissue specimens such as in the skin in disseminated gonococcal infection (arthritis-dermatitis syndrome).

Genital infection in males

After a 3- to 5-day incubation period, most infected men have sudden onset of burning, frequent urination, and a yellow, thick, purulent urethral discharge (Figure 10-1). Some men do not develop symptoms for 5 to 14 days and then complain only of mild dysuria with a mucoid urethral discharge as observed in nongonococcal urethritis. Some men, 5% to 50%, never develop symptoms and become carriers for months, acting, as do asymptomatic women, as major contributors to the ongoing gonorrhea epidemic.[1,2] Infection may spread to the prostate, seminal vesicles, and epididymis, but presently these complications are uncommon because most symptomatic men are treated.

Diagnosis. The diagnosis can be confirmed without culture in men with a typical history of acute urethritis by finding in urethral exudate gram-negative intracellular diplococci within polymorphonuclear leukocytes. Urethral culture is indicated when the Gram stain is negative, in tests of cure, or as a test for asymptomatic urethral infection. Material for culture is obtained by inserting a bacteriologic wire loop or a sterile calcium alginate swab approximately 2 cm into the anterior urethra. No attempt should be made to insert the larger cotton-tipped swabs contained in standard culture kits.

Figure 10-1
Gonorrhea. Yellow, thick, purulent urethral discharge appears 3 to 5 days after exposure to an infected individual.

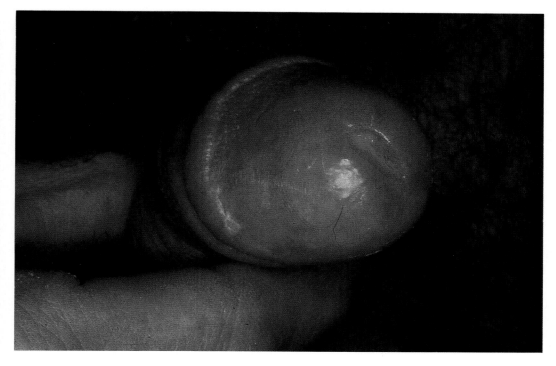

Genital infection in females

Female genital gonorrhea has traditionally been described as an asymptomatic disease, but symptoms of urethritis and endocervicitis may be elicited from 40% to 60% of the women.[3] Urethritis begins with urinary frequency and dysuria after a 3- to 5-day incubation. These symptoms are of variable intensity. Pus may be seen exuding from the red external urinary meatus or after "milking" the urethra with a finger in the vagina.

Endocervical infection may present with a nonspecific pale yellow vaginal discharge, but in many cases this is not detected or is accepted as being a normal variation. The cervix may appear normal or it may show marked inflammatory changes with cervical erosions and pus exuding from the os.

Skene's glands, which lie on either side of the urinary meatus, exude pus if infected.

Bartholin's ducts, which open on the inner surfaces of the labia minora at the junction of their middle and posterior thirds near the vaginal opening, may, if infected, show a drop of pus at the gland orifice. After occlusion of the infected duct, the patient complains of swelling and discomfort while walking or sitting. A swollen, painful Bartholin's gland may be palpated as a swollen mass deep in the posterior half of the labia majora.

Salpingitis. Salpingitis or pelvic inflammatory disease (PID) occurs in approximately 2% to 17% of women with gonorrhea.[4] In two-thirds of the cases the onset occurs during or directly after menstruation. The disease may be acute, subacute, or chronic.

- Acute PID: Symptoms of acute PID are diffuse low abdominal pain concentrated in the iliac fossae with elevated temperature, white blood cell count, and sedimentation rate.
- Subacute PID: Symptoms of subacute PID are diffuse, poorly localized abdominal pain or aching in the groin or lower back with normal or slightly elevated temperature varying in time and intensity.
- Chronic PID: Chronic PID has no abdominal symptoms but is possibly associated with sterility or disturbances of menstruation.

Lower abdominal pain intensified by moving the cervix from side to side during manual examination is a characteristic sign. Etiologic agents include *N gonorrhoeae, Chlamydia trachomatis,* anaerobic bacteria (including *Bacteroides* and gram-positive cocci), facultative gram-negative rods such as *E coli, Actinomyces israelii,* and *Mycoplasma hominis.*[5-7] In the individual patient it is often impossible to differentiate among these agents. The presence of an intrauterine contraceptive device may predispose to tubal infection. If gonorrhea is not suspected, the diagnosis may not be made until laparotomy for suspected appendicitis. Previously inflamed fallopian tubes predispose to sterility and ectopic pregnancy.

Diagnosis

Gram stain. The diagnosis of acute urethritis can be made with a high degree of certainty if gram-negative intracellular diplococci are found in the purulent exudate from the urethra. Fifty percent of the cases of endocervical gonorrhea can be diagnosed by a carefully interpreted gram-stained smear of the endocervical canal.[8] *Neisseria* species (e.g., *N catarrhalis* and *N sicca*) inhabit the female genital tract; thus the diagnosis is considered only if gram-negative diplococci are present within polymorphonuclear leukocytes.

Culture is the most reliable technique for establishing the presence of endocervical infection. However, the diagnosis will be missed in 10% of cases if reliance is exclusively on culture.[8] An endocervical culture is taken by initially localizing the cervix with a water-moistened nonlubricated speculum. Excess cervical mucus is most easily removed with a cotton ball held in a ring forceps. A sterile cotton-tipped swab is inserted into the endocervical canal, moved from side to side, and allowed to remain in place for 10 to 30 seconds before inoculating onto appropriate media. A culture of the anal canal need only be performed if there are anal symptoms, a history of rectal sexual exposure, or followup of treated gonorrhea in women.

Rectal gonorrhea

Rectal gonorrhea is acquired by rectal intercourse. Women with genital gonorrhea may also acquire rectal gonorrhea from contamination of the anorectal mucosa by infectious vaginal discharge. A history of rectal intercourse is the most important clue to the diagnosis, since the symptoms and signs of rectal gonorrhea are, in most cases, relatively nonspecific.[9,10] Anoscopic examination of homosexual men reveals generalized exudate in 54% of culture-positive patients and 37% of culture-negative patients.[11] Many infected patients have normal-appearing rectal mucosae. These figures emphasize what is generally observed: the specificity of the most common signs and symptoms of rectal gonorrhea is low. Some patients do report pain on defecation, blood in the stools, pus on undergarments, or intense discomfort while walking.

Diagnosis. Anal culture should be considered for symptomatic male homosexuals and symptomatic females who have engaged in rectal intercourse. Gonococcal proctitis does not involve segments of bowel beyond the rectum. The area of infection is about 2.5 cm within the anal canal in the pectinate lining of the crypts of Morgagni. To obtain culture material, an anoscope is unnecessary. Insert a sterile cotton-tipped swab approximately 2.5 cm into the anal canal. (If the swab is inadvertently pushed into feces, use another swab to obtain specimen.) Move the swab from side to side in the anal canal to sample crypts; allow 10 to 30 seconds for absorption of organisms onto the swab.

Gram stain is unreliable because of the presence of numerous other bacteria.

Gonococcal pharyngitis

Gonococcal pharyngitis is acquired by penile-oral exposure and rarely by cunnilingus or kissing. Possibility of infection is increased when the penis is inserted deep into the posterior pharynx as practiced by most homosexuals. The majority of cases are asymptomatic, and the gonococcus can be carried for months in the pharynx without being detected.[12] In those having symptoms, complaints range from mild sore throat to severe pharyngitis with diffuse erythema and exudates.[13]

Diagnosis. Culture is most productive if exudates are present. *N meningitidis* is a normal inhabitant of the pharynx; consequently, sugar utilization tests are necessary on *Neisseria* species isolated from the pharynx to determine accurately if infectious organisms are present.

Gram stain is useful only if exudate is present and must, therefore, be interpreted with caution to avoid confusion with other *Neisseria* species.

Disseminated gonococcal infection (arthritis-dermatitis syndrome)

Two percent of all recognized cases of gonorrhea disseminate from any of the previously described primary sites. Patients may be infected with a specific organism that tends to produce an asymptomatic infection, is highly sensitive to penicillin, and additionally is more likely to disseminate.[14] There is

no evidence that dissemination is more likely from the pharynx. Dissemination was formerly much more common in women, but presently men and women in some areas are affected equally. The risk of systemic infection increases during second and third trimester of pregnancy and during menstruation. The disease may evolve through three phases.

In the bacteremic phase symptoms include chills and fever for a few days accompanied by pain, redness, and swelling of three to six small joints without effusion. This occurs usually in the hands and wrists, with pain in the tendons of the wrist and fingers.[15] Chills and fever terminate as the rash appears on the extensor surfaces of the hands and dorsal surfaces of the ankles and toes. The total number of lesions is usually less than ten. The skin lesions begin as tiny red papules or petechiae that either disappear or evolve through a vesicular (Figure 10-2) and pustular stage, developing a gray necrotic and then hemorrhagic center (Figure 10-3). The central hemorrhagic area is the embolic focus of the gonococcus. These lesions heal in a few weeks.

The quiescent stage may be nonexistent or it may last for 2 to 3 weeks.

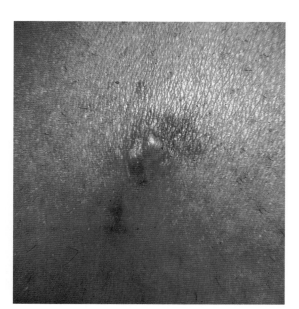

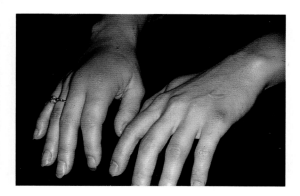

Figure 10-2
Gonococcal septicemia. There is erythema and swelling of the joints on the right hand. A single vesicle is present on the left hand.

Figure 10-3
Gonococcal septicemia. A more advanced lesion than that shown in Figure 10-2. The base has become hemorrhagic and necrotic.

In the septic joint phase, usually one or two large joints are affected, most frequently the knee and ankle. The affected joint is hot, painful, and swollen and movement is restricted. Permanent joint changes may occur.

Reiter's syndrome (urethritis, arthritis, conjunctivitis, and keratodermia blennorrhagica, a psoriasis-like eruption) may be confused with disseminated gonorrhea. The arthritis of Reiter's syndrome, however, may be chronic and recurrent and does not respond to antibiotic therapy.

Other less common complications of dissemination include endocarditis, myocarditis, and meningitis.

Diagnosis. Gram stain of the skin lesions is performed on the pus obtained by unroofing the pustule. Blood cultures are usually positive only during the first few days of the bacteremic phase, and the rate of isolation is low. Multiple samples should be grown in trypticase soy broth. Mucosal surfaces of the urethra, endocervix, pharynx, and anus should be cultured. The diagnosis of septic arthritis is supported by finding an elevated leukocyte count, poor mucin clot, and elevated protein in the aspirated joint fluid. Less than 50% of joint cultures are positive for N gonorrhoeae.[16] Fluorescent antibody testing (not available in every laboratory) may be performed on joint exudate and smears from skin lesions if the diagnosis is suspected, but identification has not been made by other means.

Treatment of gonococcal infection*
Uncomplicated infection in adults: recommended regimens†

Tetracycline hydrochloride: 500 mg by mouth 4 times a day for 7 days (total dose 14 gm). Other tetracyclines are not more effective than tetracycline HCl. All tetracyclines are ineffective as a single-dose therapy. Doxycycline hyclate 100 mg by mouth twice a day for 7 days may be substituted for tetracycline.

Advantages	Disadvantages
1. Effective against co-existing chlamydial infections	1. Requires compliance with multiple doses
	2. May encourage the emergence of tetracycline-resistant strains if the regimen is not strictly followed
	3. Ineffective against ano-rectal gonococcal infections in men
	4. Ten percent failure rate in women[17]

OR

Amoxicillin/ampicillin: Amoxicillin (3 gm) or ampicillin (3.5 gm) with 1 gm probenecid by mouth.

Advantages	Disadvantages
1. Single-dose treatment	1. Ineffective against chlamydial infections
	2. Ineffective against ano-rectal and pharyngeal gonococcal infections

OR

Aqueous procaine penicillin G: 4.8 million units injected intramuscularly at two sites with 1 gm probenecid by mouth.

Advantages	Disadvantages
1. Single-dose therapy	1. Injection
	2. Possible procaine reaction
	3. Possible penicillin anaphylaxis
	4. Ineffective against chlamydia infections

Special note. Tetracycline or aqueous procaine penicillin G (APPG) is the preferred therapy for pharyngeal gonococcal infection. Pharyngeal infection is not effectively treated by either the amoxicillin or ampicillin regimens.

A homosexual man with uncomplicated gonococcal infection should be treated with aqueous procaine penicillin G (4.8 million units) plus 1 gm of probenecid. If he is allergic to penicillin, use spectinomycin (2 gm IM in one injection). Both these regimens provide adequate treatment for urethral and anorectal gonococcal infection. However, spectinomycin is ineffective in the treatment of pharyngeal gonococcal infection.

Other considerations. Patients other than homosexual men who are allergic to penicillins or probenecid should be treated with oral tetracycline or doxycycline as described above. Penicillin-allergic patients who cannot tolerate tetracyclines can be treated with spectinomycin HCl (2 gm IM in one injection).

Patients with incubating syphilis (seronegative without clinical signs of syphilis) are likely to be cured by all the above regimens except spectinomycin. All patients treated for gonorrhea should have a serologic test for syphilis.

Patients with gonorrhea who also have syphilis or are established contacts of syphilis patients should be given additional treatment appropriate to the stage of syphilis.

Treatment of sexual partners. Men and women exposed to gonorrhea should be examined, cultured, and treated at once with one of the regimens described above.

Followup. Followup cultures should be obtained from the infected sites 4 to 7 days after completion of treatment. In addition, cultures should be ob-

*From Center for Disease Control: Morbidity and Mortality Weekly Report Supplement **31**(25), Aug 20, 1982.
†The order of presentation does not indicate preference.

tained from the rectum of all women who have been treated for gonorrhea.

Treatment failures. The patient in whom gonorrhea persists after treatment with one of the non-spectinomycin regimens described above should be treated with 2 gm of spectinomycin IM. Recurrent gonococcal infections after treatment with the recommended schedules may result from reinfection and indicate a need for improved contact tracing and patient education. Since penicillinase-producing *Neisseria gonorrhoeae* (PPNG) infection is a cause of treatment failure, posttreatment isolates should be tested for penicillinase production.

Drugs not recommended. Although long-acting forms of penicillin (such as benzathine penicillin G) are effective in the treatment of syphilis, they have no place in the treatment of gonorrhea. Oral penicillin preparations such as penicillin V are not recommended for the treatment of gonococcal infection.

Penicillinase-producing *Neisseria gonorrhoeae*

Patients with proven PPNG infection or those who are likely to have acquired gonorrhea in areas of high PPNG prevalence and their sexual partners should receive spectinomycin (2 gm IM in a single injection). Tetracycline may be added to treat co-existent chlamydial infection.[17] Patients with positive cultures after spectinomycin therapy should be treated with cefoxitin (2 gm IM in a single injection) plus probenecid (1 gm by mouth); *or* cefotaxime (1.0 gm IM in a single injection) without probenecid. A daily single dose of nine tablets of trimethoprim/sulfamethoxazole (80 mg/400 mg) for 5 days should be used to treat pharyngeal gonococal infection resulting from PPGN. Spectinomycin and cefoxitin are ineffective in pharyngeal infection.

Gonococcal infections in pregnancy

All pregnant women should have endocervical cultures for gonococci as an integral part of the prenatal care at the first visit. A second culture late in the third trimester should be obtained from women at high risk for gonococcal infection.

Drug regimens of choice are amoxicillin or ampicillin, each with probenecid as described above. Women who are allergic to penicillin or probenecid should be treated with spectinomycin (2.0 gm IM). Erythromycin in the dosage recommended under chlamydial infection can be added to treat coexistent chlamydial infection.[17]

Disseminated gonococcal infection

Treatment schedules. Hospitalization is usually indicated, especially for those who cannot reliably comply with treatment, have uncertain diagnosis, or who have purulent joint effusions or other complications.

There are several, acceptable treatment schedules for the gonococcal arthritis-dermatitis syndrome.

Aqueous crystalline penicillin G: 10 million units IV per day until improvement occurs, followed by amoxicillin 500 mg or ampicillin 500 mg by mouth 4 times a day to complete at least 7 days of antibiotic treatment

OR

Amoxicillin/ampicillin: amoxicillin 3 gm or ampicillin 3.5 gm by mouth, each with probenecid 1 gm followed by amoxicillin 500 mg or ampicillin 500 mg by mouth 4 times a day for at least 7 days.

OR

Tetracycline HCl: 500 mg by mouth 4 times a day for at least 7 days. Tetracycline HCl should not be used for complicated gonococcal infection in pregnant women.

OR

Cefoxitin/cefotaxime: either give cefoxitin 1 gm or cefotaxime 500 mg 4 times a day IV for at least 7 days (treatment of choice for disseminated infections caused by PPGN)

OR

Erythromycin: 500 mg by mouth 4 times a day for at least 7 days.

Special considerations. Open drainage of joints other than the hips is not indicated. Inraarticular injection of antibiotics is unnecessary.

Meningitis and endocarditis

Meningitis and endocarditis caused by the gonococcus require high-dose intravenous penicillin therapy. Optimal duration of therapy is unknown, but most authorities treat patients for 1 month. Therapy of penicillin-allergic patients must be individualized.

Acute PID

Treatment regimens active against the broadest range of pathogens should be used for endometritis, salpingitis, parametritis, and peritonitis.

Hospitalization and inpatient treatment. Many experts recommend that all patients with PID be hospitalized for treatment.

Rationale for selection of antimicrobials. The treatment of choice is not established. No single agent is active against the entire spectrum of pathogens. Several antimicrobial combinations do provide a broad spectrum of activity against the major pathogens in vitro, but many have not been adequately evaluated for clinical efficacy in PID. Following are some examples of combination regimens that have broad activity against major pathogens in PID.

Regimen 1

Doxycycline: 100 mg IV twice a day.

PLUS

Cefoxitin: 2.0 gm IV four times a day.

Continue drugs IV for at least 4 days and for at least 48 hours after patient defervesces. Continue doxycycline 100 mg by mouth twice a day after discharge from the hospital to complete 10 to 14 days of therapy.

Comment. This regimen provides optimal coverage for *N gonorrhoeae,* including PPNG and *C trachomatis.* It may not provide optimal treatment for anaerobes, pelvic mass, or PID associated with an intrauterine device.

Regimen 2

Clindamycin: 600 mg IV 4 times a day.

PLUS

Gentamicin or tobramycin: 2 mg/kg IV followed by 1.5 mg/kg IV 3 times a day in patients with normal renal function.

Continue drugs intravenously for at least 4 days and for at least 48 hours after the patient defervesces. Continue clindamycin 450 mg by mouth 4 times a day after discharge from the hospital to complete 10 to 14 days of therapy.

Comment. This regimen provides optimal activity against anaerobes and facultative gram-negative rods but may not provide optimal activity against *C trachomatis* and *N gonorrhoeae.*

Regimen 3

Doxycycline: 100 mg IV twice a day.

PLUS

Metronidazole: 1 gm IV twice a day.

Continue intravenous drugs for at least 4 days and at least 48 hours after the patient defervesces. Then continue both drugs at same dosage orally to complete 10 to 14 days of therapy.

Comment. This regimen provides excellent coverage for anaerobes and *C trachomatis.* Both drugs can be continued for oral therapy. Activity against some strains of *N gonorrhoeae,* including PPNG, and some facultative gram-negative rods is not optimal.

Ambulatory treatment. When the patient is not hospitalized, one of the following combination regimens is recommended.

Cefoxitin: 2 gm IM; *or* amoxicillin: 3 gm by mouth; *or* ampicillin; 3.5 gm by mouth; *or* aqueous procaine penicillin G: 4.8 million units IM at two sites; each along with probenecid 1 gm by mouth.

FOLLOWED BY

Doxycycline: 100 mg by mouth twice a day for 10 to 14 days.

Tetracycline HCl 500 mg by mouth 4 times a day can also be used, but is less active against certain anaerobes and requires more frequent dosing; both represent drawbacks in treatment of PID.

Comment. Cefoxitin or an equivalently effective cephalosporin plus doxycycline (or tetracycline) is active against *N gonorrhoeae,* including PPNG, and *C trachomatis.* PPNG-associated PID is not adequately treated with the combination of either amoxicillin, ampicillin, or aqueous procaine penicillin plus doxycycline.

Management of sexual partners. All persons who are sexual partners of patients with PID should be examined and treated promptly with a regimen effective against uncomplicated gonococcal and chlamydial infection.

Followup. All patients treated as outpatients should be clinically reevaluated in 48 to 72 hours. Those not responding favorably should be hospitalized. For test of cure, a culture should be done to determine whether pathogens initially isolated remain.

Intrauterine device. The IUD is a risk factor for the development of PID. Although the exact effect of removing an IUD on the response of acute salpingitis to antimicrobial therapy and on the risk of recurrent salpingitis is unknown, removal of the IUD is recommended soon after antimicrobial therapy has been initiated. When an IUD is removed, contraceptive counseling is necessary.

Nongonococcal Urethritis (NGU)

Nongonococcal urethritis (nonspecific urethritis) and cervicitis are the most common sexually transmitted diseases in the United States. The diagnosis, as the name implies, is one of exclusion, since routine diagnostic tests for identifying the number of possible infecting organisms are not as yet available. The obligate intracellular bacteria *Chlamydia trachomatis* causes 40% to 50% of all cases of NGU. *Ureaplasma urealyticum* (formerly called T-strain mycoplasma) may be responsible for a large percentage of the cases of NGU, although this has not been proved.

In many cases a source of infection cannot be identified. Epidemiologic control is difficult because, as is characteristic of gonorrhea, many of those infected have no symptoms. Previously, *C trachomatis* infections were considered self-limited because most patients became asymptomatic in a few months without treatment. Chlamydial organisms have the ability to exist in the host for years in a latent or subclinical form, and it is possible that the individual remains infectious after overt symptoms have resolved.[18]

NGU in males. In males urethritis begins with dysuria and urethral discharge. Gonococcal urethritis occurs 3 to 5 days after sexual contact and produces a burning, yellow, thick to mucopurulent ure-

TABLE 10-1

COMPARISON OF NONGONOCOCCAL AND GONOCOCCAL URETHRITIS

	Nongonococcal urethritis	Gonococcal urethritis
Incubation period	7-28 days	3-5 days
Onset	Gradual	Abrupt
Dysuria	Smarting feeling	Burning
Discharge	Mucoid or purulent	Purulent
Gram stain of discharge	Polymorphonuclear leukocytes	Gram-negative intracellular diplococci

thral discharge. NGU begins 7 to 28 days after sexual contact with a smarting sensation while urinating and a mucoid discharge. Table 10-1 compares the two forms of urethritis. C trachomatis causes at least two-thirds of the acute "idiopathic" epididymitis in sexually active men under the age of 35.[19]

NGU in females. The signs and symptoms in females are even more nonspecific. Nongonococcal cervicitis is asymptomatic or begins as a mucopurulent endocervical exudate[20] or as a mucoid vaginal discharge. There is no proof that chlamydiae cause cervical erosions, but cervical erosions may provide more sites for replication of chlamydiae, which apparently cannot infect squamous cells of the vagina or the intact outer or peripheral surfaces of the cervix. C trachomatis has been implicated as a cause of nongonococcal pelvic inflammatory disease and Reiter's syndrome.

Nongonococcal urethritis may be symptomatic or asymptomatic with varying degrees of dysuria and urinary urgency and frequency. C trachomatis is the most common cause of acute urethral syndrome (dysuria and pyuria without conventional bacterial urinary tract infection) in sexually active women.

Diagnosis. The diagnosis is made by confirming the presence of urethritis and excluding gonococcal infection. First, make a Gram stain of the urethral discharge. The presence of polymorphonuclear leukocytes confirms the diagnosis of urethritis, and the absence of gram-negative intracellular diplococci suggests that urethritis is nongonococcal. Material for the Gram stain is most effectively obtained at least 4 hours after urination. For those patients with urethral symptoms, but without a discharge, polymorphonuclear leukocytes may be demonstrated from material obtained by a sterile calcium alginate swab inserted about 2 cm beyond the urethral meatus.

Secondly, culture urethral discharge for N gonorrhoeae. Cultures for C trachomatis are presently available at some hospitals. C trachomatis must be isolated in tissue culture rather than on a conventional bacterial agar plate. If possible, cultures should be obtained from sexual contacts of men with NGU and from pregnant women who might transmit the organism to the fetus during birth, causing neonatal conjunctivitis.

Treatment. The tetracyclines are the treatment of choice. Tetracycline may cause abdominal symptoms, and minocycline may cause dizziness or ataxia. Erythromycin is used during pregnancy or for those patients who cannot tolerate tetracycline. Erythromycin is used to treat patients who have persistent symptoms of NGU after being treated with one of the tetracyclines. Persistent disease may indicate the presence of a tetracycline-resistant Ureaplasma urealyticum organism.

Penicillin, ampicillin, cephalosporins, aminoglycosides, and metronidazole are ineffective. Sulfamethoxazole trimethoprim will eradicate C trachomatis but not U urealyticum.

Treatment regimens include the following:

Tetracycline: 500 mg orally 4 times a day for 7 days.[21]

Minocycline or doxycycline: 100 mg orally every 12 hours for 7 days.[22]

Erythromycin succinate, stearate, or base: 500 mg orally 4 times a day for 7 days.

Management of sexual partners. All persons who are sexual partners of patients with NGU should be examined and promptly treated with one of the above regimens.

Followup. Patients should be advised to return if symptoms persist or recur.

Persistent or recurrent NGU. Recurrent NGU may result from failure to treat sexual partners. Patients with persistent or recurrent objective signs of urethritis after adequate treatment of the patient and partners warrant further evaluation for less common causes of urethritis.

Syphilis

Syphilis is a human infectious disease caused by the bacteria *Treponema pallidum.* The disease is transmitted by direct contact with a lesion during the primary or secondary stage, in utero by the transplacental route, or during delivery as the baby passes through an infected canal. Like the gonococcus, this bacterium is fragile and dies when removed from the human environment. Unlike the gonococcus, *T pallidum* may infect any organ, causing an infinite number of possible clinical presentations; thus the old adage, "he who knows syphilis knows medicine."

Untreated syphilis may pass through three stages, beginning with infectious cutaneous primary and secondary stages, which may terminate without further sequel or evolve into a latent stage lasting for months or years before the now-rare tertiary stage. Tertiary syphilis is marked by the appearance of cardiovascular, neurologic, and deep cutaneous complications. Syphilis is more common in those who have sexual contact with numerous persons, such as prostitutes and homosexuals.

T pallidum, the organism responsible for syphilis, is a very small spiral bacteria (spirochete) whose form and corkscrew rotation motility can be observed only by dark field microscopy (Figure 10-4). The Gram stain cannot be used, and the bacteria have never been cultured.

Primary syphilis

Primary syphilis, characterized by a cutaneous ulcer, is acquired by direct contact with an infectious lesion of the skin or the moist surface of the mouth, anus, or vagina. From 10 to 90 days (average 21 days) after exposure a primary lesion, the chancre, develops at the site of initial contact. Chancres are usually solitary, but multiple lesions are not uncommon. The lesion begins as a papule that erodes, forming an 0.3- to 2-cm, painless-to-tender, indolent ulcer with a clean nonpurulent base (Figure 10-5). The rim of the ulcer is smooth, regular, sharply defined, and elevated. The entire lesion is indurated. Painless, firm regional lymphadenopathy occurs 1 to 2 weeks after the onset of the chancre in most patients. Without treatment the chancre heals with scarring in 3 to 6 weeks. Painless vaginal and anal lesions may never be detected (Figures 10-6 and 10-7). The differential diagnosis includes ulcerative genital lesions such as chancroid, herpes progenitalis, aphthae (Behcet's syndrome), and traumatic ulcers such as those that occur with biting (Table 10-2).

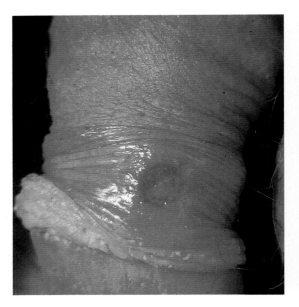

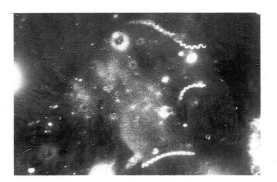

Figure 10-4
Treponema pallidum. *The organism responsible for syphilis is seen here photographed through a dark-field microscope. (Courtesy Centers for Disease Control, Atlanta, Ga.)*

Figure 10-5
Primary syphilis. A syphilitic chancre is an ulcer with a clean nonpurulent base and a smooth regular sharply defined border.

TABLE 10-2   DIFFERENTIAL DIAGNOSIS AND TREATMENT OF GENITAL ULCERATIONS

Disease	Chancroid	Granuloma inguinale	Lymphogranuloma venereum (LGV)	Primary syphilis	Herpes simplex
Etiology	*Hemophilus ducreyi*	*Calymmatobacterium (Donovania) granulomatis*	*Chlamydia*	*Treponema pallidum*	*Herpesvirus hominis*
Incubation period	12 hours to 3 days	3-6 weeks	3 days to several weeks	3 weeks	3-10 days
Initial lesion	Single or multiple, round to oval, deep ulcers with irregular outlines, ragged and undermined borders and a purulent base; lesions are tender	Soft, nontender papule(s) that forms irregular ulcer with beefy-red, friable base and raised, "rolled" border	Evanescent ulcer (rarely seen)	Nontender, eroded papule with clean base and raised, firm, indurated borders; multiple lesions occasionally seen	Primary lesions are multiple, edematous, painful erosions with yellow-white membranous coating; recurrent episodes may have grouped vesicles on an erythematous base
Duration	Undetermined (months)	Undetermined (years)	2-6 days	3-6 weeks	Primary 2-6 weeks; recurrent 7-10 days
Site	Genital or perianal	Genital, perianal, or inguinal	Genital, perianal, or rectal	Genital, perianal, or rectal	Genital or perianal
Regional adenopathy	Unilateral or bilateral tender, matted, fixed, adenopathy that may become soft and fluctuant	Subcutaneous perilymphatic granulomatous lesions that produce inguinal swellings and are not lymphadenitis (pseudobuboes)	Unilateral or bilateral firm, painful inguinal adenopathy with overlying "disky skin"; may become fluctuant and develop "grooves in the groin"	Unilateral or bilateral firm, movable, nonsuppportive, painless inguinal adenopathy	Bilateral, tender inguinal adenopathy, usually present with primary vulvovaginitis and may or may not be present with recurrent genital lesions
Diagnostic tests	Smear, culture, or biopsy of lesion; smear from aspirated unruptured lymph node	Biopsy; touch preparation from biopsy stained with Giemsa	LGV complement fixation test; culture	Dark-field examination, VDRL, FTA-ABS	Tzanck smear; culture
Treatment					
Drug of choice	Erythromycin, 500 mg qid for 10 days or longer	Tetracycline, 500 mg qid for 3 weeks	Tetracycline, 500 mg qid for 3 weeks	Benzathine penicillin G, 2.4 million units IM; repeat in 1 week	Symptomatic
Alternative drug	Trimethoprim/sulfamethoxazole, double-strength tablet (160/800 mg) bid 10 days or longer	Trimethoprim/sulfamethoxazole, double-strength tablet (160/800 mg) bid for 3 weeks Streptomycin, 1 gm bid for 3 weeks	Sulfisoxazole, 4 gm initially, then 1 gm qid for 3 weeks Erythromycin, 500 mg qid for 2 weeks	Tetracycline, 500 mg qid for 2 weeks	

Adapted from Margolis RJ, Hood AF: Chancroid: diagnosis and treatment, J Am Acad Dermatol **6**:496, 1982.

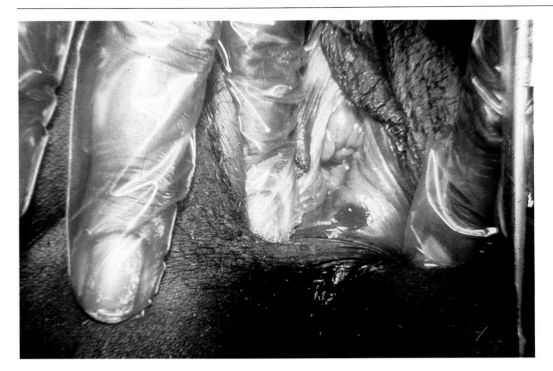

Figure 10-6
*Primary syphilis. A chancre in the vagina.
(Courtesy Centers for Disease Control, Atlanta,
Ga.)*

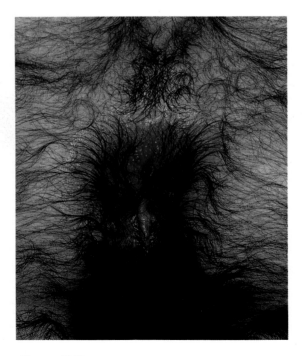

Figure 10-7
*Primary syphilis. A large chancre on the anus of
a male homosexual.*

Secondary syphilis

Secondary syphilis is characterized by mucocutaneous lesions, a flu-like syndrome, and generalized adenopathy. Patients may be acutely ill or have signs and symptoms so subtle they go undetected. Asymptomatic dissemination of *T pallidum* to all organs occurs as the chancre heals and the disease proceeds to resolve in approximately 75% of cases (Figure 10-8).[23] In the remaining 25% the clinical signs of the secondary stage begin approximately 6 weeks (range, 2 weeks to 6 months) after the chancre appears and last for 2 to 10 weeks. Cutaneous lesions are preceded by a flu-like syndrome (sore throat, headache, fever, hoarseness, muscle aches, meningismus, and loss of appetite) and generalized painless lymphadenopathy. Hepatosplenomegaly may be present. In some cases lesions of secondary syphilis appear before the chancre heals. The distribution and morphology of the skin and mucosal lesions are varied and may be confused with numerous other skin diseases. As with most other systemic cutaneous diseases, the rash is usually bilaterally symmetric (Figures 10-9 and 10-10).

Course of disease and blood tests

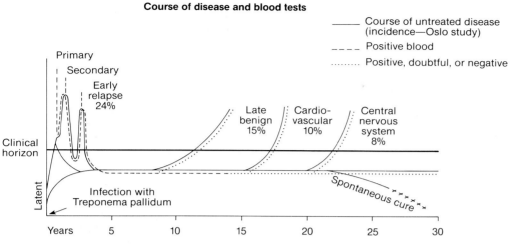

Figure legend:
_____ Course of untreated disease (incidence—Oslo study)
_ _ _ _ Positive blood
.... Positive, doubtful, or negative

Figure 10-8
The natural history of untreated acquired syphilis.
*(From South Med J **26**:18, 1933; incidence from*
*Clark EG, Danbolt N: J Chron Dis **2**:311, 1955.)*

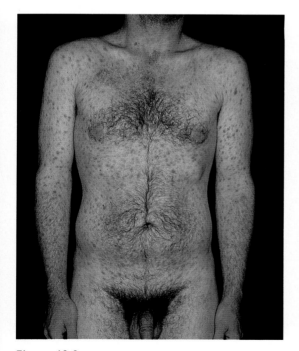

Figure 10-9
Secondary syphilis. Numerous lesions are present on all body surfaces.

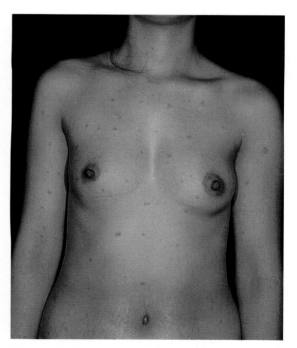

Figure 10-10
Secondary syphilis. A few oval lesions are present on the trunk. Initial diagnosis was pityriasis rosea.

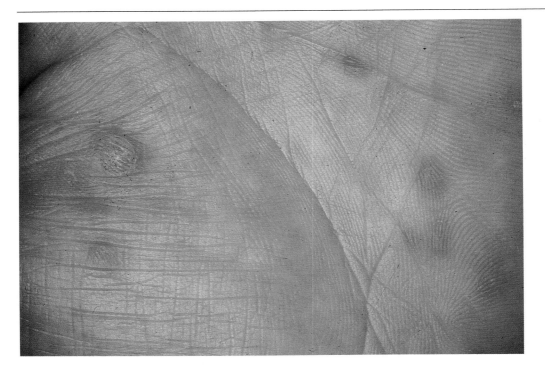

Figure 10-11
Secondary syphilis. Lesions on the palms and soles occur in a majority of patients with secondary syphilis. The coppery color resembling that of a clean-cut ham is characteristic of secondary syphilis.

Figure 10-12
Secondary syphilis. "Moth eaten" alopecia of the scalp.

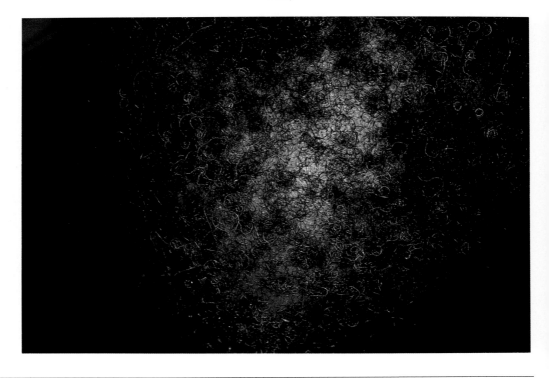

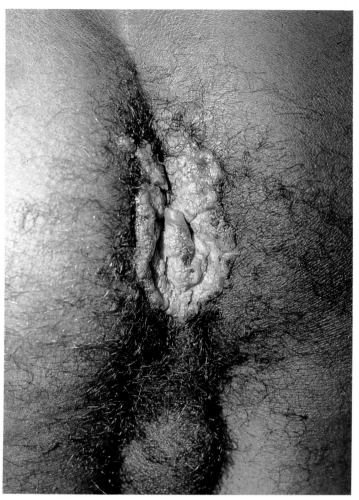

Figure 10-13
Secondary syphilis. Moist anal wart-like papules (condylomata lata) are highly infectious.

The lesions of secondary syphilis have certain characteristics that differentiate them from other cutaneous diseases.[24-26] Lesions are noninflammatory, develop slowly, and may persist for weeks or months. Pain or itching is minimal or absent. There is a marked tendency to polymorphism with various types of lesions present simultaneously, unlike other eruptive skin diseases in which the morphology of the lesions is uniform. The color is characteristic, resembling a "clean-cut ham" or having a coppery tint. Lesions may assume a variety of shapes, including round, elliptical, or annular. The eruption may be limited and discrete, profuse, generalized, or more or less confluent and may vary in intensity.

The types of lesions in approximate order of frequency are maculopapular, papular, macular, annular papular, papulopustular, and psoriasiform. Annular lesions are most frequently seen in blacks. Lesions occur on the palms, soles, or both in a majority of patients with secondary syphilis (Figure 10-11). Unlike the pigmented melanotic macules frequently seen on the palms and soles of older blacks, lesions of secondary syphilis of the palms and soles are isolated, oval, slightly raised, erythematous, and scaly. Temporary irregular ("moth eaten") alopecia of the beard, scalp, or eyelashes may occur (Figure 10-12). Moist, anal wart-like papules (condylomata lata) are highly infectious (Figure 10-13). Lesions may appear on any mucous membrane. All cutaneous lesions of secondary syphilis are infectious; therefore, if you don't know what it is, don't touch it. The differential diagosis is vast. The commonly observed diseases that may be confused with secondary syphilis are pityriasis rosea (especially if the herald patch is absent), guttate psoriasis (psoriasis that appears suddenly with numerous small papules and plaques), lichen planus, tinea versicolor, and exanthematous drug and viral eruptions.

Latent syphilis

Latent syphilis is characterized by positive serologic results with no clinical signs and is classified as being early or late. The latent stage is defined as a period following active infection in which signs and symptoms are absent, but the serology remains positive; a patient is said to have latent disease if a positive serology (not a false positive test) is discovered without evidence of active disease. By convention, early latent syphilis is latent syphilis of 1 year or less and late latent syphilis is syphilis of more than 1 year's duration. Patients in the early latent stage may be infectious. They may also relapse into primary and secondary disease, progress to tertiary syphilis, or enter an inactive period in which no further signs or symptoms develop and the positive serologic findings decrease, and finally results become negative (Figure 10-8).

Tertiary syphilis

A small number of untreated or inadequately treated patients will develop systemic disease, including cardiovascular disease, central nervous system lesions, and systemic granulomas (gummas).[27,28]

Congenital syphilis

T pallidum can be transmitted by an infected mother to the fetus in utero. Because of the barrier imposed by the early developing placenta, *T pallidum* cannot infect the fetus until after the fourth month of pregnancy. The fetus is at greatest risk when maternal syphilis is of less than 2 years' duration. The potential for the mother to infect the fetus diminishes but never disappears in late latent stages.[29]

Early congenital syphilis. In early congenital syphilis, fetal stigmata presenting before the age of 2 include eruptions characteristic of secondary syphilis (unlike the lesions of acquired disease, they may be vesicular or bullous); fissures at the lips, perianal areas, and vulva; rhinitis with highly infectious nasal discharge; nontender generalized adenopathy; meningitis; hepatosplenomegaly; alopecia; iritis; and osteochondritis with tenderness in the limbs during the first year of life.

Late congenital syphilis. Symptoms and signs of late congenital syphilis[30,31] become evident after age 5. The most important signs are interstitial keratitis, synovitis (Clutton's joint), eighth nerve deafness, frontal bossae (bony prominences of the forehead), short maxilla, high palatal arch, "Hutchinson's teeth" (peg-shaped upper central incisors of the permanent dentition that appear after age 6) (Figure 10-14), saddle nose, mulberry molars (more than four small cusps on a narrow first lower molar of the second dentition), and Higoumenakis' sign (enlargement of the sternoclavicular portion of the clavicle).

Syphilis serology

Two classes of antibodies are produced in response to infection with *T pallidum;* these are nonspecific antibodies measured by the Venereal Disease Research Laboratory (VDRL) and rapid plasma reagin (RPR) tests and specific antibodies measured by the fluorescent treponemal antibody absorption (FTA-ABS) test (Table 10-3).[32]

VDRL and RPR. Antibodies (reagins of the IgM and IgG rather than IgE class) are directed against lipoidal antigens and are measured by the VDRL or RPR tests or any of the modifications of these flocculation tests. Most can give quantitative as well as qualitative results and, therefore, can be used to monitor response to therapy. These tests are used for screening and have a high degree of sensitivity (positive in most patients with syphilis), but relatively low specificity (positive in patients without syphilis). A rising titer indicates active disease; the titer falls in response to treatment. Biologic false-positive reactions to nontreponemal tests (range, 3% to 20%) are defined as a positive nontreponemal antibody test in patients in whom the FTA-ABS is negative (see Table 10-4).[33-38]

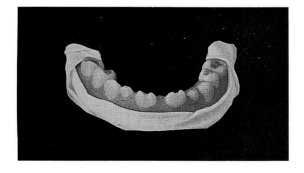

Figure 10-14
Late congenital syphilis. Hutchinson's teeth (peg-shaped upper central incisors of permanent dentition).

TABLE 10-3

SENSITIVITY OF SEROLOGIC TESTS IN THE STAGES OF SYPHILIS (PERCENT POSITIVE)*

Test	Primary	Secondary	Latent	Tertiary	Screening
VDRL†	72	100	73	77	86
FTA-ABS‡	91	100	97	100	99

*From Griner PF, Mayewski AJ, Mushlin AI, et al: Application of principles. Ann Intern Med **94**(part 2):585, 1981.
†Specificity variable by stage and proportion of population tested with chronic and autoimmune diseases. Specificity in screening general population approximately 97%.
‡Specificity for all stages probably 98% to 99%, including those with biologic false positives on nontreponemal test.

TABLE 10-4

DISEASES THAT RESULT IN POSITIVE REACTIONS TO TESTS ALTHOUGH PATIENTS DO NOT HAVE SYPHILIS (FALSE-POSITIVE REACTIONS)

Nontreponomal tests	FTA-ABS
Viral infection	Pyodermas
Collagen-vascular disease	Skin neoplasms
Acute or chronic illness	Acne vulgaris and rosacea
Pregnancy	Mycoses
Recent immunization	Crural ulceration
Heroin addiction	Psoriasis
Leprosy	Systemic lupus erythematosus (LE), discoid LE, drug-induced LE
Malaria	Pregnancy
	Drug addiction
	Herpes genitalis (not confirmed)
	LE, scleroderma, rheumatoid arthritis (atypical beaded fluorescence pattern)

About two-thirds of patients with false positive reactions will become seronegative in 6 months (acute reactors), and the remaining one-third will have persistent elevation of their titers (chronic reactors). Undiluted serum containing a high titer of nonspecific antibody, as occurs in secondary syphilis, may result in a negative flocculation test. This is called the prozone phenomenon and occurs because the large quantity of antibody occupies all of antigen sites and prevents flocculation. The laboratory may perform flocculation tests on diluted serum in anticipation of this problem.

FTA-ABS. Specific treponemal antigen tests such as the commonly used FTA-ABS measure antibody directed against *T pallidum.* They are more sensitive and more specific than the nontreponemal tests but are not used for screening because of cost and technical reasons. The FTA-ABS results are reported as nonreactive, borderline, and reactive (1+ to 4+). A 2% incidence of false positive reactions has been found to be most common at the borderline or 1+ reaction level (see Table 10-4).[36-38] An atypical beaded fluorescent pattern may be found in patients with systemic lupus erythematosus (SLE), scleroderma, and rheumatoid arthritis. An FTA-ABS reported as a beaded pattern may be the first indication that a patient will evolve symptoms of SLE. The FTA-ABS is performed when the VDRL or RPR is positive and in patients with clinical evidence of syphilis for whom the nontreponemal test is negative.

Treatment of syphilis*

Early syphilis. This includes primary, secondary, and early latent syphilis of less than 1 year's duration.

Benzathine penicillin G: 2,400,000 units IM immediately, to be repeated in 7 days for a total of 4,800,000 units.[39] NOTE: this schedule differs from the CDC recommendation.

Patients sensitive to penicillin

Tetracycline: 500 mg orally 4 times daily for 12 days.

Doxycycline: 100 mg orally 2 times daily for 12 days.

Minocycline: 100 mg orally 2 times daily for 12 days.

Erythromycin: 500 mg orally 4 times daily for 12 days.

The drug of choice in the treatment of syphilis is *benzathine penicillin G.* Spectinomycin should *not* be used in the treatment of syphilis; patients sensitive to penicillin should be treated with the alternate drugs listed above.

Patients with their first attack of primary syphilis will have a nonreactive rapid plasma reagin circle card (RPR-CT) test within 1 year. Patients with secondary syphilis will have a nonreactive RPR-CT test within 2 years. Patients with early latent syphilis of less than 1 year will be seronegative within 4 years.

Syphilis of more than 1 year's duration except "neurosyphilis." This includes latent syphilis of 1 year or longer and late tertiary stages, including mucocutaneous, osseous, visceral, and cardiovascular involvement.

Benzathine penicillin G: 2,400,000 units IM immediately, to be repeated in 7 days for a total of 4,800,000 units. NOTE: this schedule differs from the CDC recommendation.

Procaine penicillin G in aqueous suspension: 600,000 units IM daily or every other day for 10 doses.

Patients sensitive to penicillin

Tetracycline: 500 mg orally 4 times daily for 12 days.

Doxycycline: 100 mg orally 2 times daily for 12 days.

Minocycline: 100 mg orally 2 times daily for 12 days.

Erythromycin: 500 mg orally 4 times daily for 12 days.

There is no objection to administering larger doses of the above drugs, but smaller doses are unacceptable. In 75% of cases studied patients who had a first attack of latent syphilis of 1 to 4 years' duration and who were treated with the above regimens had a nonreactive RPR-CT in 5 years. In patients with late latent syphilis, 45% were seronegative in 5 years, and the remainder were Wasserman- or reagin-fast. A cerebrospinal fluid (CSF) examination is not performed unless patient has neurological or psychiatric signs and symptoms.

Neurosyphilis

Benzathine penicillin G: 2,400,000 units IM at weekly intervals for not less than 3 weeks (total of 7.2 million units).

Patients sensitive to penicillin

Tetracycline: 500 mg orally 4 times daily for at least 20 days.

Doxycycline: 100 mg orally 2 times daily for at least 20 days.

Minocycline: 100 mg orally 2 times daily for at least 20 days.

Erythromycin: 500 mg orally 4 times daily for at least 20 days.

Syphilis in pregnancy

Benzathine penicillin G: 2,400,000 units IM immediately, to be repeated in 7 days for a total of 4,800,000 units.

Patients sensitive to penicillin

Tetracycline: 500 mg orally 4 times daily for 12 days.[39] NOTE: this schedule differs from the CDC recommendation.

Doxycycline: 100 mg orally 2 times daily for 12 days.

Any pregnant woman with a positive blood test for syphilis and no history of treatment should be treated prophylactically, pending the results of a diagnostic workup.

Erythromycin is not recommended in pregnancy. Although effective for the mother, erythromycin will not pass the placenta in sufficient concentration to protect the fetus. Thus, congenital syphilis has occurred in a mother given 30 gm of erythromycin over 15 days. The Massachusetts Public Health Service recommends that infants born to mothers treated with erythromycin for early syphilis should be retreated with penicillin.

Early congenital syphilis. This appears in children less than 2 years of age. A CSF examination is not required before treatment.

Procaine penicillin G in aqueous suspension: 100,000 to 250,000 units/kg (2.2 lb) of body weight intramuscularly, divided into 10 doses. For practical purposes, 100,000 units of procaine penicillin G in aqueous suspension intramuscularly daily for 10 days, for total of 1 million units.

Benzathine penicillin G: 100,000 units/kg (2.2 lbs) of body weight intramuscularly, either as a single injection or divided into 2 doses a week apart.

Children 2 to 10 years receive half the adult dose of penicillin.

Children sensitive to penicillin receive erythromycin at half the adult dose.

*From Massachusetts Department of Public Health, Division of Communicable, and Venereal Diseases, Nicholas J. Fiumara, M.D., M.P.H., Director.

TABLE 10-5

USE OF NONTREPONEMAL SEROLOGIC TESTS IN FOLLOWUP AFTER TREATMENT OF SYPHILIS

Stage	Followup interval
Early syphilis (less than 1 year)	3, 6, 12 months after treatment
Late syphilis (more than 1 year)	2 years after treatment
Neurosyphilis	Blood and cerebrospinal fluid levels every 6 months for 3 years after treatment
Retreatment	Cerebrospinal fluid level

Reinfection syphilis. Treatment schedules are the same as for the initial infection.
Contacts of patients with early syphilis
Benzathine penicillin G: 2.4 million units IM if RPR-CT is nonreactive.
Patients sensitive to penicillin
Tetracycline, 500 mg orally 4 times daily for at least 7 days.

Posttreatment evaluation of syphilis

Frequency of followup serologic tests. All patients treated for syphilis must be followed to assess the effectiveness of initial treatment. Quantitative nontreponemal tests (VDRL or RPR) are obtained at certain intervals after treatment (Table 10-5).[32] Retreatment should be considered for any patient who has a sustained fourfold increase in titer or when an initially high titer fails to show a fourfold decrease within a year.[32]

Serologic responses to treatment
Primary, secondary, and early latent syphilis. All patients with primary syphilis treated with the recommended schedules will become seronegative in 1 year; those with secondary syphilis treated with the recommended schedules will become seronegative in 2 years[40] (Figure 10-15). The speed at which seronegativity occurs after treatment for secondary syphilis is related to the type of rash initially present (i.e., macular, maculopapular, papular, or pustular) (Figure 10-16).[41] Patients treated for early latent syphilis will become seronegative within 4 years. The lower the serologic titer before treatment, the quicker the blood test result will revert to normal.[42]

Patients with treated secondary syphilis who fail to achieve seronegativity within 2 years are those who become reinfected as evidenced by a recurrence of the rash or a fourfold or greater increase in the serologic titer, those who had acquired or congenital syphilis before infection, or those who had a chronic biologic false-positive reaction before the current infection.

Late latent syphilis. One study reveals that 44% of late latent syphilis patients became seronegative within 5 years, and 56% had persistently positive reagin tests.[43] The criteria of effectiveness in the treatment of patients with late latent syphilis are reversion of the reagin blood test for syphilis from reactive to nonreactive, a fourfold or greater decrease in the reagin titer, or a fixed titer with no significant change during the period of observation.

Reinfection in primary, secondary, and latent syphilis. The titers of reagin antibody are higher than those during the first infection and the serologic responses to treatment are slower, taking about twice the time to become nonreactive as that expected after treatment of a first episode of syphilis.

Cerebral spinal fluid examination. Patients with syphilis who are not treated or are inadequately treated are at risk for developing neurosyphilis. Prevention of this complication is one of the major reasons for following the progress of the blood reagin level. A VDRL should be performed on CSF of patients with tertiary syphilis, those with symptoms of syphilitic meningitis, and those with primary or secondary syphilis with a history of probable untreated syphilis. Some authors recommend CSF examination in patients with latent syphilis, whereas others feel it is merely necessary to follow reagin levels and perform a lumbar puncture if there are neurologic or psychiatric abnormalities or the criteria listed for effective treatment are not met. Others think it is necessary to obtain only a blood FTA-ABS, since a negative blood FTA-ABS rules out the diagnosis of neurosyphilis.[44,45] No cases of neurosyphilis have been reported with a negative FTA-ABS.

The diagnosis of neurosyphilis is made with the CSF VDRL, through demonstration of lymphocytes and an increased total protein level in the CSF. The cell count is done within 2 hours of the spinal tap. Five or more lymphocytes per cubic millimeter and a total protein above 35 mg/dl are abnormal.

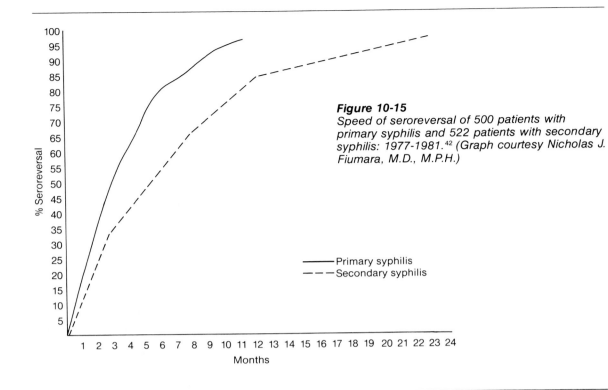

Figure 10-15
Speed of seroreversal of 500 patients with primary syphilis and 522 patients with secondary syphilis: 1977-1981.[42] *(Graph courtesy Nicholas J. Fiumara, M.D., M.P.H.)*

Figure 10-16
Speed of seroreversal of 522 patients with secondary syphilis by type of lesion: 1977-1981.[42] *(Graph courtesy Nicholas J. Fiumara, M.D., M.P.H.)*

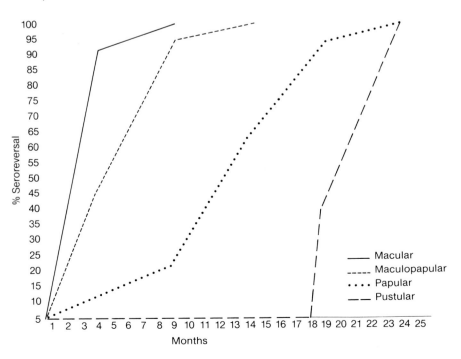

Rare Sexually Transmitted Diseases

Lymphogranuloma venereum

Lymphogranuloma venereum (LGV) is caused by several related strains of *Chlamydia trachomatis*.

Primary lesion. After an incubation period of 5 to 21 days, a small papule or viral (herpetiform) vesicle occurs on the penis, fourchette, or cervix (Figure 10-17). The lesion evolves rapidly to a small painless erosion that heals without scarring. The lesion may be so innocuous that patients may not remember it. The primary lesion is rarely seen in women.

Lymphadenopathy. Unilateral or bilateral inguinal lymphadenopathy accompanied by headache, fever, and migratory polymyalgia and arthralgia appears from 1 to 4 weeks after the primary lesion heals (Figure 10-18). In a short time the lymph nodes become tender and fluctuant and are referred to as buboes when they ulcerate and discharge purulent material. Draining buboes may persist for months. Buboes are common in men, but occur in only approximately one-third of infected females. For unexplained reasons, women develop inflammation of the perineal lymph nodes that may lead to scarring and ulceration of the labia, rectal mucosa, and vagina. Chronic edema (elephantiasis) of the female external genitalia is a late manifestation of lymphatic obstruction.

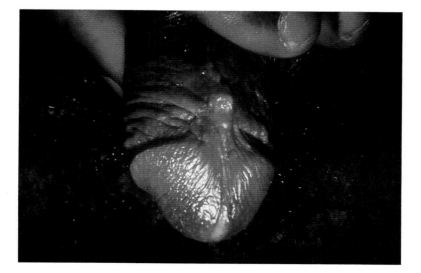

Figure 10-17
Lymphogranuloma venereum. Primary lesion consists of a small painless erosion that heals in a short time without scarring. (Courtesy Centers for Disease Control, Atlanta, Ga.)

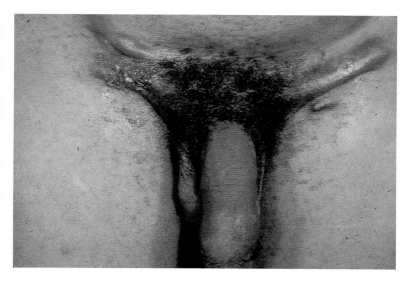

Figure 10-18
Lymphogranuloma venereum. Bilateral inguinal lymphadenopathy that discharges purulent material (buboes).

Diagnosis

Complement fixation test. The lymphogranuloma venereum complement fixation test (LGV-CFT)[46] becomes positive within 1 to 3 weeks. The antigen used is a genus-specific chlamydial group antigen that is not specific for the LGV organism; therefore, the diagnosis cannot be absolute from this test unless rising titers can be shown. A single titre of 1:32 suggests the diagnosis. A fourfold rise in titre in the presence of the clinical syndrome is considered diagnostic of chlamydial infection. However, rising titers are difficult to demonstrate because the patient is usually seen after the acute stage when the initial lesion has healed.

Micro-immunofluorescent technique. The micro-immunofluorescent (micro-IF)[47] method is a highly sensitive and specific method for determining individual serotypes of *C trachomatis*. Demonstration of a rising titer is difficult, but a single titer of 1:32 in active cases provides strong support for the diagnosis of LGV. The test is available through some state laboratories.

Culture. Chlamydia transport media are now available at most hospital laboratories. Aspirates of lymph nodes are inoculated onto transport media and then submitted for tissue culture. Cultures are seldom positive.

Frei skin test. The Frei skin test is no longer available.

Treatment

Drug regimen. The drug regimen of choice[48,49] is tetracycline HCl, 500 mg by mouth 4 times a day for at least 2 weeks.

Alternative regimens. One of the following drugs should be given for at least 2 weeks: doxycycline, 100 mg by mouth twice a day; erythromycin, 500 mg by mouth 4 times a day; sulfisoxazole, 4 gm initially, then 1 gm 4 times a day. Other sulfonamides can be used in equivalent dosage.

Lesion management. Fluctuant lymph nodes should be aspirated as needed through healthy adjacent normal skin. Incision and drainage or excision of nodes will delay healing and is contraindicated. Late sequelae such as stricture or fistula may require surgical intervention.

Chancroid

Chancroid is the most common of the minor venereal diseases. It is caused by the short gram-negative rod *Hemophilus ducreyi*. The male to female ratio of reported cases is approximately 10:1.

Figure 10-19
Chancroid. Several small painful ulcers are usually present. The base is purulent, in contrast to the chancre of syphilis.

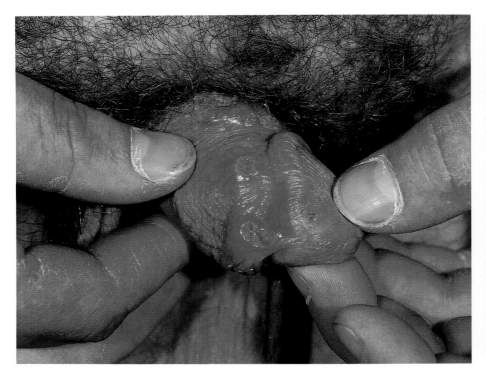

Primary state. After an incubation period of 2 to 5 days, a red papule appears at the site of contact, rapidly becomes pustular, and then ulcerates. The ulcer (soft chancre), which bleeds easily, has a red overhanging edge and a base covered by yellow-gray exudate (Figure 10-19). The ulcers are highly infectious and multiple lesions appear on the genitalia from autoinoculation. Unlike those of syphilis the ulcers may be so painful that some patients refuse the manipulation necessary to obtain culture material. Untreated cases may resolve spontaneously or, more often, progress to cause deep ulceration (Figure 10-20), severe phimosis, and scarring. Systemic symptoms, including anorexia, malaise, and low-grade fever, are occasionally present. Women may have lesions on the labia, cervix, or anus or have no detectable lesions and be asymptomatic carriers.

Lymphadenopathy. Unilateral or bilateral inguinal lymphadenopathy develops in approximately 50% of untreated patients beginning approximately 1 week after the onset of the initial lesion. The nodes then resolve spontaneously or suppurate and break down.

Diagnosis. Dark-field microscopic examination should be done to rule out syphilis. Stained smears of the ulcer or aspirated buboes are the quickest way of determining the diagnosis; however, preparation and interpretation is difficult. Smears taken from the surface areas are of little use. Material is obtained by drawing the flat surface of a toothpick under the undermined border of the ulcer. The cellular debris is then smeared on a glass slide and gently fixed with heat. A Gram stain shows pus cells with gram-negative coccobacilli in parallel arrays (school-of-fish arrangement) (Figure 10-21). Bacteria may be intercellular. H ducreyi may also be demonstrated with Wright's, Giemsa, or Unna-Pappenheim stains.

The histology of chancroid is specific, but the biopsy procedure is so painful that other means of confirming the diagnosis should first be utilized.

This organism cannot be cultured on routine medium. ECA-V (enriched chocolate agar with vancomycin),[50,51] available from Difco, is a sensitive medium for primary isolation of H ducreyi, but it is not stocked routinely in most hospital laboratories. The exudate from the ulcer must be inoculated directly onto the plate, not onto transport media.

For autologous culture media[52] a sample of 5 to 10 ml of the patient's blood is placed in a sterile tube

Figure 10-20
Chancroid. Ulcers have coalesced during a 4-week period without treatment.

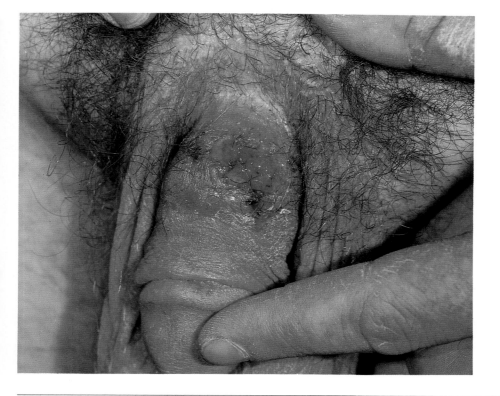

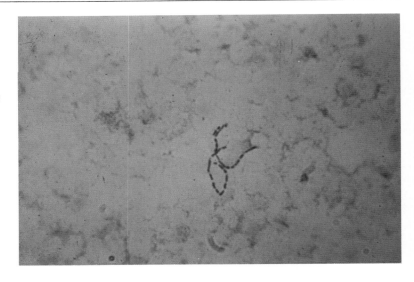

Figure 10-21
Chancroid. A Wright stain of
the purulent material of the
base of the ulcer shows a chain
of coccobacilli. (Couresty
Centers for Disease Control,
Atlanta, Ga.)

and allowed to clot at room temperature (22° C).
This autologous medium is inoculated with serous
exudate from an ulcer and incubated at 35° C for 48
hours in a 5% CO_2-enriched atmosphere. At 48
hours a Gram stain is performed on the autologous
blood; if positive, it shows clusters and parallel rows
of Gram-negative rods. ECA-V culture medium is
more sensitive than autologous culture medium for
the isolation of H ducreyi.

Treatment. Drug regimens are erythromycin,
500 mg by mouth 4 times a day,[53] or trimethoprim/
sulfamethoxazole, a double-strength tablet (160/
800 mg) by mouth twice a day.[54] Therapy should be
given for a minimum of 10 days and continued until
ulcers and lymph nodes have healed.

Antimicrobial susceptibility testing should be
done on H ducreyi isolated from patients who do not
respond to the recommended therapies.

Granuloma inguinale

Granuloma inguinale (donovanosis) is a chronic,
superficial, ulcerating disease of the genital, inguinal, and perianal areas caused by the gram-negative rode Calymmatobacterium granulomatis. The
incubation period is unknown, but 40 days incubation is suspected. The disease begins as a papule,
nodule, or ulcer on the genitalia and then evolves
into a painless, broad superficial ulcer with a beefy
red, granulating texture raised above the skin surface (Figure 10-22). The ulceration spreads con-
tiguously to the genitocrural and inguinal folds in
males and the perineal and perianal areas in females. It remains confined to areas of moist stratified epithelium, sparing the columnar epithelium of
the rectal area. No regional adenopathy is found, as
with lymphogranuloma venereum and chancroid.

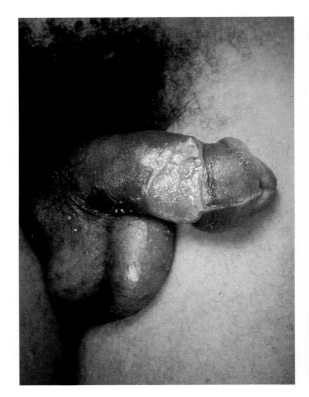

Figure 10-22
Granuloma inguinale. A painless broad superficial
ulcer with a beefy red texture is raised above the
skin surface. (Courtesy Nicholas J. Fiumara, M.D.,
M.P.H.)

Diagnosis. Organisms are sometimes more easily demonstrated in stained smears than in histopathologic sections. A piece of tissue is obtained by curetting deeply beneath the active extending border of the ulcer. Part of the specimen is sent for histopathology. A thin section is cut from the remaining fragments of tissue and crushed firmly between two glass slides or smeared across the slide. Wright's stain is added and diluted in 1.5 minutes with phosphate buffer (pH 6.4). Mononuclear cells contain blue to deep purple pleomorphic rods surrounded by clear or pink capsules (Donovan's bodies).

For histopathology, special silver stains are necessary to demonstrate the organisms in tissue. Culture requires yolk-sac inoculation and is not practical.

Treatment. The following regimens are listed in the order of preference. The minimum duration of treatment is 21 days. However, treatment should be continued until all lesions have completely healed.[55] Treatments are tetracycline, 0.5 gm orally 4 times a day; trimethoprim (160 mg) or sulfamethoxazole (800 mg) tablets 2 times a day[56]; streptomycin, 1 gm IM twice daily; or chloramphenicol, 0.5 gm orally 3 times a day.

Relapses after apparent cure occasionally occur, and such recurrent lesions may become resistant to medication. Under such circumstances, switching to another antibiotic generally has been found to be effective.

REFERENCES

1. Handsfield HH, Lipman TO, Harnish JP, et al: Asymptomatic gonorrhea in men. N Engl J Med **290**:117, 1974.
2. Fiumara NJ: Gonorrhea and nongonococcal urethritis. Cutis **27**:258, 1981.
3. Barlow D, Phillips I: Gonorrhea in women: diagnostic, clinical and laboratory aspects. Lancet **1**:761, 1978.
4. Eschenbach DA, Holms KK: Acute pelvic inflammatory disease: current concepts of pathogenesis, etiology, and management. Clinic Obstet Gynecol **18**:35, 1975.
5. Eschenback DA, Buchanan TM, Pollock HM, et al: Polymicrobial etiology of acute pelvic inflammatory disease. N Engl J Med **293**:166, 1975.
6. Taylor-Robinson D, McCormack WM: The genital mycoplasmas. N Engl J Med **302**:1003, 1980.
7. Mårdh P-A, Ripa T, Svensson L, et al: Chlamydia trachomatis infection in patients with acute salpingitis. N Engl J Med **296**:1377, 1977.
8. Wiesner PJ: Gonorrhea. Cutis **27**:249, 1981.
9. Kilpatrick ZM: Gonorrheal proctitis. N Engl J Med **287**:967, 1972.
10. Catterall RD: Anorectal gonorrhoea. Proc R Soc Med **55**:871, 1962.
11. Lebedeff DA, Elliott HB: Rectal gonorrhea in men: diagnosis and treatment. Ann Intern Med **92**:463, 1980.
12. Wiesner PJ, Tronca E, Bonin P, et al: Clinical spectrum of pharyngeal gonococcal infection. N Engl J Med **288**:181, 1973.
13. Fiumara NJ: Pharyngeal infection with neisseria gonorrhoeae. Sex Transm Dis **6**:264, 1979.
14. Felman YM, Nikitas JA: Disseminated gonococcal infection. Cutis **27**:140, 1981.
15. Brogadir SP, Schimmer BM, Myers AR: Spectrum of the gonococcal arthritis-dermatitis syndrome. Semin Arthritis Rheum **8**:177, 1979.
16. Holmes KK, Counts GW, Beaty HN: Disseminated gonococcal infection. Ann Intern Med **74**:979, 1971.
17. Stam WE, Guinan ME, Johnson C, et al: Effect of treatment regimens for Neisseria gonorrhoeae on simultaneous infection with Chlamydia trachomatis. N Engl J Med **310**:545, 1984.
18. Schachter J: Chlamydial infections. N Engl J Med **298**:428, 1978.
19. Berger RE, et al: Chlamydia trachomatis as a cause of acute "idiopathic" epididymitis. N Engl J Med **298**:301, 1978.
20. Brunham RC, Paavonen J, Stevens CE, et al: Mucopurulent cervicitis: the ignored counterpart in women of urethritis in men. N Engl J Med **311**:1, 1984.
21. Bowie WR, et al: Tetracycline in nongonococcal urethritis: comparison of 2 g and 1 g daily for 7 days. Br J Vener Dis **56**:332, 1980.
22. Bowie WR, et al: Therapy for nongonococcal urethritis: double-blind randomized comparison of two doses and two durations of minocycline. Ann Intern Med **95**:306, 1981.
23. Clark EG, Danbolt N: The Oslo study of the natural course of untreated syphilis. J Chronic Dis **2**:311, 1955.
24. Gooddard PB: Ricord's illustrations of venereal disease. Philadelphia, 1851, A Hart, Late Carey and Hart.
25. Felman YM, Nikitas JA: Secondary syphilis. Cutis **29**:322, 1982.
26. Syphilis: A synopsis. Public Health Service Publication No. 1660. Washington, DC. 1968, US Government Printing Office.
27. Kampmeier RH: Late and congenital syphilis. Symposium on Sexually Transmitted Diseases. Dermatol Clin **1**:23, 1983.
28. Luxon LM: Neurosyphilis (review). Int J Dermatol **19**:310, 1980.
29. Paley PS: Syphilis in pregnancy. NY State J Med **37**:585, 1937.
30. Robinson RCV: Congenital syphilis: review article. Arch Dermatol **99**:599, 1969.
31. Fiumara NJ, Lessell S: Manifestations of late congenital syphilis. Arch Dermatol **102**:78, 1970.
32. Griner PF, Mayewski AJ, Mushlin AI, et al: Application of principles. Ann Intern Med **94**(part 2):585, 1981.
33. Rhodes AR, Legar AFH: False-positive reactions to the nontreponemal tests. In Dermatology in general medicine. Second edition. Fitzpatrick TB, et al editors. New York, 1979, McGraw-Hill.
34. Catterall RD: Systemic disease and the biologic false positive reaction. Br J Vener Dis **48**:1, 1972.
35. British Cooperative Clinical Group: Acute and chronic biologic false positive reactors to serologic tests for syphilis. Br J Vener Dis **50**:428, 1974.

36. Gibowski M, Neumann E: Non-specific positive test results to syphilis in dermatological diseases. Br J Vener Dis **56**:17, 1980.
37. Chapel T, Jeffries CD, Brown WJ, et al: Influence of genital herpes on results of fluorescent treponemal antibody absorption test. Br J Vener Dis **54**:299, 1978.
38. Drew FL, Sarandria JL: False positive FTA-ABS in pregnancy. J Am Vener Dis Assoc **1**:165-166, 1975.
39. Fiumara NJ: Therapy guidelines for sexually transmitted diseases (letter). J Am Acad Dermatol **9**:600, 1983.
40. Fiumara NJ: Treatment of primary and secondary syphilis: serological response. JAMA **243**:2500, 1980.
41. Fiumara NJ: Infectious syphilis. Symposium on Sexually Transmitted Disease. Dermatol Clin **1**: 1983.
42. Fiumara NJ: Treatment of early syphilis of less than a year's duration. Sex Transm Dis **5**:85, 1978.
43. Fiumara NJ: Serologic responses to treatment of 128 patients with late latent syphilis. Sex Transm Dis **6**:
44. Harris AD, Bossak HM, Deacon WE, et al: Comparison of the fluorescent treponemal antibody test with other tests for syphilis on cerebrospinal fluids. Br J Vener Dis **36**:178, 1960.
45. Duncan WP, Jenkins TW, Parham CE: Fluorescent treponemal antibody-cerebrospinal fluid (FTA-CSF) test: a provisional technique. Br J Vener Dis **48**:97, 1972.
46. Schachter J: Chlamydial infections. N Engl J Med **298**:428, 1978.

47. Wang S-P, Grayston JT: Immunologic relationship between genital tric, lymphogranuloma venereum, and related organisms in a new microtiter indirect immunofluorescence test. Am J Ophthalmol **70**:367, 1970.
48. Felman YM, Nikitas J: Lymphogranuloma venereum. Cutis **25**:264, 1980.
49. Knight AA, David VC: Treatment of venereal lymphogranuloma with sulfonamides. JAMA **112**:527, 1939.
50. Sottnek FO, et al: Isolation and identification of Haemophilus ducreyi in a clinical study. J Clin Microbiol **12**:170, 1980.
51. Borchers SL: Treatment of chancroid (letter to the editor). J Am Acad Dermatol **8**:128, 1983.
52. Borchardt KA, Hoke AW: Simplified laboratory technique for diagnosis of chancroid. Arch Dermatol **102**: 189, 1970.
53. Carpenter JL, Back A, Gehle D, et al: Treatment of chancroid with erythromycin. Sex Transm Dis **8**:192, 1981.
54. Fitzpatrick JE, Tyler H, Gramstad ND: Treatment of chancroid: comparison of sulfamethoxazole-trimethoprim with recommended therapies. JAMA **26**: 1804, 1981.
55. Felman YM, Nikitas JA: Granuloma inguinale. Cutis **27**:364, 1981.
56. Rosen T, Tschen JA, Ramsdell W, et al: Granuloma inguinale. J Am Acad Dermatol **11**:433, 1984.

ADDITIONAL READING

Holmes KK, Mårdh P-A, Sparling PF, Wiesner PJ, editors: Sexually transmitted diseases. New York, 1984, McGraw-Hill Book Co.

Chapter Eleven

Superficial Fungal Infections

Dermatophyte Fungal Infections

The dermatophytes include a group of fungi (ringworm) that have the ability to infect and survive only on dead keratin, i.e., the top layer of the skin (stratum corneum or keratin layer), hair, and nails. They cannot invade the dermis or subcutaneous tissue or infect any internal organ. Dermatophytes are responsible for the vast majority of skin, nail, and hair fungal infections. They are classified in several ways.

Classification. The ringworm fungi belong to three genera: *Microsporum, Trichophyton,* and *Epidermophyton.* There are several species of *Microsporum* and *Trichophyton* and one of *Epidermophyton.*

Place of origin. The anthropophilic dermatophytes grow only on human skin, hair, or nails. The zoophilic varieties originate from animals but may infect humans. Geophilic dermatophytes live in soil but may infect humans.

Type of inflammation. The inflammatory response to dermatophytes varies. In general, zoophilic and geophilic dermatophytes elicit a brisk inflammatory response on skin and in hair follicles. The inflammatory response to anthropophilic fungi is usually mild.

Type of hair invasion. Some species are able to infect the hair shaft. Microscopic examination of infected hairs will show fungal spores and hyphae either in the hair shaft or both inside and on the surface. The endothrix pattern consists of fungal hyphae inside the hair shaft, while the ectothrix pattern is fungal hyphae inside and on the surface of the hair shaft.

Spores of fungi are either large or small. The type of hair invasion is further classified as large or small spore ectothrix or large spore endothrix.

The dermatophytes, or ringworm fungi, produce disease patterns that vary with the location and species. Learning the numerous patterns of disease produced by each species is complicated and unnecessary because all dermatophytes respond to the same topical and oral agents. It is important to be familiar with the general patterns of inflammation in different body regions and to be able to interpret accurately a potassium hydroxide wet mount preparation of scale, hair, or nails. Species identification by culture is necessary only for scalp, inflammatory skin and some nail infections.

Clinically, dermatophyte infections have traditionally been classified by body region. Tinea means fungus infection. The term tinea capitis, for example, indicates dermatophyte infection of the scalp.

Diagnosis

Potassium hydroxide wet mount preparation. The single most important test for the diagnosis of dermatophyte infection is the direct microscopic visualization of the branching hyphae in keratinized material. Scale is obtained by holding a #15 surgical blade perpendicular to the skin surface and smoothly but firmly drawing the blade with several short strokes against the scale. If an active border is present, the blade is drawn along the border at right angles to the fringe of scale. If the blade is drawn from the center of the lesion out and parallel to the active border, some normal scale may also be included. The small fragments of scale are placed on a microscope slide and gently separated; a coverslip is applied. Potassium hydroxide (10% or 20% solution) is applied with a toothpick or eye dropper to the edge of the coverslip and allowed to run under by capillary action. The preparation is gently heated under a low flame, then pressed to facilitate

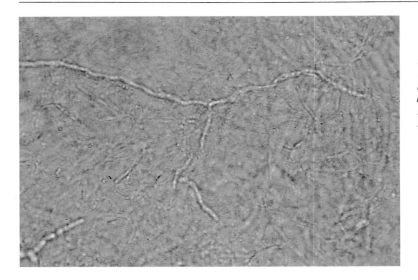

Figure 11-1
Fungal hyphae. A potassium hydroxide wet mount. The identifying characteristics are branching and a filamentous structure uniform in width.

Figure 11-2
A drop of ink added to the potassium hydroxide wet mount will accentuate hyphae. (Courtesy Dr. Lenor Haley, Centers for Disease Control.)

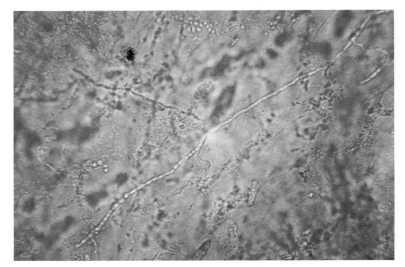

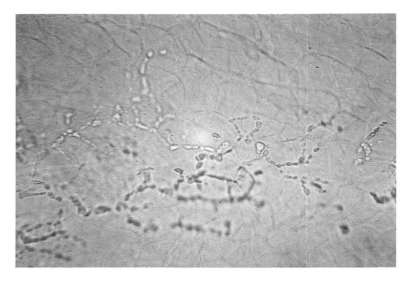

Figure 11-3
Mosaic artifact. Lipid droplets appearing in a single-file line between epithelial cells simulated fungal hyphae in potassium hydroxide wet mounts. Heat encourages cell separation and the artifact disappears. (Courtesy Dr. Lenor Haley, Centers for Disease Control.)

separation of the epithelial cells and fungal hyphae. Potassium hydroxide dissolves material binding cells together, but does not distort the epithelial cells or fungi. Lowering the condenser of the microscope and dimming the light enhances contrast, making hyphae easier to identify.

Study the preparation carefully by scanning the entire area under the coverslip at low power. The presence of hyphae should be confirmed by examination with the 40× objective. Slightly rotating the focusing knob back and forth is helpful in visualizing the entire segment of the hyphae, which may be at different depths. It is not uncommon to find only one small fragment of scale containing many hyphae, with none in the remainder of the preparation. Study the entire preparation carefully.

Nail plate keratin is thick and difficult to digest. The nail plate can be adequately softened by leaving the fragments along with several drops of potassium hydroxide in a watch glass covered with a Petri dish for 24 hours. Hair specimens require no special preparation or digestion and can be examined immediately.

The interpretation of potassium hydroxide wet mounts takes experience. Dermatophytes appear as translucent branching rod-shaped filaments (hyphae) of uniform width with lines of separation (septa) spanning the width at irregular intervals (Figures 11-1 and 11-2). The uniform width and characteristic bending and branching distinguish hyphae from hair and other debris. Hair tapers at the tip. Some hyphae contain a single-file line of bubbles in their cytoplasm. Hyphae may fragment into round or polygonal fragments that look like spores. Hyphae may be seen in combination with scale or floating free in the potassium hydroxide.

Confusion may arise with the so-called mosaic artifact produced by lipid droplets appearing in a single-file line between cells, especially from specimens taken from the palms and soles (Figure 11-3). These will disappear when the cells are further separated by additional heating and pressure. Although spores and branching and short nonbranching hyphae are seen in superficial candida infections and tinea versicolor, only branching hyphae are seen in dermatophyte infections. Longitudinal rod-shaped potassium hydroxide crystals that simulate hyphae may appear if the wet mount is heated excessively.

Culture. It is usually not necessary to know the species of dermatophyte infecting skin because the same oral and topical agents are active against all of them. Fungal culture is necessary for hair and nail fungal infections. Scalp hair infections in children may originate from an animal that carries a typical species of dermatophyte. The animal can then be traced and treated or destroyed to prevent further infection of other humans. Nail plate, especially of the toenails, may be infected with nondermatophytes, such as the saprophytic mold *Scopulariopsis,* which do not respond to griseofulvin. Identification of the genus of fungus responsible for nail plate infection is therefore necessary before embarking on a 6- to 12-month course of griseofulvin.

The two types of culture media used most often for isolation and identification are Dermatophyte Test Medium (DTM) and Sabouraud's dextrose agar. Both media contain antibiotics to inhibit the growth of bacteria and nonpathogenic fungi. Many hospital laboratories lack the experience to interpret fungal cultures and send them outside for analysis. Alternatively, many hospitals and individual practitioners now rely on DTM for faster but slightly less accurate results. DTM is a commercially available medium supplied in vials ready for direct inoculation. The yellow medium, which contains the indicator phenol red, turns red in the presence of the alkaline metabolic products of dermatophytes, but remains yellow in the presence of the acid metabolic products of nonpathogenic fungi. Species identification is possible with DTM. Material to be cultured can be sent directly to a laboratory because, unlike many bacteria, fungi will remain viable for days in scale and hair without being inoculated onto media.

Wood's light examination. Light rays with a wavelength above 365 nm are produced when ultraviolet light is projected through a Wood's filter. Hair, but not the skin of the scalp, will fluoresce with a blue-green color if infected with *Microsporum canis* or *Microsporum audouini.* The rarer *Trichophyton schoenleini* will produce a paler green fluorescence of infected hair. All other dermatophytes that infect hair will not fluoresce. Fungal infections of the skin do not fluoresce, except for tinea versicolor which fluoresces a pale white-yellow. Erythrasma, a noninflammatory pale brown scaly eruption of the toe webs, groin, and axillae caused by the bacteria *Corynebacterium minutissimum,* shows a brilliant coral-red fluorescence with the Wood's light. Wood's light examination should be performed in a dark room with a high intensity instrument.

Tinea of the foot

The feet are the most common area infected by the dermatophytes (tinea pedis, athlete's foot). Shoes promote warmth and sweating, which encourages fungal growth. Fungal infections of the feet are common in adult males, uncommon in women, and rare in children. The occurrence of tinea pedis seems to be inevitable in immunologically predisposed individuals regardless of elaborate precautions taken to avoid the infecting organism. Locker room floors contain few fungal elements and are probably not an important source of infection.[1] White socks do nothing to prevent tinea pedis. Once established, the individual becomes a carrier and is more susceptible to recurrences. There are many different clinical presentations of tinea pedis.

Clinical presentations

Toe web infection. Tight-fitting shoes compress the toes, creating a warm moist environment in the webs suited to fungal growth. The web between the fourth and fifth toe is most commonly involved, but all webs may be infected. The web can become fissured or white, macerated, and soggy (Figure 11-4). Itching is most intense when the shoes and socks are removed. Extension out of the web space onto the plantar surface or the dorsum of the foot is common. The extending lesion may have the appearance of the typical chronic ringworm type of scaly advancing border or may be an acute vesicular eruption. Identification of fungal hyphae in the macerated skin of the toe webs may be difficult.

Chronic scaly infection of the plantar surface. This is a particularly chronic form of tinea, which is resistant to treatment. The entire sole is usually infected and covered with a fine silvery-white scale (Figures 11-5 to 11-7). The skin is pink, tender, or pruritic. The hands may be similarly infected. It is rare to see both palms and soles infected simultaneously; rather, the pattern is two feet and one hand or two hands and one foot infected.

Acute vesicular tinea pedis. A highly inflammatory fungal infection may occur, particularly in people who wear occlusive shoes. This acute form of infection often originates from a more chronic web infection. A few or many vesicles evolve rapidly on the sole or on the dorsum of the foot. The vesicles may fuse into bullae (Figure 11-8) or remain as collections of fluid under the thick scale of the sole and never rupture through the surface. Secondary bacterial infection occurs commonly in eroded areas after bullae rupture. Fungal hyphae are difficult to identify in severely inflamed skin. Specimens for potassium hydroxide examination should be taken from the roof of the vesicle.

A second wave of vesicles may follow shortly in the same areas or at distant sites such as the arms, chest, and along the sides of the fingers. These itchy sterile vesicles represent an allergic response to the fungus and are termed a dermatophytid or id reaction. They subside when the infection is controlled. At times the id reaction is the only clinical manifestation of a fungus infection. Careful examination of these patients may show an asymptomatic fissure or area of maceration in the toe webs.

Treatment. Toe web infections will respond to the various topical creams and lotions listed in

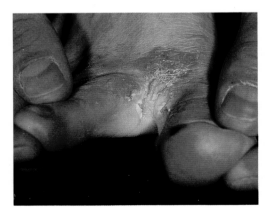

Figure 11-4
Tinea pedis (toe web infection). The toe web space contains macerated scale. Inflammation has extended from the web area onto the dorsum of the foot.

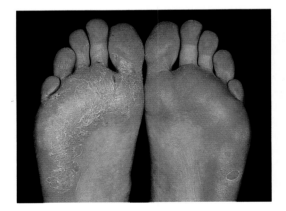

Figure 11-5
Tinea pedis. Web spaces and plantar surfaces of one foot have been inflamed for years; the other foot remains clear.

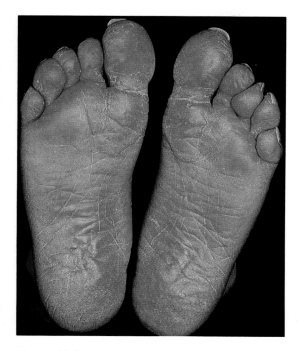

Figure 11-6
Tinea pedis. The entire plantar surfaces of both feet is thickened, tan colored, and covered with a fine white scale.

Table 11-1. Recurrence is prevented by wearing wider shoes and expanding the web space with a small strand of lamb's wool (Dr. Scholl's Lamb's Wool). Powders, not necessarily medicated, applied to the feet, rather than the shoes absorb moisture. Wet socks should be changed.

Tinea of the plantar surface responds slowly to topical therapy and may require griseofulvin for adequate control (Table 11-4). The recurrence rate is high, and additional treatment can be withheld until symptoms return.

Acute vesicular tinea pedis responds to Burow's wet compresses applied for 30 minutes several times each day. Griseofulvin should be started (Table 11-4), and topical antifungal agents applied once the macerated tissue has been dried. Lotrisone may provide rapid suppression of inflamed lesions. Secondary bacterial infection is treated with oral antibiotics. A vesicular id reaction sometimes occurs at distant sites during an inflammatory foot infection. Wet dressings and Group V topical steroids and occasionally prednisone, 20 mg twice a day, for 8 to 10 days are required for control of id reactions.

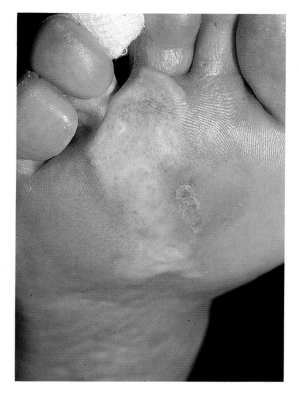

Figure 11-8
Acute vesicular tinea pedis. Inflammation appeared abruptly in a patient with chronic toe web infection after wearing heavy wet boots for several hours.

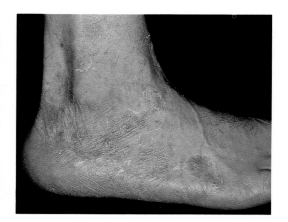

Figure 11-7
Tinea pedis. This patient has chronic inflammation of the soles that periodically flares on the dorsum and ankle.

TABLE 11-1

TOPICAL AGENTS ACTIVE AGAINST DERMATOPHYTES AND CANDIDA

Generic name	Brand name	Cream size (gm)	Lotion (ml)
Ciclopirox olamine	Loprox	15, 30, 90	
Clotrimazole	Lotrimin Mycelex	15, 30, 45, 90	10, 30
Clotrimazole, betamethasone dipropionate	Lotrisone*	15, 45	
Econazole	Spectazole	15, 30, 85	
Haloprogin	Halotex	15, 30	10, 30
Miconazole	Monistat-Derm	15, 30, 85	30, 60

*A preparation containing an antifungal agent and potent topical steroid; it is useful for inflamed fungal infections. Potent topical steroids should be used only for short durations in intertriginous areas such as the groin.

Tinea of the groin

Tinea of the groin (tinea cruris, jock itch) occurs often in the summer months after sweating or wearing wet clothing and in the winter months after wearing several layers of clothing. The predisposing factor, as with many other types of superficial infection, is the presence of a warm, moist environment. Men are affected much more frequently than women. Children rarely develop tinea of the groin. Itching becomes worse as moisture accumulates and macerates this intertriginous area.

The lesions are often bilateral and begin in the crural fold. A half-moon-shaped plaque forms as a well-defined scaling and sometimes vesicular border advances out of the crural fold onto the thigh (Figure 11-9). The skin within the border turns red-brown, is less scaly, and may develop red papules (Figure 11-10). Acute inflammation may appear after wearing occlusive clothing for an extended period (Figure 11-11). The infection occasionally migrates to the buttock and gluteal cleft area. Involvement of the scrotum is unusual, unlike candida in which it is common. Specimens for potassium hydroxide examination should be taken from the advancing scaling border.

Topical steroid creams are frequently prescribed for inflammatory skin disease of the groin and will modify the typical clinical presentation of tinea. The eruption may be much more extensive and the advancing scaly border may not be present. Red papules sometimes appear at the edges and center of the lesion (Figure 11-12). This modified form (tinea incognito) may not be immediately recognized as tinea; the only clue is the history of a typical half-moon-shaped plaque treated with cortisone cream. Scale, if present, contains numerous hyphae.

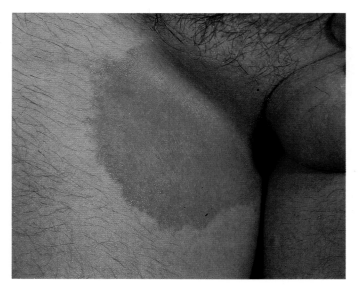

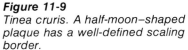

Figure 11-9
Tinea cruris. A half-moon–shaped plaque has a well-defined scaling border.

Figure 11-10
Tinea cruris. A half-moon–shaped plaque is inflamed over the entire surface.

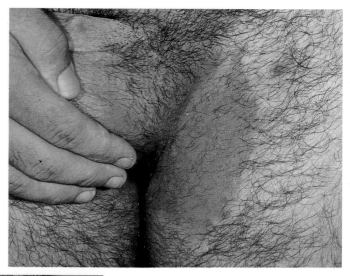

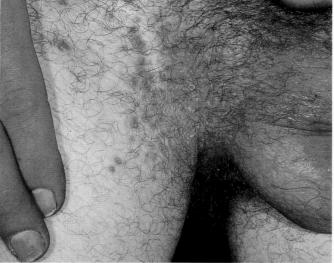

Figure 11-11
Tinea cruris. An acute dermatophyte infection occurred after working in a hot environment for an extended period. This presentation is indistinguishable from an acute candida infection.

Figure 11-12
Tinea incognito. Red papules and pustules appeared suddenly in the groin after application of a topical steroid to an area infected with dermatophytes.

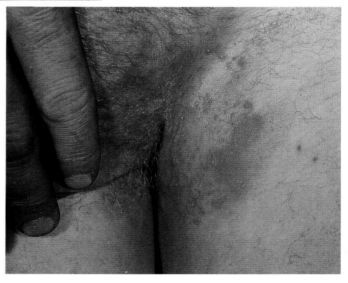

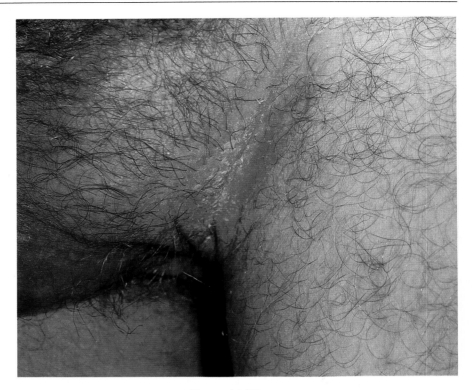

Figure 11-13
Intertrigo. A tender red plaque with a moist macerated surface extends to an equal extent onto the scrotum and thigh.

Differential diagnosis

Intertrigo. A red macerated half-moon-shaped plaque, resembling tinea of the groin and extending to an equal extent onto the groin and down the thigh, forms after moisture accumulates in the crural fold (Figure 11-13). The sharp borders touch where the opposed skin surfaces of the groin and thigh meet. Obesity predisposes to this inflammatory process, which may be infected with a mixed flora of bacteria, fungi, and yeast. Painful longitudinal fissures occur in the crease of the crural fold (Figure 11-14). Groin intertrigo recurs after treatment unless weight and moisture are controlled. Psoriasis and seborrheic dermatitis of the groin may mimic intertrigo; see the section on candida intertrigo.

Erythrasma. This bacterial infection *(Corynebacterium minutissimum)*[2] may be confused with tinea cruris because of the similar half-moon-shaped plaque (Figure 11-15). Erythrasma differs in that it is noninflammatory, is uniformly brown and scaly, has no advancing border, and fluoresces coral-red with the Wood's light. Tinea of the groin does not fluoresce. Gram stain of the scale shows gram-positive rod-like organisms in long filaments. However, the scale is difficult to fix to a slide for Gram stain. One technique is to strip the scale with clear tape, then carefully stain the tape-scale preparation. Erythrasma responds equally well to either erythromycin orally, 250 mg 4 times a day for 2 weeks, or topical erythromycin (A/T/S, Staticin, EryDerm) applied twice daily for 2 weeks. The topical erythromycins contain alcohol and may be irritating when applied to the groin.

Treatment. Tinea of the groin will respond to any of the topical antifungal creams listed in Table 11-1. Lesions may appear to respond quickly, but creams should be applied twice a day for at least 10 days. Moist intertriginous lesions may be contaminated with dermatophytes, fungus, or bacteria. Antifungal creams with activity against candida and dermatophytes (miconazole, etc.) are applied and covered with a cool wet Burow's compress for 20 to 30 minutes 2 to 6 times daily until macerated wet skin has been dried. The wet dressings are discontinued when the skin is dry, but the cream is continued for at least 14 days or until all evidence of the fungal infection has disappeared. Any residual inflammation from the intertrigo is treated with a Group V to VII topical steroid 2 times a day for a specified time (e.g., 10 days). Prescribe a limited amount of topical steroid cream to discourage long-term use. Inflamed lesions may also be treated initially with Lotrisone. Absorbent powders, not necessarily medicated (Z-Sorb, etc.), will help to control moisture but should not be applied until the inflammation is gone.

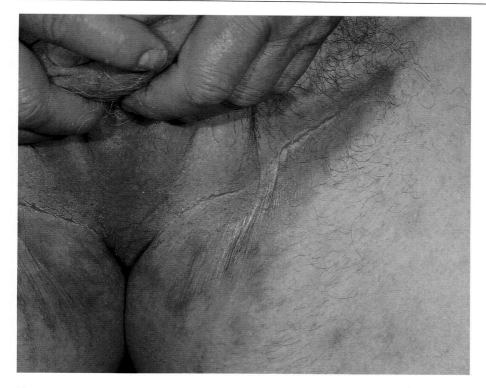

Figure 11-14
Intertrigo. An advanced case with deep longitudinal fissuring in the crural fold.

Figure 11-15
Erythrasma. A bacterial infection (Corynebacterium minutissimum). *The diffuse brown scaly plaque resembles tinea cruris.*

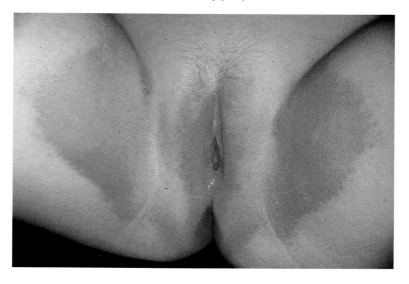

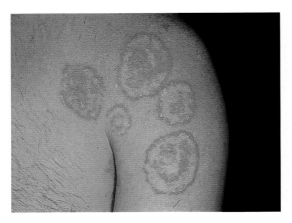

Figure 11-16
Tinea corporis. A classic presentation with an advancing red scaly border. The reason for the designation "ringworm" is obvious.

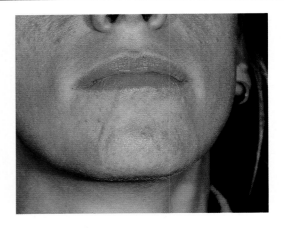

Figure 11-17
Tinea of the face. Sharply defined borders extend from the lip to the chin. The central area is hypopigmented.

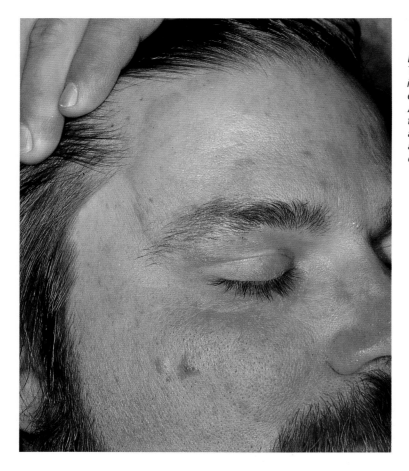

Figure 11-18
Tinea of the face. The plaque involves the forehead and central portion of the face. A sharp border occurs on the temple, across the lateral aspect of the eyebrow, and across the midportion of the cheek.

Tinea of the body and face

Tinea of the face (excluding the beard area in men), trunk, and limbs is called tinea corporis (ringworm of the body). The disease is seen at all ages and is more common in warm climates. There is a broad range of presentations, with lesions varying in size, degree of inflammation, and depth of involvement. This variability is explained by differences in host immunity and species of fungus.

Round annular lesions. In classic ringworm, lesions begin as flat, scaly spots, which then develop a raised border that extends out at variable rates in all directions. The advancing scaly border may have red raised papules or vesicles. The central area becomes brown or hypopigmented and less scaly as the active border progresses outward (Figures 11-16 to 11-18). However, it is not uncommon to see several red papules in the central area. There may be just one ring that grows to a few centimeters in diameter and then resolves or several annular lesions than enlarge to cover large areas of the body surface (Figures 11-19 and 11-20). These larger lesions tend to be mildly itchy or asymptomatic. They may reach a certain size and remain for years with no tendency to resolve. Clear central areas of the larger lesions are yellow-brown and usually contain several red papules. The borders are serpiginous or annular and quite irregular.

Pityriasis rosea and multiple small annular lesions of tinea corporis may appear to be similar. However, the scaly ring of pityriasis rosea does not reach the edge of the red border as it does in tinea. Other distinguishing features of pityriasis rosea include rapid onset of lesions and localization to the trunk. Tinea from cats may appear suddenly as multiple round-to-oval plaques on the trunk and extremities.

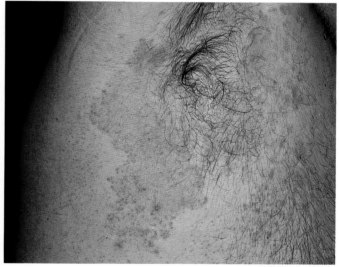

Figure 11-19
Tinea corporis. The border areas are fairly distinct and contain red papules. The central area is light brown and scaly.

Figure 11-20
Tinea corporis. A huge plaque remained fixed in location for several months.

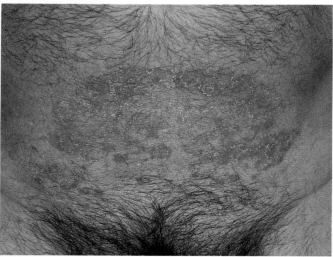

Deep inflammatory lesions. Zoophilic fungi such as *Trichophyton verrucosum* from cattle may produce a highly inflammatory skin infection.[3] The infection is more common in the north, where cattle are confined in close quarters during the winter. The round intensely inflamed lesion has a uniformly elevated red, boggy, pustular surface. The pustules are follicular and represent deep penetration of the fungus into the hair follicle (Figure 11-21). Secondary bacterial infection can occur. The process ends with brown hyperpigmentation and scarring (Figure 11-22). A fungal culture will help to identify the animal source of the infection.

A distinctive form of inflammatory tinea called Majocchi's granuloma and caused by *Trichophyton rubrum* (Figure 11-23) was originally described on the lower legs of women who shave, but it is also seen on men and at other sites.[4] The primary lesion is a follicular papulopustule or inflammatory nodule, thus the term granuloma. Lesions are single or multiple and discrete or confluent. The area involved covers a few to 10 cm and may be red and scaly, but it is not as intensely inflamed as the process just described. The border may not be well defined. Skin biopsy with special stains for fungi are required for diagnosis if hyphae cannot be demonstrated in scale or hair.

Treatment. The superficial lesions of tinea corporis respond to the antifungal creams described in Table 11-1. Lesions usually respond after 2 weeks of twice daily application, but treatment should be continued for at least 1 week after resolution of the infection. Extensive superficial lesions or those with red papules respond more predictably to 3 weeks of oral therapy (Table 11-4). The recurrence rate is high for those with extensive superficial infections. Deep inflammatory lesions require 1 to 3 or more months of oral therapy. Inflammation can be reduced with Burow's wet compresses, and bacterial infection is treated with the appropriate antibiotics. Some authors believe that oral or topical antifungal agents do not alter the course of highly inflammatory tinea (e.g., tinea verrucosum), since the intense inflammatory response destroys the organisms. However, griseofulvin is safe and there are few who would withhold such therapy.

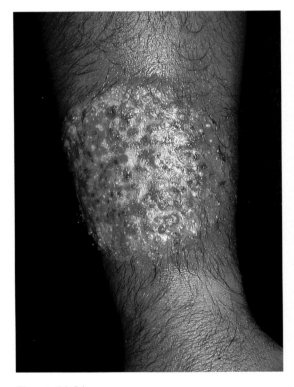

Figure 11-21
Trichophyton verrucosum. *A zoophilic fungi from cattle that causes intense inflammation in humans.*

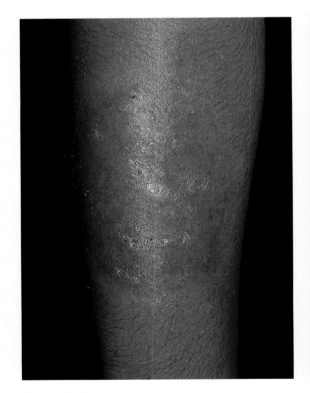

Figure 11-22
Trichophyton verrucosum. *The deep inflammatory infection has caused brown hyperpigmentation and scarring. The hair follicles were destroyed.*

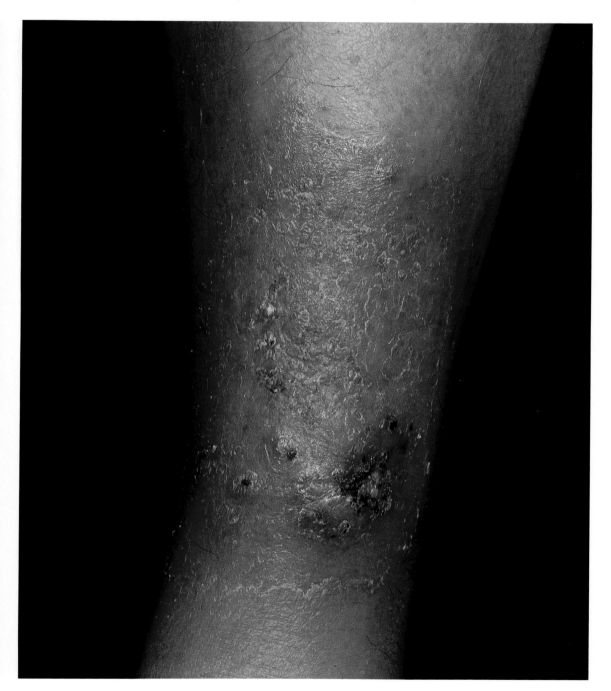

Figure 11-23
Majocchi's granuloma (Trichophyton rubrum). *A deep follicular fungal infection most often located on the lower legs of women.*

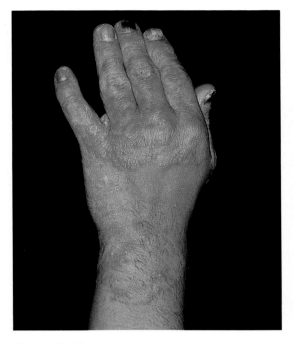

Figure 11-24
Tinea of the hand and wrist. The infected areas are red with little or no scale. Note infection of the fingernails.

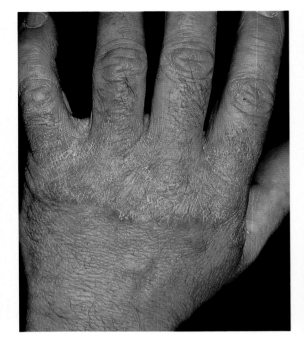

Figure 11-25
Tinea of the hand. There is a well defined red border. Scaling is present, in contrast to the case illustrated in Figure 11-24.

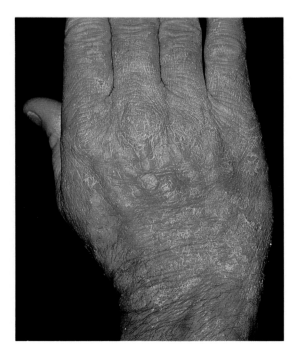

Tinea of the hand

Tinea of the dorsal aspect of the hand (tinea manuum) has all of the features of tinea corporis; tinea of the palm has the same appearance as the dry, diffuse, keratotic form of tinea on the soles (Figures 11-24 to 11-26). The dry keratotic form may be asymptomatic and the patient may be unaware of the infection, attributing the dry thick scaly surface to hard physical labor (Figure 11-27). Tinea of the palms is frequently seen in association with tinea pedis. The usual pattern of infection is to have one foot and two hands or two feet and one hand involved. Fingernail infection often accompanies infection of the dorsum of the hand or palm. Treatment is the same as for tinea pedis; as with the soles, a high recurrence rate can be expected for palm infection.

Figure 11-26
Tinea of the hand. There is diffuse erythema and scaling simulating contact dermatitis. Compare this presentation with the case of tinea pedis in Figure 11-7.

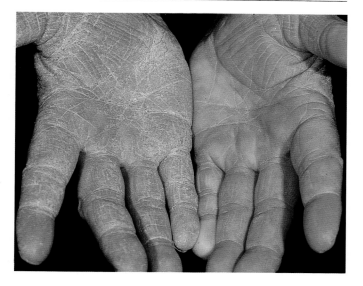

Figure 11-27
Tinea of the palm. The involved palm is thickened, very dry, and scaly. The patient is often unaware of the infection and feels that these changes are secondary to dry skin or hard physical labor.

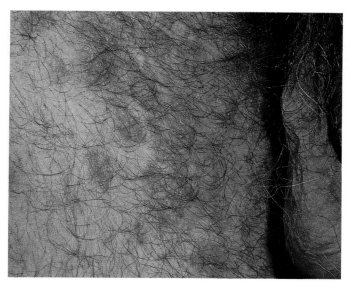

Figure 11-28
Tinea incognito. A Group IV topical steroid was applied to the area of tinea cruris for 3 weeks. Characteristic features of tinea are missing.

Tinea incognito

Fungal infections treated only with topical steroids often lose some of their characteristic features. Topical steroids decrease inflammation and give the false impression that the rash is improving while the fungus actually flourishes secondary to cortisone-induced immunologic changes. Treatment is stopped, the rash returns, and memory of the good initial response prompts reuse of the steroid cream, but by this time the rash has changed. Scaling at the margins may be absent. Diffuse erythema, diffuse scale, scattered pustules or papules, and brown hyperpigmentation may all result (Figures 11-12 and 11-28). A well-defined border may not be present and a once-localized process may have expanded greatly. The intensity of itching is variable. Tinea incognito is most often seen in the groin and on the face and dorsal aspect of the hand.[5] Tinea infections of the hands are often misdiagnosed as eczema and treated with topical steroids. Hyphae are easily demonstrated, especially a few days after discontinuing use of the steroid cream.

Tinea of the scalp

Tinea of the scalp (tinea capitis) is a disease that occurs almost exclusively in prepubertal children. The infection has several different presentations. The infection originates from contact with a pet or an infected person. Each animal is associated with a limited number of fungal species; therefore, an attempt should be made to identify the fungus by culture to help locate and treat a possible animal source. Unlike other fungal infections, tinea of the scalp may be contagious by direct contact or from contaminated clothing; this provides some justification for briefly isolating those with proven infection. A systematic approach is presented for the clinical and laboratory investigations of tinea capitis (Table 11-2). The inflammatory response to infection is variable. Noninflammatory tinea of the scalp is illustrated in Figure 11-29. A severe inflammatory reaction with a boggy indurated tumor-like mass that exudes pus is called a kerion (Figure 11-30). It represents a hypersensitivity reaction to fungus and heals with scarring and some hair loss (Figure 11-31). The hair loss is less than would be expected from the degree and depth of inflammation.

Differential diagnosis. Seborrheic dermatitis and psoriasis may be confused with tinea of the scalp. A particular form of seborrheic dermatitis in children called tinea amiantacea is frequently misdiagnosed as tinea. A localized 2- to 8-cm patch of large brown polygonal-shaped scales adheres to the scalp and mats the hair. The matted scale grows out attached to the hair (see Figure 8-24). There is little or no inflammation.

Treatment. Griseofulvin is the treatment of choice. Patients with tinea capitis should be treated 2 weeks beyond the time when cultures and potassium hydroxide preparations become negative. This generally requires at least 4 weeks of treatment (see Table 11-4). Continuous daily treatment is desirable, but unreliable patients can be treated with a single 4-gm dose of microsized griseofulvin that has been pulverized and mixed with food. This single dose schedule gives a high cure rate in noninflammatory tinea capitis.[6] A few authors have suggested suppressing the inflammation of a kerion with oral or intralesional steroids.[7] Although this seems reasonable, there has been little experience with this practice.

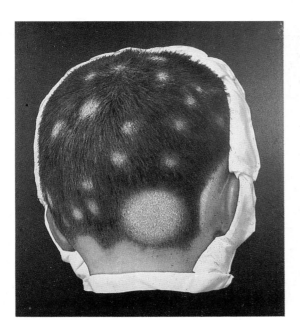

Figure 11-29
Tinea capitis ("gray patch ringworm").
Noninflammatory tinea of the scalp.

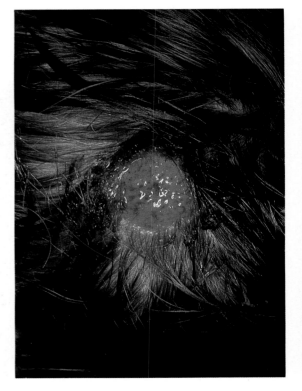

Figure 11-30
Tinea capitis. A severely inflammatory boggy
indurated tumor-like mass (kerion).

Figure 11-31
Tinea capitis. A huge kerion healed after 2 months of treatment with griseofulvin. The scalp is scarred, and hair follicles have been destroyed.

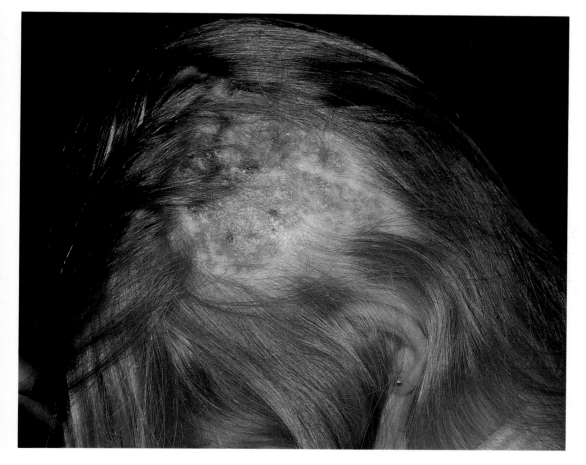

TABLE 11-2

SYSTEMATIC APPROACH TO INVESTIGATION OF TINEA CAPITAS

DETERMINE CLINICAL PRESENTATION

Most forms of tinea capitis present with one or several round patches of scale or alopecia. Inflammatory lesions would, even if untreated, tend to resolve spontaneously in a few months; the noninflammatory infections are more chronic.

Patchy alopecia + fine dry scale + no inflammation
    Short stubs of broken hair ("gray patch ringworm")
        M audouini (Figure 11-29)
    Hairs broken off at surface ("black dot ringworm")
        T tonsurans (most common), *T violaceum*

Patchy alopecia + swelling + purulent discharge
    M canis, T mentagrophytes (granular), *T verrucosum*

Kerion is a severe inflammatory reaction with boggy induration. Any fungus but especially
    M canis, T mentagrophytes (granular), *T verrucosum* (Figures 11-22 and 11-30)

WOOD'S LIGHT EXAMINATION

Blue-green fluorescence of hair—only *M canis* and *M audouini* have this feature. Scale and skin do not fluoresce.

POTASSIUM HYDROXIDE WET MOUNT OF PLUCKED HAIRS

The pattern of hair invasion is characteristic for each species of fungus. Hairs that can be removed with little resistance are best for evaluation.

Large spore endothrix pattern-chains of large spores (densely packed) within the hair, "like a sack full of marbles."
    T tonsurans, T violaceum (Figure 11-32)

Large spore ectothrix pattern-chains of large spores inside and on the surface of the hair shaft and visible with the low power objective
    T verrucosum, T mentagrophytes (Figure 11-33)

Small spore ectothrix—small spores randomly arranged in masses inside and on the surface of the hair shaft, not visible with the low power objective. Looks like a stick dipped in maple syrup and rolled in sand.
    M canis, M audouini

IDENTIFICATION OF SOURCE AFTER SPECIES IS VERIFIED BY CULTURE

Anthropophilic (parasitic on humans)—infection from other humans
    M audouini, T tonsurans, T violaceum

Zoophilic (parasitic on animals)—infection from animals or other infected humans
    M canis—dog, cat, monkey
    T mentagrophytes (granular)—dog, rabbit, guinea pig, monkey
    T verrucosum—cattle

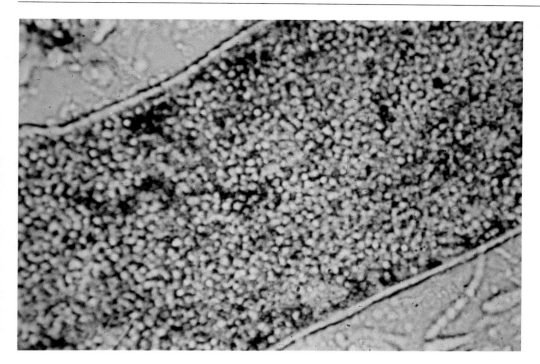

Figure 11-32
Large spore endothrix pattern of hair invasion.
T tonsurans *("a sack of marbles").*

Figure 11-33
Large spore ectothrix pattern of hair invasion.
T verrucosum.

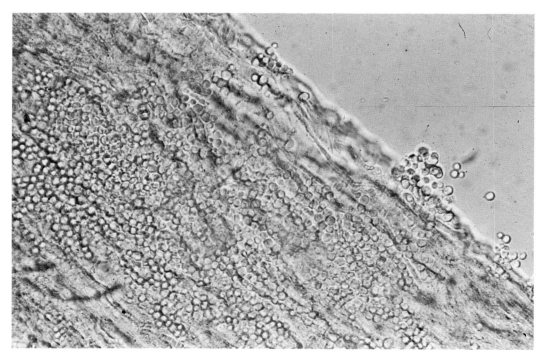

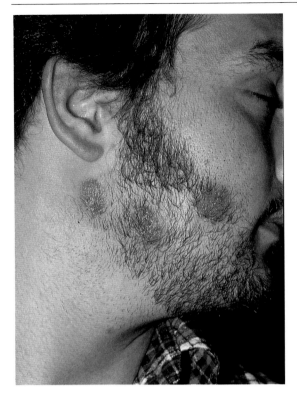

Figure 11-34
Tinea barbae. Inflamed areas are indurated and eroded on the surface. Hairs may be painlessly removed. Removal of beard hair in bacterial infections is usually painful.

Figure 11-35
A potassium hydroxide wet mount of a plucked hair from the patient in Figure 11-34. Numerous hyphae surround the base of the hair shaft.

Tinea of the beard

Fungal infection of the beard area (tinea barbae) should be considered when inflammation occurs in this area. Bacterial folliculitis and inflammation secondary to ingrown hairs (pseudofolliculitis) are common. However, it is not unusual to see patients who have finally been diagnosed as having tinea after failing to respond to several courses of antibiotics. A positive culture for staphylococcus does not rule out tinea, in which purulent lesions may be secondarily infected with bacteria. Like tinea capitis, the hairs are almost always infected and easily removed. The hairs in bacterial folliculitis resist removal.

Superficial infection. This pattern resembles the annular lesions of tinea corporis. The hair is usually infected.

Deep follicular infection. This pattern clinically resembles bacterial folliculitis except that it is slower to evolve and is usually restricted to one area of the beard. Bacterial folliculitis spreads rapidly over wide areas after shaving. Tinea begins insidiously with a small group of follicular pustules. The process becomes confluent in time with the development of a boggy, erythematous, tumor-like abscess covered with dense superficial crust (Figure 11-34). Hairs may be painlessly removed at almost any stage of the infection and examined for hyphae (Figure 11-35). Zoophilic *T mentagrophytes* and *T verrucosum* are the most common pathogens. Species identification by culture will help identify the possible animal reservoir of infection.

Treatment. Treatment is the same as that for tinea capitis. Griseofulvin is required because creams will not penetrate to the depths of the hair follicle.

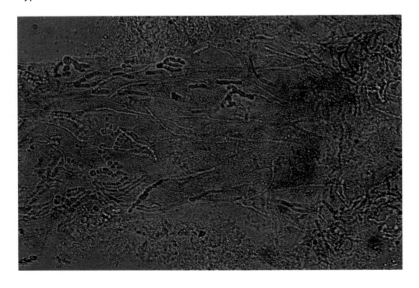

TABLE 11-3

OVER-THE-COUNTER TOPICAL AGENTS ACTIVE AGAINST DERMATOPHYTES

Generic name	Brand name	Cream size (gm)	Lotion (ml)
Miconazole	Micatin*	15, 30	
Tolnaftate	Tinactin*	15	10
Undecylenic acid	Desenex*	0.9 oz	1.5 oz

*Powder and aerosol are available.

TABLE 11-4

GRISEOFULVIN: TREATMENT GUIDELINES

Site of involvement	Duration of treatment	Dosage for ultramicrosize form (mg/kg/day)
Scalp	4-8 weeks	7-10
Skin	2-4 weeks	5-7
Palms and soles	8-12 weeks	5-7
Fingernails	4-9 months	7-10
Toenails	6-18 months	10-15

Treatment of fungal infections

Topical preparations. A variety of preparations is commercially available. Recent studies have shown that undecylenic acid (Desenex, etc.) may be almost as effective for treating dermatophyte infections as all of the newer agents.[8] Most of the medicines are available as creams or lotions; some are available as powders or aerosols. They are effective for all dermatophyte infections except for deep inflammatory lesions of the body and scalp. They have no effect on tinea of the nail. Creams or lotions should be applied twice a day until the infection is clear. Tables 11-1 and 11-3 list the available topical agents.

Systemic agents. Griseofulvin is active only against dermatophytes. The drug has been available for over 20 years and has proved to be safe. Headache is the most common complaint; it usually occurs during the first few days of treatment and may disappear as treatment is continued. A trial at a lower dose level is warranted for those with headache lasting more than 48 hours. Patients with persistant headache after a trial at a lower dose will need alternative treatment. Bone marrow suppression, once attributed to griseofulvin, probably never occurs and routine complete blood counts are not necessary. Gastrointestinal upset, urticaria, photosensitivity, and morbilliform skin eruptions have been reported. Griseofulvin activates hepatic enzymes that cause degradation of warfarin and other drugs.[9] Appropriate steps should be taken if combined treatment is used.

Dosage. The dosage should be adequate. Reported treatment failures are probably a result of using too small a dose rather than resistant organisms.

Griseofulvin. Griseofulvin has a sustained blood level so that a once or twice a day schedule is adequate. The medication is best absorbed when taken with food containing fat or with whole milk.[10] Two preparations are available—microsize and ultramicrosize. The newer ultramicrosized forms are better absorbed and require about 50% to 70% of the dose of the microsized form. Many brands are available in both forms. The supply is microsize 125 mg, 250 mg, and 500 mg tablets, and for adults and children, the dosage is 10 mg/kg/day. In ultramicrosize the supply is 125-, 165-, 250-, and 330-mg tablets. The recommended dosage and duration of therapy for the ultramicrosize form is listed in Table 11-4.

Ketoconazole. Ketoconazole is an oral imidazole with a wider spectrum of action than griseofulvin. It is active against dermatophytes,[11] candida,[12] tinea versicolor, and deep fungal infections[13] such as histoplasmosis. Preliminary studies indicate that it is more effective than griseofulvin for resistant areas such as the toenails.[14] Toxicity is minimal, although there are some reports of hepatitis with jaundice and elevated liver enzymes.[15] One study reported that gynecomastia occurred in 5% of male patients treated with ketoconazole.[16] As of this time ketaconazole is approved by the FDA only for candida and deep fungal infections, for which the dosage is 200 to 400 mg once a day.

Candidiasis (Moniliasis)

The yeast-like fungus *Candida albicans* and a few other *Candida* species are capable of producing skin, mucous membrane, and internal infections. The organism lives with the normal flora of the mouth, vaginal tract, and gut and reproduces by the budding of oval yeast forms. Pregnancy, oral contraception, antibiotic therapy, diabetes, skin maceration, topical steroid therapy, certain endocrinopathies, and factors related to depression of cell-mediated immunity may allow the yeast to become pathogenic and produce budding spores and elongated cells (pseudohyphae) or true hyphae with septate walls. The pseudohyphae and hyphae are indistinguishable from dermatophytes in potassium hydroxide preparations (Figure 11-36). Culture results must be interpreted carefully because the yeast is part of the normal flora in many areas.

The yeast infects only the outer layers of the epithelium of mucous membrane and skin (the stratum corneum). The primary lesion is a pustule, the contents of which dissect horizontally under the stratum corneum and peel it away. Clinically, this process results in a red denuded glistening surface with a long, cigarette paper–like, scaling, advancing border. The infected mucous membranes of the mouth and vaginal tract accumulate scale and inflammatory cells that develop into characteristic white or white-yellow curdy material.

Figure 11-36
Candida albicans. *A potassium hydroxide wet mount of skin scrapings showing both elongated pseudohyphae and budding spores.*

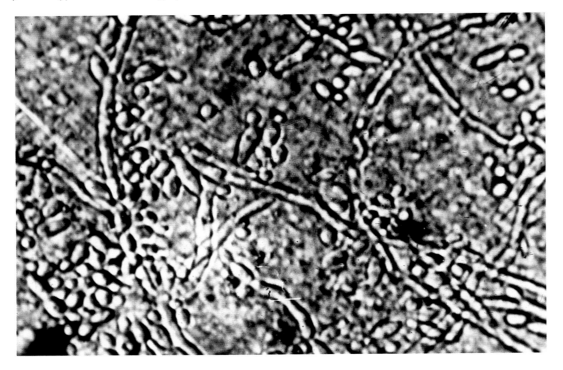

Yeast grows best in a warm moist environment; therefore, infection is usually confined to the mucous membranes and intertriginous areas. The advancing infected border usually stops when dry skin is reached.

Candidiasis of normally moist areas

Candidiasis affects normally moist areas such as the vagina, the mouth, and the uncircumcised penis. In the vagina it causes vulvovaginitis; in the mouth, it causes thrush, and in the uncircumcised penis, it causes balanitis.

Vulvovaginitis

Candida is present in the normal flora of the vaginal tract and rectum in some women. Heat and moisture are increased under large folds of fat and occlusive undergarments. Symptoms may worsen a few days before menstruation. Candida, which often coexists with trichomonas infection, usually begins with vaginal itching and/or a white thin-to-creamy discharge. Symptoms may resolve spontaneously after several days or they may progress. The vaginal mucous membranes and external genitalia become red, swollen, and sometimes eroded. They are covered with a thick, white, crumbly discharge, which becomes more copious during pregnancy. The infection may spread onto the thighs and anus, producing a tender red skin surface with discrete pustules, called satellite lesions, ahead of the advancing border. The diagnosis is confirmed by a potassium hydroxide preparation of the discharge.

Therapeutic goals include elimination of the fungus and correction of predisposing factors. Patients with recurrent disease should be advised to lose excess weight and wear loose-fitting cotton undergarments. Reducing the number of yeast in the gastrointestinal tract with nystatin and attempting to restore normal flora with *Lactobacillus* preparations may be useful in the resistant case.

Miconazole (Monistat 7 vaginal cream). One applicator is administered intravaginally once at bedtime for 7 days. The course should be continued for another 7 days if symptoms have not subsided. Similar cure rates have been reported when inserts were used twice a day for 3 days.

Clotrimazole (Gyne-Lotrimin vaginal tablets or Mycelex-G). Gyne-Lotrimin tablets (seven tablets per package) or Mycelex-G (1% vaginal cream in a 45-gm tube or seven tablets per package) are available. The tablet or cream is inserted intravaginally at bedtime with the plastic applicator. The course should be continued for another 7 days if signs or symptoms persist. Cream is useful if the external areas are also infected. The cream will run out and coat the vulva; cream may also be applied directly from the 45-gm tube. Enough cream is supplied for both external and internal application.

Nystatin (Mycostatin vaginal tablets). One tablet is placed with the applicator high in the vaginal tract twice a day for 2 weeks. The duration of treatment is extended if signs or symptoms persist. Although nystatin must be used longer than miconazole or clotrimazole, it is still an effective and safe medicine.

Gentian violet. This purple dye has been used for years and is a safe effective agent that has both antiyeast and antibacterial activity. A sanitary napkin will prevent staining of clothing. Gentian violet may be useful in resistant cases in which long periods of treatment are required. A number of preparations are available, such as GVS (0.4% in a water-washable base; 12 vaginal inserts with applicator), Hyva (2 mg/tablet, 14 or 28 tablets with applicator), and Genapax (5 mg/tampon in a package of 12 tampons). They should be used once or twice a day for at least 7 days or until symptoms have cleared.

Ketoconazole (Nizoral). Studies have shown oral ketoconazole (available as Nizoral in a 200-mg oral tablet) is as effective as miconazole vaginal creams in eradicating the yeast, but the recurrence rate may be higher with ketoconazole.[17,18]

Treating resistant cases. Some women have repeated or ongoing infection even after several courses of intravaginal antiyeast therapy. Recontamination from the rectal area may be the cause. The number of yeast in the gastrointestinal tract can be reduced by giving one or two tablets of nystatin (Mycostatin oral tablets 500,000 units per tablet) 3 times a day for 2 weeks. Intravaginal antiyeast creams or tablets are used simultaneously. *Lactobacillus* preparations (Lactinex tablets or granules or Bacid capsules) given during and after the treatment period may help to restore the normal flora. Other predisposing factors for recurrence should be ruled out. Oral contraceptives may have to be discontinued.

Oral candidiasis

Candida albicans may be transmitted to the infant's oral cavity during passage through the birth canal. It constitutes part of the normal mouth flora in many adults.

Infants. Oral candidiasis in children is called thrush. Healthy newborn infants, especially if premature, are susceptible. Thrush in older infants usually occurs in the presence of predisposing factors such as antibiotic treatment or debilitation. Thrush in the healthy newborn is a self-limited infection, but should be treated to avoid interference with feeding. The infection presents as a white, creamy exudate or white, flaky, adherent plaques. The underlying mucosa is red and sore. The mother should be examined for vaginal candidiasis.

Adults. Oral candidiasis in the adult occurs for several reasons and clinically is found in a variety of acute and chronic forms. Extensive oral infection may occur in diabetics, patients with depressed cell-mediated immunity, the elderly, and patients with cancer (especially leukemia). Inhalant steroids may also cause infection.

The acute process is similar to the infantile infection. The tongue is almost always involved (Figure 11-37). Infection may spread into the trachea or esophagus and cause painful erosions, presenting as dysphagia, or on to the skin at the angles of the mouth (perlèche). A specimen may be taken by gently scraping with a tongue blade. Pseudohyphae are easily demonstrated. In other cases the oral cavity may be red, swollen, and sore with little or no exudate (Figure 11-38). In this instance pseudo-hyphae are often difficult to find and treatment may have to be started without laboratory verification.

Chronic infection appears as localized, firmly adherent plaques with an irregular, velvety surface on the buccal mucosa. They may occur from the mechanical trauma of cheek biting, pipe smoking, or irritation from dentures. A biopsy is indicated to rule out leukoplakia if organisms cannot be demonstrated.

Localized erythema and erosions with minimal white exudate may result from candida infection beneath dentures and is commonly called "denture sore mouth." The border is usually sharply defined. Hyperplasia with thickening of the mucosa occurs if the process is long lasting. The gums and hard palate are most frequently involved. Organisms may be difficult to find.

Nystatin oral suspension. For infants, treatment is 2 ml of nystatin oral suspention 4 times a day (1 ml in each side of the mouth). For adults, the dose is 4 to 6 ml 4 times a day (with one-half of the dose in each side of the mouth) retained in the mouth as long as possible before swallowing. Treatment is continued for 48 hours after symptoms have disappeared; a 10-day course is typical. The oral suspension is useful for infants, but less effective for adults, probably because the liquid may not come in contact with the entire surface of the oral cavity. The medication is very expensive.

Mycelex troches. Children and adults are effectively treated by slowly dissolving a clotrimazole (Mycelex) troche in the mouth 5 times each day for 14 days.

Figure 11-37
Oral candidiasis. On the sides of the tongue are white plaques on an erythematous base.

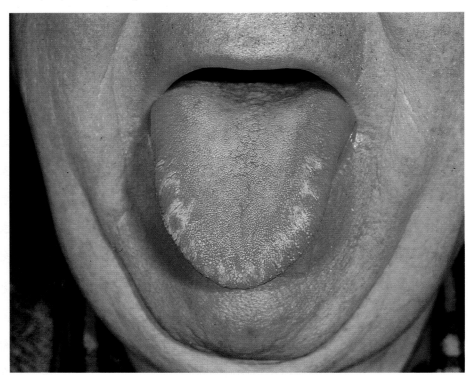

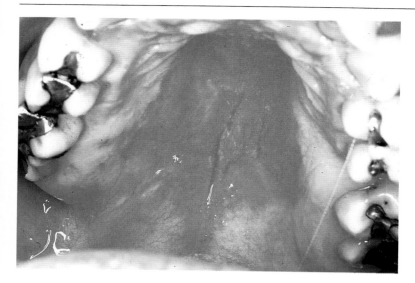

Figure 11-38
Oral candidiasis. The hard palate is red and swollen.

Gentian violet. Gentian violet is available from Purepac as a 1% or 2% aqueous solution in a 1-oz bottle. The oral cavity of infants or adults is painted with this purple solution twice a day. The medicine lasts longer than nystatin when applied directly to the affected areas and is probably more effective; unfortunately, it spreads easily to clothing and produces stains. Irritation may occur if swallowed; therefore, the 1% solution should be used in children.

Ketoconazole (Nizoral). Preliminary studies of this drug were promising; ketoconazole (Nizoral, 200-mg tablets) may be the drug of choice in resistant cases.[19-21]

Candida balanitis

The uncircumsized penis provides the warm moist environment ideally suited for yeast infection, but the circumsized male is also at risk. Tender, pinpoint red papules and pustules appear on the glans and shaft of the penis and may occur after intercourse with an infected female. The pustules rupture quickly under the foreskin and may not be noticed (Figure 11-39). A typical picture of 1- to 2-mm white, doughnut-shaped, possibly confluent rings is seen after the pustules break. Some cases never evolve pustules and the multiple red papules may be transient, resolving without treatment. The infection may occur and persist without sexual exposure.

Treatment. The eruption responds quickly to twice daily applications for 10 days of any of the creams listed in Table 11-1. Relief is almost immediate, but treatment should be continued for 10 days. Topical steroid creams (Groups VI and VII) may be used with antifungal agents when inflamma-

tion is intense. Each preparation is applied twice each day but not simultaneously. Topical steroid creams when used as the only therapeutic agent will give temporary relief by suppressing inflammation, but the eruption will rebound and worsen, sometimes even before the cortisone cream is discontinued.

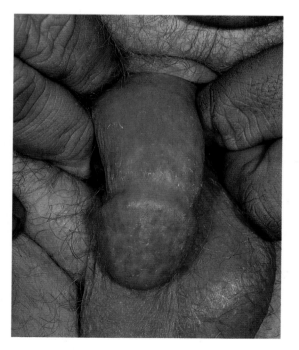

Figure 11-39
Candida balanitis. Multiple red round erosions are present on the glans and shaft of the penis.

Candidiasis of large skin folds

Candidiasis of large skin folds (candida intertrigo) occurs under pendulous breasts, between overhanging abdominal folds, in the groin and rectal area, and in the axillae. Skin folds (intertriginous areas in which skin touches skin) contain heat and moisture, providing the environment suited for yeast infection. Hot humid weather, tight or abrasive underclothing, poor hygiene, and other inflammatory diseases occurring in the skin folds (e.g., psoriasis) make a yeast infection more likely. The clinical presentation is similar in all cases. A red moist glistening base extends to or just beyond the limits of the opposing skin folds. The advancing border is long and sharply defined from normal skin and is led by an ocean wave–shaped fringe of macerated scale (Figures 11-40 and 11-41). The characteristic pustule of candidiasis is not observed in intertriginous areas because it is macerated away as soon as it forms. Pinpoint pustules do appear outside the advancing border and are an important diagnostic feature when present (Figure 11-42). There is a tendency for painful fissuring in the skin creases.

Treatment. Eradication of the yeast infection must be accompanied by maintenance of dryness in the area. A cool wet Burow's compress is applied for 20 to 30 minutes several times each day to promote dryness. Antifungal cream is applied in a thin layer twice a day until the rash clears. Some of these medicines are also available in lotion form, but the liquid base may cause stinging when applied to intertriginous areas. Monistat-Derm lotion (miconazole) is the least irritating. Topical steroid creams (Groups VI and VII) may be used with antifungal agents when inflammation is intense. Each preparation is applied twice each day but not simultaneously. Compresses should be continued until the skin remains dry. Heat from a gooseneck lamp held several inches away from the involved site is sometimes useful to enhance drying. An absorbent powder, not necessarily medicated, such as Z-Sorb may be applied after the inflammation is gone. The powder absorbs a small amount of moisture and acts as a dry lubricant, allowing skin surfaces to slide freely, thus preventing moisture accumulation in a potentially stagnant area.

Figure 11-40
Candidiasis of the axillae. A prominent fringe of scale is present at the border.

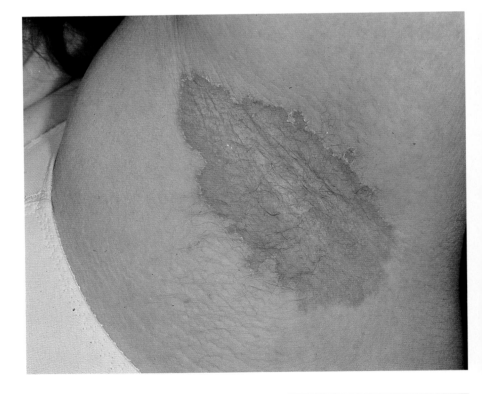

Figure 11-41
Candida intertrigo. The overhanging abdominal fold and groin area are infected in this obese patient.

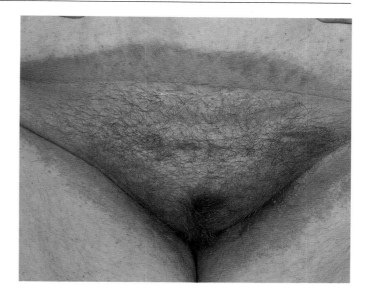

Figure 11-42
Candida intertrigo. An acute infection. The fringe of scale is present on the opposing borders. There are numerous satellite pustules beyond the intertriginous area.

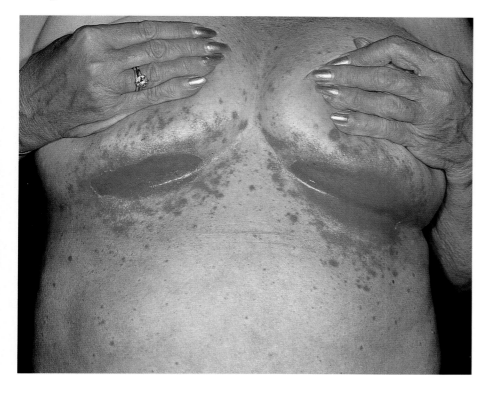

Diaper candidiasis

An artificial intertriginous area is created under a wet diaper, predisposing to a yeast infection with the characteristic red base and satellite pustules as described above (Figure 11-43). Diaper dermatitis is often treated with steroid combination creams that also contain antibiotics. Although these creams may contain the antiyeast agent nystatin, its concentration may not be sufficient to control the yeast infection. The cortisone component may alter the clinical presentation and prolong the disease. A nodular granulomatous form of candidiasis in the diaper area presenting as dull, red, irregularly shaped nodules, sometimes on a red base, has recently been described and may represent an unusual reaction to candida or a candida infection modified by steroids (Figure 11-44).[22] Every effort should be made to identify the organism and treat appropriately.

Treatment. Maintain dryness by changing the diaper frequently or leaving it off for short periods. Apply antifungal creams twice a day until the eruption is clear, about 10 days. Some erythema from irritation may be present after 10 days; this can be treated by alternately applying 1% hydrocortisone cream followed in a few hours by creams active against yeasts (Table 11-1). Apply each agent 2 times a day. Baby powders may help to prevent recurrence by absorbing moisture.

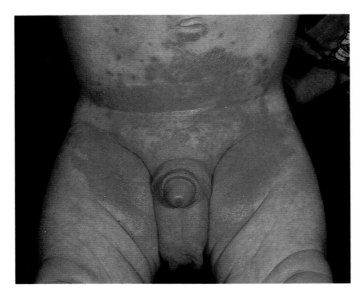

Figure 11-43
Diaper candidiasis. The skin folds are deeply erythematous. The urethral meatus is infected and numerous satellite pustules are on the lower abdominal area.

Figure 11-44
Nodular candidiasis of the diaper area. Red nodules are present on a red base and beyond the diffusely inflamed area. The patient had been treated with a cream containing corticosteroids, neomycin, and antifungal agents.

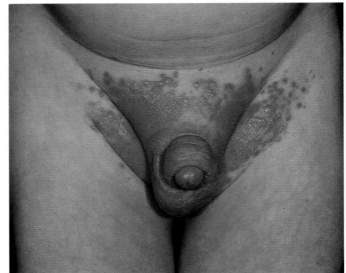

Candidiasis of small skin folds

Finger and toe webs. Web spaces are like small intertriginous areas. Cooks, bartenders, dishwashers, dentists, and others who work in a moist environment are at risk. White, tender, macerated skin erodes, revealing a pink moist base (Figures 11-45 and 11-46). Candida infection of the toe webs occurs most commonly in the narrow interspace between the fourth and fifth toes, where it may coexist with dermatophytes and gram-negative bacteria. Clinically and in potassium hydroxide preparations, candida and dermatophyte infection may appear identical. Macerated white scale becomes thick and adherent. Diffuse candidiasis of the webs and feet is unusual. Both areas are treated with any of the anti-

fungal creams or lotions listed in Table 11-1. Strands of lamb's wool (Dr. Scholl's lamb's wool) can be placed between the toe webs to separate and promote dryness.

Angles of the mouth. Angular cheilitis or perlèche, an inflammation at the angles of the mouth, can occur at any age. Patients may believe they have a vitamin B deficiency. Yeast and bacteria may be involved in the process. Lip licking or biting the corners of the mouth causes perlèche in the young. Continued irritation may lead to eczematous inflammation. A moist intertriginous space forms as skin folds appear at the angles of the mouth with advancing age. Capillary action draws fluid from the mouth into the fold, creating the nec-

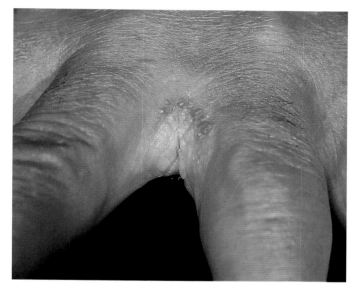

Figure 11-45
Candida of the finger web. The acute phase with maceration of the web. Pustules are present at the border.

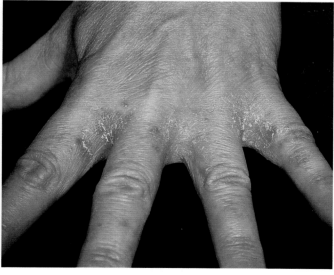

Figure 11-46
Candidiasis of the finger webs. All webs are infected except the wide space between the thumb and index finger.

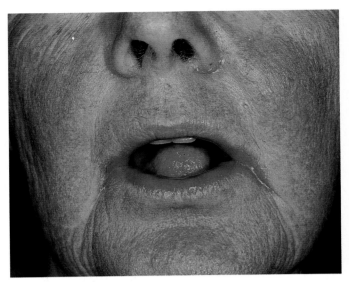

Figure 11-47
Angular cheilitis (perlèche). Skin folds at the angles of the mouth are red and eroded.

essary conditions for infection. Poorly fitting dentures may stimulate excess salivation.

The infection starts as a sore fissure in the depth of the skin fold (Figure 11-47). Erythema, scale, and crust form at the sides of the fold. Patients lick and moisten the area in an attempt to prevent further cracking. This attempt at relief only aggravates the problem and may lead to eczematous inflammation, staphylococcal infection, or hypertrophy of the skin fold.

Treatment consists of applying antifungal creams (Table 11-1), followed in a few hours by a Group V steroid cream with a nongreasy base (such as Aristocort-A 0.1%) until the area is dry and free of inflammation. Thereafter, a thick protective lip balm such as Chap Stick is applied frequently.

Chronic mucocutaneous candidiasis

The syndrome chronic mucocutaneous candidiasis occurs with a variety of endocrine and immunologic deficiencies associated with the inability of T lymphocytes to react to candida antigen.[23] The disease usually begins in early childhood with yeast infections of the fingernails, mouth, and skin. The hypertrophic fingernail infection is characteristic and is rarely seen as an isolated phenomenon without the other stigmata of this syndrome (see the chapter on nail disease). Thick yeast-infected crusted masses occur in the scalp and sometimes on the skin. The entire oral cavity is lined with white adherent debris. Systemic candidiasis is rare. Ketoconazole is now the treatment of choice.[24]

Tinea Versicolor

Tinea versicolor is a common fungal infection of the skin caused by the lipophilic yeast *Pityrosporon orbiculare (Malassezia furfur)*. The organism is part of the normal skin flora and appears in highest numbers in areas with increased sebaceous activity. Excess heat and humidity, predisposing genetic factors, or Cushing's syndrome produced by disease or corticosteroid therapy may lower the patient's resistance and allow this normally nonpathogenic resident to proliferate in the upper layers of the stratum corneum. Whether the disease is contagious or not is unknown. The disease may occur at any age, but is much more common during the years of higher sebaceous activity (i.e., adolescence and young adulthood). Some individuals, especially those with oily skin, may be more susceptible.

Clinical presentation. The individual lesions and distribution are highly characteristic. Lesions begin as multiple small circular macules of various colors (white, pink, or brown) which enlarge radially (Figures 11-48 to 11-51). The lesions may be hyperpigmented in blacks. The color is uniform in each individual. The lesions may be inconspicuous in fair complected individuals during the winter. White hypopigmentation becomes more obvious as unaffected skin tans. The lack of tanning used to be attributed to the sunscreening effect of the slightly thick scaly stratum corneum, but inhibition of tyrosinase in skin melanocytes has been proposed as the reason for the relative lack of pigmentation. The upper trunk is most commonly affected, but spread

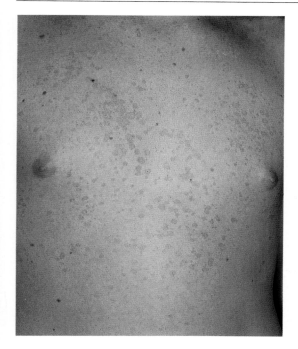

Figure 11-48
*Tinea versicolor. Numerous circular scaly lesions.
The eruption is light brown or fawn colored in fair
complected untanned skin.*

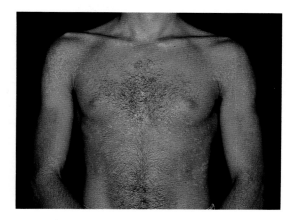

Figure 11-49
*Tinea versicolor. Numerous circular lesions. The
infected areas appear white in dark complected
or tanned skin.*

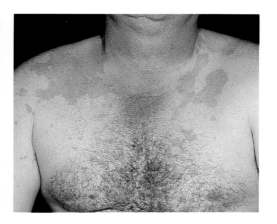

Figure 11-50
*Tinea versicolor. Broad confluent scaly patches in
a fair skinned individual.*

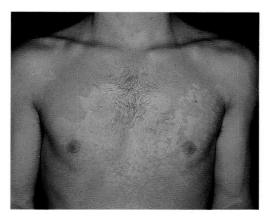

Figure 11-51
*Tinea versicolor. Broad confluent scaly patches in
a patient with a dark tan.*

to the upper arms, neck, and abdomen is not unusual. Involvement of the face, dorsal hands, and legs can occur. The eruption may itch if inflammatory, but it is usually asymptomatic. The disease may vary in activity for years, but diminishes or disappears with advancing age. The differential diagnosis includes vitiligo, pityriasis alba, seborrheic dermatitis, secondary syphilis, and pityriasis rosea.

Diagnosis. A powdery scale that may not be obvious on inspection can easily be demonstrated by scraping lightly with a #15 surgical blade (Figure 11-52). Potassium hydroxide examination of the scale shows numerous hyphae that tend to break into short rod-shaped fragments intermixed with round spores in grape-like clusters, giving the so-called spaghetti-and-meatballs pattern (Figure 11-53). Wood's light examination shows irregular pale yellow-to-white fluorescence that fades with improvement. Culture is possible but rarely necessary.

Treatment. Griseofulvin is not active against tinea versicolor. A variety of medicines will eliminate the fungus, but relief is usually temporary and recurrences are common. Patients must understand that the hypopigmented areas will not disappear immediately after treatment. Sunlight will accelerate repigmentation after treatment. The inability to produce powdery scale by scraping with a #15 surgical blade indicates the fungus has been reduced or eradicated. Fungal elements may be retained in frequently worn garments that are in contact with the

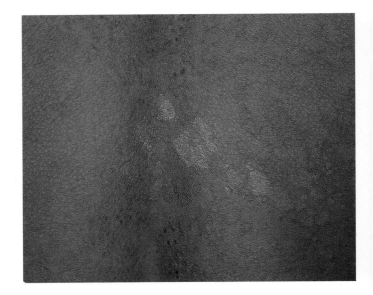

Figure 11-52
Tinea versicolor in a black patient. The central area was scraped with a #15 surgical blade to demonstrate white powdery scale.

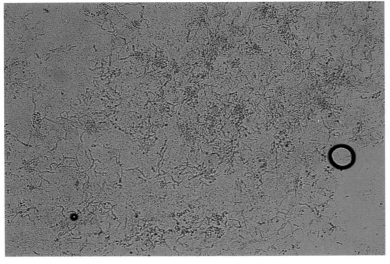

Figure 11-53
Tinea versicolor. A potassium hydroxide wet mount. A low power view showing numerous short broad hyphae and clusters of budding cells, which have been described as having the appearance of "spaghetti and meatballs."

skin; discarding or boiling such clothing might decrease the chance of recurrence. Patients without obvious involvement who have a history of multiple recurrences might consider repeating a treatment program just before the summer months to avoid uneven tanning.

Medication

Selenium sulfide suspension 2.5%. Available as Selsun or Exsel, the suspension is applied to the entire skin surface from the lower posterior scalp area down to the thighs, left on for 10 minutes, and then washed off; this is repeated once each day for 7 consecutive days.[25] There are many suggested variations of this treatment schedule.

Sodium thiosulfate 25%. Sodium thiosulfate (Tinver lotion, 5-oz bottle) is applied twice a day to the entire involved area for 2 weeks. This preparation is effective and inexpensive, but some patients object to the odor.

Miconazole and related agents. Miconazole, available as Monistat-Derm cream (85-gm tube), clotrimazole (Lotrimin or Mycelex cream, 90-gm tube), econazole (Spectazole cream, 85-gm tube), or ciclopirox olamine (Loprox, 90-gm tube) is applied once a day for 2 weeks to the entire affected areas. The cream is odorless and nongreasy, but expensive.

Keratolytic soaps. Sal acid soap (Stiefel) may be useful in preventing recurrences for patients who can tolerate the drying effect.

Ketoconazole. A 4-week, double-blind study showed that ketoconazole, 200 mg/day, produced a clinical and mycologic cure in 97% of patients. Follow-up after 1 year revealed that 64% of patients given ketoconazole were still clear.[26] Ketoconazole is not as yet FDA approved for treating tinea versicolor.

REFERENCES

1. Baer RL: The biology of fungus infections of the feet. JAMA 197:1017, 1966.
2. Montes LF, Black SH: Fine structure of diphtheroids of erythrasma. J Invest Dermatol 48:342, 1967.
3. Powell FC, Muller SA: Kerion of the glabrous skin. J Am Acad Dermatol 7:490, 1982.
4. Jones HE: Therapy of superficial fungal infection. Med Clin North Am 66:873, 1982.
5. Ive FA, Mark SR: Tinea incognito. Br Med J 3:149, 1968.
6. Oskoi J: Intermittent use of griseofulvin in tinea capitis. Cutis 21:689, 1978.
7. Kahn G: Kerion treatment (letters to the editor). Pediatrics 61:501, 1978.
8. Landau JW: Commentary: undecylenic acid and fungus infections. Arch Dermatol 119:351, 1983.
9. Sande MA, Mandell GL: Antimicrobial agents. In the Pharmacological basis of therapeutics, sixth edition. New York, 1980, Macmillan Publishing Co.
10. Ginsburg CM, McCracken CH Jr, Petruska M, et al: The effect of feeding on the bioavailability of griseofulvin in children. J Pediatr 102:309, 1983.
11. Robertson MH, Rich P, Parker F, et al: Ketoconazole in griseofulvin-resistant dermatophytosis. J Am Acad Dermatol 6:224, 1982.
12. Horsburgh CR, Kirkpatrick CH: Long-term therapy of chronic mucocutaneous candidiasis with ketoconazole: experience with twenty-one patients. Am J Med 70(1B):23, 1983.
13. Drouhet E, DuPont B: Laboratory and clinical assessment of ketaconazole in deep-seated mycoses. Am J Med 70(1B):30, 1983.
14. Heel RC, Broaden RN, Carmine A, et al: Ketoconazole: A review of its therapeutic efficacy in superficial and systemic fungal infections. Drugs 23:1, 1982.
15. Janssen PAJ, Symoens J: Hepatic reactions during ketoconazole treatment. Am J Med 70(1B):80, 1983.
16. DeFelice R, Johnson DG, Galgiani JN: Gynecomastia with ketoconazole. Antimicrob Agents Chemother 19:1073, 1981.
17. Creatsas G, Zissis NP, Lolis D: Ketoconazole: a new antifungal agent, in vaginal candidiasis. Curr Ther Res 28:121, 1980.
18. Fregoso-Duenas F: Ketoconazole in vulvovaginal candidosis. Rev Infect Dis 2:620, 1980.
19. Meunier-Carpentier F: Treatment of mycoses in cancer patients. Am J Med 74(1B):74, 1983.
20. Cauwenbergh G, Casneuf J, DeLoore F, et al: Ketoconazole treatment of candidosis in neonates and infants. In Twenty-first Interscience Conference on Antimicrobial Agents and Chemotherapy. Chicago, November 4-6, 1981.
21. Heel RC: Oral candidiasis (thrush). In Ketoconazole in the management of fungal diseases. New York, 1982, Adis Press.
22. Hamada T: Granuloma intertriginosum infantum (granuloma glutaele infantum) (letters to the editor). Arch Dermatol 111:1072, 1975.
23. Fitzpatrick CH, Rich RR, Bennett JE: Chronic mucocutaneous candidiasis: model-building in cellular immunity. Ann Intern Med 74:955, 1971.
24. Rosenblatt HM, Stiehm ER: Therapy of chronic mucocutaneous candidiasis. Am J Med 70(1B):20, 1983.
25. Sánchez JL, Torres VM: Double-blind efficacy study of selenium sulfide in tinea versicolor. J Am Acad Dermatol 11:235, 1984.
26. Savin RC: Systemic ketoconazole in tinea versicolor: A double-blind evaluation and 1-year follow-up. J Am Acad Dermatol 10:824, 1984.

Chapter Twelve

Warts, Herpes Simplex, and Other Virus Infections

Warts

Warts are benign epidermal neoplasms caused by at least six antigenically distinct human papilloma viruses.[1] Different viruses cause different types of warts. They commonly occur in children and young adults, but may appear at any age. Their course is highly variable. Most resolve spontaneously in weeks or months; others may last years or a lifetime. Warts are transmitted simply by touch; it is not unusual to see warts on adjacent toes ("kissing lesions"). Warts commonly appear at sites of trauma, on the hands, in periungual regions from nail biting, and on plantar surfaces.

Individual variations in cell-mediated immunity may explain differences in severity and duration. Warts occur more frequently, last longer, and appear in greater numbers in patients with atopic dermatitis or lymphomas and those taking immunosuppressive drugs.[2]

Some types of warts respond quickly to routine therapy, whereas others are resistant. It should be explained to patients that warts often require several treatment sessions before a cure is realized. Because warts are confined to the epidermis, they can be removed with little, if any, scarring. Treatment should be conservative to avoid scarring. A hand with many scars is not worth trading for lesions that undergo spontaneous resolution.

Warts obscure normal skin lines; this is an important diagnostic feature. When skin lines are reestablished, the wart is gone. Warts vary in shape and location and are managed in several different ways.

Common warts

Common warts (verruca vulgaris) begin as smooth, flesh-colored papules and evolve into dome-shaped, gray-brown hyperkeratotic growths with black dots on the surface (Figure 12-1). The black dots, which are thrombosed capillaries, are a useful diagnostic sign and may be exposed by paring the hyperkeratotic surface with a #15 surgical blade. The hands are the most commonly involved area, but warts may be found on any skin surface. Generally, the warts are few, but it is not unusual for common warts to become so numerous that they become confluent and obscure large areas of normal skin.

Treatment. Topical salicylic acid preparations, liquid nitrogen, or light electrocautery are the best methods for initial therapy. Blunt dissection is used for resistant or large lesions. (See Chapter 27 for surgical techniques.) The technique for application of salicylic acid is described in the treatment section for plantar warts.

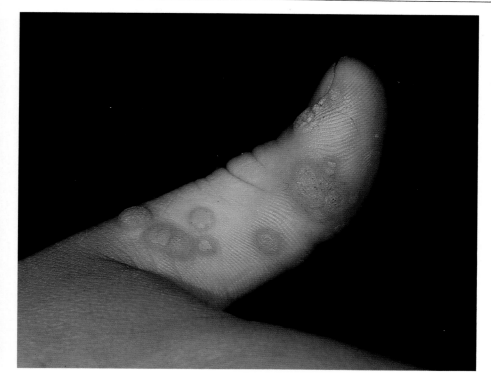

Figure 12-1
Common warts with thrombosed vessels (black dots) on the surface.

Filiform and digitate warts

These growths consist of a few or several finger-like, flesh-colored projections emanating from a narrow or broad base. They are most commonly observed around the mouth, eyes, and ala nasi (Figure 12-2).

Treatment. Filiform and digitate warts are the easiest warts to treat. Those with a narrow base do not require anesthesia. A firm base is created by retracting the skin on either side of the wart. A curette is then firmly drawn across the base, removing the wart with one stroke. Bleeding is controlled with gauze pressure rather than by using painful Monsel's solution. This technique is particularly useful in young children who refuse local anesthesia with a needle. Light electrocautery is a useful alternative.

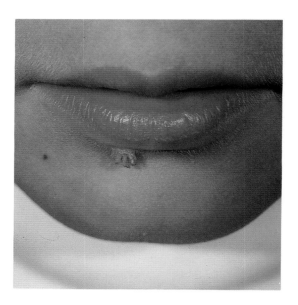

Figure 12-2
Filiform wart with finger-like projections.

Flat warts

Flat warts (verrucae plana) are pink, light brown or light yellow, slightly elevated, flat-topped papules that vary in size from 0.1 to 0.3 cm. There may be only a few, but generally they are numerous. Typical sites of involvement are the forehead (Figure 12-3), around the mouth (Figure 12-4), the backs of the hands, and shaved areas such as the beard area in men and the lower legs in women. A line of flat warts may appear as a result of scratching these sites.

Treatment. Flat warts present a special therapeutic problem. Their duration may be lengthy and they may be highly resistent to treatment. In addition, they are generally located in cosmetically important areas where aggressive, scarring procedures are to be avoided. Treatment may be started with tretinoin (Retin-A) cream, 0.05% or 0.1%, ap-

plied at bedtime over the entire involved area.[3] The frequency of application is subsequently adjusted in order to produce a fine scaling with mild erythema. Treatment may be required for weeks or months. Freezing individual lesions with liquid nitrogen or exercising a very light touch with the electrocautery needle may be performed for patients who are concerned with cosmetic appearance and desire quick results. Treatment with 5-fluorouracil cream (Efudex 5%) applied once or twice a day for 3 to 5 weeks may produce dramatic clearing of flat warts; it is worth the attempt if other measures fail.[4] Persistent hyperpigmentation may occur after 5-fluorouracil use. This result may be minimized by applying the ointment to individual lesions with a cotton-tipped applicator. Warts may reappear in skin inflamed by 5-fluorouracil.

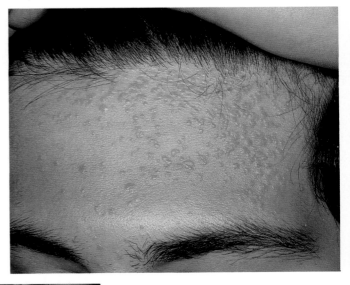

Figure 12-3
Flat warts.

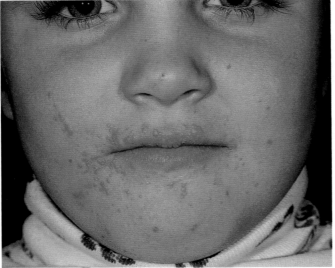

Figure 12-4
Flat warts. The wart virus has been inoculated into a scratch line, producing a linear lesion.

Genital warts

Genital warts (condylomata acuminata or venereal warts), or any warts in moist areas, are pale pink with numerous discrete narrow-to-wide projections on a broad base. The surface is smooth or velvety and moist and lacks the hyperkeratosis of warts on glabrous skin (Figures 12-5 to 12-7). They may coalesce in the rectal or perineal area to form a large cauliflower-like mass. Warts spread rapidly over moist areas and may, therefore, be symmetric on opposing surfaces of the labia or rectum (Figures 12-8 and 12-9). Whether common warts can be the source of genital warts is unknown although they are usually caused by different antigenic types of virus. Warts may extend into the vaginal tract and rectum, requiring a speculum or sigmoidoscope for visualization and treatment.

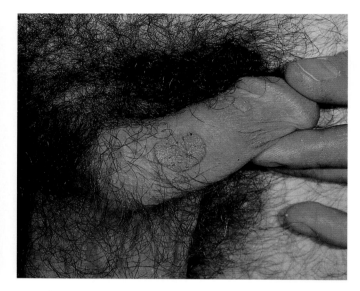

Figure 12-5
Broad-based wart on the shaft of a penis.

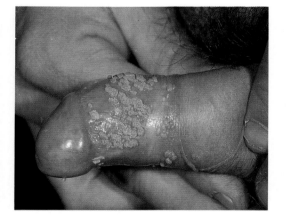

Figure 12-6
Multiple small warts under the foreskin. Multiple inoculations occur on a moist surface.

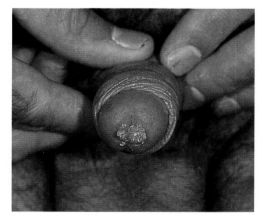

Figure 12-7
Wart at the urethral meatus.

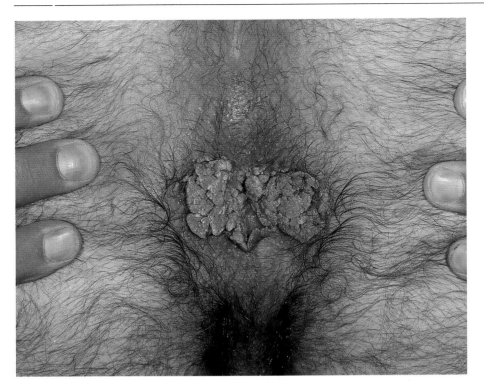

Figure 12-8
Mass of warts on opposing surfaces of the anus.

Figure 12-9
Massive inoculation of warts on the vulva.

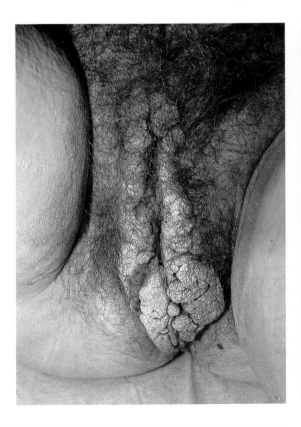

Dome-shaped or hair-like projections called pearly penile papules appear on the corona of the penis in up to 10% of males. These small angiofibromas are normal variants, but are sometimes mistaken for warts. No treatment is required (Figures 12-10 and 12-11).

Treatment

Podophyllum resin. Moist genital warts are most efficiently treated with 20% podophyllum resin in compound tincture of benzoin applied with a cotton-tipped applicator.

The entire surface of the wart is covered with the solution and the patient remains still until the solution dries, about 2 mintues. Powdering the wart after treatment may help to avoid contamination of normal skin with the irritating resin. The medicine is removed by washing 1 hour later. The patient is retreated in 1 week. The podophyllum may then remain on the wart for 4 to 6 hours if little or no inflammation followed the first treatment.

Overenthusiastic initial treatment can result in intense inflammation and discomfort lasting for days. Because the procedure is simple, it is tempting to allow home treatment, but in most cases this should be avoided. Very frequently the patient will overtreat and cause excessive inflammation by applying podophyllum on normal skin. To avoid extreme discomfort, treat only part of a large warty mass in the perineal and rectal area. Warts on the shaft of the penis do not respond as successfully to podophyllum as do warts on the glans or under the foreskin; consequently, electrosurgery or cryosurgery should be used if two or three treatment sessions with podophyllum fail. Many warts will disappear after a single treatment. Alternate forms of therapy should be attempted if there is no improvement after five treatment sessions.

Warning. Systemic toxicity occurs from absorption of podophyllum. Paresthesia, polyneuritis, paralytic ileus, leukopenia, thrombocytopenia, coma, and death have occurred when large quantities of podophyllum were applied to extensive areas or allowed to remain in contact with the skin for an extended time.[5] Treat only limited areas during each session. Very small quantities should be used in the mouth, vaginal tract, or rectosigmoid. A stillborn child delivered after 2.5 ml of a 25% solution of podophyllum was applied to the vulva of an 18-year-old woman in her 34th week of pregnancy.[6]

Alteration of histopathology. Podophyllum can produce bizarre forms of squamous cells that can be mistaken for squamous cell carcinoma. The pathologist must be informed of the patient's exposure to podophyllum when a biopsy of a previously treated wart is submitted.

Electrosurgery. One or two warts on the shaft of the penis are best treated with conservative electrosurgery rather than by subjecting the patient to repeated sessions with podophyllum. Large unresponsive masses of warts around the rectum or vulva may be treated by scissor excision of the bulk of the mass, followed by electrocautery of the remaining tissue down to the skin surface.[7] Removal of a very large mass of warts is a painful procedure and is best performed under general or spinal anesthesia in the operating room.

Cryosurgery. Liquid nitrogen applied with a cotton applicator is very effective for treating smaller genital warts. Warts on the shaft of the penis and vulva respond very well with little or no scarring. Cryosurgery of the rectal area is painful.

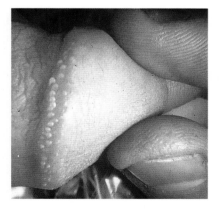

Figure 12-10
Pearly penile papules (dome-shaped). An anatomic variant of normal found on the corona of the penis. They are sometimes mistaken for warts. No treatment is required.

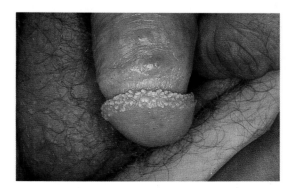

Figure 12-11
Pearly penile papules (hair-like). An anatomic variant on the corona. They are sometimes mistaken for warts.

Plantar warts

Patients refer to warts on any surface as a plantar wart. Plantar warts frequently occur at points of maximum pressure, over the heads of the metatarsal bones, or on the heels. A thick painful callus forms in response to pressure and the foot is repositioned while walking. This may result in distortion of posture and pain in other parts of the foot, leg, or back. A little wart can cause a lot of trouble.

Warts may appear anywhere on the plantar surface. A cluster of many warts that appears to fuse is referred to as a mosaic wart (Figure 12-12).

Differential diagnosis. Corns or clavi over the metatarsal heads are frequently mistaken for warts. The two entities can be easily distinguished by paring the callus with a #15 surgical blade. Warts lack skin lines crossing their surface; they do have centrally located black dots that will bleed with additional paring.

Clavi or corns also lack skin lines crossing the surface, but they have a hard, painful, well-demarcated, translucent central core (Figure 12-13). The core or kernel can easily be removed by inserting the point of a #15 surgical blade into the cleavage plane between normal skin and the core, holding the scalpel vertically, and smoothly drawing the blade circumferentially. The hard kernel is freed by drawing the blade horizontally through the base to reveal a deep depression (Figure 12-14). Pain is greatly relieved by this simple procedure. Lateral pressure on a wart causes pain, but pinching a plantar corn is painless.

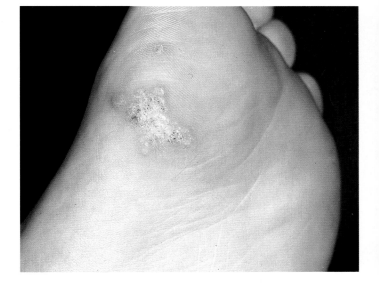

Figure 12-12
Plantar wart. Fusion of numerous small warts to form a mosaic wart.

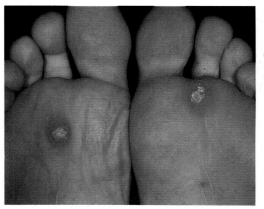

Figure 12-13
Corns (clavi) on the plantar surface are frequently mistaken for warts.

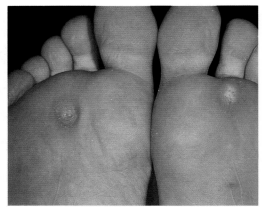

Figure 12-14
Plantar surface depicted in Figure 12-13 with soft and hard callus removed from corns to reveal a deep depression.

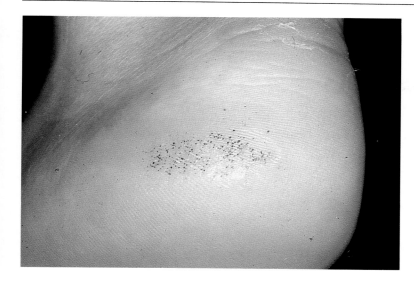

Figure 12-15
Black heel. Trauma causes capillaries to shear, resulting in a group of black dots; appearance may be confused with warts.

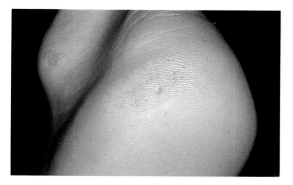

Figure 12-16
Paring the skin over the black dots in Figure 12-15 reveals normal skin lines, proving that a wart is not present.

Figure 12-17
Warts in the process of undergoing spontaneous resolution will suddenly turn black and, when pared with a blade, feel soft and amorphous.

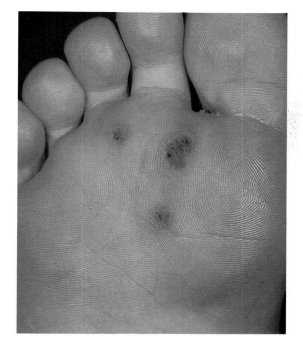

Black heel. A cluster of blue-black dots (ruptured capillaries) may appear on the heel or anywhere on the plantar surface after the shearing trauma of sports that involve sudden stops or position changes (Figure 12-15). At first glance this may be confused with a wart, but closer examination reveals normal skin lines, and paring does not cause additional bleeding (Figure 12-16). The condition resolves spontaneously in a few weeks.

Black warts. Warts in the process of undergoing spontaneous resolution, particularly on the plantar surface, may turn black and feel soft when pared with a blade (Figure 12-17).

Treatment. Plantar warts do not require therapy as long as they are painless. Although their number may increase, it is sometimes best simply to explain the natural history of the virus infection and wait for resolution rather than subject the patient to a long treatment program. Minimal discomfort can be relieved by periodically removing the callus with a blade or pumice stone. Painful warts must be treated. A technique should be used that does not cause scarring. Scars on the soles of the feet may be painful and a lasting source of discomfort.

Keratolytic therapy (salicylic acid and lactic acid paint). Keratolytic therapy with salicylic acid and lactic acid paint (Duofilm, Ti Flex, Viranol) is conservative initial therapy for plantar warts. The treatment is nonscarring and relatively effective, but it requires persistent application of medication once each day for many weeks.

The wart is pared with a blade, pumice stone, or sandpaper (emery board). The affected area is soaked in warm water to hydrate the keratin surface; this facilitates penetration of the medicine. A drop of solution is applied with the glass rod applicator and allowed to dry. Additional solution is added as needed to cover the entire surface of the wart. Penetration of the acid mixture is enhanced if the treated wart is covered with a piece of adhesive tape. Inflammation and soreness may follow tape occlusion, requiring periodic interruption of treatment; consequently, the patient may be satisfied with the longer, more comfortable process of simply applying the solution at bed time. White pliable keratin forms in a few days and should be pared with a blade or worn away with abrasives such as sandpaper or a pumice stone. Ideally, the white keratin should be removed to expose pink skin. To accomplish this result, an occasional visit to the office may be necessary.

Keratolytic therapy (40% salicylic acid plasters). This is a safe, nonscarring treatment similar to the previous process, with the exception that in this case the salicylic acid has been incorporated into a pad. The 40% salicylic acid plasters are particularly useful in treating mosaic warts covering a large area.

The plaster is cut to the size of the wart. The backing of the plaster is removed and the sticky surface is applied to the wart and secured with tape. The plaster is removed in 24 to 48 hours, the pliable white keratin is reduced in the manner previously described, and another plaster is applied. The treatment requires many weeks, but it is effective and less irritating than salicylic acid and lactic acid paint. Pain is relieved because a large amount of keratin is removed during the first few days of treatment. The 40% plasters are available in 3- by 4-inch sheets called Mediplast. The cost is about $1 per sheet.

Blunt dissection. Blunt dissection is a surgical alternative that is fast, effective (90% cure rate), and usually nonscarring. It is superior to both electro-desiccation-curettage and excision because normal tissue is not disturbed.[8,9] (See Chapter 27 for surgical techniques.)

Chemotherapy. For years a variety of acids has been successfully administered to treat plantar warts. This technique is occasionally used to treat warts that have recurred after treatment with other techniques; it is sometimes used as initial therapy. Like keratolytic therapy, repeated application is required. Home application of acids is too dangerous; therefore, weekly or biweekly visits to the office are required. A number of acids may be used. Bichloracetic acid is commercially available; it is made by Kahlenberg.

To begin treatment, pare the excess callus. Protect the surrounding area with petrolatum. Coat the entire lesion with acid and work the acid into the wart with a sharp toothpick. Repeat the above procedure every 7 to 10 days.

Formalin. This technique is rarely used, but may be considered for resistant cases. Mosaic warts or other large involved areas may be treated with daily soaking for 30 minutes in 4% formalin solution.[10] The firm fixed tissue is pared before subsequent soaking. There is a risk of inducing sensitization to formalin by this procedure. Since formalin is used in wash-and-wear clothing, allergy to these materials would be particularly troublesome.

Cryosurgery. Cryosurgery on the sole may produce a deep, painful blister and interfere with mobility. Repeated light applications of liquid nitrogen are preferred to aggressive treatment.

Immunotherapy. Immunotherapy has been reported as being successful for treatment of resistant warts.[11,12] However, this treatment is controversial because the chemical used, dinitrochlorobenzene (DNCB), is theoretically carcinogenic. The safety of this procedure is being evaluated. The use of other sensitizers such as *Rhus* antigen (poison ivy) has been suggested as a safer alternative.

The technique is as follows: Sensitize the patient by applying[13] 0.15 ml of a 2% acetone solution of DNCB to the upper arm; cover with a Band-Aid for 24 hours. For the majority of patients a spontaneous flare from cell-mediated immunity will arise in approximately 7 to 10 days. Wait for 2 weeks and then proceed to test those patients who did not flare with a patch test of 0.1% DNCB in acetone.

Sensitized patients are treated with either 0.1% or 1% DNCB in petrolatum, depending on the degree of reaction during testing. The treated wart is covered with paper tape for 48 hours. The treatment is repeated weekly and the concentration is adjusted to maintain erythema without excessive pruritus, erythema, or edema. Treatment may require continuation for 3 or 4 months. Warts in other areas may be treated similarly.

Subungual and periungual warts

Subungual and periungual warts (Figure 12-18) are more resistant to both chemical and surgical methods of treatment than are warts in other areas. A wart next to the nail may simply be the tip of the iceberg; much more of the wart may be submerged under the nail. The tips of the fingers and toes are a confined area. Therapeutic measures that cause inflammation and swelling, such as cryosurgery, may produce considerable pain. Aggressive cryosurgery over superficial nerves on the volar or lateral aspects of the proximal phalanges of the fingers has caused neuropathy.[14] Permanent nail changes may occur if the nail matrix is frozen.

Treatment

Cantharidin. Cantharidin (Cantharone) causes blister formation at the dermoepidermal junction, but will not cause scarring. Adverse effects are postinflammatory hyperpigmentation, painful blistering, and dissemination of warts to the area of blistering.

In treatment the solution is applied to the surface and allowed to dry. The patient is seen 1 week later for evaluation. Blisters are opened, and the remaining wart is retreated. If blistering did not occur, then cantharidin is applied in one to three layers and covered with tape for 48 hours. Each layer should be dry before the next application of cantharidin.

The treatment is effective in some patients, but some warts do not respond to repeated applications.

Keratolytic preparations. The same procedures described for treating plantar warts with salicylic acid and lactic acid paint and salicylic acid plasters are useful for periungual warts.

Blunt dissection. When conventional measures fail, blunt dissection offers an excellent surgical alternative.[9] (See Chapter 27 on surgical technique.) Local anesthesia is induced with 2% lidocaine without epinephrine, injected around and under small warts. A digital block is required for larger warts. Hemostasis during the procedure is maintained by firm pressure over the digital arteries or with a rubber band tourniquet. The nail should be removed only if the wart is very large and imbedded. The procedure is exactly the same as described for blunt dissection of plantar warts.

Tape occlusion. This is a technique of unproven efficacy that may be worth attempting for children for whom a conservative approach is desired.[15] To completely cover the wart, the tip of the finger is wrapped with tape. The tape remains in place for 6 days, is removed at home, and is then reapplied in a similar manner 12 hours later; it remains in place for another 6 days. The patient is seen 2 weeks after the initial visit and the wart is treated with a drop of liquified phenol or bichloracetic acid (Kahlenberg) and the finger is again occluded in the aforementioned manner. The process is repeated until the wart is gone.

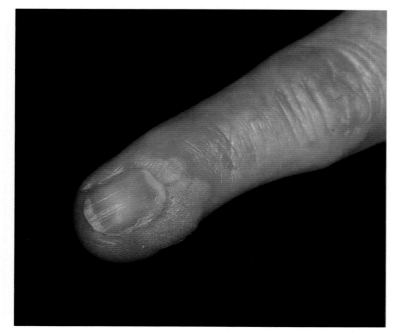

Figure 12-18
Periungual wart. Wart may extend under the nail.

Molluscum Contagiosum

Clinical manifestations. Molluscum contagiosum is a virus infection of the skin characterized by discrete, 2- to 5-mm, slightly umbilicated, flesh-colored, dome-shaped papules (Figure 12-19). It spreads by autoinoculation, by scratching, or by touching a lesion. The areas most commonly involved are the face (Figure 12-20), trunk, axillae, and extremities in children and the pubic and genital areas in adults. Lesions are frequently grouped. There may be few or many covering a wide area. Unlike warts, the palms and soles are not involved. It is not uncommon to see erythema and scaling at the periphery of single or several lesions (Figure 12-21). This may be the result of inflammation from scratching or it may be a hypersensitivity reaction. Lesions spread to inflamed skin, such as areas of atopic dermatitis. The individual lesion begins as a smooth, dome-shaped, white-to-flesh-colored papule. With time the center becomes soft and umbilicated. Most lesions are self-limiting and will spontaneously clear in 6 to 9 months; however, they may last much longer

Diagnosis. The diagnosis can be easily established by laboratory methods. The virus infects epithelial cells, creating very large intracytoplasmic inclusion bodies and disrupting cell bonds by which epithelial cells are generally held together. These highly characteristic inclusions can be readily demonstrated either by a potassium hydroxide examination or in a fixed and stained biopsy specimen (Figure 12-22). Rapid confirmation can be made by removing a small lesion with a curette and placing it with a drop of potassium hydroxide between two microscope slides. The preparation is gently heated and then crushed with firm pressure. Larger umbilicated papules may have a soft center, the contents of which can be obtained by scooping with a needle. This material contains only infected cells and can be examined directly in a heated potassium hydroxide preparation. The infected cells are dark and round and disperse easily with slight pressure, whereas normal epithelial cells are flat and rectangular and tend to remain stuck together in sheets. Stained biopsy specimens show a mass of very large eosinophilic round intracytoplasmic inclusion bodies.

Treatment. Treatment must be individualized. Conservative nonscarring methods should be used for children who have many lesions. Genital lesions in adults should be definitively treated to prevent spread by sexual contact. New lesions that were too small to be detected may appear after treatment and may require additional attention.

Curettage. Small papules can be quickly removed with a curette and without local anesthesia. Bleeding is controlled with gauze pressure. Monsel's solution is painful to use in an unanesthetized

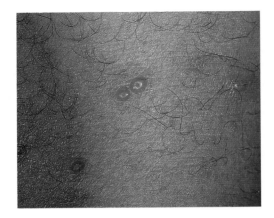

Figure 12-19
Molluscum contagiosum. Individual lesions are 2- to 5-mm, flesh-colored, dome-shaped umbilicated papules.

area. Curettage is useful when there are a few lesions because it provides the quickest, most reliable treatment. A small scar may form; therefore, this technique should be avoided in cosmetically important areas.

Cryosurgery. Cryosurgery is the treatment of choice in patients who do not object to the pain. Touch the papule lightly with a nitrogen-bathed cotton swab until the advancing white frozen border has progressed down the side of the papule to form a 1-mm halo on the normal skin surrounding the lesion. This should take about 5 seconds. This conservative method will destroy most lesions in one to three treatment sessions at 1- or 2-week intervals and it rarely produces a scar.

Tretinoin. Tretinoin (Retin-A) cream (0.05% or 0.1%) or gel (0.01% or 0.025%) should be applied once or twice daily to individual lesions. Weeks or months may be required. This method is useful for children whose parents are anxious for some type of treatment.

Salicylic acid and lactic acid paint (Duofilm). Duofilm applied each day without tape occlusion may cause irritation and encourage resolution.

Cantharidin. Apply a small drop of cantharidin (Cantharone) over the surface of the lesion and avoid contaminating normal skin. Lesions may clear without scarring. Occasionally, new lesions will appear at the site of the blister created by cantharidin.

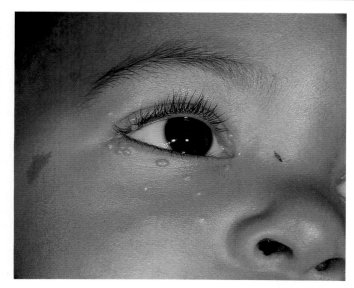

Figure 12-20
Molluscum contagiosum. Inoculation around the eye, a typical presentation for children.

Figure 12-21
Molluscum contagiosum. A single lesion became inflamed and disappeared 10 days later.

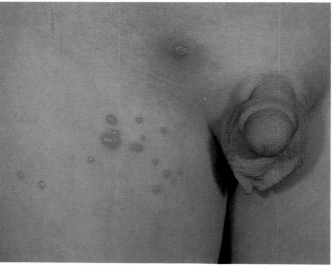

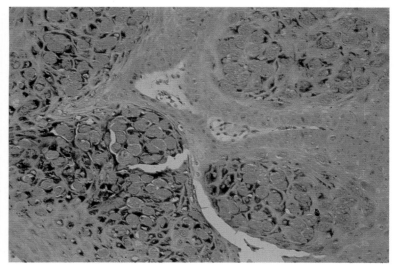

Figure 12-22
Molluscum contagiosum. Eosinophilic intracytoplasmic inclusion bodies.

Herpes Simplex

Herpes simplex is a virus infection caused by two different virus types (type 1 and type 2), which can be distinguished in the laboratory.[16,17] Type 1 is generally associated with oral infections, and type 2 with genital infections. Type 1 genital infections and type 2 oral infections are becoming more common, possibly as a result of oral-genital sexual contact. Both types seem to produce identical patterns of infection. Many infections are asymptomatic and evidence of previous infection can be detected only by an elevated antibody titer. Herpes simplex virus (HSV) infections have two phases, primary infection, after which the virus becomes established in a nerve ganglion, and the secondary phase, characterized by recurrent disease at the same site.[18] Infections can occur anywhere on the skin. Infection in one area does not protect the patient from subsequent infection at a different site. Lesions are intraepidermal and usually heal without scarring.

Primary infection. Many primary infections are asymptomatic and can be detected only by a rising antibody titer. Like most virus infections, the severity of disease increases with age. The virus may be spread from respiratory droplets, direct contact with an active lesion, or virus-containing fluid such as saliva or cervical secretions in patients with no evidence of active disease. Symptoms occur from 3 to 7 or more days after contact. Tenderness, pain, mild paresthesias, or burning occur before the onset of lesions at the site of inoculation. Localized pain, tender lymphadenopathy, headache, generalized aching, and fever are characteristic prodromal symptoms. However, some patients have no prodromal symptoms. Grouped vesicles on an erythematous base appear and subsequently erode. The vesicles in primary herpes simplex are more numerous and scattered than in the recurrent infection. Mucous membrane lesions will accumulate exudate while skin lesions form a crust. Lesions last 2 to 6 weeks unless secondarily infected and heal without scarring. During this primary infection, the virus enters the nerve endings in the skin directly below the lesions and ascends through peripheral nerves to dorsal root ganglia where it apparently remains in a latent stage.

Recurrent infection. Local skin trauma (ultraviolet light exposure, chapping, abrasion, etc.) or systemic changes (menses, fatigue, fever, etc.) reactivate the virus, which then travels down the peripheral nerves to the site of initial infection and causes the characteristic focal recurrent infection. Recurrent infection is not inevitable. Many individuals have a rise in antibody titer and never experience recurrence. The prodromal symptoms, lasting 2 to 24 hours, resemble those of the primary infection. Within 12 hours, a group of lesions evolve rapidly from an erythematous base to form papules and then vesicles. The dome-shaped tense vesicles rapidly umbilicate. In 2 to 4 days they rupture, forming aptha-like erosions in the mouth and vaginal area or erosions covered by crusts on the lips and glabrous skin. Crusts are shed in about 8 days to reveal a pink reepithelialized surface. In contrast to the primary infection, systemic symptoms and lymphadenopathy rarely occur unless there is secondary infection.

Laboratory diagnosis. It is vitally important to document genital herpes simplex in pregnant women and cutaneous herpes in newborn infants. Consequently, in these instances, suspicious vesicular and eroded lesions should be cultured. In all other forms, the clinical presentation is usually so characteristic that an accurate diagnosis can be made by inspection. A number of laboratory procedures are available if confirmation is desired.

Tzanck smear. A Tzanck smear should be performed on an intact vesicle. It is prepared by carefully removing the roof of the vesicle and scraping the underlying moist skin and the underside of the roof of the vesicle with a #15 surgical blade. The material is smeared onto a glass slide and allowed to air dry or is dried with an alcohol lamp. Tap water, 0.5 ml, and Giemsa tissue stain, 0.5 ml, are mixed in a small syringe. The slide is then flooded with the staining solution over a sink. After 30 to 40 seconds the slide is thoroughly rinsed in tap water and air dried.[18a] The slide is examined directly, or mounting medium and a cover slip are applied if a permanent smear is required. Giant cells with 2 to 15 nuclei are the characteristic finding. A positive Tzanck smear confirms the diagnosis of herpetic infection; however, a negative result does not rule it out.[19] Material from lesions of herpes zoster produces identical results.

Papanicolaou smear. The interpretation of this presentation requires experience. The nucleus has a ground glass appearance during the primary infection and contains the more characteristic irregular eosinophilic nuclear inclusions during the recurrent infection.

Culture. Culture for herpes virus is now a routine procedure for pregnant women with a history of genital herpes simplex. Collection kits (e.g., Virocult) are available in most hospitals or can be obtained from independent laboratories. The kits must be stored at 2° to 6° C and reach room temperature before using. Cotton-tipped swabs should not be used because they leach substances toxic to the virus. Specimens to be shipped must be packed in dry ice and frozen to at least −20° C.

The swabs are inoculated onto human diploid fibroblasts in tissue culture and incubated at 35° C for 5 days. Cultures are examined daily and, if cytopathogenic effects are observed, the cells are harvested and stained by a direct fluorescent antibody technique. Results may be available 24 hours after incubation is initiated. This procedure allows the differentiation of HSV from varicella/zoster and most HSV isolates can be characterized as type 1 or 2.

Viral cultures are expensive.

Technique. It is essential that the lesion to be sampled is active. Early lesions that have not yet eroded and lesions that are resolving (usually 5 days or more) are not generally productive for culture.

For accessible lesions, as on the external genitalia, moisten two viral collection swabs with saline. Swab the lesion gently and discard swab. Squeeze the lesion gently, swab again with a second swab, and place the entire swab in a transport tube.

For the vaginal canal or cervix, scrape the active lesion or, if screening, the transitional zone of the cervix with a metal curette and transfer the scrapings to the transport medium.

For shingles or chickenpox, lance an active vesicle, collect the exudate with a swab from the viral collection kit, and place the entire swab in a transport tube.

Histopathology. An intact vesicle should be biopsied. The histologic picture is characteristic but not unique for herpes simplex.

Immunofluorescence. Smears and biopsy specimens can be studied with this technique, which is useful if virus cannot be cultured.[20] This technique is rarely used.

Serology. A fourfold increase in neutralizing antibody during a 2-week period supports the diagnosis of primary herpes simplex.[21] Recurrences produce little change in antibody titer.

Treatment. A number of measures can be taken to relieve discomfort and promote healing. These are described in the following sections. There is no treatment that will prevent recurrence. Acyclovir (Zovirax), an antiviral drug active against herpes viruses, is available for both topical and intravenous administration. The ointment is approved for the management of initial herpes genitalis and in limited nonlife-threatening mucocutaneous herpes simplex virus infections in immunocompromised patients. The intravenous form is approved for initial and recurrent mucosal and cutaneous herpes simplex infections in immunocompromised adults and children and for severe initial clinical episodes of herpes genitalis in patients who are not immunocompromised. The drug decreases the duration of viral excretion, new lesion formation and vesicles and promotes rapid healing. Since acyclovir is new, more experience is required before all of its potential is realized.

Oral herpes simplex

Primary infection. Primary oral herpes simplex (primary gingivostomatitis and recurrent herpes labialis) infection occurs most commonly in children between ages 1 and 5. The incubation period is 3 to 12 days. Although most cases are mild, some are severe. Sore throat and fever may precede the onset of painful vesicles occurring anywhere in the oral cavity. The vesicles rapidly coalesce and erode with a white, then yellow, superficial, purulent exudate. Pain interferes with eating, and tender cervical lymphadenopathy develops. Fever subsides in 3 to 5 days and oral pain and erosions are usually gone in 2 weeks; in severe cases, they may last for 3 weeks.

Recurrent infection. Recurrent oral herpes simplex can appear as a localized cluster of small ulcers in the oral cavity, but the most common presentation is eruptions on the vermilion border of the lip (recurrent herpes labialis) (Figures 12-23 to 12-25). Fever (fever blisters), upper respiratory infections (cold sores), and exposure to ultraviolet light, among other things, may precede the onset. The course of the disease is the same as that in other areas.

Treatment. A number of treatment modalities have been tried for herpes on the vermilion border. There is as yet no oral or topical medication that will prevent the recurrent disease. Measures can be taken to delay recurrence and promote rapid healing.

The lips should be protected from sun exposure with opaque creams such as zinc oxide or with sun-blocking agents incorporated into a lip balm (Chap-Stick 15). Topical epinephrine (Adrenalin) solution 1:1000 in a 30-ml bottle is available from Parke-Davis. Application every few minutes during the prodromal itching phase may abort an episode.[22] A cool Burow's compress will decrease erythema and debride crusts to promote healing.

Lubricating creams may be applied if lips become too dry, but petrolatum-based ointments applied directly to an erosion may delay healing.

Figure 12-23
Herpes simplex labialis. Typical presentation with tense vesicles appearing on the lips and extending onto the skin.

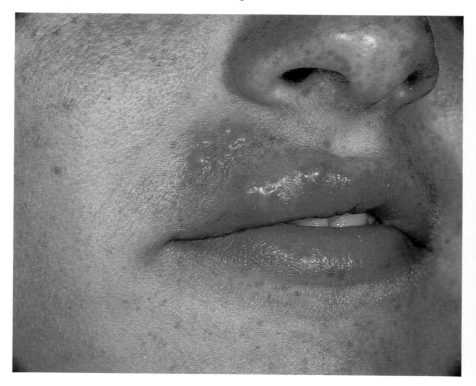

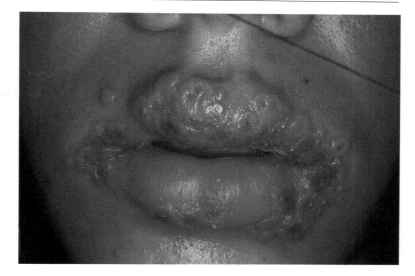

Figure 12-24
Herpes simplex labialis. Extensive involvement of the lips with umbilicated vesicles.

Figure 12-25
Herpes simplex labialis. Extensive involvement in an immunosuppressed patient.

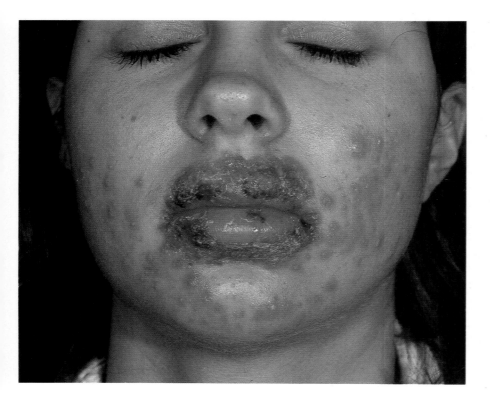

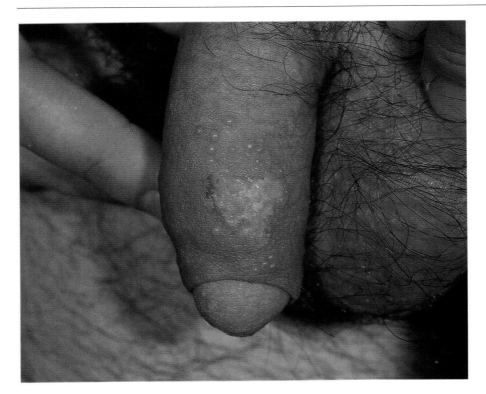

Figure 12-26
Primary herpes simplex of the penis. A group of vesicles has ruptured, leaving an erosion. Tense vesicles are at the periphery.

Genital herpes simplex

Herpes simplex infection of the penis (herpes progenitalis) (Figures 12-26 to 12-28), vulva (Figure 12-29), and rectum (Figure 12-30) is pathophysiologically identical to herpes infection in other areas. Rarely seen a few decades ago, it has reached epidemic proportions, possibly as a result of increased sexual promiscuity. The public is well informed about the increased risk of cervical cancer, the method of transmission, the potential for harm to the infected newborn, and the incurability of this relatively new disease. Recurrences cannot be predicted, but they often follow sexual intercourse. Sexual encounters are delayed or avoided for fear of becoming infected with or transmitting the disease. The psychological implications are obvious.

Genital herpes is primarily a disease of young adults. Both antigenic types 1 and 2 infect the genital area.[23] The virus can be cultured for approximately 5 days from active genital lesions and the lesions are almost certainly infectious during this time.[24] Whether disease can be transmitted by asymptomatic carriers is an unsettled question.

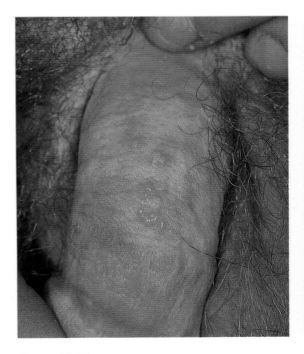

Figure 12-27
Recurrent herpes simplex. A small group of vesicles on an erythematous base. A few smaller vesicles show slight umbilication.

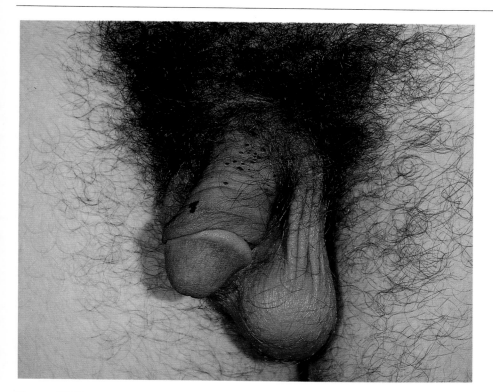

Figure 12-28
Herpes simplex penis. Scattered small crusts on the shaft of the penis. The diagnosis should be suspected even though primary lesions are absent.

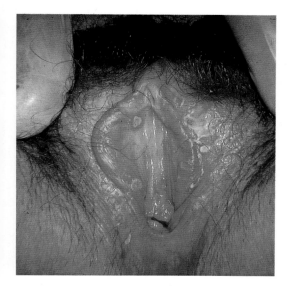

Figure 12-29
Herpes simplex vulva. Scattered erosions covered with exudate.

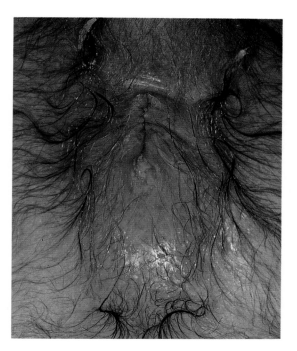

Figure 12-30
Herpes simplex anus. Numerous erosions of a primary infection after anal intercourse.

Male patients develop infections from contact with females who have no obvious disease. The infection may have been acquired from an active cervical infection or from cervical secretions of a female who chronically carries the virus. The data on whether males are asymptomatic carriers are conflicting.

Primary infection. Virus infections spread easily over moist surfaces. Wide areas of the female genitalia may be covered with painful erosions (Figure 12-29). Inflammation, edema, and pain may be so extreme that urination is interfered with and catheterization is required. The patient may be immobilized and require bed rest at home or in the hospital.

Males develop a similar pattern of extensive involvement with edema and possible urinary retention, especially if uncircumcised. The eruption frequently extends onto the pubic area, possibly spread from secretions during sexual contact. The anal area may be involved after anal intercourse (Figure 12-30).

Recurrent infection. Recurrent infection in females may be so minor or hidden from view in the vagina or cervix that it is unnoticed. This may explain why some males who develop primary disease are not aware of the source.

Prevention. Virus can be recovered from the eroded lesions for approximately 5 days[24] from the onset, but sexual contact should be avoided until reepithelialization is complete. Male (urethra) and female (cervix) asymptomatic carriers can probably transmit the infection at any time. The use of spermicidal foams and condoms should be recommended for patients with a history of recurrent genital herpes. For sexual partners who have both had genital herpes, protective measures are probably not necessary if both partners carry the same virus type (one partner infected the other) and active lesions are not present. Remember that having herpes in one area does not protect one from acquiring the infection in another location. Contact should be avoided when active lesions are present.

Treatment

Cool compresses. Extensive erosion on the vulva and penis may be treated with silver nitrate $\frac{1}{8}$% or Burow's compresses applied for 20 minutes several times daily. This effective local therapy reduces edema and inflammation, macerates and debrides crust and purulent material, and relieves pain. The legs may be supported with pillows under the knees to expose the inflamed tissues and promote drying.

Acyclovir. Primary genital infections of limited extent may be treated with acyclovir ointment (Zovirax) applied every 3 hours 6 times daily for 7 days.[25] The ointment may be applied before and after wet compresses or may be applied as the only treatment for limited primary infections.

Primary genital infections that are severe may be treated intravenously with acyclovir.[26] The dosage is 5 mg/kg infused at a constant rate over 1 hour every 8 hours for 7 days in adults with normal renal function. This schedule will decrease the duration of viral excretion, new lesion formation, and duration of vesicle formation and will promote rapid healing. Oral acyclovir is also effective for primary genital herpes[27] and markedly reduces but does not completely prevent recurrences of genital herpes and does not influence the long-term natural history of the disease.[27a] The safety and efficacy of orally administered acyclovir in the suppression of frequent episodes of genital herpes have been established only for up to 6 months. Chronic suppressive therapy is most appropriate when the benefits of such a regimen outweigh known or potential adverse reactions.

Lubrication. Occlusive ointments such as petroleum jelly should not be applied to eroded lesions. Light lubricating body lotions are soothing when inflammation subsides and tissues become dry.

Women with multiple eroded lesions on the labia will experience great discomfort while urinating. Pain can be avoided by sitting in a tub of water and urinating while holding the labia apart.

Herpes simplex in the newborn

Herpes simplex in the newborn is presently a rare disease, but the incidence can be expected to increase as the number of infected young women increases. The mortality rate is about 50% and many survivors have ocular or neurologic complications. The infection is acquired during passage through the birth canal or from virus that has ascended past the ruptured membranes. Transplacental infection during pregnancy with associated birth defects is very rare. The major concern is infection transmitted at birth. Premature infants are at greatest risk. The most serious form of neonatal herpes simplex is disseminated disease. The incubation period is about 6 days, but can vary from hours after birth to 3 weeks.[28]

Approximately 50% of those developing disseminated disease will have cutaneous involvement.[29] Vesicles on the scalp may be the first sign of infection. The vesicles are larger and more diffuse than in adults. They may occur on the cornea, oral cavity, or anywhere on the skin; the eruption may resemble impetigo. Dissemination is usually accompanied by central nervous system signs, but infection of nearly every organ in the body has been reported. Dissemination is not inevitable and the infection may be localized to the skin or central nervous system.

Management. Women at greatest risk are those who have been exposed to or have had an active infection during pregnancy. Cultures from these women should be obtained from the cervix each week starting at 32 weeks. It is safest to start at this early date in order to have data available in case of premature delivery. A swab is taken from the cervical os and any eroded lesion in the genital area and inoculated onto transport media (e.g., Virocult). Positive cultures may be obtained in 24 to 72 hours, but may not appear for 5 days. Many hospitals do not culture for virus infections; consequently, time should be alloted for transport by mail. Women with an infection before becoming pregnant who have no clinical signs of infection during pregnancy should have several Pap smears interpreted by a cytologist experienced with the cellular changes induced by herpes virus infection. Some recommend weekly cultures, starting at 32 weeks, of any women with a previous infection, although clinical signs of disease have been absent during pregnancy. The number of positive cultures will be low in this group of women. If cultures are positive near the time of delivery, cesarean section should be performed. The virus can rapidly pass to the fetus once membranes have ruptured and the protective effect of cesarean delivery is negligible if not performed within 4 to 6 hours.

Treatment. The infected infant should be treated with vidarabine intravenously.[30] Acyclovir is currently under investigation for treatment of neonatal herpes infection.

Cutaneous herpes simplex

Herpes simplex may appear on any skin surface (Figures 12-31 and 12-32). The clinical presentation has been previously described. It is important to identify all of the characteristic features when attempting to differentiate cutaneous herpes from other vesicular eruptions. Dentists or nurses risk developing herpes of the fingertip (herpetic whitlow), which can resemble a group of warts or bacterial infection (Figure 12-33). Herpes simplex of the lumbosacral region or trunk may be very difficult to differentiate from herpes zoster, with the diagnosis becoming apparent only at the time of recurrence. Herpes simplex of the buttock areas seems to be more common in women (Figure 12-34).

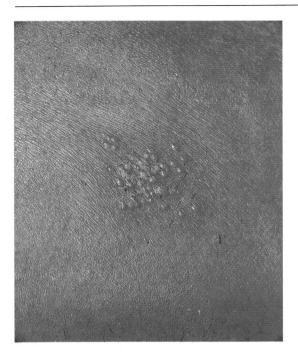

Figure 12-31
Herpes simplex of the skin. Uniform size of the vesicles helps differentiate this from herpes zoster, in which vesicles vary in size.

Figure 12-32
Herpes simplex skin. Crusts have replaced the vesicles in this localized lesion.

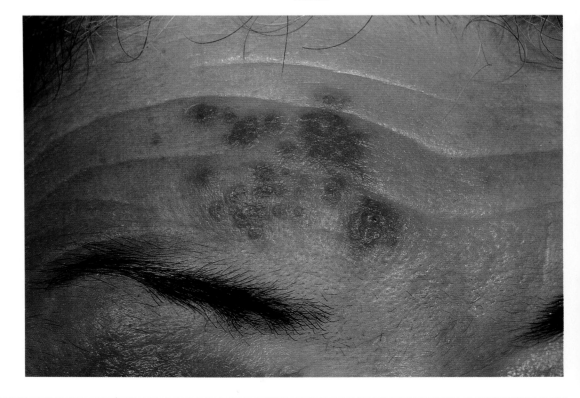

Figure 12-33
Herpes simplex of the finger (herpetic whitlow). Inoculation followed examination of a patient's mouth.

Figure 12-34
Herpes simplex of the buttocks. Infection of this location is seen more frequently in women.

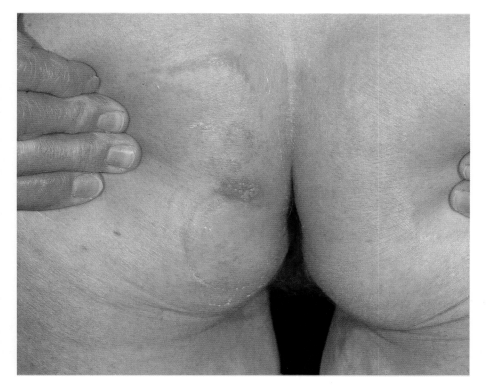

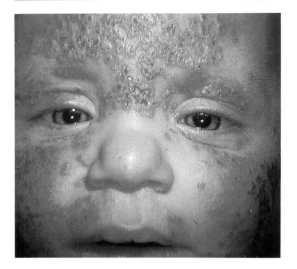

Figure 12-35
Eczema herpeticum. Numerous umbilicated vesicles of the face.

Eczema herpeticum

Certain atopic infants and adults may develop a diffuse form of cutaneous herpes simplex known as eczema herpeticum (Kaposi's varicelliform eruption). The disease is most common in areas of active or recently healed atopic dermatitis, particularly the face, but normal skin can be involved.[31] About 10 days after exposure, numerous vesicles develop, become pustular, and umbilicate markedly (Figure 12-35). Secondary staphylococcal infection commonly occurs. New crops of vesicles may appear during the following weeks. High fever and adenopathy occur 2 to 3 days after the onset of vesiculation. The fever subsides in 4 to 5 days in uncomplicated cases and the lesions evolve in the typical manner (Figure 12-36). Recurrent disease is milder and usually without constitutional symptoms.

Treatment. Eczema herpeticum is managed with cool, wet compresses, similar to diffuse genital herpes simplex. Intravenous acyclovir should be particularly helpful in attenuating this virulent disease.

Figure 12-36
Eczema herpeticum. First crop of lesions has formed crusts; a new lesion has appeared on the ear.

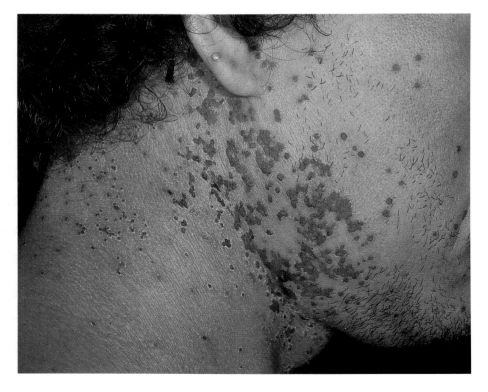

Varicella

Varicella or chickenpox is a highly contagious viral infection which, during epidemics, affects the majority of urban children before puberty. Transmission is by airborn droplets or vesicular fluid. The systemic symptoms, extent of eruption, and complications are greater in adults; thus some parents intentionally expose their young children. Patients with defective cell-mediated immunity or those using immunosuppressive drugs, especially systemic corticosteroids, will have a prolonged course with more extensive eruptions and a greater incidence of complications. An attack of chickenpox usually confers life-long immunity.

Clinical course. The incubation period averages 15 days, with a range of 9 to 23 days. The prodromal symptoms in children are absent or consist of low fever, headache, and malaise, which appear directly before or with the onset of the eruption. In adults, symptoms consisting of fever, chills, malaise, and backache are more severe and occur 2 to 3 days before the eruption.

Eruptive phase. The rash begins on the trunk (centripetal distribution) (Figure 12-37) and spreads to the face and extremities. The extent of involvement varies considerably. Some children have so few lesions that the disease goes unnoticed. Older children and adults have a more extensive eruption involving all areas, sometimes with lesions too numerous to count.

Figure 12-37
Chickenpox. Numerous lesions on the trunk (centripetal distribution).

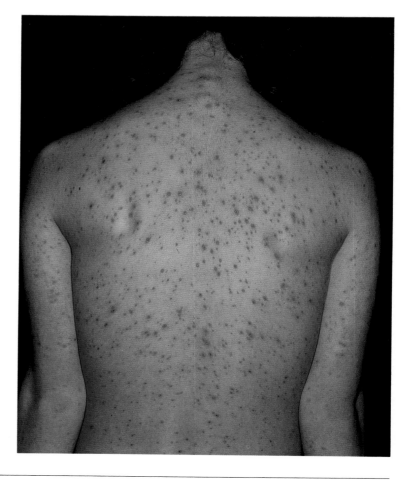

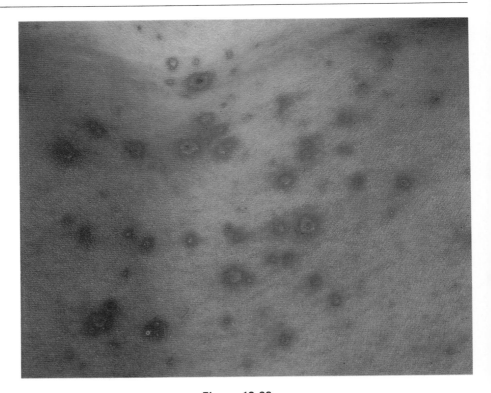

Figure 12-38
Chickenpox. Unique lesions showing a thin-walled vesicle on an irregular red base ("dewdrop on a rose petal").

The lesion starts as a 2- to 4-mm red papule, which develops an irregular outline (rose petal) as a thin-walled clear vesicle appears on the surface (dew drop). This lesion, "dew drop on a rose petal," is highly characteristic (Figure 12-38). The vesicle becomes umbilicated and cloudy and breaks in 8 to 12 hours to form a crust as the red base disappears. Fresh crops of additional lesions undergoing the same process occur in all areas at irregular intervals during the following 3 to 5 days, giving the characteristic picture of intermingled papules, vesicles, pustules, and crusts (Figure 12-39). Moderate to intense pruritus is usually present during the vesicular stage. The degree of temperature elevation parallels the extent and severity of the eruption and varies from 101° to 105° F. The temperature returns to normal when the vesicles have disappeared. Crusts fall off in 7 days (range, 5 to 20 days) and heal without scarring. Secondary infection or excoriation extends the process into the dermis, producing a crater-like pockmark scar. Vesicles often form in the oral cavity and vagina and rupture quickly to form multiple aphtha-like ulcers.

Complications. Adults develop viral pneumonia, which in most cases is asymptomatic and can be detected exclusively by roentgenogram.[32] Cough, dyspnea, and chest pain indicate progressive disease that, in rare cases, may be fatal.

Chickenpox in the immunocompromised patient

Patients with cancer or patients who are taking immunosuppressive drugs, particularly systemic corticosteroids, have extensive eruptions and more complications and may develop hemorrhagic chickenpox and disseminated infection (Figure 12-40).[33] With hemorrhagic chickenpox (also called malignant chickenpox), the lesions are numerous and often bullous and bleeding occurs in the skin at the base of the lesion. The bullae turn dark brown and then black as blood accumulates in the blister fluid. Patients usually have high fever and delirium and may develop convulsions and coma. They frequently bleed from the gastrointestinal tract and mucous membranes. Pneumonia with hemoptysis commonly occurs. The mortality rate was 71% in one series.[34]

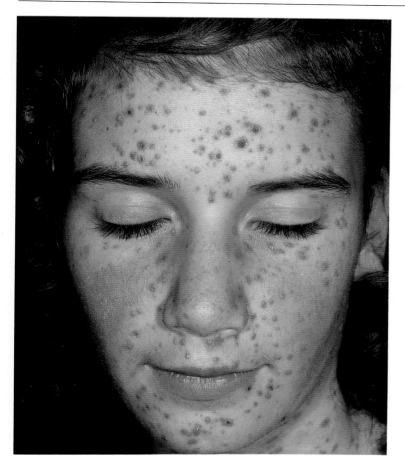

Figure 12-39
Chickenpox. Lesions present in all stages of development.

Figure 12-40
Hemorrhagic chickenpox. Numerous vesicular and bullous lesions with hemorrhage at the base.

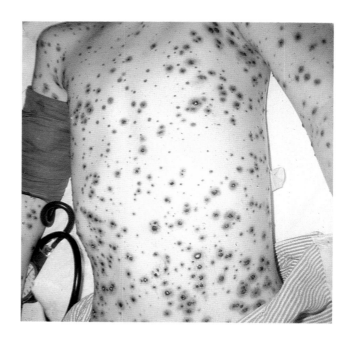

Congenital and neonatal chickenpox

Maternal varicella

First trimester. Women who acquire chickenpox during the early months of pregnancy may deliver a child with multiple congenital anomalies.[35] This syndrome is so rare that accurate rates of fetal infection during maternal infection have not been established. Therefore, parents can be informed only that fetal damage is possible if the mother is infected during the early months of pregnancy.

Second trimester. Maternal varicella in the middle months of pregnancy may result in undetected fetal chickenpox. The newborn child who has already had chickenpox is at risk for developing herpes zoster (shingles). This may explain why some infants and children develop herpes zoster without the expected history of chickenpox.

Near birth. If the mother has varicella 2 to 3 weeks before delivery, the fetus may be infected in utero and may be born with or develop lesions 1 to 4 days after birth.[36] Transplacental maternal antibody protects the infant and the course is usually benign. There is a high incidence of disseminated varicella in the infant when the mother's eruption appears 1 to 4 days before delivery or the child's eruption appears 5 to 10 days after birth. In this situation the virus was either acquired transplacentally or from contact with maternal lesions during birth; there was insufficient time to receive adequate maternal antibody. The infant is immunologically incapable of controlling the infection and is at great risk of developing a disseminated disease. These infants should be given zoster immune globulin (ZIG) or gamma globulin if ZIG is not available.[37]

Laboratory diagnosis. In questionable cases, virus can be cultured from vesicular fluid. (See the section on herpes virus for culture technique). A rise in complement-fixing antibody titer will give a retrospective diagnosis. Obtain serum from the acute stage as early as possible in the course of the disease and serum from the chronic stage 2 or more weeks later. Cytologic smear (Tzanck smear) as described for the diagnosis of herpes simplex and biopsy of a lesion are also helpful. A chest roentgenogram should be obtained if respiratory symptoms develop. The white blood cell count is variably elevated; it is necessary to obtain it only if the disease progresses.

Treatment. Bland antipruritic lotions (e.g., Sarna, menthol and phenol) provide symptomatic relief. Antihistamines (hydroxyzine) may help control excoriation. Oral antibiotics active against streptococcus and staphylococcus are indicated for control of infected lesions. Aspirin should be avoided because of the possible relationship between varicella and Reye's syndrome. ZIG has been used to modify the course of varicella in high risk children (susceptible newborn infants, corticosteroid-treated children, and children with leukemia).[38]

Herpes Zoster

Herpes zoster or shingles, a cutaneous viral infection generally involving the skin of a single dermatome (Figure 12-41), infects approximately 3% of the population. It is considered to result from reactivation of varicella virus that entered the cutaneous nerves during an earlier episode of chickenpox, traveled to the dorsal root ganglia, and remained in a latent form. Age, immunosuppressive drugs, lymphoma, fatigue, emotional upsets, and radiation therapy have been implicated in reactivating the virus, which subsequently travels back down the sensory nerve, infecting the skin. Some patients, particularly children with zoster, have no history of chickenpox. They may have acquired chickenpox by the transplacental route. Although reported, herpes zoster acquired by direct contact with a patient having active varicella or zoster is rare.[39] After contact with such patients, infections are more likely to result from reactivation of latent infection.

Varicella zoster virus can be cultured from vesicles during an eruption; it may also cause chickenpox in those not previously infected.

The predisposition in the elderly for the development of herpes zoster is considered to be a consequence of diminishing immunologic function. The elderly are also at greater risk in developing segmental pain, which can continue for months after the skin lesions have healed.

Figure 12-41
Dermatome areas. (From Pharm-Dex, Everdale Communications, Denville, New Jersey.)

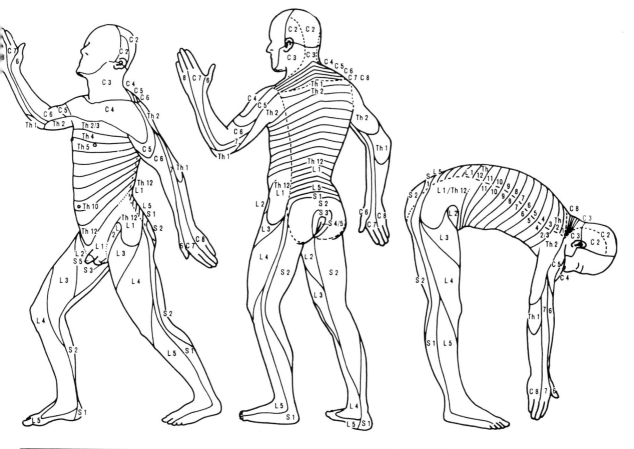

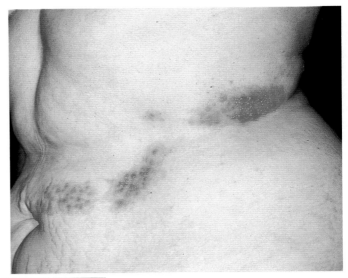

Figure 12-42
Herpes zoster. A common presentation with involvement of a single thoracic dermatome.

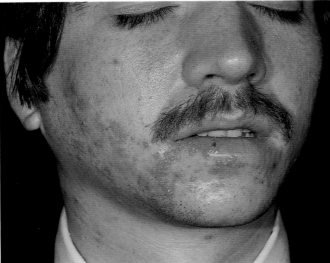

Figure 12-43
Herpes zoster. Unilateral single-dermatome distribution involving the mandibular branch of the fifth nerve.

Figure 12-44
Herpes zoster. An extensive eruption with vesicles involving more than one dermatome.

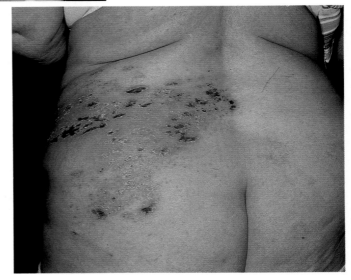

Clinical presentation. Preeruptive pain, itching, or burning, generally localized to the dermatome, precedes the eruption by 4 to 5 days. The pain may simulate pleurisy, myocardial infarction, or abdominal disease and present a difficult diagnostic problem until the characteristic eruption provides the answer. Preeruptive tenderness or hyperesthesia throughout the dermatome is a useful predictive sign.

"Zoster sine herpete" refers to acute segmental neuralgia without a cutaneous eruption.[41] Constitutional symptoms of fever, headache, and malaise may precede the eruption by several days. Regional lymphadenopathy may be present. Segmental pain and constitutional symptoms gradually subside as the eruption appears. Prodromal symptoms may be absent, particularly in children.

Eruptive phase. Although generally limited to the skin of a single dermatome (Figures 12-42 and 12-43), the eruption may involve one or two adjacent dermatomes (Figure 12-44). Occasionally, a few vesicles appear across the midline. Eruption is rare in bilaterally symmetric or asymmetric dermatomes. Approximately 50% of patients with uncomplicated zoster will have a viremia, with the appearance of 20 to 30 vesicles scattered over the skin surface outside the affected dermatome. Possibly because chickenpox is centripetal (located on the trunk), the thoracic region is affected in two-third of herpes zoster cases. An attack of herpes zoster does not confer lasting immunity and it is not abnormal to have two or three episodes in a lifetime.

The eruption begins with red, swollen plaques of various sizes and spreads to involve part or all of a dermatome (Figure 12-45). The vesicles arise in

Figure 12-45
Herpes zoster. Diffuse involvement of a dermatome in a 13-year-old male.

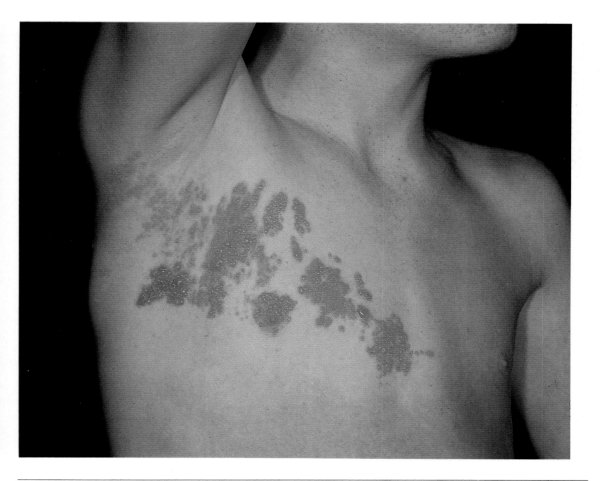

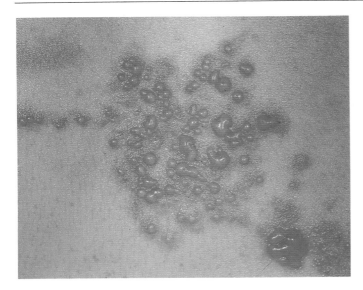

Figure 12-46
Herpes zoster (same patient as in Figure 12-45). A group of vesicles that vary in size. Vesicles of herpes simplex are of uniform size.

Figure 12-47
Herpes zoster. Vesicles become umbilicated.

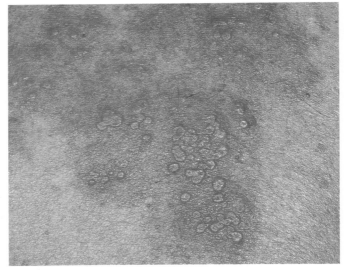

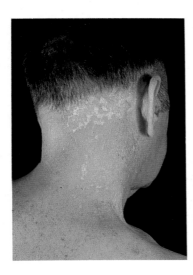

Figure 12-48
Herpes zoster. Several linear scars localized to a dermatome.

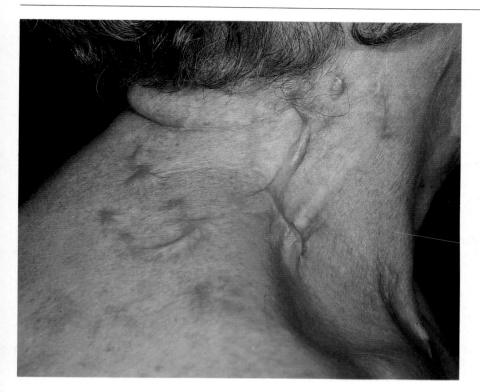

Figure 12-49
Herpes zoster. Hypertrophic scars. Plastic surgery was required to improve mobility in the neck.

clusters from the erythematous base and become cloudy with purulent fluid. The vesicles vary in size, in contrast to the cluster of uniformly sized vesicles noted in herpes simplex (Figure 12-46). Successive crops continue to appear for 7 days. Vesicles either umbilicate (Figure 12-47) or rupture before forming crust, which falls off in 2 to 3 weeks. Elderly or debilitated patients may have a prolonged and difficult course. For them, the eruption is typically more extensive and inflammatory, occasionally resulting in hemorrhagic blisters, skin necrosis, secondary bacterial infection, or extensive scarring (Figure 12-48), which is sometimes hypertrophic or keloidal (Figure 12-49).

Syndromes

Ophthalmic zoster. The ophthalmic division of the trigeminal nerve divides into the frontal, lacrimal, and nasociliary nerves just before it passes through the superior orbital fissure. Involvement of any branch of this nerve is called herpes zoster ophthalmicus. It is involved in 8% to 56% in various series.[40,41] With ophthalmic zoster the rash may extend from eye level to the vertex of the skull but does not cross the midline (Figure 12-50). Herpes

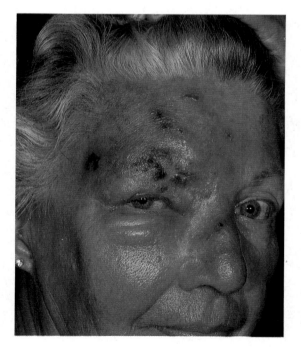

Figure 12-50
Herpes zoster (ophthalmic zoster). Involvement of the first branch of the fifth nerve.

TABLE 12-1

OCULAR COMPLICATIONS IN 86 PATIENTS WITH HERPES ZOSTER OPHTHALMICUS*

Complication	No. of patients
Lid involvement	
Entropion with trichiasis of upper lid	5
Ptosis	1
Cicatricial ectropion with exposure of cornea	2
Scarring of both upper and lower lids	3
TOTAL	11
Corneal involvement	
Acute epithelial keratitis	
Pseudodendritic keratitis	7
Punctate epithelial keratitis	12
Mucous plaques	2
TOTAL	19†
Acute anterior stromal infiltrates	7
Disciform keratitis	17
Sclerokeratitis	2
Neurotrophic keratitis	10
Late dendritic keratitis	1
Peforation	1
TOTAL	47†
Scleral involvement	
Episcleritis (recurrent)	1
Scleritis	3
TOTAL	4
Canalicular scarring	2
Uveitis	
Diffuse	33
Localized	2
Sectorial iris atrophy	15
TOTAL	37†
Glaucoma (secondary)	10
Persistent	2
Cataract	7
Neuro-ophthalmic involvement	
Cranial nerve palsy	3
Contralateral hemiplegia	2
Segmental cerebral arteritis	2
TOTAL	7
Postherpetic neuralgia	15

*From Womack LW, Liesegang TJ: Complications of herpes zoster ophthalmicus. Arch Ophthalmol **101**:44, 1983. By permission of Mayo Foundation.
†Some patients had more than one manifestation of involvement.

zoster ophthalmicus may be confined to certain branches of the trigeminal nerve. The tip and side of the nose and eye are innervated by the nasociliary branch of the trigeminal nerve. Vesicles on the side or tip of the nose (Hutchinson's sign) occurring during an episode of zoster are associated with the most serious ocular complications, including conjunctival, corneal, scleral, and other ocular diseases, although this is not invariable. Involvement of the other sensory branches of the trigeminal nerve are most likely to yield periocular involvement but spare the eyeball[38,42] (Table 12-1).

Ramsay Hunt syndrome. Varicella zoster of the geniculate ganglion is called the Ramsay Hunt syndrome. There may be unilateral loss of taste on the anterior two-thirds of the tongue and vesicles on the tympanic membrane, external auditory meatus, concha, and pinna. Involvement of the motor division of the seventh cranial nerve causes unilateral facial paralysis. Recovery from the motor paralysis is generally complete, but residual weakness is possible.

Sacral zoster (S2, S3, or S4 dermatomes). A neurogenic bladder with urinary hesitancy or retention has been reported to be associated with zoster of the sacral dermatomes S2, S3, or S4.[43] Migration of virus to the adjacent autonomic nerves is responsible for these symptoms.

Complications

Dissemination. Patients with Hodgkin's disease are uniquely susceptible to herpes zoster. Furthermore, 15% to 50% of zoster patients with active Hodgkin's disease have disseminated disease involving the skin, lungs, and brain; 10% to 25% of those patients will die.[44] In patients with other types of cancer, death from zoster is unusual.

Motor paresis. Weakness in the muscle group associated with the infected dermatome may be observed before, during, or after an episode of herpes zoster. This weakness results from involvement of the lower motor neurons by the virus. Patients in the sixth to eighth decades are most commonly affected.

Necrosis, infection, and scarring. Elderly, malnourished, debilitated, or immunosuppressed patients tend to have a more virulent and extensive course. The entire skin area of a dermatome may be lost after diffuse vesiculation. Large adherent crusts promote infection and increase the depth of involvement. Scarring, sometimes hypertrophic or keloidal (see Figure 12-49), will follow.

Postherpetic neuralgia. Pain can persist in a dermatome for months or years after the lesions have disappeared. The pain is often severe, intractable, and exhausting. The patient protects areas of hyperesthesia to avoid the slightest pressure, which activates another wave of pain. There is a yearning for a few hours of sleep, but sharp paroxysms of lancinating pain invade the mind and the patient is again awakened. Despair and sometimes suicide occur if hope and encouragement are not provided.

The majority of patients under 30 experience no pain. By age 40, the risk of prolonged pain for longer than 1 month increases to 33%. By 70 years, the risk increases to 74%. Postherpetic neuralgia is more common and persists longer in cases of trigeminal nerve involvement. The degree of pain is not related to the extent of involvement within a dermatome nor to the number of vesicles present. The mechanism of pain has not been explained.

Differential diagnosis

Herpes simplex. The diagnosis of herpes zoster is usually obvious. Herpes simplex can be extensive, particularly on the trunk. It may be confined to a dermatome and possess many of the same features of zoster (zosteriform herpes simplex). The vesicles of zoster vary in size, while those of simplex are uniform within a cluster. A later recurrence will prove the diagnosis.

Poison ivy. A group of vesicles may be mistaken for poison ivy (Figure 12-51).

"Zoster sine herpete." Neuralgia within a dermatome without the typical rash can be confusing.[41] A concurrent rise in varicella-zoster complement fixation titers has been demonstrated in a number of such cases.

Cellulitis. The eruption of zoster may never evolve to the vesicular stage. The red, inflamed, edematous or urticarial-like plaques may appear infected, but they usually have a fine cobblestone surface indicative of a cluster of minute vesicles. A skin biopsy shows characteristic changes.

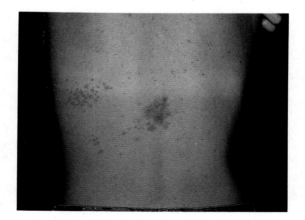

Figure 12-51
Herpes zoster in a young woman. The diagnosis of poison ivy was suspected, but the Tzanck smear was positive in this unilateral cluster of vesicles.

Laboratory diagnosis. The laboratory methods for identification are the same as for herpes simplex. Tzanck smears, skin biopsy (Figure 12-52), complement-fixation titers, vesicular fluid immuno-fluorescent antibody stains, and culture of vesicle fluid are some of the studies to consider.

Treatment

Suppression of inflammation and infection. Burow's solution can be used in a wet compress. The compresses applied 20 minutes 3 times a day will macerate the vesicles, remove serum and crust, and suppress bacterial growth. A whirlpool with Betadine solution is particularly helpful in removing the crust and serum that occur with extensive eruption in the elderly.

Attenuation of the acute phase with acyclovir. Acyclovir has exhibited effective results in inducing more rapid disappearance of pain, collapse of vesicles, disappearance of inflammation, and acceleration of scab formation. There is no effect on the subsequent development of postherpetic neuralgia, including patients who had immediate pain relief.[45-47]

Prevention of postherpetic neuralgia. The use of systemic steroids during the early acute phases of herpes zoster to prevent postherpetic neuralgia remains controversial. Several reports have indicated that the incidence of pain is significantly reduced if systemic corticosteroids are given during the early eruptive stages of herpes zoster.[48,49] Systemic corticosteroids have no effect on postherpetic neuralgia when the lesions have healed. The risk of dissemination is reported to be minimal if patients with malignant disease or immunologic deficiencies are excluded from treatment. This prophylactic treatment should be considered for those patients at greatest risk for developing postherpetic neuralgia, patients over age 60, or those with trigeminal nerve involvement. The recommended schedule is prednisone 20 mg 3 times a day for 7 days, 20 mg twice a day for 7 days, and 20 mg each morning for 7 days.

Treatment of postherpetic neuralgia.[50] Oral analgesics should be used as needed. Addiction is a potential problem. Major tranquilizers such as chlorpromazine 25 mg 4 times a day may be effective in a limited number of patients.[50,51]

One report claims attenuation or elimination of pain in both the eruptive stage and for postherpetic neuralgia with the following simple technique.[52] Inject 0.5% lidocaine to a total of 4 to 5 ml per patient into the subcutaneous tissue through the skin at the most painful sites. For patients with intolerable pain or necrotic herpes zoster, 2.0 ml of 1% lidocaine is injected deep into the proximal area, innervating the herpes zoster lesions. Injections are repeated every 4 to 5 days as needed. Others have claimed substantial relief with a similar schedule using subcutaneous injections through the affected skin with a combination of lidocaine and triamcinolone.[53,54] The mixture is prepared by diluting triamcinolone 10 mg/5 ml with equal parts 1% lidocaine.

Rhizotomy, or surgical separation of pain fibers by a neurosurgeon, may be considered in extreme cases where no therapy has been helpful and the pain is intolerable and persistent.

These patients can be miserable for several months. Emotional support is as important as other therapeutic measures.

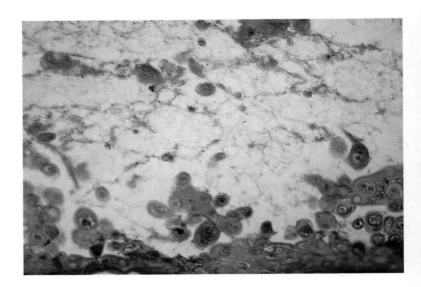

Figure 12-52
Herpes zoster. A skin biopsy showing multinucleated giant cells at the base of a vesicle.

Hand, Foot, and Mouth Disease

Hand, foot, and mouth disease, which has no relation to hoof and mouth disease in cattle, is one of the most distinctive disease complexes caused by the coxsackievirus. This contagious disease may occur as an isolated phenomenon or may occur in epidemic form; it is more common among children.

Clinical presentation. The incubation period is 4 to 6 days. There may be mild symptoms of low grade fever, sore throat, and malaise for 1 or 2 days. Twenty percent of patients develop submandibular or cervical lymphadenopathy or both.

Eruptive phase. The oral lesions, present in 90% of cases, are generally the presenting sign. Aphtha-like erosions varying from a few to 10 or more appear anywhere in the oral cavity and are most frequently small and asymptomatic (Figure 12-53). The cutaneous lesions, which occur in about two-thirds of patients, appear less than 24 hours after the enanthem. They begin as 3- to 7-mm red macules, which rapidly become pale, white, oval vesicles with a red areola. There may be a few inconspicuous lesions or there may be dozens. The vesicles occur on the palms, soles (Figure 12-54), dorsal aspects of the fingers and toes, and occasionally on the face, buttocks, and legs. They heal in about 7 days, usually without crusting or scarring.

Differential diagnosis. When cutaneous lesions are absent, the disease may be confused with aphthous stomatitis. The oral erosions of hand, foot, and mouth disease are usually smaller and more uniform. The vesicles of herpes appear in clusters and those of varicella endure for a longer time; they always crust. Both varicella and herpes have multinucleated giant cells in smears taken from the moist skin exposed when a vesicle is removed (Tzanck smear). Giant cells are not present in lesions of hand, foot, and mouth disease.

Treatment. Symptomatic relief and reassurance are all that is required.

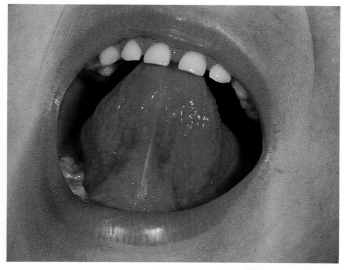

Figure 12-53
Hand, foot, and mouth disease. Aphtha-like lesions in the mouth of a young boy.

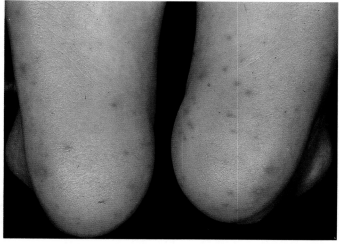

Figure 12-54
Hand, foot, and mouth disease. A cluster on the soles of a young boy. The pale, white, oval vesicles with a red areola are a distinguishing feature of this disease.

REFERENCES

1. Dvoretzky I, Lowy DR: Infections by human papillomavirus (warts). Am J Dermatopathol 4:85, 1982.
2. Morison WL: Viral warts, herpes simplex and herpes zoster in patients with secondary immune deficiencies and neoplasms. Br J Dermatol 92:625, 1975.
3. Coskey R: Warts and their therapy. Dermatology March 1981, p 19.
4. Lockshin NA: Flat facial warts treated with fluorouracil. Arch Dermatol 115:929-1030, 1979.
5. Fisher AA: Severe systemic and local reactions to topical podophyllum resin. Cutis 28:233, 1981.
6. Perez-Figaredo RA, Baden HP: The pharmacology of podophyllum. Prog Dermatol 10:1, 1976.
7. Robinson JK: Extirpation by electrocautery of massive lesions of condyloma acuminatum in genito-perineo-anal region. J Dermatol Surg Oncol 6:733, 1980.
8. Pringle WM, Helms BC: Treatment of plantar warts by blunt dissection. Arch Dermatol 108:79, 1973.
9. Habif TP, Graf FA: Extirpation of subungual and periungual warts by blunt dissection. J Dermatol Surg Oncol 7:553, 1981.
10. Domonkos AN, Arnold HL, Odom RB: Andrews' diseases of the skin, seventh edition. Philadelphia, 1981, WB Saunders Co.
11. Eriksen K: Treatment of the common wart by induced allergic inflammation. Dermatologica 160:161, 1980.
12. Dunagin WG, Millikan LE: Dinitrochlorobenzene immunotherapy for verrucae resistant to standard treatment modalities. J Am Acad Dermatol 6:40, 1982.
13. Saunders BB, Smith KW: Dinitrochlorobenzene immunotherapy of human warts. Cutis 27:389, 1981.
14. Nix TE: Liquid-nitrogen neuropathy. Arch Dermatol 92:185, 1965.
15. Litt JZ: Don't excise—exorcise, treatment for subungual and periungual warts. Cutis 22:673, 1978.
16. Nahmias AJ, Chiana WT, Del Buono I, et al: Typing of herpes virus hominis strains by a direct immunofluorescent technique. Proc Soc Exp Biol Med 132:386, 1969.
17. Nahmias AJ, Roizman B: Infection with herpes-simplex viruses 1 and 2 (First part). N Engl J Med 289:667, 1973.
18. Baringer JR: Recovery of herpes simplex virus from human sacral ganglions. N Engl J Med 291:828, 1974.
18a. Wheeland RG, Burgdorf WHC, Hoshaw RA: A quick Tzanck smear. J Am Acad Dermatol 8:258, 1983.
19. Solomon AR, Rasmussen JE, Varani J, et al: The Tzanck smear in the diagnosis of cutaneous herpes simplex. JAMA 251:633, 1984.
20. Hitchcock G, Randell PL, Wishart MM: Herpes simplex lesions of the skin diagnosed by immunofluorescence technic. Med J Aust 2:280, 1974.
21. Raeb B, Lorincz AL: Genital herpes simplex: concepts and treatment. J Am Acad Dermatol 5:249, 1981.
22. Robinson JK, Spencer SK: Treatment of recurrent herpes simplex. Arch Dermatol 114:1096, 1978.
23. Kalinyak JE, Fleagle G, Docherty J: Incidence and distribution of herpes simplex virus types 1 and 2 from genital lesions in college women. J Med Virol 1:175, 1977.
24. August MJ, Nordlund JJ, Hsuing GD: Persistence of herpes simplex virus types 1 and 2 in infected individuals. Arch Dermatol 115:309, 1979.
25. Corey L, et al: A trial of topical acyclovir in genital herpes simplex virus infections. N Engl J Med 306:1313, 1982.
26. Mindel A, Adler MW, Sutherland S, et al: Intravenous acyclovir treatment for primary genital herpes. Lancet 1:697, 1982.
27. Bryson YJ, Dillon M, Lovett M, et al: Treatment of first episodes of genital herpes simplex virus infections with oral acyclovir: a randomized double-blind controlled trial in normal subjects. N Engl J Med 308:916, 1983.
27a. Douglas JM, Critchlow C, Benedetti J, et al: A double-blind study of oral acyclovir for suppression of recurrences of genital herpes simplex virus infection. N Engl J Med 310:1551, 1984.
28. Jarratt M: Herpes simplex infection in the newborn. Dermatology, April 1979, p 51.
29. Nahmias AJ, Josey WE, Naib Z: Significance of herpes simplex virus infection during pregnancy. Clin Obstet Gynecol 15:929, 1972.
30. Hirsch MS, Schooley RT: Treatment of herpes virus infections. N Engl J Med 309:1034, 1983.
31. Wheeler CE, Abele DC: Eczema herpeticum: primary and recurrent. Arch Dermatol 93:162, 1966.
32. Triebwasser JH, Harris RE, Bryant ER, et al: Varicella pneumonia in adults: report of seven cases and a review of the literature. Medicine 46:409, 1967.
33. Close GC, Houston IB: Fatal haemorrhagic chickenpox in a child on long-term steroids. Lancet 2:480, 1981.
34. Feldman S, Hughes WT, Daniel CB: Varicella in children with cancer: seventy-seven cases. Pediatrics 56:388, 1975.
35. Wheller TH: Varicella and herpes zoster: changing concepts of the natural history, control, and importance of a not-so-benign virus. N Engl J Med 309:1434, 1983.
36. Krugman S, Katz SL: Infectious diseases of children. St. Louis, 1981, C.V. Mosby Co.
37. Evans EB, Pollock TM, Craddock-Wilson JE, et al: Human anti-chickenpox immunoglobulin in the prevention of chickenpox. Lancet 1:354, 1980.
38. Liesegang, TJ: The varicella-zoster virus: systemic and ocular features. J Am Acad Dermatol 11:165, 1984.
39. Daniel SU WP, Muller SA: Herpes zoster: case report of possible accidental inoculation. Arch Dermatol 112:1755, 1976.
40. Hope-Simpson RE: The nature of herpes zoster: a long-term study and a new hypothesis. Proc R Soc Med 58:9, 1965.
41. Lewis GW: Zoster sine herpete. Br Med J 2:418, 1958.
42. Womack LW, Liesegang TJ: Complications of herpes zoster ophthalmicus. Arch Ophthalmol 101:42, 1983.
43. Weaver SM, Kelly AP: Herpes zoster as a cause of neurogenic bladder. Cutis 29:611, 1982.
44. Mazur MH, Dolin R: Herpes zoster at the NIH: a 20-year experience. Am J Med 65:738, 1978.

45. Bean B, Braun C, Balfour HH: Acyclovir therapy for acute herpes zoster. Lancet **2**:118, 1982.
46. Peterslund NA, et al: Acyclovir in herpes zoster. Lancet **2**:827, 1981.
47. Selby PJ, Powles RL, Janeson B, et al: Parenteral acyclovir therapy for herpes virus infections in man. Lancet **2**:1267, 1979.
48. Keczkes K, Basheer AM: Do corticosteroids prevent post-herpetic neuralgia? Br J Dermatol **102**:551, 1980.
49. Eaglstein WN, Katz R, Brow JA: The effects of early corticosteriod therapy on the skin eruption and pain of herpes zoster. JAMA **211**:1681, 1970.
50. Thiers MD: Unusual treatments for herpesvirus infections. II. Herpes zoster. J Am Acad Dermatol **8**:433, 1983.
51. Kramer P: The management of post-herpetic neuralgia with chlorprothixene. Surg Neurol **15**:102, 1981.
52. Ogata A, et al: Local anesthesia for herpes zoster. J Dermatol **7**:161, 1980.
53. Epstein E: Treatment of herpes zoster and postzoster neuralgia by subcutaneous injection of triamcinolone. Int J Dermatol **20**:65, 1981.
54. Epstein E: Triamcinolone-procaine in the treatment of zoster and postzoster neuralgia. California Med **115**:6, 1971.

Chapter Thirteen

Exanthems

Measles
Scarlet fever
Rubella
Erythema infectiosum
Roseola infantum
Infectious mononucleosis
Enteroviruses: ECHO and Coxsackie viral
    exanthems
Exanthematous drug eruptions

The word exanthem means a skin eruption that bursts forth or blooms. Exanthematous diseases are characterized by widespread, symmetric, erythematous, discrete or confluent macules and papules that initially do not form scale. This appears to be one of the few instances in which the term maculopapular is an appropriate descriptive term. Other lesions such as pustules, vesicles, and petechiae may form, but most of the exanthematous diseases begin with red macules or papules. Widespread red eruptions such as guttate psoriasis or pityriasis rosea may have a similar beginning and are often symmetric, but these conditions have characteristic types of scale and are therefore referred to as papulosquamous eruptions. Diseases with exanthems may be caused by bacteria, viruses, or drugs. Most have a number of characteristic features such as the primary lesion, distribution and duration, and systemic symptoms. Some are accompanied by oral lesions referred to as enanthems.

Exanthems were previously consecutively numbered according to their historical appearance and description. These were first disease, measles; second disease, scarlet fever; third disease, rubella; fourth disease, "Dukes' disease" (probably coxsackie or ECHO virus); fifth disease, erythema infectiosum; and sixth disease, roseola infantum.

Measles

Measles (rubeola or morbilli) is a highly contagious viral disease transmitted by contact with droplets from infected individuals, usually children. Most cases have a benign course, but encephalitis occurs in 1 of 2000 individuals[1]; survivors frequently have permanent brain damage and mental retardation. Death, predominantly from respiratory and neurologic causes, occurs in 1 of every 3000 reported cases of measles.[2] The risk of death is known to be greater for infants and adults than for children and adolescents. Measles occurring during pregnancy may affect the fetus. Most commonly, this involves premature labor, moderately increased

rates of spontaneous abortion, and low-birth-weight infants.[3] Results of one study in an isolated population suggested that measles infection in the first trimester of pregnancy was associated with an increased rate of congenital malformation.[4] Before measles vaccine was available, more than 400,000 measles cases were reported each year in the United States. In 1980 there were about 3,000 reported cases. In the prevaccine era, most measles cases affected preschool and young school-age children. In 1980 more than 60% of cases in which the age was known occurred among persons 10 years or older.

Lifelong immunity is established with a single injection of live measles virus vaccine given at approximately 15 months of age. Susceptible persons include those who were vaccinated between 1963 and 1967 with inactivated vaccine, patients given live measles virus vaccine before their first birthday, and those patients who have never had measles. Prior recipients of killed measles vaccine may develop atypical measles syndrome when exposed to natural measles and should be revaccinated with live measles virus vaccine.

Clinical course

Typical measles. Typical measles (Figure 13-1) has an incubation period of 10 or 11 days, with a range from 7 to 14 days. Prodromal symptoms of severe, brassy cough, coryza, conjunctivitis, photophobia, and fever appear 3 to 4 days before the exanthem and increase daily in severity. Koplik's spots, blue-white spots with a red halo, appear on the buccal mucous membrane opposite the premolar teeth 24 to 48 hours before the exanthem and remain for 2 to 4 days.

Eruptive phase. The rash begins on the face and behind the ears, but in 24 hours it spreads to the trunk and extremities (Figure 13-2). It reaches maximum intensity simultaneously in all areas with constitutional symptoms in approximately 3 days and fades in 5 to 10 days. The rash consists of slightly elevated maculopapules that vary in size from 0.1 to 1 cm and vary in color from dark red to purplish. They are frequently confluent on both the face and body, a feature that is such a distinct characteristic

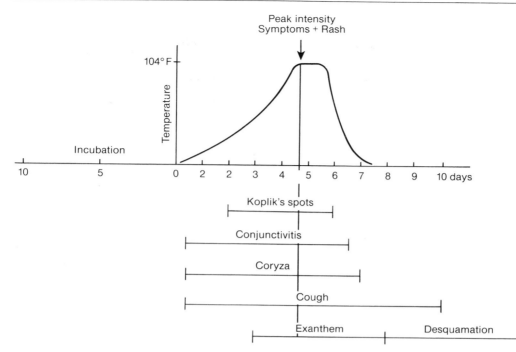

Figure 13-1
Measles. Evolution of the signs and symptoms.

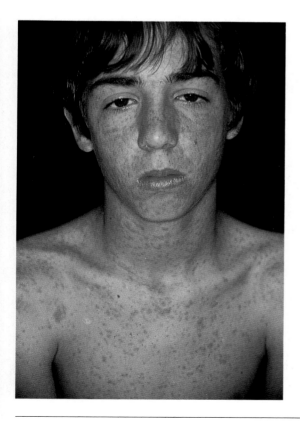

Figure 13-2
Measles. Early eruptive stage with involvement of the face and trunk. Eruption has become confluent on the face.

of measles that eruptions of similar appearance in other diseases are termed morbilliform (Figure 13-3). The early rash blanches on pressure; the fading rash is yellowish-brown with a fine scale and does not blanch. Supportive treatment is the only necessity, unless complications such as bacterial infection or encephalitis appear.

Prevention. Live measles virus vaccine is administered at approximately 15 months of age; at least 95% of vaccine recipients develop measles antibody after a single dose. The most commonly used test for measurement of immunity to measles is the hemagglutination-inhibition (HI) test. Most immune individuals will have measles HI antibody levels of greater than 4.

Sporadic epidemics of measles continue to appear. Cases are rare in those previously immunized and in those who have experienced previous infection with measles. During outbreaks the immunity status of exposed individuals should be determined. Susceptible patients should be vaccinated. Measles vaccine may provide protection if given within 72 hours of exposure. During outbreaks, infants as young as 6 months of age may be vaccinated when exposure to measles is likely. Infants under 12 months of age should receive single-antigen measles vaccine rather than measles-mumps-rubella vaccines. Such infants should be revaccinated when they are about 15 months old.

Immune globulin may also be used to prevent or modify measles in infants and may be especially indicated for susceptible household contacts of measles patients (particularly if under 1 year of age) for whom the risk of complication is highest. The recommended dose is 0.25 ml/kg (0.11 ml/lb) of body weight (maximum dose, 15 ml) intramuscularly, within 6 days of exposure.

Atypical measles. Atypical measles occurs in adolescents and young adults. As with typical measles, there is a prodromal period accompanied by conjunctivitis, coryza, cough, and Koplik's spots. After a 3- to 5-day prodromal period, the rash begins on the wrists and ankles as a mildly pruritic maculopapular rash. It extends to the palms and soles and the hands and feet are often swollen. The temperature rises to 41° C, and within 2 to 5 days the rash gradually spreads centripetally to involve the extremities and torso.[5] The face is usually spared. The rash may become vesicular, prupuric, and hemorrhagic. Pulmonary consolidation and pleural effusions may occur. The illness is self-limited and clears in 2 weeks. Mild desquamation of the palms and soles may follow.

Figure 13-3
Measles. Maculopapules on the trunk have become dark colored and confluent, a characteristic appearance of measles. Rashes of similar appearances are termed morbilliform.

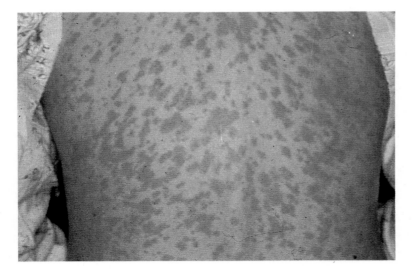

Scarlet Fever

Scarlet fever (scarlatina) is an endemic contagious disease produced by a streptococcal erythrogenic toxin. The circulating toxin is responsible for the rash and systemic symptoms. The infection may originate in the pharynx or skin and is most common in children who lack immunity to the toxin. Scarlet fever was a feared disease in the nineteenth and early twentieth centuries, when the disease was more virulent, but presently scarlet fever is usually benign.

Clinical course. In the clinical course of scarlet fever (Figure 13-4), there is an incubation period of 2 to 4 days.

Prodromal and eruptive phase. The sudden onset of fever and pharyngitis is followed shortly by nausea, vomiting, headache, and abdominal pain. The entire oral cavity may be red, and the tongue is covered with a yellowish-white coat through which red papillae protrude. Diffuse lymphadenopathy may appear just before the onset of the eruption. The systemic symptoms continue until the fever subsides. The rash begins around the neck and face and spreads in 48 hours to the trunk and extremities; the palms and soles are spared (Figure 13-5). The face is flushed except for circumoral pallor, while all other involved areas exhibit a vivid scarlet hue with innumerable pinpoint papules that

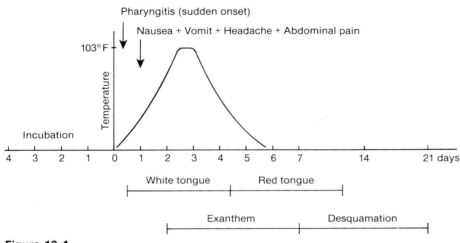

Figure 13-4
Scarlet fever. Evolution of signs and symptoms.

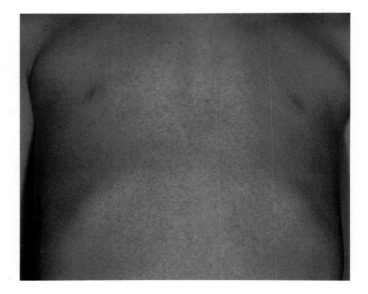

Figure 13-5
Scarlet fever. Early eruptive stage on the trunk showing numerous pinpoint red papules.

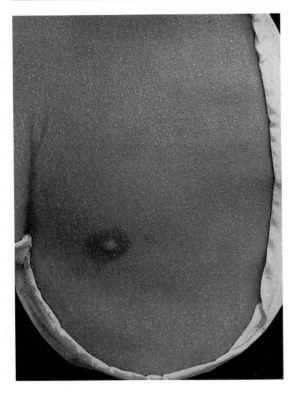

Figure 13-6
Scarlet fever. Fully evolved eruption. Numerous papules giving a sandpaper-like texture to the skin.

give a rough sandpaper quality to the skin (Figure 13-6). The rash is more limited and less dramatic in milder cases. Linear petechiae (Pastia's lines) are characteristic; they are found in skin folds, particularly the antecubital fossa and inguinal area. The tongue sheds the white coat to reveal a red, raw, glazed surface with engorged papillae (Figure 13-7).

The fever and rash subside and desquamation more pronounced than in any of the eruptive fevers appears. It begins on the face, where it is sparse and superficial, progresses to the trunk, often with a circular punched-out appearance, and finally spreads to the hands (Figure 13-8) and feet (Figure 13-9) where the epidermis is the thickest. Clinically, the hands and feet appear normal during the initial stages of the disease. Large sheaths of epidermis may be shed from the palms and soles in a glove-like cast, exposing new and often tender epidermis beneath. A transverse groove may be produced in all of the nails (Beau's lines) (Figure 13-10). The pattern of desquamation of the palms and soles and grooving of the nails is such a distinct characteristic of scarlet fever that it is helpful in making retrospective diagnosis in cases where the eruption was minimal. A rising antistreptolysin-O titer constitutes additional supporting evidence for a recent infection. Desquamation is generally complete in 4 weeks, but may last for 8 weeks.

Treatment. Various drugs are available for treatment. They include benzathine penicillin G (single injection): under 60 lb, 600,000 units; over 60 lb, 1.2 million units; penicillin V (10-day oral course): under 60 lb, 125 mg 4 times a day; over 60 lb, 250 mg 4 times a day; oral erythromycin (child, 40 mg/kg/day; adult, 250 mg 4 times a day).

Figure 13-7
Scarlet fever. Portions of the white coat remain in the center but the remainder of the tongue is red with engorged papillae ("strawberry tongue").

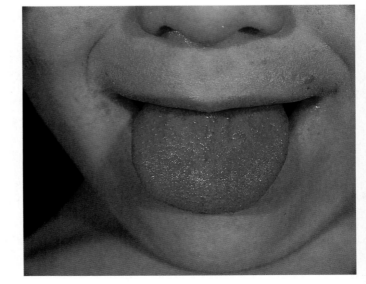

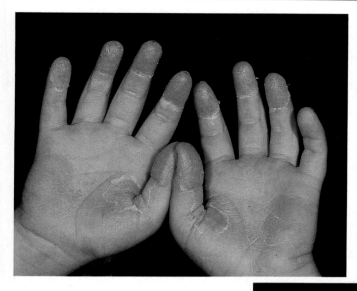

Figure 13-8
Scarlet fever. Desquamation of the hands.

Figure 13-9
Scarlet fever. Desquamation of the feet.

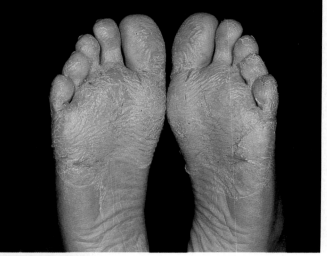

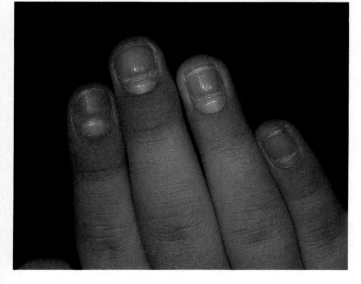

Figure 13-10
Scarlet fever. Beau's lines: transverse grooves on all nails several weeks after skin signs of scarlet fever have cleared.

Rubella

Rubella (German measles, 3-day measles), a benign, contagious, viral disease spread by the respiratory route, is most common in children and young adults. The incidence has decreased since the introduction of rubella vaccine, which is given along with mumps and measles vaccine in a single injection at the age of 15 months.

Pregnant women who have rubella early in the first trimester may transmit the disease to the fetus, which may consequently develop a number of congenital defects (congenital rubella syndrome).[6] Presently, most women who plan a pregnancy have rubella hemagglutination-inhibition titer measured. Many women have had a subclinical infection and already have an adequate titer. Those women with no evidence of previous infection should be immunized and then warned that pregnancy must be avoided for 2 months, during which time attenuated virus may be present in the tissues. Women of unknown immune status who conceive and are subsequently exposed to rubella or develop an exanthem that in any way resembles rubella should have an hemagglutination-inhibition titer measured immediately and 7 to 14 days later. If infection is likely and therapeutic abortion is unacceptable, then passive immunization with immune serum globulin (0.25 mg/lb) should be given. The value of this prophylactic treatment is unknown.

Clinical course. In the clinical course of rubella (Figure 13-11) there is an incubation period of 18 days, with a range of 14 to 21 days.

Prodromal phase. Mild symptoms of malaise, headache, and moderate temperature elevation may precede the eruption by a few hours or a day. Children are usually asymptomatic. Lymphadenopathy, characteristically postauricular, suboccipital, and cervical, may appear 4 to 7 days before the rash and may be maximal at the onset of the exanthem. In 2% of cases, petechiae on the soft palate occur late in the prodromal phase or early in the eruptive phase.

Eruptive phase. The eruption begins on the neck or face and in hours spreads to the trunk and extremities. The lesions are pinpoint to 1-cm, round or oval, pinkish or rosy red, macules or maculopapules. The color is less vivid than that of scarlet fever and lacks the blue of violaceous tinge seen in measles (Figure 13-12). The lesions are usually discrete, but may be grouped or coalesce on the face or trunk. The rash fades in 24 to 48 hours in the same order in which it appeared and may be followed by a fine desquamation. Arthritis, affecting primarily the phalangeal joints of adult females, may occur in the prodromal period and may last for 2 to 3 weeks after the rash has disappeared.[7] No treatment is required.

Figure 13-11
Rubella. Evolution of signs and symptoms.

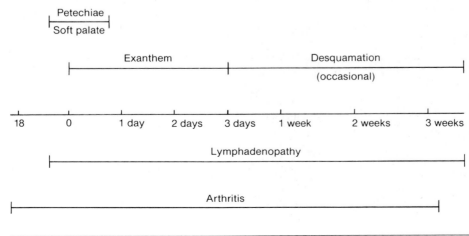

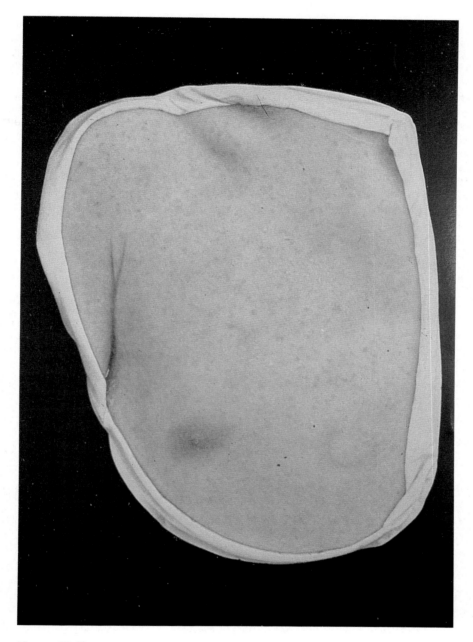

Figure 13-12
Rubella. Pink oval maculopapules lack the rich
color of scarlet fever and measles.

Erythema Infectiosum

Erythema infectiosum (fifth disease) is probably caused by a virus. It is relatively common and mildly contagious and appears sporadically or in epidemics in children over the age of 3 and in young adults.

Clinical course. In the clinical course of erythema infectiosum (Figure 13-13) there is an incubation period of 4 to 14 days.

Prodromal symptoms. Symptoms are usually mild or absent. Pruritus, low-grade fever, malaise, and sore throat precede the eruption in about 10% of cases. Lympadenopathy is absent. Older individuals may complain of joint pain.

Eruptive phase. There are three distinct overlapping stages.

Facial erythema ("slapped cheek"). Red papules on the cheeks rapidly coalesce in hours, forming red, slightly edematous, warm, erysipelas-like plaques, which are symmetric on both cheeks and spare the nasolabial fold and the circumoral region. The "slapped cheek" appearance fades in 4 days.

Net pattern erythema. This unique characteristic eruption with erythema in a fishnet-like pattern begins on the extremities about 2 days after the onset of facial erythema and extends to the trunk and buttock, fading in 6 to 14 days (Figure 13-14). At times, the exanthem begins with erythema and does not become characteristic until irregular clearing takes place. Livedo reticularis has a similar net-like pattern, but does not fade quickly.

Recurrent phase. The eruption may fade and then reappear in previously affected sites on the face and body during the next 2 to 3 weeks. Temperature changes, emotional upsets, and sunlight may stimulate recurrences. The rash fades without scaling or pigmentation. There may be a slight lymphocytosis or eosinophilia.

Treatment. Parents need only to be assured that this unusual extensive eruption will fade and will not require treatment.

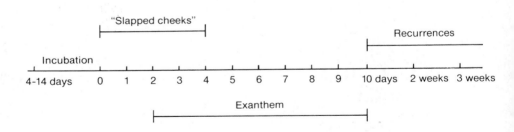

Figure 13-13
Erythema infectiosum. Evolution of signs and symptoms.

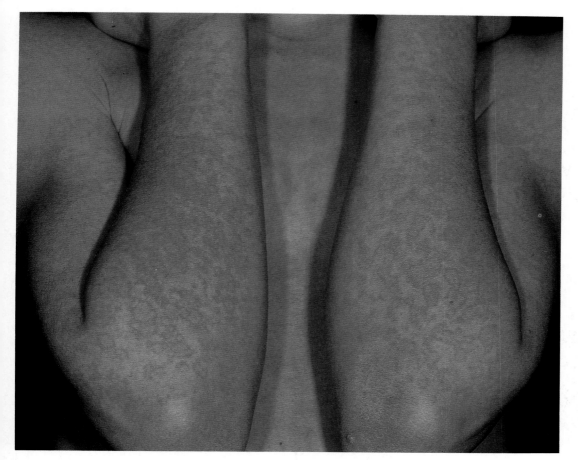

Figure 13-14
*Erythema infectiosum. Net-like pattern of
erythema.*

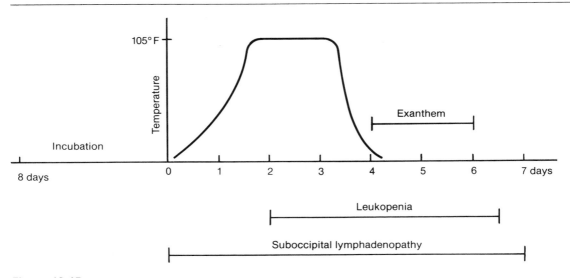

Figure 13-15
Roseola infantum. Evolution of signs and symptoms.

Figure 13-16
Roseola infantum. Pale pink macules may appear first on the neck.

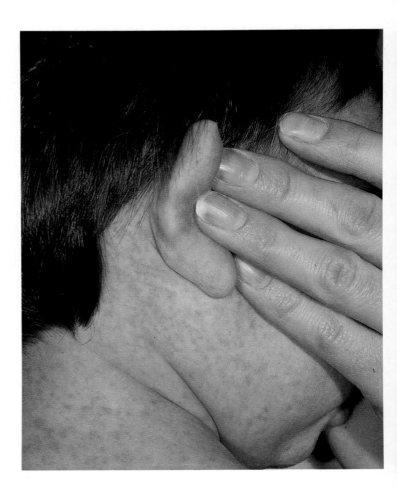

Roseola Infantum

Roseola infantum (exanthem subitum, "sudden rash"; sixth disease) is probably caused by a virus. Most cases are asymptomatic or occur without a rash. The disease is sporadic and the majority of cases occur in patients between the ages of 6 months and 4 years. The development of high fever as seen in roseola is worrisome, but the onset of the characteristic rash is reassuring.

Clinical course. In the clinical course of roseola infantum (Figure 13-15), there is an incubation period of 8 days, with a range of 5 to 15 days.

Prodromal symptoms. There is a sudden onset of high fever of 103° to 106° F with few or minor symptoms. Most children appear inappropriately well for the degree of temperature elevation, but they may experience slight anorexia or one or two episodes of vomiting. Seizures, probably febrile, sometimes occur. Mild to moderate lymphadenopathy, usually in the occipital regions, begins at the onset of the febrile period and persists until after the eruption has subsided. Leukocytosis develops at the onset of fever, but leukopenia with a relative lymphocytosis appears as the temperature increases and persists until the eruption fades.

Eruptive phase. The rash begins as the fever subsides. Numerous pale pink almond-shaped macules appear on the trunk and neck, become confluent, and then fade in a few hours to 2 days without scaling or pigmentation (Figures 13-16 and 13-17). The exanthem may resemble rubella or measles, but the pattern of development, distribution, and associated symptoms of these other exanthematous diseases are different.

Treatment. Control temperature with aspirin and provide reassurance.

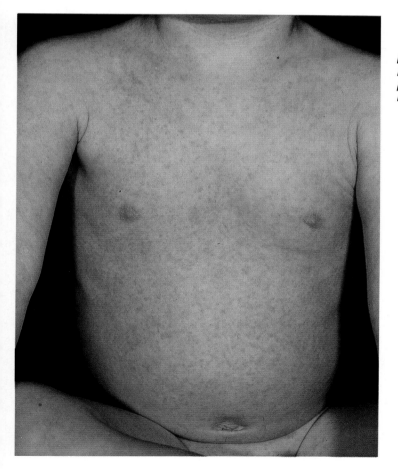

Figure 13-17
Roseola infantum. Numerous pale pink almond-shaped macules.

Infectious Mononucleosis

Infectious mononucleosis, caused by the Epstein-Barr virus, may result in a morbilliform eruption indistinguishable from that of other viral exanthems in about 3% to 15% of cases. Most infections are probably subclinical. Transmission appears to occur by direct contact. The incubation period is from 33 to 49 days.

Clinical features. In the clinical course (Figure 13-18) headache and malaise are followed by fever of 101° to 104° F. Sore throat (80% of cases) and membranous tonsillitis (20% of cases) develop a few days later, followed shortly by petechiae of the soft and hard palate (25% of cases), cervical or generalized lymphadenopathy, and splenomegaly. Hepatomegaly and icteric hepatitis may occur. The exanthem, if it occurs, appears on the fourth to sixth day. A macular or maculopapular morbilliform eruption appears on the trunk or upper arms and may involve the face and, less frequently, the distal extremities. Sometimes the eruption resembles scarlet fever or may be urticarial.[8] The exanthem fades in a few days. Most symptoms will subside in 3 weeks, but fatigue lasting for several more weeks may occur, especially in adults. A majority of patients with infectious mononucleosis who are treated with ampicillin will develop a generalized morbilliform eruption 5 to 8 days after starting ampicillin ("typical ampicillin rash").[9]

Laboratory diagnosis. A heterophile antibody titer of greater than 1:128 is considered significant. In one study, 38% of patients showed a significant level at 1 week, 60% by 2 weeks, and 80% by 3 weeks.[10] A rapid slide test (mono test) has a low incidence of false reactions and a high degree of specificity. There is usually a white blood cell count of 10,000, but it may be greater than 40,000, with lymphocytosis and atypical lymphocytes. The throat should be cultured to rule out streptococcal pharyngitis.

Treatment. Treatment is symptomatic. Avoid use of ampicillin because of the high incidence of skin eruptions. Protect the patient from abdominal trauma during the next 6 months to prevent possible damage to an enlarged spleen.

Figure 13-18
Infectious mononucleosis. Evolution of signs and symptoms.

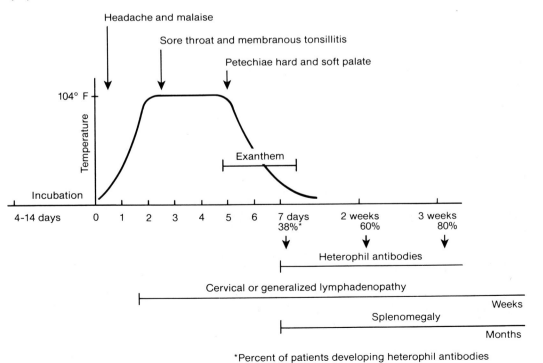

*Percent of patients developing heterophil antibodies

Enteroviruses: ECHO and Coxsackie Viral Exanthems

The previously described diseases characteristically display a predictable set of signs and symptoms. Roseola and erythema infectiosum are relatively common. Many physicians will never see measles, German measles, or scarlet fever. The most common exanthematous eruptions are caused by the enteroviruses ECHO and Coxsackie. A large number of these viruses may cause a skin eruption. Some of these eruptions are characteristic of the virus type, but in most cases one must be satisfied with the diagnosis of "viral rash." In many cases drug eruptions cannot be distinguished from the nonspecific exanthems of these enteroviruses.

Clinical presentation

Systemic symptoms. Many symptoms are possible, such as fever, nausea, vomiting and diarrhea, along with typical viral symptoms of photophobia, lymphadenopathy, sore throat, and possibly encephalitis.

Exanthem. The rash may appear at any time during the course of the illness and is usually generalized. Lesions are erythematous maculopapules with areas of confluence, but may be urticarial, vesicular, and sometimes petechial (Figures 13-19 and 13-20). The palms and soles may be involved. The eruptions are more common in children than in adults. In most cases the rash fades without pigmentation or scaling.

Treatment. Treatment consists of relieving symptoms.

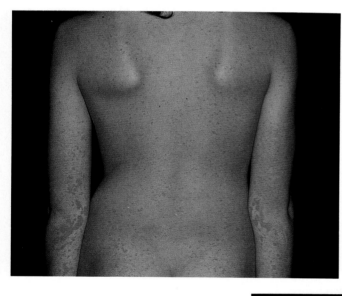

Figure 13-19
Viral exanthem. Symmetric erythematous maculopapular eruption.

Figure 13-20
Viral exanthem. Diffuse erythematous papular eruption involving the entire cutaneous surface.

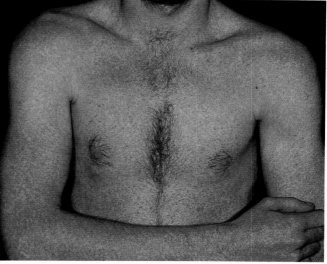

Exanthematous Drug Eruptions

Exanthematous drug eruptions commonly resemble viral rashes. The most common presentation consists of symmetric, morbilliform, discrete or confluent erythematous maculopapules on the trunk; less commonly, they appear on the face, extremities, palms, and soles. The rash appears 1 week after starting the drug and fades in 1 to 3 weeks. The rash may be scarletina-form, urticarial, petechial, vesicular, or bullous. Prutitus is mild to severe. Itching of the palms is characteristic of drug eruptions. Ampicillin is the most common drug to cause eruption; reactions to it will be described.

Ampicillin rash. Two types of skin reactions occur; these are an urticarial reaction mediated by skin-sensitizing antibody and a much more common exanthematous maculopapular reaction for which no allergic basis can be established.[11] Ampicillin or other penicillins should not be given to patients who have had previous urticarial reactions while taking ampicillin. Ampicillin may be given safely to patients who have previously had a maculopapular ampicillin rash. There is a marked increase in exanthema-tous ampicillin eruptions when ampicillin is given during the course of certain viral infections (e.g., infectious mononucleosis and cytomegalovirus), in patients with adult lymphocytic leukemia, and when given simultaneously with allopurinol.

Clinical presentation. The rash begins 5 to 9 days (range, 1 day to 4 weeks) after initiation of ampicillin and may occur after the drug is terminated. The rash starts on the trunk as a mildly pruritic, red, maculopapular, sometimes confluent eruption and in hours spreads symmetrically to the face and extremities (Figure 13-21). The palms, soles, and mucous membranes are spared. The rash begins to fade in 3 days and is gone in 6 days, even if ampicillin is continued.

Management. No treatment is required for the maculopapular eruption. If the nature of a previous reaction is unknown and there is no adequate substitute drug, then skin tests with ampicillin, major determinants penicilloyl-polylysine (PPL; Pre-Pen), and a minor determinant (diluted penicillin G or sodium penicilloate) should be undertaken.

Figure 13-21
Drug eruption (ampicillin). Asymmetric confluent maculopapular eruption.

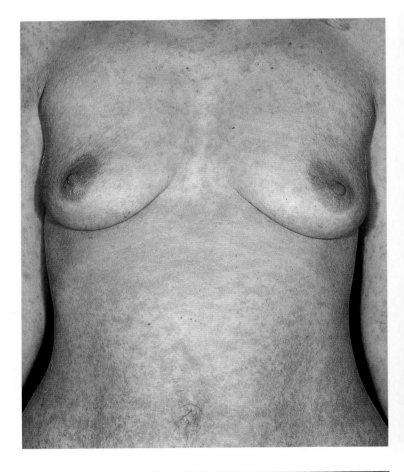

REFERENCES

1. Tidstrom B: Complications in measles with special reference to encephalitis. Acta Med Scand **184:**411, 1968.
2. Recommendation of the Immunization Practices Advisory Committee: Measles prevention. Morbidity and Mortality Weekly Report **31**(17):May 7, 1982.
3. Siegel M, Fuerst HT: Low birth weight and maternal virus disease: a prospective study of rubella, measles, mumps, chickenpox, and hepatitis. JAMA **197:**680, 1966.
4. Jespersen CS, Littauer J, Sagild U: Measles as a cause of fetal defects. Acta Paediatr Scand **66:**367, 1977.
5. Martin DB, Weiner LB, Nieburg PI, et al: Atypical measles in adolescents and young adults. Ann Intern Med **90:**877, 1979.
6. Bellanti JA, Arnstein MS, Olson LC, et al: Congenital rubella. Am J Dis Child **110:**464, 1965.
7. Judelson RG, Wyll SA: Rubella in Bermuda: termination of an epidemic by mass vaccination. JAMA **223:**401, 1973.
8. Karzon DT: Infectious mononucleosis. Adv Pediatr **22:**231, 1976.
9. Levene G, Baker H: Ampicillin and infectious mononucleosis. Br J Dermatol **80:**417. 1978.
10. Niederman JC: Heterophil antibody determinations in a series of 166 cases of infectious mononucleosis listed according to various stages of the disease. Yale J Biol Med **28:**629, 1956.
11. Kraemer MJ, Smith AL: Rashes with ampicillin. Pediatr Rev **1:**197, 1980.

Chapter Fourteen

Infestations and Bites

Scabies

Human scabies is a contagious disease caused by the mite *Sarcoptes scabiei* var *hominis.* Dogs and cats may be infested by almost identical organisms; these may sometimes be a source of human infestation. Incidence figures show that epidemics occur about every 30 years and last 15 years, with the greatest number of cases occurring at the midpoint in time. The reason for the occurrence of this disease in epidemics and its duration for a particular interval is unknown. In the past scabies has been attributed to poor hygiene. Most contemporary cases, however, appear in individuals with adequate hygiene who are in close contact with numbers of individuals such as school children. Blacks rarely acquire scabies; the reason is unknown.

Anatomical features, life cycle, and immunology. The adult mite is $\frac{1}{3}$ mm long and has a flattened oval body with wrinkle-like transverse corrugations and eight legs (Figure 14-1). The first two pairs of legs bear claw-shaped suckers and the two rear pairs end in long trailing bristles. The digestive tract fills a major portion of the body and is readily observed when the mite is seen in cross-section of histologic specimens (Figures 14-2).

Infestation begins when a fertilized female mite arrives on the skin surface. Within the hour the female excavates a burrow in the stratum corneum (dead horny layer); during her 30-day life cycle this burrow reaches from several millimeters to a few centimeters in length. The burrow does not enter the underlying epidermis except in the case of hyperkeratotic Norwegian scabies, a condition in which retarded, immunosuppressed, or elderly patients develop scaly thick skin in the presence of thousands of mites. Eggs laid at the rate of two or three a day (Figure 14-3) and fecal pellets (scybala) are deposited in the burrow behind the advancing female. Scybala are dark oval masses easily visualized with the eggs when burrow scrapings are examined under the microscope. Scybala may act as an irritant and be responsible for some of the itching. The larvae hatch, leave an egg casing in the burrow, and reach maturity in 14 to 17 days The adult mites copulate and repeat the cycle. Therefore, 3 to 5 weeks after infestation only a few mites are present. Understanding this life cycle assists in explaining why patients experience few if any symptoms during the first month after contact with a infested individual. After a number of mites (usually less than 20) have reached maturity and have spread by scatching or migration, the initial minor localized itch evolves into intense generalized pruritus.

A hypersensitivity reaction rather than a foreign body response may be responsible for the lesions; this may delay recognition of symptoms of scabies. Some patients infested with scabies develop elevated IgE titers, eosinophilia, and an immediate type hypersensitivity reaction to an extract prepared from female mites.[1] IgE levels fall within a year after infestation. Eosinophilia returns to normal shortly after treatment. The fact that patients develop symptoms much more rapidly when reinfested supports the claim that symptoms and lesion of scabies are the result of a hypersensitivity reaction.

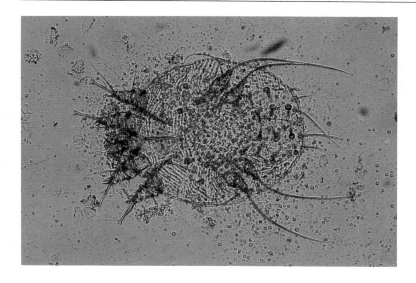

Figure 14-1
Sarcoptes scabiei *in a potassium hydroxide wet mount. (×40.)*

Figure 14-2
Sarcoptes scabiei. *Cross section of a mite in the stratum corneum.*

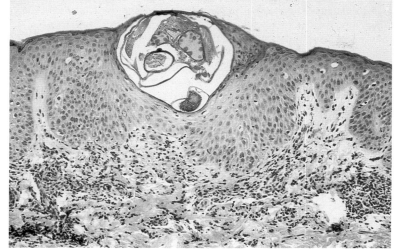

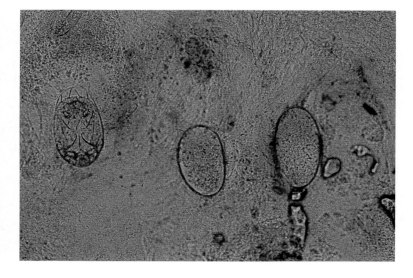

Figure 14-3
Sarcoptes scabiei. *Eggs containing mites. A potassium hydroxide wet mount. (×40.)*

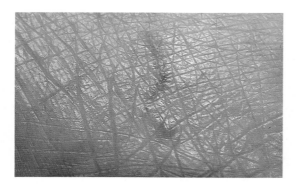

Figure 14-4
Scabies. An S-shaped burrow with a tiny vesicle at one end.

Clinical manifestations. Transmission of scabies occurs after direct skin contact with an infected patient. Whether the mite can be acquired from infested clothing or bed linen is not known. A mite that leaves human skin can survive for 24 to 36 hours at room conditions.[2] Mites survive up to 7 days in mineral oil microscopic slide mounts.

The disease begins insidiously. Symptoms are minor at first and are attributed to a bite or dry skin. Scratching destroys burrows and removes mites, providing initial relief. The patient remains comfortable during the day but itches at night. Nocturnal pruritus is highly characteristic of scabies. Scratching spreads mites to other areas and after 6 to 8 weeks the once localized area of minor irritation has become a widespread intensely pruritic eruption.

The most characteristic features of the lesions of scabies are pleomorphism and a tendency to remain discrete and small. Primary lesions are soon destroyed by scratching.

Primary lesions. Mites are found in burrows and at the edge of vesicles, but rarely in papules.

Burrow. The linear, curved, or S-shaped burrow is approximately as wide as #2 suture material and is 2 to 15 mm in length. They are pink-white and slightly elevated. A vesicle or the mite seen as a black dot may often be visualized at one end (Figure 14-4). Scratching destroys burrows, so that they do not appear in some patients. Burrows are most likely to be found in the finger webs, wrists, sides of the hands and feet, penis, buttocks, scrotum, and in infants, in palms and soles.

Vesicle and papule. Vesicles are isolated, pinpoint, and filled with serous rather than purulent fluid. The fact that they remain discrete is a key point in differentiating scabies from other vesicluar diseases such as poison ivy. The finger webs are the most likely area in which to find intact vesicles (Figure 14-5). Infants may have vesicles or pustules on the palms and soles. Small discrete papules may represent a hypersensitivity reaction and rarely contain mites.

Secondary lesions. Secondary lesions result from infection or are created by scratching. They often dominate the clinical picture. Pinpoint erosions are the most common secondary lesions. Pustules are a sign of secondary infection (Figure 14-6). Scaling and erythema and all stages of eczematous inflammation occur as a response to excoriation or from irritation caused by overzealous attempts at self-medication (Figure 14-7). Nodules occur in covered areas such as the buttock, groin, scrotum, penis, and axillae. The 5- to 10-mm indolent red nodules sometimes have a slightly eroded surface, especially on the glans penis (Figure 14-8). Nodules may persist for weeks or months after the mites have been eradicated.

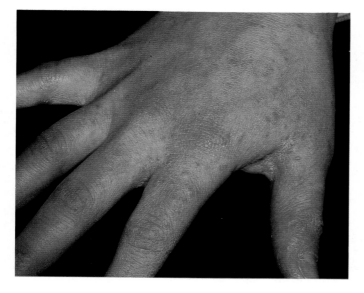

Figure 14-5
Scabies. Tiny vesicles and papules in the finger webs and back of the hand.

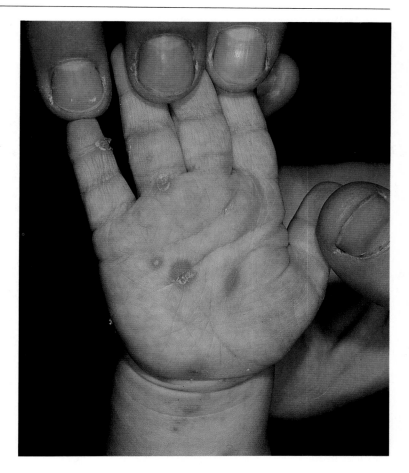

Figure 14-6
Scabies. Pustules on the palms of an infant. Note the papular lesions on the wrist.

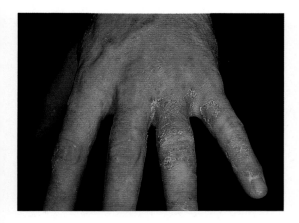

Figure 14-7
Scabies. Pinpoint erosions are present on the back of the hands. Eczematous inflammation and infection are present on the fourth and fifth fingers, a response to chronic excoriation.

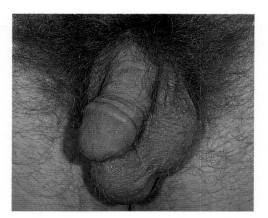

Figure 14-8
Scabies. Burrow is located near the tip of the glans. Nodules are present on the shaft and scrotum.

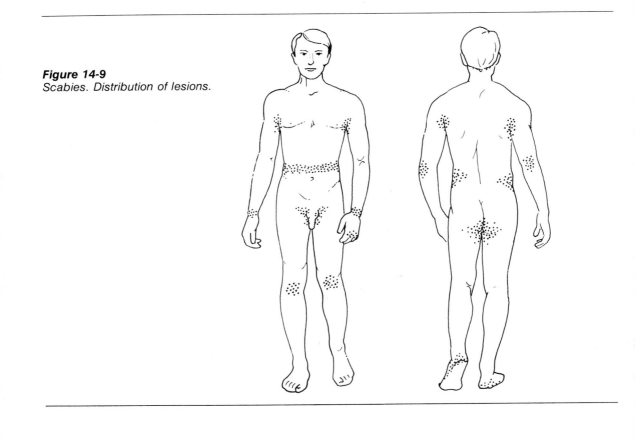

Figure 14-9
Scabies. Distribution of lesions.

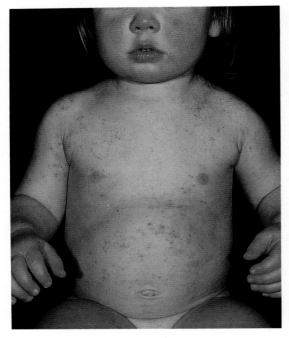

Figure 14-10
Diffuse scabies in an infant. The face is clear.
The lesions are most numerous around the
axillae, chest, and abdomen.

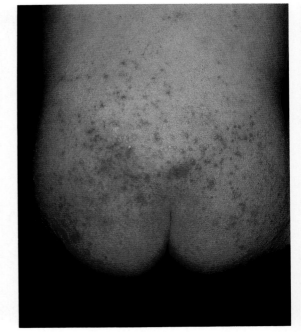

Figure 14-11
Scabies. Diffuse infestation of the buttock area.

Distribution. Lesions of scabies are typically found in the finger webs, wrists, extensor surfaces of the elbows and knees, sides of the hands and feet, axillary areas, buttocks, waist area, and around the ankles (Figure 14-9 to 14-11). In the male the penis and scrotum are usually involved; in the female, the breast including the areola and nipple may be infested. Lesions often vesicular or pustular may be most numerous on the palms and soles of infants. The scalp and face are rarely involved in adults, but occasionally are infested in infants.

The number and type of lesions and extent of involvement vary greatly among patients. Some patients will experience a few itchy vesicles in the finger webs early in the course of their disease. Many patients in these early stages attempt self-treatment and are encouraged by the relief obtained from over-the-counter antipruritic lotions. Topical steroids offer greater relief, but mask the progressive disease by suppressing inflammation. Delay of proper treatment allows the eruption to extend into all of the characteristic areas and beyond, onto the trunk, arms, legs, and occasionally the face. Extensive involvement is often accompanied by erythema, scaling, and infection. Infants and children develop diffuse scabies more often than do adults. Symptoms vary from periods of nocturnal pruritus to constant frantic itching. Untreated scabies can last for months or years.

Infants. Infants more frequently than adults have widespread involvement. This may occur because the diagnosis is not suspected and proper treatment is delayed while medication is given for other suspected causes of itching such as dry skin, eczema, and infection (Figure 14-12). Infants occasionally are infested on the face and scalp, a pattern rarely seen in adults. Vesicles are common on the palms and soles; this is a highly characteristic sign of scabies in infants (Figure 14-13). Nodules may be seen in the axillae and diaper area.

The elderly. Elderly patients have few cutaneous lesions, but itch severely. The decreased immunity associated with advanced age may allow the mites to multiply and survive in great numbers. They have few cutaneous lesions other than excoriations, dry

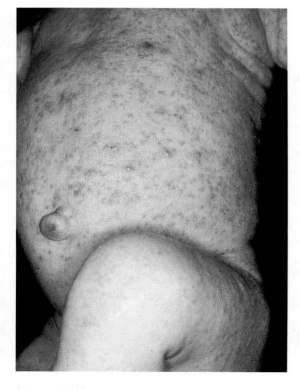

Figure 14-12
Scabies in an infant. Diffuse involvement in an infant who was initially treated with topical steroids.

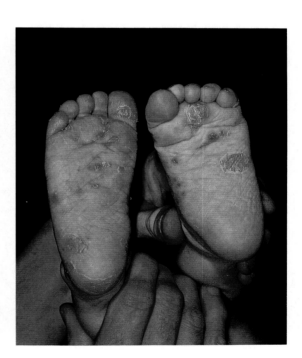

Figure 14-13
Scabies. Infestation of the palms and soles is common in infants. The vesicular lesions have all ruptured.

TABLE 14-1

SIGNS AND SYMPTOMS OF SCABIES

Nodules on the penis and scrotum
Rash present for 4 to 8 weeks, which has suddenly become worse
Pustules on the palms and soles of infants
Nocturnal itching
Generalized severe itching
Pinpoint erosions and crusts on the buttock
Vesicles in finger webs
Diffuse eruption with sparing of the face
Patient who became better then worse after treatment with topical steroids
Rash present in several members of the same family
Patient (especially infants) whose rash becomes more extensive despite treatment with antibiotics and topical medications

skin, and scaling, but they experience intense itching. Entire nursing home populations may be infested. A skin scraping from any scaling area may show numerous mites in all stages of development.

The retarded. Retarded patients, especially those with Down's syndrome, may develop diffuse thick scaling and crusts on the hands and feet and diffuse erythema and scaling on the face, neck, scalp, and trunk; this is the so-called Norwegian scabies. Itching may be absent or severe. A lack of immunity or indifference to pruritus has been suggested as reason for the development of this distinct clinical picture.

Diagnosis. The diagnosis is suspected when burrows are found or a patient has typical symptoms or characteristic lesions and distribution (Table 14-1). A definite diagnosis is made when any of the following products are obtained from burrows or vesicles and identified microscopically: mites, eggs, egg casings (hatched eggs), or feces (scybala).

Burrow identification. Initially, observe the areas most apt to contain burrows. Burrows may be enhanced for better visualization by touching the surface with a drop of mineral or immersion oil or dyeing the burrow by touching the area with a blue or black fountain pen or felt tip pen and removing the surface ink with an alcohol swab. The burrow absorbs the ink and is highlighted as a dark line (Figure 14-14). The accentuated lesions are smoothly scraped away with a #15 (curved) scalpel blade and transferred to a glass microscope slide for examination.

Papules and vesicles. Nonexcoriated papules and vesicles may be sampled but will not usually contain the eggs and egg casings found in an established burrow.

Sampling techniques and slide mount preparation. Various techniques are available for obtaining diagnostic material. In most cases the suspected lesion can be sampled easily with a #15 surgical blade by shaving or scraping and transferring the material to a microscope slide for direct examination.

Mineral oil mounts. A drop of mineral oil may be placed over the suspected lesion before removal. Skin scrapings will adhere, feces are preserved, and the mite remains alive and motile in clear oil. Squamous cells will not separate when heated in a clear oil mount and mites under a clump of squamous cells may be missed.

Potassium hydroxide wet mounts. The scrapings are transferred directly to a glass slide, a drop of potassium hydroxide is added, and a coverslip is applied. If diagnostic material is not found, the preparation is gently heated and the coverslip is pressed to separate squamous cells. Feces remain intact for short periods but may be dissolved quickly when the mount is heated.

Skin biopsy is rarely necessary to make the diagnosis.

Treatment and management. Controversy exists about the safety of the various preparations available to treat scabies. Lindane, the most effective scabicide, has been the point of greatest dispute because of reports of neurotoxicity in infants after systemic absorbtion through the skin.[3] Further evaluation of these very few case reports revealed that lindane has been misused substantially.[4]

Lindane. Lindane is the generic name for the chemical gamma benzene hexachloride, a compound chemically similar to an agricultural pesticide also referred to as lindane. Kwell and Scabene are brand names for 1% lindane lotion. Kwell is also

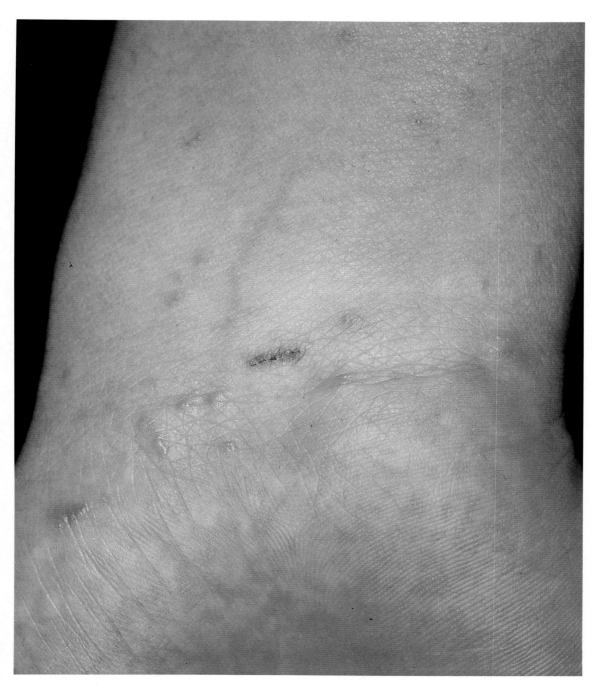

Figure 14-14
*Felt-tipped pen ink has penetrated and
highlighted a burrow. The ink is retained after the
surface is wiped clean with an alcohol swab.*

available as cream and shampoo. When used properly, lindane is the most effective scabicide and should in most cases be used as the drug of first choice for treating scabies. Explicit instructions must be given with the medication. Patients are repulsed by the thought of having "bugs" on their body and want to be cured immediately. They reason that if a little medication is good, a lot is better. Overuse leads to side effects. One application of lindane is highly effective. Lindane should be used with caution in pregnant women. Lindane is a fat-soluble chemical and may be present in the milk of nursing mothers. Babies should be bottle-fed during treatment of mothers and for several days thereafter. The following recommendations provide a 98% cure rate.

Apply lindane lotion to all skin surfaces below the neck. For adults 1 oz of the 1% lotion is usually adequate. Lindane is applied to the face if evidence for infestation in that area is present. Reapply lindane to the hands if hands are washed. A hot soapy bath is not necessary before application. Moisture increases the permeability of the epidermis and increases the chance for systemic absorption. Infants should have lindane applied during the day and then be fully clothed and observed to prevent licking of treated sites. If licking cannot be prevented, consider using sulfur instead of lindane.

Wash 8 to 12 hours[5] after application. Explain to patients that it is normal to continue to itch for days or weeks after treatment and that further application of lindane is not only dangerous but worsens itching by causing irritation. Apply bland lubricants for itching.

Inform patients that lindane is safe when used as directed but that lindane is toxic, penetrates the skin, and causes convulsions when overused. Tell them that sufficient quantities have been prescribed, without refills to preclude overuse. They should return for evaluation if itching does not gradually subside or if a rash appears. Patients should be warned against taking lindane orally.

Crotamiton. Crotamiton (Eurax lotion) has been offered as a safe alternative to lindane. The toxicity of crotamiton is unknown. Reported cure rates for once-a-day application for 5 days range from 50% to 100%.[6] Crotamiton may have antipruritic properties, but this has been questioned.

Sulfur. Sulfur has been used to treat scabies for over 150 years. The pharmacist mixes 6% (range, 5% to 10%) precipitated sulfur in petrolatum. The compound is applied to the entire body below the neck once each day for 3 days. The patient is instructed to bathe 24 hours after each application. Sulfur applied in this manner is very effective, but these preparations are messy, have an unpleasant odor, and stain. Sulfur in petrolatum was considered to be safer than lindane for treating infants, but the

safety of lindane when used properly has been established; sulfur preparations need be used only if patients object to using lindane.

Management of complications

Eczematous inflammation and pyoderma. Although there is little evidence that lindane will be absorbed in greater quantity through inflamed skin, it seems prudent to control secondary changes before the application of this scabicide. Patients with signs of infection should be started on appropriate oral antibiotics. A Group V topical steroid may be applied 3 times a day to all red scaling lesions for a day or two before the application of lindane.

Postscabietic pruritus. Itching usually decreases substantially 24 hours after treatment with lindane and then gradually decreases during the following week or two. Patients with persistent itching may be treated with oral antihistamines and, if inflamed, with topical steroids.

Nodular scabies. Persistent nodular lesions are treated with intralesional steroids (e.g., triamcinolone 10 mg/ml).

Environmental management. Intimate contacts and all family members in the same household should be treated.[7] The role of clothing that has touched infected skin in the transmission of scabies is probably minimal; however, it is difficult to convince patients of that fact. Patients should be instructed to wash in a normal washing machine cycle all clothing, towels, and bed linen that have touched the skin. It is not necessary to rewash clean clothing that has not yet been worn. Emphasize that coats, furniture, rugs, floors, and walls do not need to be cleaned in any special manner.

Pediculosis

Infestation with lice is called pediculosis. Lice are acquired through close personal contact and contact with objects such as combs, hats, clothing, and bed linen. Diagnosis is made by visualizing the lice or its eggs and treatment with lindane or pyrethrins is effective.

Biology and life cycle. Lice are called ectoparasites because they live on, rather than in, the body. They are classified as insects because they have six legs. Three kinds of lice infest humans; these are *Pediculus humanus* var *capitis* (head louse), *Pediculus humanus* var *corporis* (body louse), and *Phthirus pubis* (pubic or crab louse).

All three have similar anatomic characteristics. Each is a small (less than 2 mm), flat, wingless insect with three pairs of legs located on the anterior part of the body directly behind the head. The legs terminate in sharp claws that are adapted for feeding and permit the louse to grasp and firmly hold on to hair or clothing. The body louse is the largest and is similar in shape to the head louse (Figure 14-15).

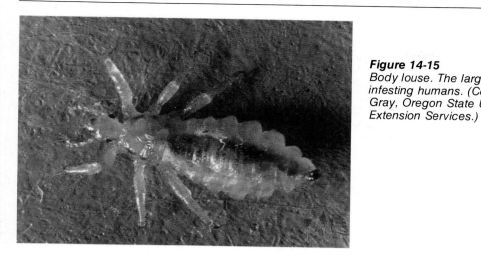

Figure 14-15
Body louse. The largest of three lice infesting humans. (Courtesy Ken Gray, Oregon State University Extension Services.)

The crab louse is the smallest, with a short oval body, which with its prominent claws resembles a sea crab (Figure 14-16).

Lice feed approximately five times each day by piercing the skin with their claws, injecting irritating saliva, and sucking blood. They do not become engorged like ticks, but are more easily identified after feeding, when they become rust-colored from the ingestion of blood. Lice feces can be seen on the skin as small rust-colored flecks. Saliva and possibly fecal material can induce a hypersensitivity reaction and inflammation. Lice are active and can travel quickly, which explains why they can be transmitted so easily. They can live 2 or more days off the human body. The life cycle from egg to egg is about 1 month. The female lays approximately six eggs or nits each day. The louse incubates, hatches, and reaches maturity in about 18 days. Nits are 0.8 mm long and are firmly cemented to the base of hair shafts close to the skin in order to acquire adequate heat for incubation (Figure 14-17). Nits that are detached from the host may remain viable for up to 1 month. Nits are extremely difficult to remove from the hair shaft.

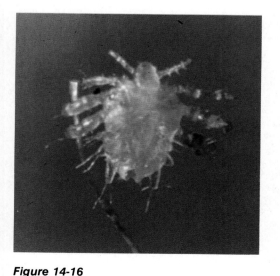

Figure 14-16
Crab louse has a short body and large claws used to grasp hair. (Courtesy Ken Gray, Oregon State University Extension Services.)

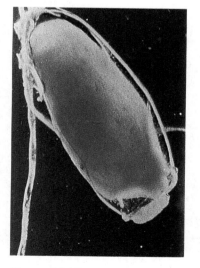

Figure 14-17
Louse egg (nit) is cemented to a hair shaft. (Courtesy Reed & Carnick, Piscataway, NJ.)

Clinical manifestations

Pediculosis capitis. Lice infestation of the scalp is most common in children. More girls than boys are afflicted; American blacks rarely have head lice.[8] Head lice can be found anywhere on the scalp, but are most commonly seen on the back of the head and neck and behind the ears (Figure 14-18). Scratching causes inflammation and secondary bacterial infection, with pustules, crusting, and cervical adenopathy. Posterior cervical adenopathy without obvious disease should make one think of lice. The eyelashes may be involved, causing redness and swelling. Examination of the posterior scalp shows few adult organisms but many nits. Nits are cemented to the hair; dandruff scale is easily moved along the hair shaft. Live nits fluoresce and can be detected easily by Wood's light examination, a technique especially useful for rapid examination of a large group of children.

Pediculosis pubis. Pubic lice are the most contagious sexually transmitted problem known. Up to 30% of patients infested with pubic lice have one or more other sexually transmitted disease.[9] The chance of acquiring pubic lice from an infested partner is over 90%, whereas the chance of acquiring syphilis or gonorrhea from one sexual exposure with an infected partner is only about 30%. Blacks are affected as frequently as whites. The pubic hair

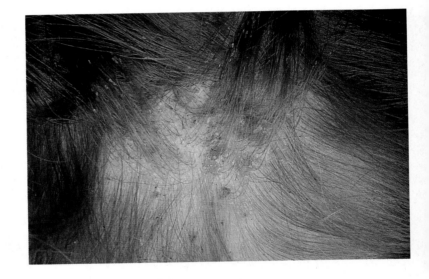

Figure 14-18
Pediculosis capitis. A heavy infestation with secondary pyoderma.

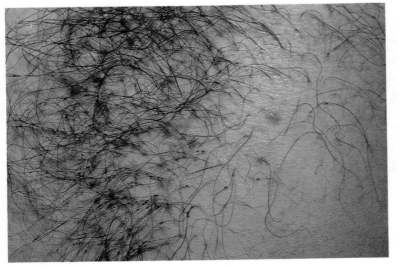

Figure 14-19
Pediculosis. Human lice can spread from the pubic area to involve the axillae.

is the most common site of infestation, but lice frequently spread to the hair around the anus. In hairy persons lice may spread to the upper thighs, abdominal area, axillae (Figure 14-19), chest, and beard. Infested adults may spread pubic lice to the eyelashes of children.

The majority of patients complain of pruritus. Many patients are aware that something is crawling on the groin, but are not familiar with the disease and have never seen lice. About one-half of patients seen have little inflammation, but those who delay seeking help may develop widespread inflammation and infection of the groin with regional adenopathy. Occasionally, gray-blue macules (maculae ceru-

leae) (Figure 14-20) varying in size from 1 to 2 cm are seen in the groin and at sites distant from the infestation. Their cause is not known, but they may represent altered blood pigment.

Pediculosis corporis. Infestation by body lice is uncommon. Typhus, relapsing fever, and trench fever are spread by body lice during wartime and in underdeveloped countries. Pediculosis corporis is a disease of the unclean. Body lice live and lay their nits in the seams of clothing (Figure 14-21) and return to the skin surface only to feed. They run and hide when disturbed and are rarely seen. Body lice induce pruritus that leads to scratching and secondary infection.

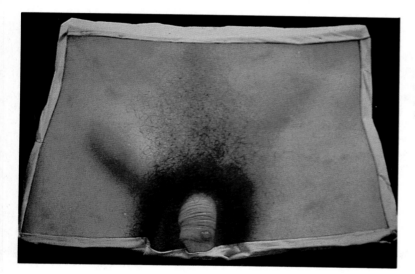

Figure 14-20
Pediculosis pubis (maculae ceruleae). Blue-gray macules can be seen with lice infestation.

Figure 14-21
Pediculosis corporis. Body lice nits laid in the seams of clothing. (Courtesy Reed & Carnick, Piscataway, NJ.)

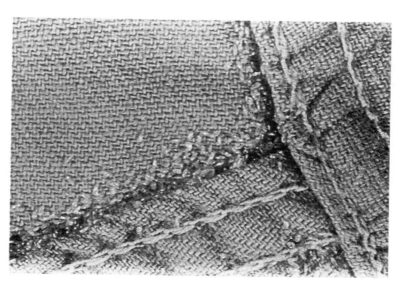

Eyelash infestation. Infestation of the eyelashes is seen almost exclusively in children. The lice are acquired from other children or from an infested adult with pubic lice. Eyelash infestation may induce blepharitis.

Diagnosis. Suspect the diagnosis when a patient complains of itching in a localized area without an apparent rash. Scalp and pubic lice will be apparent to those who carefully examine individual hairs; they are not apparent with only a cursory examination. Lice and nits can be seen easily under the microscope. Live nits fluoresce with Wood's light.

Treatment

Head, body, and pubic lice. Both lindane (Kwell) and synergized pyrethrins[10] (Rid, A-200) are effective for treating head, body, and pubic lice. Both preparations are available as shampoos or lotions. The shampoos are applied, lathered, and washed off in 5 minutes. Lotions are used for treating body and pubic hair infestation. They are applied over the entire affected area and washed off in 12 hours. Malathion lotion 0.5% (Prioderm lotion) is approved for the treatment of head lice. The lotion is sprinkled on dry hair until the hair and scalp are thoroughly wet and then allowed to dry. The scalp is shampooed 8 to 12 hours later. One application is usually sufficient, but another treatment 8 days later will kill newly hatched lice whose nits may not have come in contact with the medication during the first treatment. Pyrethrins are chemicals extracted from certain flowers and plants. Of the available insecticides, they are the least toxic to humans. They induce nervous system paralysis of insects on contact but are apparently nontoxic to humans. All preparations kill nits and lice. The dead nits will remain attached to the hair until removed. The cement holding nits to the hair shaft may be dissolved with vinegar compresses applied to the hair for 15 minutes.

Eye infestation. Several methods are used for treating eye infestation. The most practical and effective method is to place petrolatum on the fingertips, close the eyes, and rub the petrolatum slowly into the lids and brows 3 times each day for 5 days. A simple alternative is to close the eyes and apply baby shampoo to the lashes and brows with a cotton swab 3 times each day for 5 days. Some patients are so mortified by the presence of lice close to their eyes that they demand immediate removal. Have the reclining patient close the eyes, then pluck the lice from the eyelashes with forceps. Older children tolerate this simple procedure.

Physostigmine ophthalmic ointment (Eserine) is effective when applied twice each day for 2 or 3 days. However, it leaks into the eyes and induces myopia with visual blurring.

Managing epidemics. Lice infestation may rapidly spread through schools and day care centers. If many children in a class are infested, it is prudent to treat all classmates simultaneously. A message could be sent home to all parents advising them that lice have been found on many school children and that it is recommended that all classmates be treated on the same specified night with an over-the-counter pediculocidal shampoo such as A-200 or Rid. Request the child to bring the wrapper from the medication to school so that the nurse knows which preparation was used. Nits remain after proper therapy and are not a sign of treatment failure. The practice of restricting school attendance until nits are removed is unnecessary.

Caterpillar Dermatitis

Caterpillars are the larvae of butterflies or moths. Many species of caterpillars posses short hairs (setae) that can irritate the skin (Figure 14-22). Outbreaks of caterpillar dermatitis are seasonal; they occur shortly after the young caterpillars have appeared. Contact with the setae occurs by direct exposure to the caterpillar or from windblown setae.

Gypsy moth caterpillars in the northeastern United States hang from trees on long threads. Suspension in the air allows setae to float away on the wind and land on skin or clothing hung out to dry. The puss caterpillar, also known as the wooly slug, is found in the southeastern United States. It is approximately 1 inch long, and its back and sides are completely covered with fine bristles. The io moth caterpillar is found east of the Rocky Mountains. It is 2 to 3 inches long and pale green with reddish stripes. Each body segment is armed with tufts of spines. The saddleback caterpillar is found each of Texas and south of Massachusetts. It is about 1 inch long and is green and fleshy. The characteristic marking is a brown or purple saddle-shaped midback. Stout spines are located at each end and along the sides; these spines are hollow and contain a toxin.

Clinical manifestations. Erythema, papules, and vesicles may appear shortly after contact; irritation may result from mechanical stimulation or from release of irritating substances on the hairs (Figure 14-23). The sting of the puss caterpillar produces an immediate severe shooting burning pain in practically all cases. Some patients experience delayed symptoms such as itching and may develop papules and vesicles similar to insect bites 12 hours after exposure. Closed patch testing with gypsy moth caterpillar hairs revealed that when exposed to hairs these patients developed a delayed hypersensitivity response similar to that in poison ivy contact dermatitis.[11]

The distribution varies. Linear lesions are noted where caterpillars crawl on the skin. Eruptions sec-

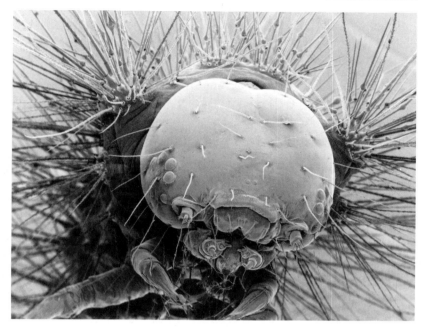

Figure 14-22
Gypsy moth caterpillar. The caterpillar is covered with numerous hair-like structures. (Courtesy Kathleen Shields, Ph.D., United States Department of Agriculture, Hamden, Conn.)

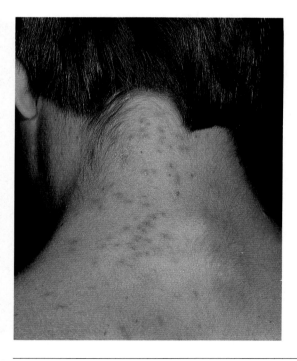

Figure 14-23
Gypsy moth dermatitis. A group of papules and vesicles occurred shortly after a gypsy moth caterpillar was dropped on the neck of this young boy.

ondary to windblown hairs that become embedded in clothing are localized around the collar region, the inside surfaces of the arms and legs, the abdominal flank, and the feet. A unique grid-like track may be left on the skin after contact with the puss caterpillar. In addition to cutaneous signs, some patients develop rhinitis, conjunctivitis, and wheezing.

Diagnosis. The diagnosis is suspected when a rash of the above description is seen in the early spring. The diagnosis can be confirmed by demonstrating caterpillar hairs on the skin surface.

The technique is as follows: The sticky side of a strip of clear tape is applied to the affected area of skin. The tape is then turned sticky side down onto a microscope slide and observed under low power. Short straight thread-like hairs are diagnostic of caterpillar dermatitis.[12]

Treatment. Most cases will resolve spontaneously within a few days to 2 weeks. For puss caterpillar stings, the immediate gentle application of adhesive or Scotch tape will help remove remaining spines. Calamine lotion may be helpful and antihistamines sometimes bring relief if used immediately. Group V topical steroids are useful for persistent or pruritic lesions. Puss caterpillar stings often produce severe pain that may require potent analgesics. Clothing should not be hung out to dry when thread-suspended caterpillars such as the gypsy moth caterpillar appear in the spring.

Spiders

Spiders are carnivorous arthropods, all of which have fangs and venom that they use to catch and immobilize or kill their prey. Most spiders are small and their fangs are too short to penetrate human skin. Spiders are not aggressive and bite only in self-defense. Spider bites may not be felt at the instant they occur. Localized pain, swelling, itching, erythema, blisters, and necrosis may occur. Most spider venoms are composed of the harmless enzyme-spreading factor hyaluronidase and a toxin that is distributed by the spreading factor. Most toxins simply cause pain, swelling, inflammation, but brown recluse spider toxin causes necrosis, and black widow spider toxin causes neuromuscular abnormalities. Spider bites are common, but of the 50 species of spiders in the United States that have been known to bite humans, only the black widow and the brown recluse spider are capable of producing severe reactions.

The diagnosis of spider bite cannot be made with certainty unless the act is witnessed or the spider is recovered.

Common spider bites

Most spider bites are felt as pain at the instant they occur. A hive-like swelling appears at the bite site and expands radially, usually for just a few centimeters; however, the swelling can sometimes reach gigantic proportions. Occasionally, two puncta or fang marks can be found on the skin surface. The warmth and deep erythema of a bite may resemble bacterial cellulitis, but the elevated hive-like swelling and small satellite hives are not characteristic of bacterial infection. A biopsy, although usually not necessary for diagnosis, may show mouth parts and intense inflammation. The lesion will resolve spontaneously, but itching and swelling can be controlled with cool compresses and antihistamines.

Black widow spider

The black widow spider, *Latrodectus mactans* ("shoe button spider"); is so named because the female attacks and then consumes her mate shortly after copulation. The black widow is found in every state except Alaska and is especially numerous in the rural south. The female has a smooth black body, long slender legs, and a red hourglass marking on the underside of the abdomen. This marking may appear as triangles, spots, or an irregular blotch. An adult female has a total length of 4 cm (Figure 14-24).

Black widow spiders live in dark sheltered areas such as crevices in old barns, lumber piles, and privies. They usually do not bite when away from the web; they are clumsy and need the web for support. The bite produces immediate pain. The subsequent reaction is minimal, with slight swelling and the appearance of a set of small red fang marks. The symptoms that follow are caused by lymphatic absorption and vascular dissemination of a neurotoxin and are collectively known as latrodectism.[13] Fifteen minutes to 2 hours after the bite, muscle cramps begin near the bite site and then progress to involve any or all of the skeletal muscles. Severe abdominal pain and spasm simulating pain following abdominal surgery are the most prominent and distressing features of latrodectism (Figure 14-25). The abdominal muscles assume a board-like rigidity, but there is slight tenderness. There is a generalized increase in the deep tendon reflexes. Other symptoms include dizziness, headache, sweating, nausea, and vomiting. The symptoms increase in severity for several hours (up to 24 hours) and then slowly subside, gradually decreasing in severity in the course of 2 or 3 days.

Residual symptoms such as weakness, tingling, nervousness, and transient muscle spasm may persist for weeks or months after recovery from the acute stage. Recovery from one serious attack usually offers complete systemic immunity to subse-

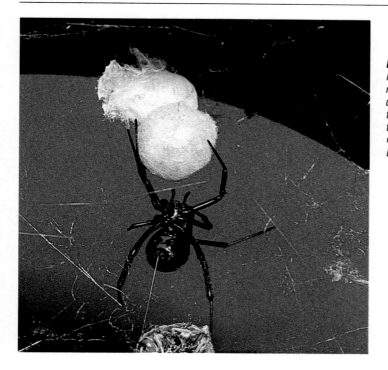

Figure 14-24
Female black widow spider with a red hourglass marking on the underside of her abdomen. Note the haphazard randomly arranged threads of the web. (Courtesy Ken Gray, Oregon State University Extension Services.)

Figure 14-25
Latrodectism. Severe abdominal muscle spasms occurring hours after a black widow spider bite.

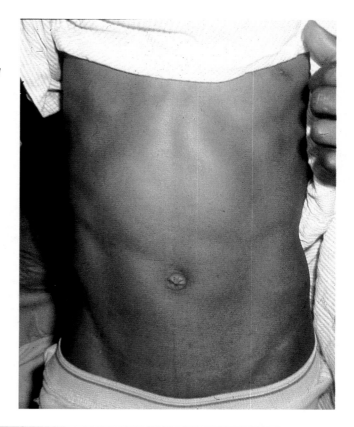

quent bites. Convulsions, paralysis, shock, and death occur in about 5% of cases, usually in the young or debilitated elderly.

Treatment

Immediate first aid. If the patient is seen within a few minutes of being bitten, ice may be applied to the bite site to help restrict the spread of venom.

Antivenin. Antivenin (*Latrodectus mactans* or black widow spider antivenin) is available from Merck Sharp and Dohme. The dose consists of the entire contents of one vial (2.5 ml) given intramuscularly or, in severe cases when the patient is under 12 or in shock, intravenously in 10 to 50 ml of saline over a 15-minute period. The antivenin is prepared from horse serum and is therefore supplied with a 1-ml vial of normal horse serum for sensitivity testing. The symptoms usually subside 1 to 3 hours after treatment; occasionally, a second dose is necessary. Treatment with antivenin may be deferred in healthy individuals between the ages of 16 and 60. These patients usually respond to muscle relaxants and recover spontaneously. In emergencies, call the local or state poison center or the department of public health for information about the closest source of antivenin.

Muscle relaxants. Among others, 1 or 2 gm of methocarbamol (Robaxin, 100 mg/ml in 10-ml vials) may be administered undiluted over a 5- to 10-minute interval. Oral doses may be used thereafter and will usually sustain the relief initiated by the injection. Calcium gluconate (10%; 10 ml IV) acts as a muscle relaxant, but Robaxin is generally considered more effective.

Analgesics. Morphine should be used with caution, since the venom is a neurotoxin and may cause respiratory paralysis.

Brown recluse spider

The brown recluse spider, *Loxosceles reclusa* ("fiddle back spider"), is small, about 1.5 cm in overall length. Its color ranges from yellowish tan to dark brown. A characteristic dark violin-shaped marking is located on the spider's back. The broad base of the violin is near the head and the violin stem points toward the abdomen, thus the name "fiddle back" (Figure 14-26). The spider is a timid recluse and lives in dark areas, under woodpiles and rocks, and inside human habitations, often in closets, behind picture frames, under porches, and in barns and basements. Its web is small, haphazard, and woven in cracks, crevices, corners. It bites only when provoked. The brown recluse is usually found in the southern half of the United States, but specimens have been found as far north as New Jersey.

The bite instantly produces sharp pain resembling a bee sting. Most bite reactions are mild and cause only minimal swelling and erythema (Figure 14-27). Severe bites may become necrotic within 4

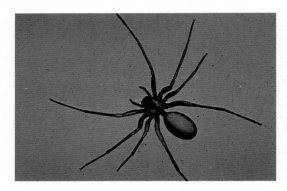

Figure 14-26
The brown recluse spider. A dark violin-shaped marking is located on the spider's back.

hours. The first and most characteristic cutaneous change in necrotic arachnidism, or loxoscelism, is rapid expansion of a tiny blue area at the bite site and a sudden increase in tenderness. At this stage the superficial skin may be rapidly infarcting and the pain is severe. The necrotizing blue macule widens and the center sinks below the normal skin surface ("sinking infarct") (Figure 14-28). The extent of the infarct is quite variable. Most patients experience localized reactions, but the depth of the necrotic tissue may extend to the muscle and over broad areas of skin, sometimes involving most of an extremity. The dead tissue sloughs, leaving a deep indolent ulcer with ragged edges. Ulcers take weeks or months to heal; scarring is significant.

A few people develop a severe progressive reaction that begins with moderate to severe pain at the bite site. Within 4 hours, the pain is unbearable and the initial erythema gives way to pallor. The victims often experience fever, chills, nausea, vomiting, weakness, joint and muscle pains, and hives or measle-like rashes within 1 or 2 days. The toxin may produce severe systemic reactions such as generalized hemolysis and renal failure, sometimes ending in death. Severe systemic reactions are rare and occur most frequently in children.

Treatment. Mild bites are treated conservatively with a cool wet compress, antihistamines, and analgesics. There is little evidence that oral and intralesional steroids decrease the severity of the progressive reaction. Early excision of necrotic areas was once believed to help prevent both the spread of the toxin and further necrosis. However, this practice is probably ineffective and should be discouraged.[14] Severe systemic loxoscelism may be treated with prednisone (1 mg/kg) given as early as possible in the development of systemic symptoms to treat hematologic abnormalities. Supportive medical treatment is required.

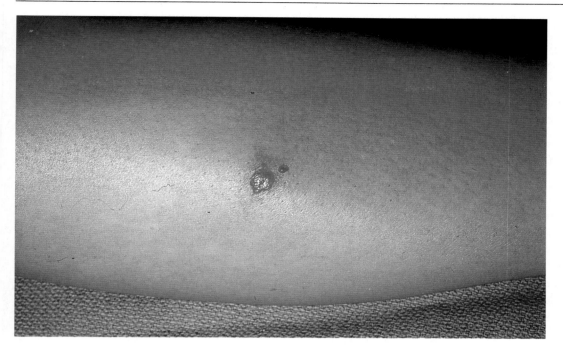

Figure 14-27
Brown recluse spider bite. Most bite reactions
are mild and cause only minimal swelling and
erythema.

Figure 14-28
Brown recluse spider bite. A severe reaction in
which infarction, bleeding, and blistering have
occurred.

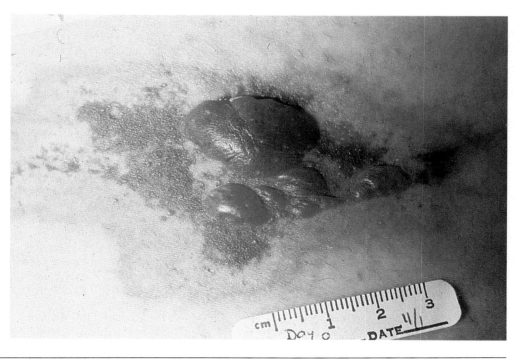

Ticks

Ticks are blood-sucking ectoparasites. Adult ticks are 1 cm in length; they have eight legs, the front two are curved forward as in crabs. The large oval or teardrop-shaped body is flat and sac-like and has a leathery outer surface. There are two families of ticks, hard and soft; they are distinguished by the consistency of their bodies. Hard ticks cause the most problems for humans. They are notable because they can inflict local reaction such as pain, erythema, and nodules; more important, they are vectors for a number of serious systemic diseases. Ticks perch on grass tips and bushes and wait for a warm-blooded host to pass by (Figure 14-29). They insert recurved teeth into the skin, produce a glue-like secretion that tightens their grip, and then proceed to suck blood (Figures 14-30 and 14-31). Hard ticks may remain attached to the host for up to 10 days, whereas soft ticks release in a few hours. The bite itself is painless, but within hours an urticarial wheal appears at the puncture site and may cause itching. Particularly in children, ticks may go unnoticed for several hours after attachment to an inconspicuous area such as the scalp. Hard ticks are vectors for most of the serious tick-borne diseases.

Types of ticks. The deer tick *(Ixodes dammini)* transmits human babesiosis and Lyme disease; it is found in areas such as Massachusetts, Connecticut, New Jersey, and the islands of coastal New England. The recent extension of this geographic range has been attributed to the proliferation of deer in North America. The spotted fever tick *(Dermacentor variabilis)* is found in most sections of the United States other than the Rocky Mountain region. Most Dermacentor ticks have white anterodorsal ornamentation. The Rocky Mountain wood tick *(Dermacentor andersoni)* is the vector for Rocky Mountain spotted fever in the west.

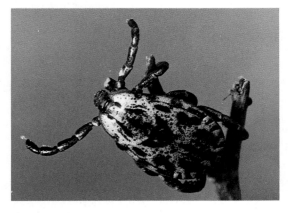

Figure 14-29
The Rocky Mountain wood tick perched on a twig waiting for a victim. (Courtesy Ken Gray, Oregon State University Extension Services.)

Diseases transmitted by ticks

Lyme disease and erythema chronicum migrans. Lyme disease and erythema chronicum migrans (ECM) are believed to be caused by a spirochete transmitted by the bite of the deer tick *(Ixodes dammini).*[15] The skin lesion ECM is the most characteristic aspect of this disease. ECM may occur as an isolated phenomenon. The lesion begins as a wheal at the bite site. Over several days the erythema expands rapidly away from the central bite punctum, centrifically forming a broad round-to-oval area of erythema measuring 5 to 10 cm (Figure 14-32). Within 1 week it clears centrally, leaving a red 1- to 2-cm ring that advances for days or weeks and may reach a diameter of 50 cm. The ring remains flat, blanches with pressure, and does not desquamate, vesiculate, or have scale at the periphery, as ringworm does. Tenderness is present and itching is minimal; 20% to 50% of cases will have multiple concentric rings. Within several days after onset of the initial skin lesion almost half of the patients develop secondary lesions, the appearance of which was similar to that of the initial lesions, but they were generally smaller, migrated less, and lacked indurated centers. These lesions were located almost anywhere except for the palms and soles. The eruptions fade within a median of 28 days (range, 1 day to 14 months).[16]

Lyme disease, named after Lyme, Connecticut, where the initial cluster of cases was reported,[17] is a syndrome that has its onset 3 to 21 days after the bite of the Ixodes tick. Cases have since been reported from all parts of the country and people of all ages are affected.

There are acute and chronic phases. The acute illness begins with malaise, fatigue, fever up to 105° F, the ECM skin lesion, headache, stiff neck, myalgias, and arthralgias. The commonest nonspecific laboratory abnormalities were a high erythrocyte sedimentation rate (53% of patients), an elevated IgM level (33%), or an increased aspartate transaminase level (19%).[16] Approximately 1 month after the acute symptoms, some patients develop one or more swollen, warm (but not red) painful joints; usually the knee is affected. Inflammation typically lasts for 1 week and may recur. Other chronic manifestations of Lyme disease include cardiac and several patterns of neurologic involvement: meningitis, encephalitis, and meningopolyneuritis (Bannwarth's syndrome). The sedimentation rate, serum cryoglobulins, and serum IgM are elevated in many patients with acute joint symptoms.

Treatment. For treatment Steere recommends oral tetracycline, 250 mg 4 times a day for at least 10 days and up to 20 days if symptoms persist or recur. In children the recommended treatment is phenoxymethyl penicillin, 50 mg/kg/day (not less than 1 gm per day or more than 2 gm per day) in

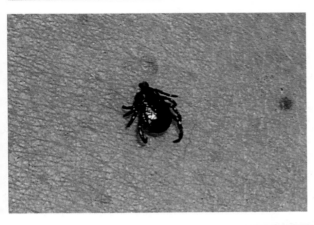

Figure 14-30
A tick, just after fixation to the skin.

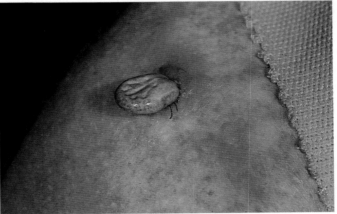

Figure 14-31
A blood-engorged tick. The bite site is red and swollen.

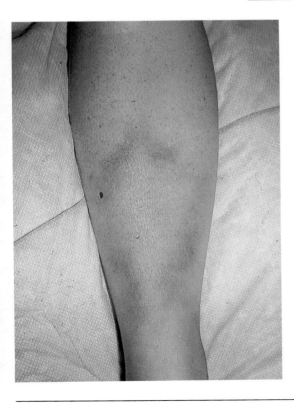

Figure 14-32
Erythema chronicum migrans. Broad oval area of erythema has slowly migrated from the central area.

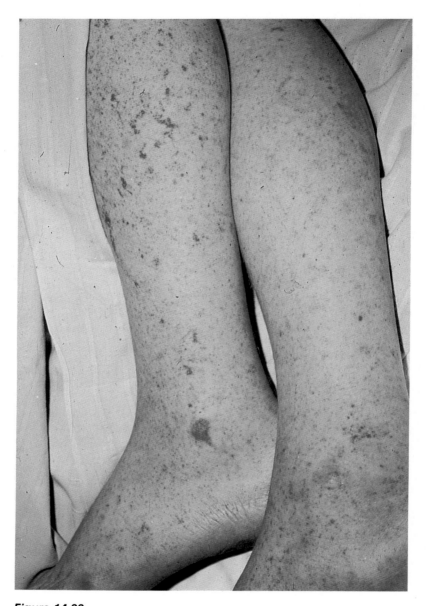

Figure 14-33
Rocky Mountain spotted fever. A generalized
petechial eruption that involves the entire
cutaneous surface including the palms and soles.

divided doses for the same duration, or in case of penicillin allergy, erythromycin, 30 mg/kg/day in divided doses for 15 or 20 days.[17]

Major late manifestations of Lyme disease—meningoencephalitis, myocarditis, or recurrent attacks of arthritis—were unusual after appropriate early antibiotic therapy. Neurologic abnormalities of Lyme disease respond to intravenous penicillin, 20 million units per day for 10 days.[18]

Rocky Mountain spotted and spotless fever. The name Rocky Mountain spotted fever was coined to describe a disease first observed in the Bitter Root Valley of western Montana. The disease occurs in many areas of the United States. Rocky Mountain spotted fever is caused by *Rickettsia rickettsii* and is transmitted by tick bite. The principal vector in the eastern United States is *Dermacentor variabilis;* in the West, it is the *Dermacentor andersoni.* The disease occurs in the spring and summer months when the ticks are active.

Ticks must be attached for 6 or more hours to transmit the disease. One week (range, 3 to 21 days) after the bite there is abrupt onset of fever, severe headache, myalgia, and arthralgia. The rash typically begins on the fourth day, erupting first on the wrists and ankles. In hours it involves the palms and soles, then becomes generalized. The rash is discrete, macular, and blanches with pressure at first; it becomes petechial in 2 to 4 days (Figure 14-33). The rash is extremely difficult to see in blacks. In approximately 10% of cases the rash does not appear; the disease is then referred to as Rocky Mountain spotless fever.[19] Rashless disease is much more common in adults. Splenomegaly is present in one-half the cases. The fever subsides in 2 to 3 weeks and the rash, if present, fades with residual hyperpigmentation. Although the overall mortality rate fluctuates between 3% and 7%, the untreated mortality may be in excess of 30%. Death usually results from visceral and central nervous system dissemination leading to irreversible shock.[20] Many of those who die have a fulminant course and are dead in 1 week. Interstitial nephritis is found in most cases at autopsy.

Laboratory diagnosis. Complete blood counts are usually normal. The blood urea nitrogen may be elevated, indicating prerenal azotemia or interstitial nephritis. Acute and convalescent serum may be drawn for specific complement fixation titers, but are useful only for confirmation of the diagnosis. These tests are performed at the Centers for Disease Control in Atlanta, Georgia; the serum may be forwarded by state health departments. Blood and tissue cultures may be performed at centers equipped for such procedures. Immunofluorescence studies on blood and tissue are sensitive and highly specific.

Treatment. Tetracycline and chloramphenicol are extremely effective and should be given in full doses. Any adult in an endemic geographic area during the summer months who develops fever, myalgia, and headache should be considered for a therapeutic trial of tetracycline for Rocky Mountain spotless fever.[19]

Tick bite paralysis. Tick bite paralysis probably results from a toxin in tick saliva that is injected while feeding. The disease is most common in children, especially girls with long thick hair. The tick, which hides in the scalp, groin, or other inconspicuous areas, must be attached for about 5 days before symptoms appear. The patient complains of fatigue, irritability, and leg paresthesias, followed within 24 hours by loss of coordination and an ascending paralysis. There is no pain or fever in the early stages. Death from respiratory failure can occur if the tick is not found and removed. Recovery follows 24 hours after the tick is detached. Tick bite paralysis is most commonly seen in the Pacific northwest and is caued by *Dermacentor andersoni.*

Removing ticks. Ticks should not be removed by direct finger contact because of the danger of contracting a rickettsial infection. Dermacentor ticks are removed by gentle steady firm traction; the mouth parts usually come away attached to the tick. *Ixodes dammini* can rarely be removed intact by manual extraction. This tick can be encouraged to release by covering it with petroleum jelly or burning its posterior section with a lighted cigarette or match. The tick's release from the host is enzyme-mediated and requires time. If the tick has not released in 10 minutes, then scrape it off. The mouth parts will remain below the skin surface. The residual parts are walled off and cause little harm; in a few cases, they may stimulate a foreign body reaction resulting in a nodule known as a tick-bite granuloma. Do not squeeze the body of the tick, since additional fluid may be injected into the skin.

Stinging Insects

Honey bees, wasps, hornets, and yellow jackets sting when confronted. A wasp, for example, will vigorously pursue nest intruders. Insect repellents such as Deet offer no protection. A firm sharp stinger is imbedded in the skin, followed immediately by secretion of venom. The honey bee stings once and dies. Its barbed stinger, glands, and viscera remain in the victim. Imbedded honey bee stingers should be flicked away with a knife or finger nail. Grasping them with fingertips will compress venom glands and make the sting worse. Stingers of other stinging insects are not barbed and remain intact, ready to be used again. The injected venom can cause a localized or generalized reaction. Reactions are classified as toxic or allergic.

Toxic reactions. Localized toxic reactions in the nonallergic individual consist of a sharp pinprick sensation at the instant of stinging, followed by moderate burning pain at the site. A red papule or wheal appears, which enlarges if scratched (Figure 14-34). The reaction subsides in hours. Multiple stings can produce a systemic toxic reaction with vomiting, diarrhea, headache, fever, muscle spasm, and loss of consciousness. More than 500 stings at one time may be fatal.

Allergic reactions. Like the toxic reaction, the local allergic reaction begins with immediate pain, but the urticarial response is exaggerated. Swelling is thick and hard, as in angioedema. The urticarial plaque may extend a few centimeters or it may involve the major part of an extremity (Figure 14-35). Swelling lasts one to several days. Forty percent of patients with generalized allergic reactions had previously had large localized reactions. The prevalence of generalized reactions to stings is between 0.4% and 0.8%. There are about 40 fatalities from stings each year in the United States. Generalized reactions begin 2 to 60 minutes after the sting. Reactions vary from generalized itching with a few hives to anaphylaxis. The symptoms of anaphylaxis include generalized itching, hives followed by short-

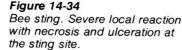
Figure 14-34
Bee sting. Severe local reaction with necrosis and ulceration at the sting site.

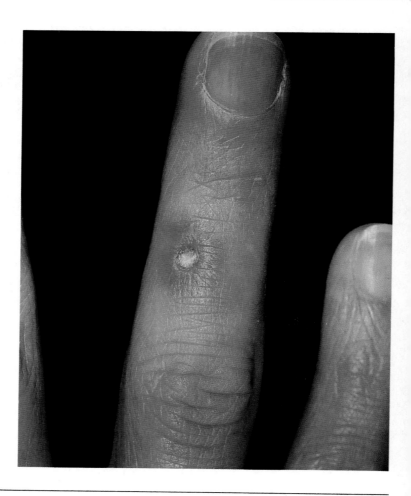

ness of breath, wheezing, nausea, and abdominal cramps. The reaction usually subsides spontaneously, but, in the unfortunate few, it progresses, with edema of the upper airway causing obstruction and death. People found dead outdoors may have had a bee sting rather than a myocardial infarction.

Diagnosis. Patients who have large localized or generalized eruptions should be tested with the venom extracts that are now substituted for whole-body extracts.[21,22] Although RAST tests are available, skin testing with species-specific pure venom is the procedure of choice for determining sensitivity. Testing and desensitization is done with venom from honeybee, yellow jacket, yellow hornet, white-faced hornet, or wasp.

Treatment. Localized nonallergic stings are treated with ice or a paste made by mixing 1 teaspoon of meat tenderizer with 1 teaspoon of water. Localized allergic reactions are treated with cool wet compresses and antihistamines. Treatment of severe generalized reactions for adults includes aqueous epinephrine 1:1000 in a dose of 0.3 to 0.5 ml administered subcutaneously and repeated once or twice at 20-minute intervals if needed. Epinephrine may be given intramuscularly if shock is imminent. If the patient is hypotensive, intravenous injections of 1:10,000 dilution may be necessary. If a severe reaction is feared, epinephrine should be administered immediately; waiting for symptoms to develop can be a dangerous practice. Kits with pre-loaded epinephrine syringes are available (e.g., Anakit, Hollister-Stier Laboratories). Highly sensitive patients should have these kits available at home and during travel. For practice, one injection of physiologic saline should be self-administered under the supervision of a physician. Shortly after administration of epinephrine, antihistamines such as diphenhydramine (Benadryl, 25 to 50 mg) are given orally or intramuscularly depending on the severity of the reaction.

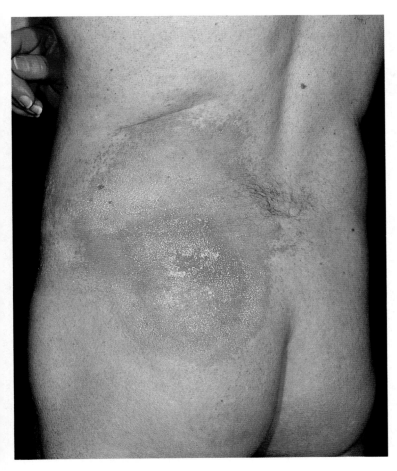

Figure 14-35
Bee sting. A huge urticarial plaque occurred within hours in this patient with a known history of bee sting allergy.

Biting Insects

Biting insects such as fleas, flies, and mosquitoes do not bite in the literal sense; rather they stab their victims with a sharp stylet covered with saliva. The sharp pain is the result of the stab; the reaction depends on the degree of sensitivity to the saliva. All are capable of transmitting infectious diseases. Biting insects seem to prefer some individuals to others. They are attracted by the warmth and moisture of humans. The patient's individual sensitivity determines the type and severity of the bite reaction. Patients who have not had previous exposure or those who have had numerous bites may show little or no response. Those who are sensitive develop localized urticarial papules and plaques immediately after the bite. The papules and plaques proceed to fade in hours and are replaced by red papules that last for days.

Papular urticaria refers to hypersensitivity bite reactions in children. Young children who are left outside unattended in the summer months may receive numerous bites. They soon become sensitized and subsequent bites will show red raised urticarial papules that itch intensely (Figure 14-36). The young child who was initially indifferent to his bites now habitually excoriates newly evolved lesions, creating crusts and infection. Chronically excoriated lesions may last for months, eventually leaving white round scars.

Fleas are tiny, red-brown, hard-bodied wingless insects capable of jumping about 2 feet. They have distinctive, laterally flattened abdomens that allow them to slip between the hairs of their hosts (Figure 14-37). They live in rugs and on the bodies of animals and may jump onto humans. Flea bites occur in a cluster or group (Figure 14-38). A tiny red dot or bite punctum may be seen at times. Bubonic plague was spread throughout Europe in the Middle Ages by fleas that had fed on infected rats.

Flies such as the horsefly, deerfly, and black fly can inflict a painful bite. The common housefly does not bite or sting.

Myiasis. If given the opportunity, flies will deposit their eggs on skin. Young children who fall asleep outside are likely victims. The larvae hatch and burrow to the subcutaneous tissue, causing a red furuncle-like mass with a hole in the center. The head of the larva rises to the surface for air about once a minute. This movement creates pain. If a patient complains of a worm in his skin, believe him; look for the central hole in a 2-cm red mass. Enlarge the hole slightly with a #11 blade and extract the maggot with forceps during one of its excursions to the surface. There is usually only one maggot in each mass. Flies lay eggs in necrotic tissue such as ulcers. Maggots quickly develop and begin feasting on dead tissue.

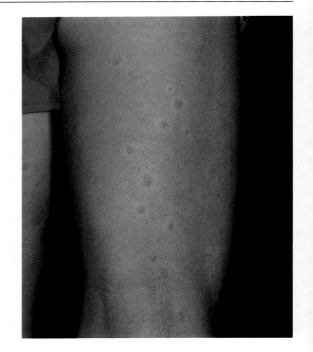

Figure 14-36
Papular urticaria. A hypersensitivity reaction to insect bites seen in children. A wheal develops at the site of each bite.

Female mosquitoes must have a blood meal before they can produce eggs. Mosquitoes usually bite late in the day. In addition to being an annoying menace for people outdoors, mosquitoes are important vectors for infectious disease. They can transmit encephalitis, filariasis, malaria, dengue, and yellow fever.

Prevention and management. Biting insects are attracted to human body odor. The most effective insect repellent available is diethyltoluamide (Deet). It is an effective repellent for most biting insects and ticks, but does not repel stinging insects. Deet blocks the ability of some biting insects to track the victim's vapor trail. It is available in most commercially available insect repellents, either alone or in combination with other chemicals that may enhance its effectiveness. Products containing deet in concentrations above 25% are the most effective. Repellents are available as liquids, sticks, sprays, and saturated pads. The sprays contain the lowest concentration of deet and are the most expensive. All exposed skin surfaces must be covered with re-

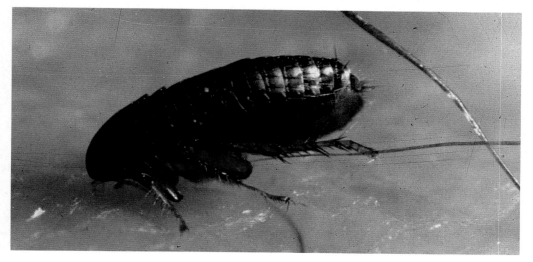

Figure 14-37
Flea. Thin wingless insects with very hard bodies and large hind legs adapted for jumping. (Courtesy Ken Gray, Oregon State University Extension Services.)

pellent; insects will seek out even small areas of skin that have not been covered. When insects begin to land on the skin, it is time for another application of Deet. Repellent may have to be applied every 2 hours in hot humid weather or it may protect up to 6 hours when the air is dry and cool.

A few reports claim that 75 to 150 mg of thiamine hydrochloride taken orally each day during the summer months protects against insect bites.[23] Others believe this has no value. Thiamine hydrochloride is safe and may be worth trying, especially in children who receive many bites.

Insect bite symptoms are treated with cool wet compresses, topical steroids, and oral antihistamines. A paste made of 1 teaspoon of meat tenderizer and 1 teaspoon of water provides symptomatic relief and discourages children from excoriating bites.

Rarely, a patient may develop a generalized reaction to fly bites. Whole-body fly extracts are available for desensitization for the rare patient who develops a generalized reaction to fly bites.

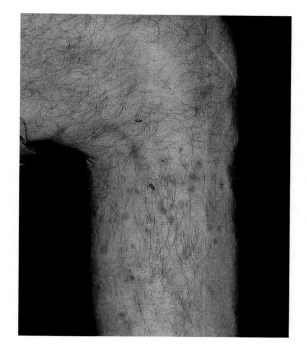

Figure 14-38
Flea bites. A cluster of bites in the knee area. This is a common site because a flea can jump no higher than about 2 feet.

Creeping Eruption

Creeping eruption (cutaneous larva migrans) is a unique cutaneous eruption caused by the aimless wandering through the skin of the hookworm larvae. *Ancylostoma braziliense* is the most common species, and most cases are found in the southeastern United States. Adult nematodes thrive in the intestines of dogs and cats, where they deposit ova that are carried to the ground in feces. The ova hatch into larvae and lie in ambush in the soil waiting for a cat or dog. In their haste to complete their growth cycle, these indiscriminate parasites may penetrate the skin of a human at the point where skin touched the soil. Workers who crawl on their backs under houses may acquire a diffuse infiltration with numerous lesions. The hookworms soon learn they they have preyed upon the wrong host. The larva penetrates into the skin in hopes of eventually reaching the intestines; however physiologic limitations in humans prevent invasion deeper than the basal area of the epidermis. The trapped larva struggles on a few millimeters to a few centimeters each day laterally through the epidermis in a random fashion, creating a tract reminiscent of the trail of a sea snail wandering aimlessly over the sand at low tide (Figure 14-39). Many larvae may be present in the same area, creating several closely approximated wavy lines. Itching is moderate to intense and secondary infection or eczematous inflammation occurs. Eosinophilia may approach 30%. The 1-cm larva stays concealed directly ahead of the advancing tip of the wavy, twisted, red-to-purple, 3-mm tract. In about 4 weeks the worm dies in the epidermis, eventually being sloughed away as the epidermis matures.

Löffler's syndrome, which is a transitory patchy infiltration of the lung, may develop with an accompanying eosinophilia of the blood and sputum.[24] This is most common in patients with severe cutaneous infestation.

Treatment. Thiabendazole (Mintezol) is vermicidal against hookworm larva. It is available in chewable tablets (500 mg) and oral suspension (500 mg/5 ml). The topical application of thiabendazole is now the treatment of choice.[25] The suspension is applied 4 times each day for 1 week. Pruritus clears in 3 days, and the tracts are inactive in 1 week. Oral antibiotics and topical steroids are prescribed if secondary infection and eczematous inflammation are present. Oral thiabendazole is effective but is associated in 40% of cases with nausea, vomiting, and dizziness. The usual dose for patients weighing less than 150 lb is 10 mg/lb; for patients weighing over 150 lb, the dose is 1.5 gm. Each dose is taken twice each day for 2 to 4 days. Freezing the advancing tip of the tract is effective, but causes unnecessary tissue destruction.

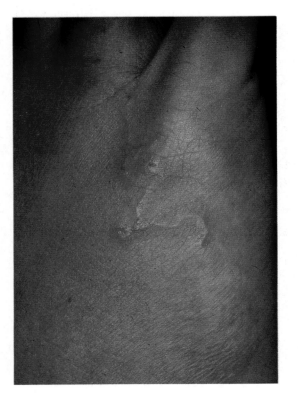

Figure 14-39
Cutaneous larva migrans. Elevated tracks that change position and shape as the larva migrates through the epidermis.

Ants

Fire ants

The fire ant entered the United States from South America and spread quickly to several states in the southeast. Fire ants are small ($1/16$ to $1/4$ inch long) and yellow to red or black with a large head containing prominent incurved jaws and a bee-like stinger on the tail. They build large mounds 1 to 3 feet in diameter. The grass at the periphery of the mound remains undisturbed and unharvested unlike that of the harvester ant mound. Fire ants are aggressive and vicious. When provoked they will attack in numbers. In an instant the ant grasps the skin with the jaws, which establishes a pivot point, then rotates and stings repeatedly, inflicting as many as 20 stings. This often results in a circle of stings with two tiny red dots in the center where the jaws were attached. The pain is immediate and sharp, like a bee sting. Pain subsides in minutes and is replaced by a wheal; 8 to 10 hours later a blister forms, the contents of which rapidly become purulent (Figure 14-40). Blisters resolve in about 10 days. Patients allergic to fire ants may have generalized reactions. Treat the bite with cool compresses, followed by application of a paste made with baking soda or meat tenderizer and water.

Harvester ants

Harvester ants are large ($1/4$ to $1/2$ inch long) red-brown, and sometimes winged. They are found in the southeastern United States where they build flat-topped raised mounds surrounded by a zone that has been cleared of grass, or harvested. The harvester ant destroys crops. When disturbed they attack in numbers and inflict vicious stings. The red bite clears in days and does not form a pustule, unlike the bite of the fire ant.

Figure 14-40
Fire ant stings. Multiple blisters in a cluster.

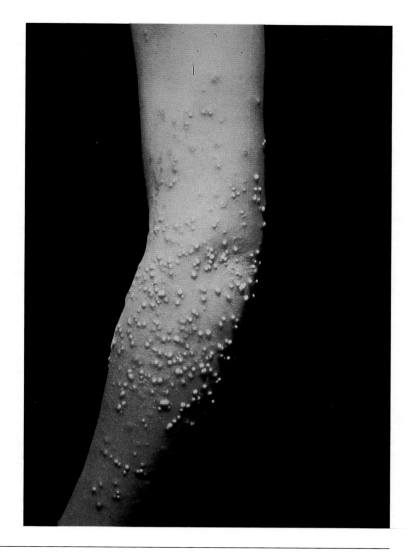

Dermatitis Associated with Swimming

Swimmer's itch

Fresh water swimmer's itch, or schistosome cercarial dermatitis, is caused by a parasite. The microscopic larvae of the parasitic flatworm schistosomes, after being released from snails, swim in the water seeking a warm-blooded host such as a duck. These larvae will penetrate human skin and die in the epidermis after producing a rash. In the United States the states surrounding the Great Lakes have the highest incidence. A more serious visceral form of the disease is present in other parts of the world.

The intensity of the eruption depends on the degree of sensitization. Some people do not develop a rash, whereas others swimming in the same water develop intense eruptions. Initial symptoms are minor after the first exposure and papules occur only after sensitization is acquired and approximately 5 to 13 days later. The typical eruption occurs with subsequent exposures. It begins as bathing water evaporates from the skin surface and cercariae begin penetrating the skin. Itching occurs for about 1 hour and is followed hours later by the development at the points of contact of discrete highly pruritic papules and occasionally pustules surrounded by erythema. They reach maximum intensity in 2 to 3 days and subside in a week. Secondary infection occurs after excoriation.

Treatment consists of relieving symptoms while the eruption is fading. Itching is controlled with antihistamines, cool compresses, and shake lotions such as calamine lotion. Intense inflammation may be suppressed with Group II through V topical steroids. Towel drying immediately after leaving the water is an effective preventative measure, since most larvae penetrate the skin as water is evaporating from it.

Seabather's eruption

Seabather's eruption usually occurs in salt water, primarily along the coast of Florida and the Gulf states. The rash occurs in areas covered by swim suits, in contrast to swimmer's itch, in which the eruption occurs on exposed areas. The cause is not known. Itchy papules or wheals resembling insect bites appear a few hours after bathing and subside in a few days or a week. Children with an extensive eruption may develop a low grade fever. Treatment is symptomatic, as with swimmer's itch.

Sea urchin dermatitis

Sea urchins are round organisms with numerous brittle, sharp, calcified spines projecting from their surface. They attach to rocks on the ocean floor. Venom-containing stalks (pedicellariae) are intermingled among the spines in some tropical species.

Contact with sea urchin spines produces an immediate burning sensation that may persist for hours. Retained spines, if not spontaneously discharged or easily removed, may have to be surgically excised. Visualization with x-ray is important before surgical exploration. Granulomatous nodules may occur weeks or months later. These represent foreign body or hypersensitivity reactions.[26] They respond to intralesional injections of triamcinolone acetonide 10 mg/ml and surgical removal of spines. Chemicals present on the sea urchin's spines are apparently responsible for a delayed reaction that occurs in some individuals; this consists of induration around the fingers and toes. This reaction lasts for weeks, may cause joint deformity, and responds to systemic antibiotics and corticosteroids.

Jellyfish and Portuguese man-of-war

There are two groups of stinging jellyfish found in the coastal waters of North America: the Portuguese man-of-war and the sea nettle. The dreaded Portuguese man-of-war has a large purple air float up to 12 cm long that rides high out of the water and is carried by the wind across the ocean. Tentacles, with their attached stinging structure, the nematocysts, trail out several feet into the water. The red or white jellyfish seen floating in large groups or washed up on the beaches of the Atlantic coast are called sea nettles. They, too, have nematocyst-bearing tentacles that measure up to 4 feet in length.

When a small organism or a human brushes against an outstretched tentacle, the object is stung. Each tentacle has numerous rings of projecting stinging cells and each cell contains a shiny oval body, the nematocyst. On the outer surface of each nematocyst is a tiny projecting trigger. Upon tactile stimulation, the nematocyst fires a thread-like whip with a hollow poisonous tip and recurved hooks on a node-like swelling at the base. The hooks hold the prey fast while the poisonous contents of the nematocyst are discharged through the thread into its body.

Stings produce immediate burning, numbness, and paresthesias. Linear papules or wheals occur where a tentacle has brushed against the skin (Figure 14-41). Lesions fade in hours or proceed to blisters and necrosis. Systemic symptoms (nausea, vomiting, headache, and muscle spasms) occur with severe or widespread stings. Anaphylactic reactions may occur in victims allergic to jellyfish venom. Recurrence of the clinical cutaneous reaction to jellyfish stings may occur within a few weeks without additional contact with the tentacles.[27]

Treatment. A tourniquet may be used to contain toxin if multiple lesions have been inflicted on an extremity. Nematocysts on tentacles may remain unfired on the skin surface and be activated by

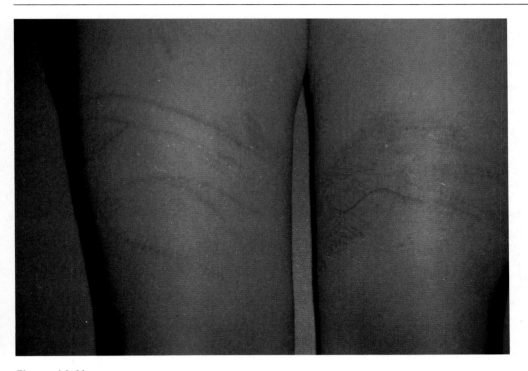

Figure 14-41
*Portuguese man-of-war stings. Linear papules
produced by nematocysts on tentacles that
brushed against the skin.*

washing with fresh water or towel drying. Attempt to
wash off tentacles and toxin by gently pouring sea
water over the afffected area. Inactivate remaining
nematocysts on the skin with alcohol (rubbing alcohol or liquor) or hot sea water. Any remaining tentacles are gently lifted off with a gloved hand. Remaining structures are removed by covering the
area with a paste made of baking soda, flour or
talcum, and sea water. The dried paste is scraped
off with a knife blade and the affected area is treated
with topical steroid creams.

Coral

Coral is formed by limestone-secreting polyps,
which become fused together, forming sharp stone-
like structures of various shapes and sizes. Coral is
encountered in the Caribbean area, including Florida, Bermuda, the Bahamas, and the West Indies,
and in the coral sea extending from Australia to
Hawaii and the Philippines. Like jellyfish, coral have
nematocysts, but these are few in number and produce minor symptoms. The most important injuries
are cuts. Itchy red wheals ("coral poisoning") occur
around the wound. Minor wounds are painful and
slow to heal and often become infected. Retained

bits of calcium may cause a delayed foreign-body
reaction. Wounds should be cleansed thoroughly to
remove bits of debris, then treated with hydrogen
peroxide.

REFERENCES

1. Falk ES: Serum IgE before and after treatment for
   scabies. Allergy **36:**167, 1981.
2. Arlian LG, Runyan RA, Achar S, et al: Survival and
   infestivity of *Sarcoptes scabiei* var. *canis* and var.
   hominis. J Am Acad Dermatol **11:**210, 1984.
3. Solomon LM, Fahrner L, Dennis PW: Gamma benzene hexachloride toxicity: a review. Arch Dermatol
   113:353, 1977.
4. Rasmussen JE: The problem of lindane. J Am Acad
   Dermatol **5:**507, 1981.
5. Shacter B: Treatment of scabies and pediculosis with
   lindane preparations: an evaluation. J Am Acad Dermatol **5:**517, 1981.
6. Cubela V, Yawalkar SJ: Clinical experience with crotamiton cream and lotion in treatment of infants with
   scabies. Br J Clin Pract **32:**229, 1978.
7. Taplin D, Arrue C, Walker JG, et al: Eradication of
   scabies with a single treatment schedule. J Am Acad
   Dermatol **9:**546, 1983.
8. Kanof NM: Of lice and man. J Am Acad Dermatol
   3:91, 1980.

9. Felman YM, Nikitas JA: Pediculosis pubis. Cutis **25:** 482, 1980.
10. Newsom JH, Flore JL Jr, Hackett E: Treatment of infestation with phthirus pubis: comparative efficacies of synergized pyrethins and gamma-benzene hexachloride. Sex Transm Dis **6:**203, 1975.
11. Beaucher WN, Farnham JE: Gypsy-moth-caterpillar dermatitis. N Engl J Med **306:**1301, 1982.
12. Shama SK, Etkind PH, Odell TM, et al: Gypsy-moth-caterpillar dermatitis. N Engl J Med **306:**1300, 1982.
13. Ferrella T, Forney RB: The black widow spider: a medical review. Dermatology p 29, March 1983.
14. Anderson PC: Necrotizing spider bites. Am Fam Pract **26:**198, 1982.
15. Steere AC, Grodzick RL, Kornblatt AN, et al: The spirochetal etiology of Lyme disease. N Engl J Med **308:** 733, 1983.
16. Steere AC, Bartenhagen NH, Craft JE, et al: The early clinical manifestations of Lyme disease. Ann Intern Med **99:**76, 1983.
17. Steere AC, Hutchinson GJ, Rohn DW, et al: Treatment of the early manifestations of Lyme disease. Ann Intern Med **99:**22, 1983.
18. Steere AC, Pachner AR, Malawista SE: Neurologic abnormalities of Lyme disease: successful treatment with high-dose intravenous penicillin. Ann Intern Med **99:**767, 1983.
19. Westerman EL: Rocky Mountain spotless fever: a dilemma for the clinician. Arch Intern Med **142:**1106, 1982.
20. Green WR, Walker DH, Cain BG: Fatal viscerotrophic Rocky Mountain spotted fever. Am J Med **64:**523, 1978.
21. Hunt KJ, Valentine MD, Sobotka AK, et al: A controlled trial of immunotherapy in insect hypersensitivity. N Engl J Med **299:**157, 1978.
22. Chipps BE, Valentine MD, Kaaey-Sobotka A, et al: Diagnosis and treatment of anaphylactic reactions to hymenoptera stings in children. J Pediatr **97:**177, 1980.
23. Marks MB: Stinging Insects: allergy implications. Pediatr Clin North Am **16:**177, 1969.
24. Guill MA, Odom RB: Larva migrans complicated by Loeffler's syndrome. Arch Dermatol **114:**1525, 1978.
25. Edelglass JW, Douglass MC, Stiefler R, et al: Cutaneous larva migrans in northern climates. J Am Acad Dermatol **7:**353, 1982.
26. Fisher AA: Atlas of aquatic dermatology. New York, 1978, Grune & Stratton, p 30.
27. Burnett JW, Cobbs CS, Kelman SN, et al: Studies of the serologic response to jellyfish envenomation. J Am Acad Dermatol **9:**229, 1983.

Chapter Fifteen

Vesicular and Bullous Diseases

Vesicles and bullae are the primary lesions in many diseases. Some are of short duration and are quite characteristic, such as poison ivy and herpes zoster. In others, such as erythema multiforme and lichen planus, a blister may or may not occur during the course of the disease. Finally, there is a group of disorders in which bullae are present almost continuously during the period of active disease. These diseases tend to be chronic and many are associated with tissue-bound or circulating antibodies. This chapter will deal with those disorders.

A blister occurs when fluid accumulates at some level in the skin. The histologic classification of bullous disorders is based on the level in the skin at which that separation occurs (Figure 15-1). Subcorneal blisters are not commonly seen intact; the very thin roof has little structural integrity and collapses. Intraepidermal blisters have a thicker roof and are more substantial, whereas subepidermal blisters have great structural integrity and can remain intact even when firmly compressed.

Granular cell layer
Bullous
  ichthyosiform
  erythroderma
Pemphigus
  foliaceus
Pemphigus
  erythematosus

Subcorneal
Candida albicans
  infection
Impetigo
Miliaria crystallina
Staphylococcal
  scalded skin
  syndrome
Subcorneal
  pustular
  dermatosis

Spinous layer
  (upper and
  mid-epidermis)
Dermatophyte
  fungous infection
Dyshidrosis
Eczematous blister
Friction blister
Insect bites and
  scabies
Miliaria rubra
Viral blisters
  (herpes simplex,
  zoster)

Spinous layer
  (lower epidermis
  and suprabasal
  area)
Benign familial
  chronic
  pemphigus
Keratosis
  follicularis
Pemphigus vulgaris
Transient
  acantholytic
  dermatosis

Basal cell area
Erythema
  multiforme
  (epidermal type)
Epidermolysis
  bullosa simplex
Fixed drug eruption
Kerosene necrosis
Lichen planus
Toxic epidermal
  necrolysis

Lamina lucida
Bullous
  pemphigoid
Cicatricial
  pemphigoid
Epidermolysis
  bullosa letalis
Herpes gestationis
Suction blister
Thermal lesions
  (burns, cold, e.g.
  liquid nitrogen)

**Basal lamina and
sublaminar
connective tissue**
Bullous dermatosis
  of hemodialysis
Bullous eruption
  of SLE
Dermatitis
  herpetiformis
Epidermolysis
  bullosa
  dystrophica
Erythema
  multiforme
  (dermal type)
Ischemic bullae
  (drug overdoses)
Lichen sclerosus et
  atrophicus
Porphyria cutanea
  tarda

**Ultrastructure of
dermoepidermal
junction**

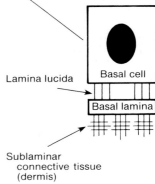

Lamina lucida — Basal cell

Basal lamina

Sublaminar
connective tissue
(dermis)

Figure 15-1
*Bullous diseases in the epidermis and
dermoepidermal junction.*

Diagnosis of Bullous Disorders

The diagnosis of many of the chronic bullous disorders can often be made on clinical grounds. These diseases have such important implications that the diagnosis should be confirmed by histology and, in many instances, by immunofluorescence.

Biopsy. A biopsy must be taken at the proper location to demonstrate the level of blister formation and the nature of the inflammatory infiltrate. Small early vesicles or inflamed skin will provide the most diagnostic features. Ruptured or excoriated lesions are of little value. A small portion of the intact skin

should be included in the biopsy specimen. Punch biopsies taken through the center of a large blister are of little value.

Level of blister formation. For blisters occurring above the basement membrane zone, the level of blister formation can be determined easily with routine studies. Blisters occurring in the dermoepidermal junction area (Figure 15-1) were once considered subepidermal in location. With the electron microscope, it has been shown that blisters may occur at different levels in that complex area. Elec-

TABLE 15-1

BULLOUS AND VASCULITIC DISORDERS—IMMUNOFLUORESCENT TESTS

	Selection of biopsy site for direct immunofluorescence	Findings on direct immunofluorescence	Circulating antibody detected by indirect immunofluorescence
Bullous pemphigoid	Erythematous perilesional skin or mucosa	IgG, C3 at DEJ* (linear)	IgG antibody present in 2/3 of cases; level does not correlate with disease activity
Cicatricial pemphigoid	Erythematous perilesional skin or mucosa	IgG, C3 at DEJ (linear)	IgG or IgM requires highly sensitive system or substrate; DEJ antibody rarely detected with routine procedures
Dermatitis herpetiformis (DH) Classical	Perilesional skin or any normal skin	IgA, C3 in clumps in the papillary dermis	None
Linear IgA disease	Perilesional skin or any normal skin	IgA at DEJ (linear)	None
Henoch-Schonlein purpura	Lesions no older than 24-48 hours	IgA, C3, fibrinogen in superficial and deep vessels	IgG occasionally found
Herpes gestationis (HG)	Erythematous perilesional skin	C3 at DEJ and IgG found in some cases	HG factor present in most cases; requires special techniques
Pemphigus, all forms except Hailey-Hailey disease	Erythematous perilesional skin	IgG and occasionally C3 in epidermal intercellular substance	Intercellular substance antibody present in most cases; reflects activity of disease
Erythema multiforme	Lesions no older than 24-48 hours	IgM, C3, fibrinogen in dermal vessel walls, cytoid bodies, and DEJ	None
Leukocytoclastic vasculitis	Lesions no older than 24-48 hours	IgG, IgM, C3, fibrinogen in cytoid bodies and/or shaggy pattern at DEJ	None
Lichen planus	Involved skin; avoid old lesions or ulcers	IgM, C3, fibrinogen in cytoid bodies and/or shaggy pattern at DEJ	None
Porphyria cutanea tarda	Intact skin, sun-exposed	IgG in or adjacent to vascular walls near the DEJ	None
Benign chronic bullous dermatosis of childhood	Erythematous perilesional skin	Same as DH or pemphigoid	Same as DH or pemphigoid

*DEJ, dermoepidermal junction.

tron microscopy is not routinely used; adequate diagnostic information can be obtained from sections stained with hematoxylin and eosin and immunofluorescence studies.

Immunofluorescence. Immunofluorescence is a laboratory technique for demonstrating the presence of tissue-bound and circulating antibodies. Most chronic bullous disorders have specific antibodies either fixed to some component of skin or circulating. Many laboratories around the country can provide this service and will supply transport media and mailing containers for tissue specimens. Freezing of specimens is no longer required.

Direct immunofluorescence. Direct immunofluorescence is designed for demonstration of tissue-bound antibody and complement. Sectioned biopsy specimens are treated with fluorescein-conjugated antisera to human immunoglobulins (IgG, IgA, IgM, IgD, and IgE), C3, and fibrin; they are then examined with a microscope equipped with a special light source. Table 15-1 shows the best sites for obtaining a biopsy for direct immunofluorescence.

Indirect immunofluorescence. Indirect immunofluorescence is used for demonstration of circulating antibodies against certain skin structures. Thin sections of animal squamous epithelium (monkey esophagus, etc.) are first incubated with the serum of the patient. Skin-reacting antibodies in the serum attach to specific components of the animal epithelium. Fluorescein-labeled antihuman IgG antiserum is then added for specific identification of the circulating antibody.

Dermatitis Herpetiformis and Linear Dermatitis Herpetiformis

Dermatitis herpetiformis (DH) is a rare, chronic, intensely burning and pruritic vesicular skin disease associated in most instances with a subclinical gluten-sensitive enteropathy and IgA deposits in the upper dermis. In hours the disease responds dramatically to sulfones, but without drugs some patients have chosen suicide as the only means of relief.

Clinical presentation. DH begins in the second to fifth decade, varies in intensity, and continues for years or a lifetime. The incidence in unknown, but DH is rarely seen in blacks or Orientals. The disease begins with a few itchy papules or vesicles that are a minor annoyance; they may be attributed to bites, scabies, or neurotic excoriation and sometimes respond to topical steroids. In time the disease evolves into the classic presentation of intensely burning urticarial papules, vesicles, and, rarely, bullae, either isolated or in groups like herpes simplex or zoster (therefore the term *herpetiformis*).

Figure 15-2
Dermatitis herpetiformis. Vesicles are symmetrically distributed on the knee. Most have been excoriated.

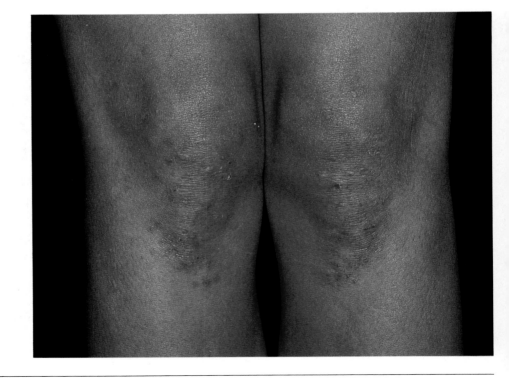

The vesicles are symmetrically distributed and appear on the elbow, knees (Figure 15-2), scalp and nuchal area, shoulders, and buttocks. They are rarely found in the mouth. The distribution may be more generalized. Destruction of the vesicles by scratching provides relief but increases the difficulty of locating a primary lesion for biopsy. Intact lesions for biopsy may be found on the back.

The symptoms vary in intensity, but most people complain of severe itching and burning. One should always think of DH when the symptom of burning is volunteered. The symptoms may precede the onset of lesions by hours and patients can frequently identify the site of a new lesion by the prodromal symptoms. Treatment does not alter the course of disease. Most patients have symptoms for years, but approximately one-third will have permanent remission.

When papules or vesicles are present, the disease may be confused with scabies, eczema, bites, and neurotic excoriations. The vesicular-bullous form is confused with bullous erythema multiforme and bullous pemphigoid.

Gluten-sensitive enteropathy

A gluten-sensitive enteropathy with patchy areas of villous atrophy and mild intestinal wall inflammation is found in a majority of patients with DH. The small intestinal changes are similar to but less severe than those found in ordinary gluten-sensitive enteropathy; symptoms of malabsorption are rarely encountered. Fewer than 20% of patients have malabsorption of fat, D-xylose, or iron. In patients with DH and ordinary gluten-sensitive enteropathy, there is a marked increase in the prevalence of the histocompatibility antigens HLA-B8/DRw3.[1] Patients with the rare form of DH, linear dermatitis herpetiformis, in which IgA is deposited in a linear fashion in the upper dermis rather than in the typical granular pattern, have no evidence of small-bowel disease and have a normal prevalence of the above histocompatibility antigens.

Lymphoma

Small-bowel lymphoma and nonintestinal lymphoma have been reported in patients with DH and celiac disease. Typical patients are those who have jejunal villous atrophy and do not adhere rigidly to a gluten-free diet. One author suggests that a gluten-free diet should be started in every DH patient with villous atrophy, even though gluten-induced abnormalities in the gut have been present for some years before diagnosis and despite the lack of epidemiological evidence that a GFD reduces the incidence of lymphoma in DH.[2]

Diagnosis

Skin biopsy. Sample new red papular lesions that have not blistered to demonstrate subepider-

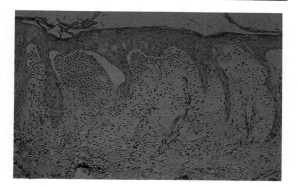

Figure 15-3
Dermatitis herpetiformis. Subepidermal clefts with microabcesses of neutrophils and eosinophils in the dermal papilla.

mal clefts of evolving vesicles (Figure 15-3) and neutrophils and eosinophils in microabscesses within dermal papillae.

Immunofluorescent studies. Skin for immunofluorescent studies is taken from adjacent normal or faintly erythematous skin because the diagnostic immunoglobulin deposits are usually destroyed during the blistering process. Most patients with dermatitis herpetiformis have granular deposits of IgA in the dermal papillae and about 10% have linear deposits of IgA in the basement membrane zone. Patients demonstrating this pattern are said to have linear dermatitis herpetiformis or linear IgA disease.

Trial of sulfones. Patients with a classic history and vesicular eruption may be given a trial of sulfone therapy if they are extremely uncomfortable. The dramatic relief of symptoms in hours or a few days supports the diagnosis of dermatitis herpetiformis.

Treatment

Dapsone or sulfapyridine. These drugs control but do not cure the disease. Dapsone is more effective than sulfapyridine. The mechanism of action is unknown but is possibly explained by lysosomal enzyme stabilization. For adults the initial dosage of dapsone is 100 to 150 mg orally each day. Itching and burning are controlled in 12 to 48 hours and new lesions gradually stop appearing. The dosage is adjusted to the lowest level that provides acceptable relief; this is usually in the range of 50 to 200 mg. Disease in some patients is controlled with 25 mg/day, whereas a few require up to 400 mg/day. Probenecid blocks the renal excretion of dapsone and rifampin increases the rate of plasma clearance. Dapsone produces dose-related hemolysis, anemia, and methemoglobinemia to some degree in all patients. A leukocyte count and hemoglobin should be checked weekly when possible for the

Figure 15-4
Bullae in a diabetic. Large bullae may appear spontaneously in diabetics.

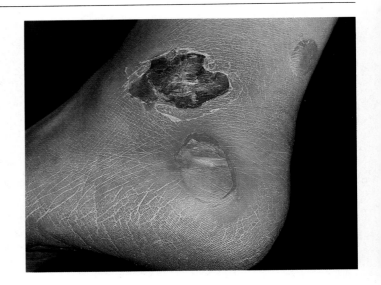

Figure 15-4
Bullae in a diabetic. Large bullae may appear spontaneously in diabetics.

first month, monthly for 6 months, and semiannually thereafter.

Methemoglobinemia, although not usually a significant problem, may cause a blue-gray cyanosis. Patients with glucose-6-phosphate dehydrogenase (G6PD) deficiency may have a profound hemolysis during sulfone or sulfapyridine therapy, and those at risk of having the deficiency (blacks, Asians, and those of Mediterranean descent) should have a G6PD level measured before starting therapy. Dapsone is usually well tolerated, but those patients developing nausea or peripheral neuropathy[3] with motor loss should have the dosage decreased or changed to sulfapyridine (starting dose, 500 to 1500 mg/day).

Gluten-free diet. Strict adherence to a gluten-free diet for at least 6 months allows most patients to begin a decrease and possibly a discontinuation of sulfone therapy. The average time required for the initial control of the rash in 12 patients on a gluten-free diet was 24 months (range, 6 to 98).[4] Although intestinal villous architecture improves, symptoms and lesions will recur in 2 to 36 weeks if a normal diet is resumed. The current evidence indicates that a gluten-free diet needs to be continued indefinitely. Patients found to have a linear IgA immunofluorescence pattern do not have villous atrophy and do not respond to a gluten-free diet.

Bullae in Diabetics

Crops of bullae may appear spontaneously on diabetics (bullosis diabeticorum), usually on the feet and lower legs. The subepidermal bullae arise from a noninflamed base, are usually multiple, and vary in size from one to several centimeters.[5] Occasionally they are huge, involving the entire dorsum of the foot or a major portion of the lower leg (Figure 15-4). The bullae are tense and rupture in about 1 week, leaving a deep painless ulcer that forms a firm adherent crust. Even if not infected, these large ulcers take many weeks to heal. Many patients will never have another episode, whereas others have recurrences. The affliction occurs most often in patients under 50 who have had diabetes for years and whose disease is frequently difficult to control.

Treatment. Ulcers may be compressed several times each day with tepid Burow's solution or silver nitrate. The clean ulcer base is painted twice each day with 2% merbromin (Mercurochrome), and the surrounding skin is cleaned with hydrogen peroxide. Firmly adherent crusts may be removed with collagenase (Santyl ointment). Loosely adherent crusts with underlying purulent material may be gently separated from the ulcer by inserting blunt-tipped scissors under the crust and cutting the fibrous adhesions.

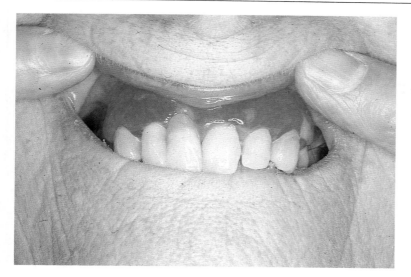

Figure 15-5
*Pemphigus vulgaris. Oral
erosions commonly occur and
may precede the onset of skin
blisters by weeks or months.*

Pemphigus

Pemphigus is a rare, lethal, intraepidermal blistering disease involving the skin and mucous membranes; it is caused by circulating IgG autoantibodies that attach to the intercellular substance of the epidermis. Many patients with pemphigus are Jewish. The mean age of onset is in the sixth decade. Lever now classifies pemphigus into two categories: pemphigus vulgaris, with pemphigus vegetans considered to be a variant, and pemphigus foliaceus, with pemphigus erythematosus designating the localized disease.[6] Pemphigus is a disease that is more heard of than seen.

Pemphigus vulgaris

Pemphigus vulgaris is the most common form of pemphigus. Oral erosions usually precede the onset of skin blisters by weeks or months (Figure 15-5). Nonpruritic skin blisters varying in size from one to several centimeters appear gradually and may be localized for a considerable length of time, but they invariably become generalized if left untreated (Figure 15-6). The blisters rupture easily because the roof, which consists only of a thin portion of the upper epidermis, is extremely fragile. Application of pressure to small intact bullae causes the fluid to dissect laterally into the midepidermal areas altered by bound IgG (Nikolsky's sign). Exposed erosions last for weeks before healing with brown hyperpigmentation, but without scarring. Death formerly resulted in all cases, usually from cutaneous infection, but now occurs in only 10% of cases, usually from complications of steroid therapy. The rare pemphigus vegetans consists of large verrucous confluent plaques localized to flexural areas.

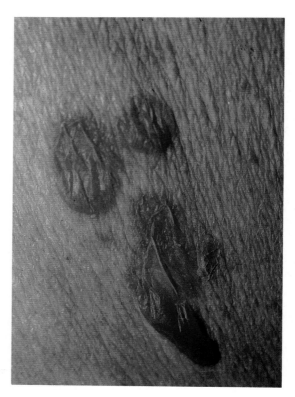

Figure 15-6
*Pemphigus vulgaris. Large flacid blisters rupture
easily to expose a glistening base.*

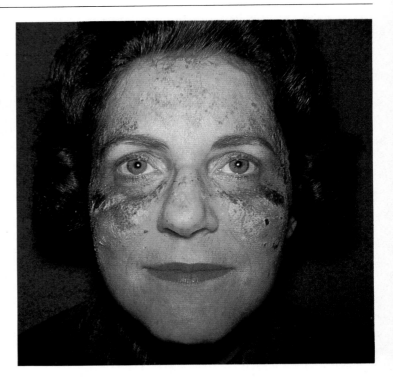

Figure 15-7
Pemphigus erythematosus. Serum and crust with occasional vesicles are present on the face in a butterfly distribution.

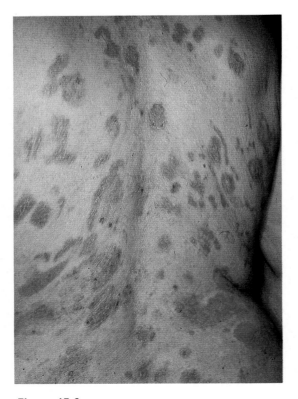

Figure 15-8
Pemphigus foliaceus. Superficial blisters ruptured, leaving oval erosions and crusts.

Pemphigus foliaceus and pemphigus erythematosus

The age of onset varies more widely in pemphigus foliaceus (PF) and pemphigus erythematosus (PE) than in pemphigus vulgaris, and there is no racial prevalence. Oral lesions are rarely present. The disease begins gradually on the face (Figure 15-7) in a "butterfly" distribution, or first appears on the scalp, chest, or upper back (Figure 15-8) as localized or broad continuous areas of erythema, scaling, crusting, and occasional bullae. IgG autoantibodies and C3 can be demonstrated high in the epidermis in the granular layer and presumably are responsible for cleft formation. The roof of this vesicle is so thin that it ruptures and is not usually observed. Serum leaks out and desiccates, forming the localized or broad areas of crust. The site of blister formation in the horizontal plane of the stratum corneum can be demonstrated in skin biopsy specimens after dislodging the upper portion of the epidermis with lateral finger pressure (Nikolsky's sign). This sign is absent in seborrheic dermatitis. PE, known also as the Senear-Usher syndrome, may actually be a combination of localized PF and systemic lupus erythematosus because many of these patients have a positive antinuclear antibody and a positive lupus band test (deposits of immunoglobulin or complement or both at the dermoepidermal junction.)[7] Both forms of the disease may evolve into a generalized eruption. The disease may last for years and may be fatal if not treated.

Pemphigus in association with other diseases

Myasthenia gravis and thymoma have been reported on many occasions in association with pemphigus, usually erythematosus.[8] Malignancy, usually of the lymphoid or reticuloendothelial system, occurs more frequently in patients with pemphigus than in normal people.[9]

Pemphigus foliaceus has been reported in approximately 5% of patients taking 500 to 2000 mg of D-penicillamine any time from 2 months to 4 years.[10] Most cases of pemphigus were mild and self-limited, resolving within weeks or sometimes months after discontinuing D-penicillamine.

Diagnosis

Skin biopsy for light microscopy. A small early vesicle or skin adjacent to a blister biopsied with a 3- or 4-mm punch shows an intraepidermal bulla, acantholysis (separation of epidermal cells near the blister after dissolution of the intercellular cement substance), and a mild to moderate infiltrate of eosinophils (Figures 15-9 and 15-10).

Direct immunofluorescence of skin. Another punch biopsy of erythematous perilesional skin is taken and deposited in transport media available from specialized laboratories around the country. These are transported unrefrigerated. IgG and, in most instances, C3 are found in the intercellular substance areas of the epidermis.

Indirect immunofluorescence. Serum IgG antibodies can be demonstrated by indirect immunofluorescence staining and are present in all forms of true pemphigus in about 75% of patients with active disease. In most cases the level of circulating intercellular substance IgG antibody reflects the activity of disease, rising during periods of activity and falling or disappearing during times of remission.

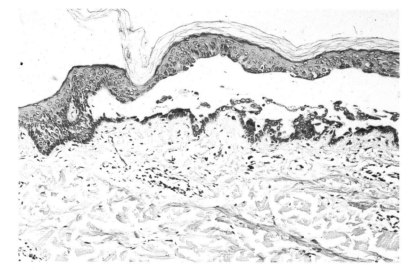

Figure 15-9
Pemphigus vulgaris. The epidermal separation occurs low in the epidermis.

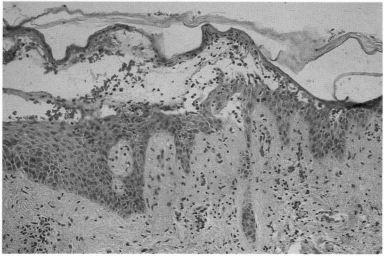

Figure 15-10
Pemphigus foliaceus. The intraepidermal separation appears high in the epidermis.

Treatment method of Walter Lever

Two treatment schedules are recommended,[11,12] the first is for patients with extensive involvement. Prednisone is given as a single dose with breakfast. The initial dose is determined by the severity of the disease and ranges from 200 to 350 mg. If no improvement occurs within 5 days, the dose should be increased by at least 60 mg. High daily doses are maintained for 5 to 10 weeks during which time all lesions will have healed or nearly healed. After completion of the high-dosage schedule, the dose of prednisone is reduced immediately to 40 mg daily for 1 week, 30 mg/day for the second week, and 25 mg/day for the third week, then to 40 mg on alternate days. At this point an immunosuppressant, usually azathioprine at a dosage of 100 mg/day, is added. The dosage of prednisone is maintained at 40 mg every other day for a year, or longer if there are persisting lesions. The dosage of prednisone is then gradually reduced during a 1-year period. Subsequently, the dosage of the immunosuppressant agent is reduced within 4 to 6 months. Lever finds that any reduction attempted more rapidly seemed to carry the risk of disease reactivation.

Patients with mild and relatively stable disease are treated initially with 40 mg of prednisone every other day and an immunosuppressant agent every day as described above. Patients whose disease flares may be advanced to the high dose prednisone schedule.

Lever warns that for the treatment of advanced diseases any dosages of prednisone between 40 mg every other day and 200 mg/day ought to be avoided. These so-called intermediate dosages often do not suppress the disease adequately. He reported that high-dose, short-term prednisone therapy is more effective and associated with fewer side effects than prolonged treatment with intermediate dosages. Most patients will remain in prolonged remission after being treated with these programs.

Other therapeutic modalities, including gold, dapsone, plasmapheresis, and intralesional corticosteroids, have been used alone or together with systemic corticosteroids.[13]

The Pemphigoid Group of Diseases

Bullous pemphigoid, herpes gestationis, and cicatricial pemphigoid are subepidermal blistering diseases with circulating IgG antibodies and basement membrane zone–bound IgG antibodies and C3.

Bullous pemphigoid

Bullous pemphigoid is a rare, relatively benign subepidermal blistering disease of unknown origin in which IgG autoantibodies are found both circulating and bound at the dermoepidermal junction. There is no racial prevalence. Pemphigoid is a disease of the elderly with most cases occurring after age 60, but cases have been reported in children.

Clinical manifestations. Oral blisters if present are mild and transient. Pemphigoid begins with a localized area of erythema or with pruritic urticarial plaques that gradually become more edematous and extensive. The amount of itching varies, but is usually moderate to severe. Within 1 to 3 weeks, the plaques turn dark red or cyanotic, resembling erythema multiforme, as vesicles and bullae rapidly appear on their surface (Figure 15-11). The eruption is usually generalized, appearing also on the palms and soles (Figure 15-12). The 1- to 7-cm bullae appear isolated or in clusters and are tense with good structural integrity, in contrast to the large, flaccid, easily ruptured bullae of pemphigus. Firm pressure on the blister will not result in extension into normal

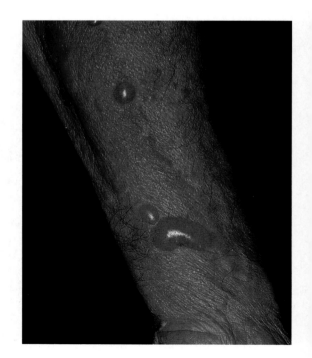

Figure 15-11
Bullous pemphigoid. Tense blisters arise from a dark red urticarial base.

skin, as is seen in pemphigus; therefore, Nikolsky's sign is negative. Most bullae rupture within a week, leaving an eroded base that, unlike pemphigus, heals rapidly.

The course is variable. Untreated pemphigoid may remain localized and undergo spontaneous remission or it may become generalized and last up to 5 years with periods of remission followed by recurrences. Throughout this impressive disease, patients remain afebrile, relatively comfortable, and ambulatory. There are a large number of case reports of malignancy occurring in patients with pemphigoid. However, no significant association with internal neoplasms was shown in one large study.[14]

Diagnosis

Skin biopsy for light microscopy. There are two important features to demonstrate in biopsies of bullous diseases: the level of cleft formation (i.e., intraepidermal or subepidermal) and the presence or absence of an inflammatory infiltrate and the type of cell present (i.e., eosinophils or neutophils). Bullae in pemphigoid may arise from inflamed (infiltrate-rich) or noninflamed (infiltrate-poor) skin; therefore, the most information will be provided by obtaining a biopsy on an early bulla on inflamed skin. Histologically, there are subepidermal bullae with eosinophils in the dermis and bullous cavity (Figure 15-13).

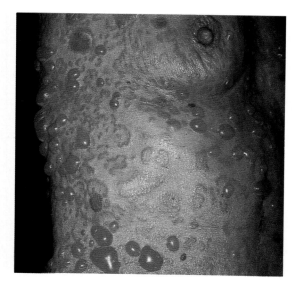

Figure 15-12
Bullous pemphigoid. Generalized eruption with tense blisters arising from an edematous erythematous annular base.

Figure 15-13
Bullous pemphigoid. A subepidermal blister contains numerous eosinophils.

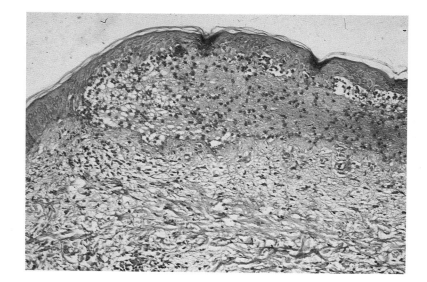

Direct immunofluorescence of skin. Another 3- or 4-mm punch biopsy of inflamed skin next to the blister is taken and submitted in special transport media. Direct immunofluorescence shows IgG and C3 in a linear band at the basement membrane zone (Figure 15-14).

Indirect immunofluorescence. Circulating IgG antibodies are present in most cases, but their level does not correlate with disease activity as it does in pemphigus.[15]

Treatment. Itching is controlled with hydroxyzine (Atarax, 10 to 50 mg every 4 hours as needed). Combined therapy with prednisone and an immunosuppressive drug such as azathioprine, methotrexate, or cyclophosphamide has made it possible to control pemphigoid effectively without having to resort to the higher dose levels of prednisone that would be required if that agent were used alone. The incidence of steroid-related side effects decreases with combined therapy.[16]

The following treatment program involves the use of azathioprine (Imuran) and prednisone.[17] The initial dose of prednisone is determined by the intensity of the disease. Patients with generalized blistering may require 180 mg or more each day; those with limited disease may be started on 40 mg/day. Azathioprine (1.5 mg/kg of body weight; usually 100 mg/day) is started at the same time. Both medications are maintained at the initial starting levels until blistering is controlled in 10 to 60 days, and then prednisone is rapidly tapered to maintenance levels (e.g., prednisone 40 mg every other day while maintaining azathioprine at 1.5 mg/kg/day). Both drugs are continued until there is no sign of new activity; duration of maintenance ranges from 4 to 24 weeks. Methotrexate and cyclophosphamide have been used in place of azathioprine.

A few patients with bullous pemphigoid respond to treatment with sulfapyridine or dapsone, and their disease can be completely controlled without the use of prednisone.

Figure 15-14
Bullous pemphigoid. Direct immunofluorescence shows IgG and C3 in a linear band at the basement membrane zone.

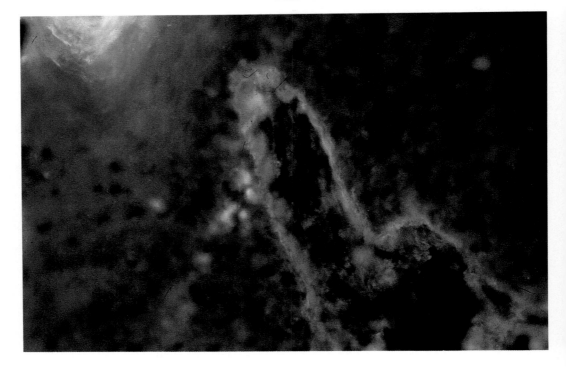

Herpes gestationis

This rare blistering disease of pregnancy is probably a variant of bullous pemphigoid. The disorder usually appears during the second trimester, but may occur from the second week to the early postpartum period. It disappears 1 or 2 months after delivery and may recur with subsequent pregnancies. The newborn fetus is most often normal, but may be delivered prematurely or as a stillbirth. The early edematous plaques occur in crops on the abdomen and extremities and coalesce into bizarre polycyclic rings covering wide areas of the skin (Figure 15-15). As with pemphigoid, the tense blisters evolve from the edematous plaques, rupture to leave slowly healing denuded areas, and heal without scarring; they do cause postinflammatory hyperpigmentation. Mucous membrane involvement is rare.

Diagnosis. Biopsy specimens taken from inflamed skin adjacent to a blister exhibit histologic features similar to pemphigoid. A band-like deposit of C3, in most cases, and IgG, in 10% of cases, can be demonstrated at the basement membrane zone by direct immunofluorescence. Circulating IgG can be detected in only a few patients by conventional indirect immunofluorescence techniques. Circulating IgG can be demonstrated in most cases with the uncommonly available test called complement indirect immunofluorescence. The so-called herpes gestationis factor can pass through the placenta and may be responsible for the transient pemphigoid-like skin lesions present in some newborns of affected mothers.[18]

Treatment. During pregnancy the patient is treated with Group II or V steroids with or without cool wet compresses. Prednisone (40 mg every day or every other day) may be required for a short time in the postpartum period.

Figure 15-15
Herpes gestationis. Blisters arise from erythematous edematous polycyclic rings.

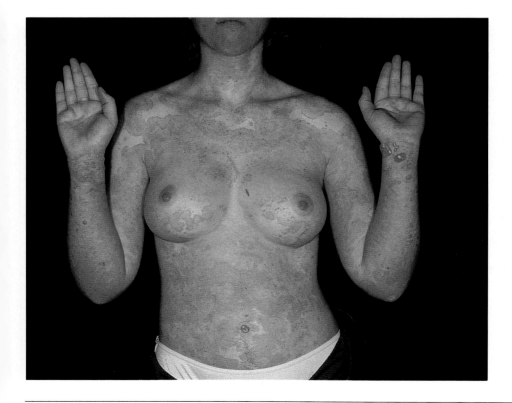

Cicatricial pemphigoid

Seen in the elderly, cicatricial pemphigoid or benign mucosal pemphigoid is a rare, chronic, subepidermal blistering and scarring disease of the mucous membranes and, occasionally, the skin. Unlike bullous pemphigoid there are few remissions. The most commonly involved moist areas, in the order of frequency, are the oral mucosa (Figure 15-16), the conjunctiva (Figure 15-17), the larynx, the genitalia, and the esophagus. Oral lesions start as vesicles, which rupture, leaving clean, noninflamed erosions that are relatively painless and do not interfere with eating. The vermillion border of the lips is spared, in contrast to pemphigus. Fibrous conjunctival adhesions become more numerous with time and in about 20% of cases lead to blindness. Hoarseness is a sign of laryngeal involvement. Fibrous adhesions and atrophy can occur on the penis, vulva, vagina, and anus. About 25% of the patients develop cutaneous lesions consisting of scattered, tense vesicles, usually on the extremities, that heal with or without scarring, or bullae arising from an erythematous base on the face and scalp that rupture, leaving a chronic erosion that eventually scars.

Diagnosis. The biopsy shows a subepidermal bulla with little inflammation. Circulating IgG antibody is occasionally found and direct immunofluorescence of perilesional mucous membrane and skin shows a linear band of IgG and C3.

Treatment. The combined treatment program described for pemphigoid may be used, except that lower doses of prednisone (e.g., 60 mg/day) are prescribed. The response is slow. In one study 24 patients were treated with dapsone (75 to 200 mg per day). Of these, 20 (83.3%) had partial or complete control with mild to no inflammatory activity.[19]

Benign chronic bullous dermatosis of childhood

Chronic bullous dermatosis of childhood is a rare, nonhereditary, subepidermal blistering disease with clinical features similar to bullous pemphigoid and dermatitis herpetiformis.[20] Large tense bullae appear in clusters on the trunk, pelvic region, and lower extremities. A significant number of patients have linear IgA deposits at the basement membrane zone, circulating IgA antibasement membrane zone antibodies, normal jejunal biopsies, and HLA–B8.[21]

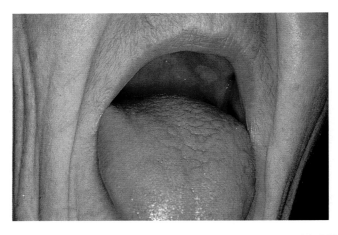

Figure 15-16
Cicatricial pemphigoid. Large oral cavity erosions.

Figure 15-17
Cicatricial pemphigoid involving the conjunctiva and surrounding skin.

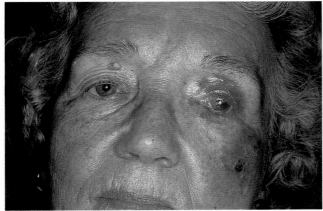

Benign Familial Chronic Pemphigus

Benign familial chronic pemphigus (Hailey-Hailey disease) is a rare, autosomal dominant, intraepidermal, nonscarring bullous disease. The disease first appears in adolescence or in early adult life, usually during the summer; it is characterized by remissions and exacerbations. Lesions develop on areas exposed to ultraviolet light (nape of the neck and back) (Figure 15-18) and on areas subject to friction and maceration (axillae and groin). Infection with staphylococci or *Candida* may also precipitate the disease. The eruption begins with a group of pruritic vesicles arising from a red or noninflamed base; they are grouped in an annular or serpiginous pattern. The vesicles rupture quickly and are replaced by an advancing rim of scale and crust similar to that seen in impetigo and tinea. The active border extends peripherally, leaving a pale hypopigmented center. New crops of vesicles appear on the border, but rupture so quickly that they may not be realized. Lesions may heal spontaneously in colder weather. Vesicles sometimes appear in intertriginous lesions, but most often the patient has moist, red, fissured, vegetating plaques that do not extend beyond the opposing skin surfaces of the groin or axillae. Intertriginous lesions are chronic and respond slowly to therapy, especially in obese patients.

Treatment

Nonintertriginous lesions. Oral antibiotics (e.g., erythromycin, dicloxacillin, or a cephalosporin) should be started, followed in 3 or 4 days by a Group III to V topical steroid. Most lesions of the back and neck respond quickly to this simple program and treatment is stopped when the lesions have healed. Sunscreens should be worn on exposed surfaces in the summer.

Intertriginous lesions. Groin and axillary lesions may be infected with bacteria and yeast. One of the above oral antibiotics is started and miconazole cream is applied to moist lesions and compressed with cool Burow's or silver nitrate solution. Compressing is discontinued once the surfaces are dry and Group V topical steroid creams are applied twice a day until lesions have healed. Chronic and unresponsive lesions have been treated successfully by excision followed by split-thickness skin grafting.

Figure 15-18
Benign familial chronic pemphigus. Erythematous annular plaques with vesicles and scale near the advancing border.

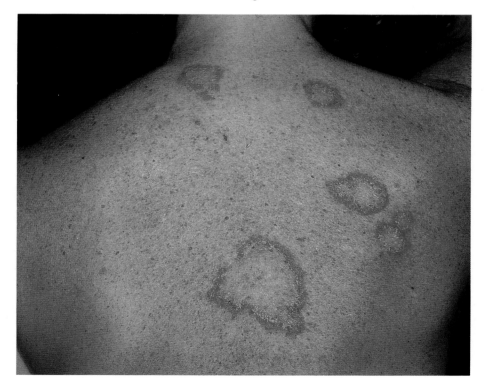

REFERENCES

1. Lawley TJ, Hall RP, Fauci AS, et al: Defective Fc-receptor functions associated with HLA-B8/Drw3 haplotype: studies in patients with dermatitis herpetiformis and normal subjects. N Engl J Med 304:185, 1981.

2. Gawkrodger DJ, Barnetson RStC: Dermatitis herpetiformis and lymphoma. Lancet 2:987, 1982.

3. Waldinger TP, Siegle RJ, Weber W et al: Dapsone induced peripheral neuropathy. Arch Dermatol 120:356, 1984.

4. Leonard J, Haffenden G, Tucker W, et al: Gluten challenge in dermatitis herpetiformis. N Engl J Med 308:816, 1983.

5. Bernstein JE, Medenica M, Soltani K, et al: Bullous eruption of diabetes mellitus. Arch Dermatol 115:324, 1979.

6. Lever WF: Pemphigus and pemphigoid: a review of the advances made since 1964. J Am Acad Dermatol 1:1, 1979.

7. Amerian ML, Ahmed AR: Pemphigus erythematosus: presentation of four cases and review of the literature. J Am Acad Dermatol 10:215, 1984.

8. Maize JC, Dobson RL, Provost TT: Pemphigus and myasthenia gravis. Arch Dermatol 111:1134, 1975.

9. Krain LS, Bierman SM: Pemphigus vulgaris and internal malignancy. Cancer 33:1091, 1974.

10. Ahmed R: Pemphigus associated with D-penicillamine, Pemphigus: current concepts. Ann Intern Med 92:396, 1980.

11. Lever WF: Pemphigus and pemphigoid: a review of the advances made since 1964. J Am Acad Dermatol 1:15, 1979.

12. Lever WF, Schaumburg-Lever G: Treatment of pemphigus vulgaris. Arch Dermatol 120:44, 1984.

13. Bystryn JC: Adjuvant therapy of pemphigus. Arch Dermatol 120:941, 1984.

14. Stone SP, Schroeter AL: Bullous pemphigoid and associated malignant neoplasms. Arch Dermatol 111:991, 1975.

15. Person JR, Rogers RS III: Bullous and cicatrical pemphigoid: clinical, histopathologic, and immunopathologic correlations. Mayo Clin Proc 52:54, 1977.

16. Feller MJ, Katz JM, McCabe JB: Successful use of cyclophosphamide and prednisone for initial treatment of pemphigus vulgaris. Arch Dermatol 114:889, 1978.

17. Ahmed AR, Maize JC, Provost TT: Bullous pemphigoid: clinical and immunologic follow-up after successful therapy. Arch Dermatol 113:1043, 1977.

18. Shornick JK, Bangert JL, Freeman RG, et al: Herpes gestationis: clinical and histologic features of twenty-eight cases. J Am Acad Dermatol 8:214, 1983.

19. Rogers RS III, Seehafer JR, Perry HO: Treatment of cicatricial (benign mucous membrane) pemphigoid with dapsone. J Am Acad Dermatol 6:215, 1982.

20. Marsden RA, MeKee PH, Bhogal B, et al: A study of benign chronic bullous dermatosis of childhood and comparison with dermatitis herpetiformis and bullous pemphigoid occurring in childhood. Clin Exp Dermatol 5:159, 1980.

21. Sweren RJ, Burnett JW: Benign chronic bullous dermatosis of childhood: a review. Cutis 29:350, 1982.

Chapter Sixteen

Connective Tissue Diseases

Lupus erythematosus
  Clinical classification
  Management of cutaneous LE
  Treatment
Dermatomyositis and polymyositis
  Dermatomyositis
  Polymyositis
Scleroderma
  Acrosclerosis
  CREST syndrome
  Diffuse systemic sclerosis
  Morphea

Lupus Erythematosus

Clinical classification

Lupus erythematosus (LE) is a multisystem disease of unknown origin characterized by the production of numerous diverse types of autoantibodies that, through immune mechanisms in various tissues, cause several combinations of clinical signs, symptoms, and laboratory abnormalities. Attempts have been made to group patients into subsets in order to define more homogeneous groups with a predictable course or response to treatment. These subsets have been defined by similar clinical features (Tables 16-1 and 16-2), laboratory abnormalities, pathologic changes, or combinations thereof. Each of these arbitrarily defined syndromes or subsets of LE is considered part of the spectrum of disease known as systemic lupus erythematosus (SLE). The subsets are redefined constantly as the pathophysiology of this complex and diverse disease is better understood.

An attempt to establish criteria for diagnosis resulted in the development of a list of the 11 most common signs and symptoms associated with SLE (Table 16-3). This was compiled by the American Rheumatism Association.[1] The presence of 4 or more of the 11 manifestations, serially or simultaneously, is considered compatible with the diagnosis of SLE. Those criteria in a modified form are illustrated by Dr. Netter in Figure 16-1.

Recently, subsets of lupus erythematosus have been defined by cutaneous manifestations present in some form in most patients having lupus.[2] The classification proposed by Gilliam and Sontheimer (Table 16-1) divides cutaneous LE into three types based upon the clinical appearance of the skin lesion. They are chronic cutaneous LE (scarring, discoid LE [DLE]), subacute cutaneous LE (SCLE), and acute cutaneous LE.

TABLE 16-1

CLASSIFICATION OF CUTANEOUS LUPUS ERYTHEMATOSUS

	Clinical forms	Clinical and laboratory features	Histologic features
DLE 15%–20%*	Localized Generalized (lesions above and below the neck) Hypertrophic	Usually localized, chronic, scarring lesions of head or neck region or both lasting months to years Usually no extracutaneous disease (5% of patients will develop SLE) Antinuclear antibodies occasionally present in low titer; anticytoplasmic antibodies not present Anti-dsDNA† antibodies rarely present Subepidermal immunoglobulin deposits commonly found in lesions (75%), but rarely present in uninvolved skin Simultaneous occurrence of severe systemic lupus erythematosus with nephritis is rare	Hydropic degeneration of the epidermal basal cell layer with focal epidermal atrophy Heavy mononuclear cell infiltrate in upper dermis, periappendageal and perivascular regions extending into the deep dermis
SCLE, 10%–15%*	Papulosquamous (psoriasiform), 8% Annular-polycyclic, 5%*	Usually widespread, nonscarring lesions with associated scaling, depigmentation, and telangiectases on face, neck, upper and extensor arms (photosensitive distribution) lasting weeks to months; lesions often exacerbated by exposure to sun Usually associated with extracutaneous disease, but severe renal or central nervous system disease uncommon Antinuclear and anticytoplasmic antibodies frequently present (60% of patients) Anti-dsDNA antibodies present in low serum concentrations in 30% of patients; hypocomplementemia rare HLA-A1, B8, and DR3 significantly increased Subepidermal immunoglobulin deposits present in only 50% of lesions and 30% of uninvolved skin	Marked hydropic changes along epidermal basal cell layer Moderate mononuclear cell infiltrate in superficial dermis only
Acute cutaneous LE, 30%–50%*	Localized, indurated erythematous lesions (malar areas of face—butterfly rash) Widespread indurated erythema (face, scalp, neck, upper chest, shoulders, extensor arms, backs of hands)	Transient (hours to days) Multisystem disease usually present; renal disease common Antinuclear antibodies usually present Anti-dsDNA antibodies present in 60%-80% of patients, often in high concentration; hypocomplementemia common Subepidermal immunoglobulin deposits commonly found in lesional (> 95%) and exposed nonlesional (75%) skin	Hydropic changes along epidermal basal layer Sparse mononuclear cell infiltrate and upper dermal edema

From Gilliam JN, Sontheimer RD: Distinctive cutaneous subsets in the spectrum of lupus erythematosus. J Am Acad Dermatol **4**:471, 1981.

TABLE 16-2

SUBSETS OF SYSTEMIC LUPUS ERYTHEMATOSUS

Clinically defined subsets	Pattern of clinical illness
1. Cutaneous LE	
a. DLE	Markedly lower incidence of severe systemic disease; excellent prognosis
b. SCLE	Mild systemic involvement; anticytoplasmic antibodies; HLA antigens B8 and DR3; good prognosis
c. Acute cutaneous LE	Active systemic LE; prognosis guarded
2. Raynaud's phenomenon	Anti-nRNP* antibodies; good prognosis
3. Vasculitis	Increased incidence of central nervous system (CNS) disease (?); poor prognosis
4. CNS disease	Poor prognosis in patients with diffuse cerebritis
5. Nephritis	Poor prognosis in patients with diffuse proliferative glomerulonephritis

From Gilliam JN, Sontheimer RD: Distinctive cutaneous subsets in the spectrum of lupus erythematosus. J Am Acad Dermatol **4:**471, 1981.
*nRNP, nuclear ribonucleoprotein.

Figure 16-1
Clinical and laboratory characteristics of systemic lupus erythematosus (SLE). (Modified from American Rheumatism Association [ARA] criteria. Copyright 1979, CIBA Pharmaceutical Company, *Division of Ciba-Geigy Corporation. Reprinted with permission from Clinical Symposia illustrated by Frank H. Netter, M.D. All rights reserved.)*

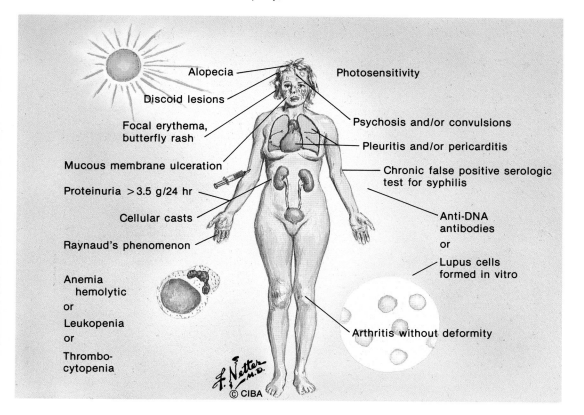

TABLE 16-3

THE 1982 REVISED CRITERIA FOR CLASSIFICATION OF SYSTEMIC LUPUS ERYTHEMATOSUS*

Criterion	Definition
1. Malar rash	Fixed erythema, flat or raised, over the malar eminences, tending to spare the nasolabial folds
2. Discoid rash	Erythematous raised patches with adherent keratotic scaling and follicular plugging; atrophic scarring may occur in older lesions
3. Photosensitivity	Skin rash as a result of unusual reaction to sunlight, by patient history or physician observation
4. Oral ulcers	Oral or nasopharyngeal ulceration, usually painless, observed by a physician
5. Arthritis	Nonerosive arthritis involving two or more peripheral joints, characterized by tenderness, swelling, or effusion
6. Serositis	Pleuritis: convincing history of pleuritic pain or rub heard by a physician or evidence of pleural effusion OR Pericarditis: documented by ECG or rub or evidence of pericardial effusion
7. Renal disorder	Persistent proteinuria greater than 0.5 gm per day or greater than 3+ if quantification not performed OR Cellular casts: may be red cell, hemoglobin, granular, tubular, or mixed
8. Neurologic disorder	Seizures: in the absence of offending drugs or known metabolic derangements, e.g., uremia, ketoacidosis, or electrolyte imbalance OR Psychosis: in the absence of offending drugs or known metabolic derangements, e.g., uremia, ketoacidosis, or electrolyte imbalance
9. Hematologic disorder	Hemolytic anemia: with reticulocytosis OR Leukopenia: less than $4,000/mm^3$ total on two or more occasions OR Lymphopenia: less than $1,500/mm^3$ on two or more occasions OR Thrombocytopenia: less than $100,000/mm^3$ in the absence of offending drugs
10. Immunologic disorder	Positive LE cell preparation OR Anti-DNA: antibody to native DNA in abnormal titer OR Anti-Sm: presence of antibody to Sm nuclear antigen OR False-positive serologic test for syphilis known to be positive for at least 6 months and confirmed by *Treponema pallidum* immobilization or fluorescent treponemal antibody absorption test
11. Antinuclear antibody	An abnormal titer of antinuclear antibody by immunofluorescence or an equivalent assay at any time and in the absence of drugs known to be associated with "drug-induced lupus" syndrome

From Tan EM, Cohen AS, Fries JS, et al: Arthritis Rheum **25**:1271, 1982.

*The proposed classification is based on 11 criteria. For the purpose of identifying patients in clinical studies, a person shall be said to have systemic lupus erythematosus if any 4 or more or the 11 criteria are present, serially or simultaneously, during any interval of observation.

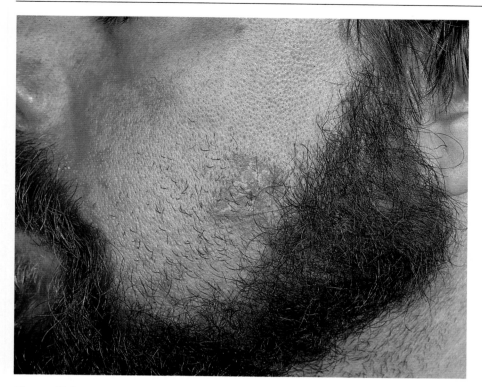

Figure 16-2
Chronic cutaneous LE (discoid LE). Well-defined elevated flat-topped hypopigmented plaques with adherent scale.

Chronic cutaneous LE (discoid LE). Patients with DLE possess a low incidence of systemic disease.[3] The disease is more common in females and it has a peak incidence in the fourth decade. Trauma and ultraviolet light exposure (with wavelengths less than 320 nm) may initiate and exacerbate lesions.

The face is the most commonly affected area, but lesions occur on any body surface. Lesions are usually asymmetrically distributed and begin as asymptomatic, well-defined, elevated, red-violaceous, 1- to 2-cm flat-topped plaques with firmly adherent scale (Figures 16-2 and 16-3). The scale penetrates into the orifices of the hair follicle. When the scale is peeled, its undersurface has the appearance of a carpet penetrated by several carpet tacks; it is called carpet tack scale (Figure 16-4). Carpet tack scale is most apparent on the face and scalp (Figure 16-5) where the follicular orifices are larger. Atrophy occurs in both the epidermis and dermis. Epidermal atrophy occurs early and gives the surface either a smooth or a wrinkled appearance. These lesions endure for months and either

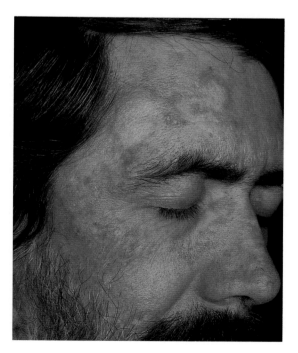

Figure 16-3
Chronic cutaneous LE (discoid LE). Lesions that are several months old are hypopigmented and atropic.

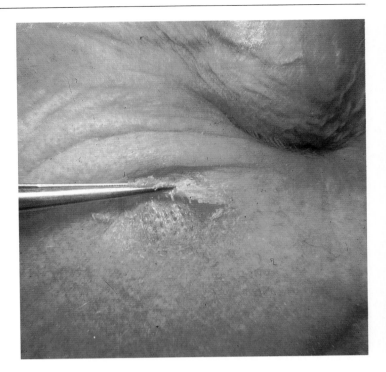

Figure 16-4
Chronic cutaneous LE (discoid LE).
Carpet tack scale created by
follicular keratin plugs.

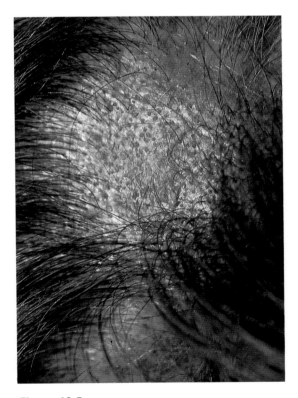

Figure 16-5
Chronic cutaneous LE (discoid LE). Prominent
follicular plugging in a plaque of discoid LE
located in the scalp.

resolve spontaneously or progress with further atrophy, ultimately forming smooth white or hyperpigmented depressed scars with telangiectasia. Occasionally, plaques become thick (hypertrophic DLE).[4] Discoid LE can cover wide areas of the face, causing disfigurement. Hypopigmentation is particularly disfiguring for blacks. The laboratory and histologic features are outlined in Tables 16-1 and 16-5.

Subacute cutaneous LE. SCLE encompasses the clinical spectrum of cutaneous LE between the chronic destructive DLE and the transient erythema of acute cutaneous LE. Like DLE, the individual lesions of SCLE may last for months; in contrast to the most chronic form of LE, they heal without scarring. SCLE has been described by a variety of terms, including superficial disseminated LE, disseminated discoid LE, subacute disseminated LE, psoriasiform LE, and maculopapular photosensitive LE. Most patients with SCLE are white females. Two morphologic varieties are a papulosquamous pattern (Figures 16-6 and 16-7) and an annular-polycyclic pattern (Figure 16-8); one will predominate. The lesions spare the knuckles (Figure 16-9), the inner aspect of the arms, the axillae, and the lateral part of the trunk.[5] Lesions are rarely seen below the waist. A subtle gray hypopigmentation and telangiectasia are frequently seen in the center of annular lesions bordered by erythema and a su-

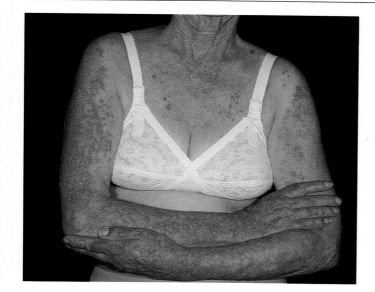

Figure 16-6
Subacute cutaneous LE (papulosquamous pattern). Lesions are confined to exposed areas on the upper half of the body.

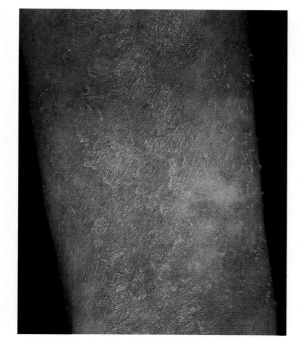

Figure 16-7
Subacute cutaneous LE (papulosquamous pattern). There is erythema, scaling, and hyperpigmentation. All of these changes are reversible.

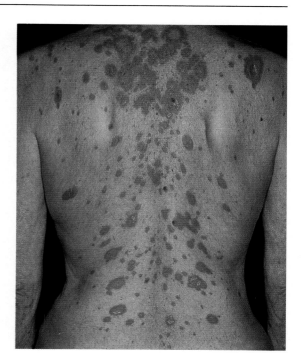

Figure 16-8
Subacute cutaneous LE (annular-polycyclic pattern). The annular plaques have an erythematous scaly border, the central area is hypopigmented, and the eruption is confined to the back and hands.

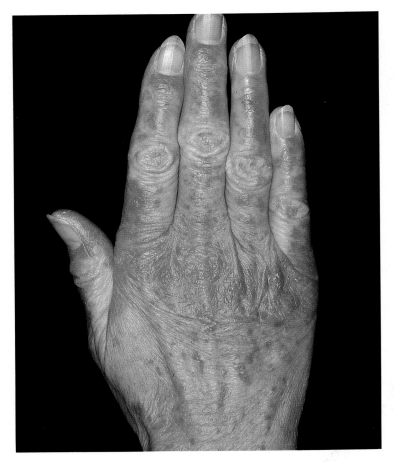

Figure 16-9
Cutaneous LE. Erythema and telangiectasia spare the knuckles, in contrast to dermatomyositis.

perficial scale. Follicular plugging, adherent scale, scarring, and dermal atrophy, characteristic of DLE, are not prominent features of SCLE. Hypopigmentation and telangiectasia become more evident as individual lesions resolve. The hypopigmentation fades after several months, but the telangiectasia may persist. The disease tends to be chronic and recurrent, lasting for years.

Other common dermatologic manifestations are diffuse, nonscarring alopecia of the scalp (59%) and photosensitivity (52%). Less frequently occurring dermatologic manifestations are mucous membrane ulcers (37%), facial telangiectasia (30%), livedo reticularis (22%), periungual telangiectasia (22%), discoid LE (19%), vasculitis (11%), and sclerosis (7%).[5]

Arthritis or arthralgia, the most frequent systemic manifestation, occurred in 74% of the patients; fever and malaise occurred in 37% of patients.[5] Central nervous system symptoms including psychoses and seizures occurred in approximately one-fifth of the patients, but were not severe. Renal involvement occurred in 11%, but was mild.

The laboratory and histologic features of SCLE are outlined in Tables 16-1 and 16-5.

Acute cutaneous LE. The rash of acute LE (ALE) consists of superficial to indurated, nonpruritic, erythematous to violaceous plaques; these occur primarily on sun-exposed areas of the face, chest, shoulders, extensor arms, and backs of hands. There may be fine scaling on the surface, but atrophy does not occur. Superficial erythematous plaques may last for a few days, becoming more intense as disease activity increases and fading with improvement in systemic symptoms. The most indurated hive-like plaques remain relatively fixed in shape and may persist for months. The classic butterfly rash over the malar and nasal area occurs in 10% to 50%[6] of patients with ALE, but it is not the most common cutaneous presentation. Erysipelas, seborrheic dermatitis, and polymorphous light eruption may occur in the central face area and may easily be confused with acute LE.

Other cutaneous signs of LE

Telangiectasia. Telangiectasia is a prominent feature of connective tissue disease. Telangiectasia

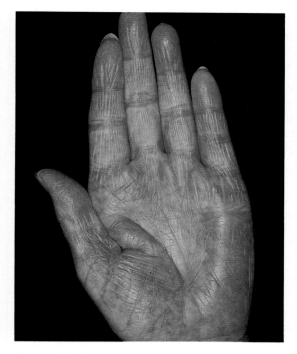

Figure 16-10
Cutaneous LE. Erythema and telangiectasia may appear on the palms.

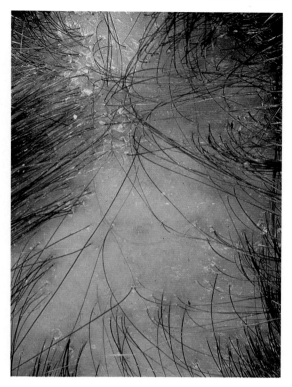

Figure 16-11
Chronic cutaneous LE (discoid LE). Scarring alopecia of the scalp, end stage disease.

occurs on the palms and fingers in associated with palmar erythema; it resembles that observed in liver disease and pregnancy (Figure 16-10). Short linear telangiectasias are a frequent finding in SLE. By use of the ophthalmoscope technique described later in this chapter, nailfold capillary microscopy, widened, tortuous, "meandering" capillary loops were reported in 53% of patients with SLE.[7] There is usually some disorganization of the capillary pattern, but avascular areas are rare (see Figure 16-20).

Alopecia. Alopecia occurs in over 20% of cases.[6] Both scarring and nonscarring alopecia occur. Nonscarring hair loss occurs more frequently in SLE, and scarring alopecia is more common in chronic cutaneous LE. In nonscarring alopecia the scalp may show focal or diffuse areas of erythema and scale similar to that seen with seborrheic dermatitis. The hair, especially in the frontal areas, becomes coarse and dry. The fragile, poorly formed shafts break, leaving patches of short unmanageable hair called "lupus hair." The scalp and hair eventually become normal as disease activity wanes.

Scarring alopecia of the scalp is a classic sign of DLE (Figure 16-11). The disease begins with scalp erythema, scale, and follicular plugging (keratotic projections from the hair follicles), followed by signs of atrophy and scarring. The skin surface becomes white, smooth, and telangiectatic and is depressed below the normal level. Hair follicles are destroyed during the inflammatory and scarring process, resulting in permanent alopecia. Hair loss is haphazard in distribution, in contrast to the nonscarring hair loss of alopecia areata. At times the scarring is minimal and the diagnosis of scarring alopecia due to LE will not be confirmed until the biopsy and immunofluorescence studies are obtained.

Urticaria. The reported incidence of urticaria or urticaria-like lesions with LE varies between 7% and 28%.[8] Urticaria is the presenting sign in approximately 5% of cases.[9] Clinically, lesions may be indistinguishable from typical hives; unlike hives, they are usually nonpruritic, persist for days, and remain relatively fixed in position. In most cases a biopsy reveals necrotizing vasculitis and the lupus band test is generally positive. Therefore, the hive-like lesions are probably a result of immune complex deposition rather than a manifestation of allergy. Some studies report a higher incidence of hypocomplementemia and renal disease in patients with urticaria-like lesions.

Vasculitis. Palpable purpuric lesions identical to those exhibited in necrotizing angiitis occur in SLE. Lesions are most common on the lower legs and may progress to ulceration.[10]

Raynaud's phenomenon. Raynaud's phenomenon occurs in 20% or more of SLE patients and may precede other signs and symptoms of SLE by months or years.[11] Progression to digital ulceration is more common in scleroderma.

Drug-induced LE. Hydralazine, procainamide, isoniazid, and, rarely, other drugs such as anticonvulsants, phenothiazines, quinidine, propylthiouracil, practolol, methyldopa, L-dopa, nitrofurantoin, and lithium carbonate can induce a lupus-like syndrome characterized by fever, arthritis or arthralgia, pleuritis, pericarditis, and sometimes rash.[12] Renal disease is rarely precipitated by these drugs. Patients with pericarditis, pleural effusions, or pulmonary infiltrates often require prednisone. They respond quickly, and prednisone can be tapered and discontinued over the course of a few months.[13]

Approximately 50% of patients treated with hydralazine or procainamide develop antinuclear antibody (ANA) within 1 year of treatment. The ANA consists of anti-single-stranded DNA (anti-ssDNA) rather than double-stranded native DNA (ds-nDNA) as in classic LE.[14] Most commonly, the onset of symptoms occurs many months after starting the drug. The symptoms generally resolve within days to weeks after the drug is discontinued and the ANA disappears.

A liver acetyltransferase enzyme inactivates these drugs. Patients can be categorized as either slow or fast acetylators. Slow acetylators may develop ANA and clinical symptoms, whereas fast acetylators rarely become symptomatic.[15] The laboratory features of drug-induced LE are elevated ANA, erythrocyte sedimentation rate (ESR), and anemia. A positive Coombs' test is commonly found in patients with procainamide and methyldopa-induced lupus. In contrast to spontaneous SLE, patients with drug-induced LE lack the following serologic abnormalities: antinative DNA (anti-nDNA), anti-Sm, and low serum complement levels.[15]

Management of cutaneous LE

Lupus is an uncommon disease that has been described extensively in the medical literature and in the lay press. Some patients are familiar with the term and fear the worst when informed of their diagnosis. Explain that the disease in the majority of patients can be controlled with existing therapy, but that periodic clinical and laboratory evaluations are necessary to monitor disease activity.

Management consists of defining the type of cutaneous subset, physical examination to document systemic symptoms, a battery of relevant blood studies as a baseline for diagnosis and later comparison as disease activity changes, biopsy of lesional skin for routine histology and immunofluorescence and, if appropriate, nonlesional skin for immunofluorescence, and topical or systemic treatment or both. A discussion of systemic symptom management is beyond the scope of this book.

TABLE 16-4

LABORATORY EVALUATION OF SLE PATIENTS

Routine tests to evaluate suspected SLE patient	Tests to further characterize disease
ANA	ESR
Anti-nDNA	Other antinuclear and anticytoplasmic antibodies (see Table 16-7)
Anti-Sm	
Serum C3, C4	Serum C2, CH50
CBC/differential	Coombs' test
Platelet count	Rheumatoid factor
VDRL (false-positive in 15% of SLE patients)	Skin biopsy of lesion (for histopathology and immunofluorescence)
Urinalysis	Skin biopsy of nonlesional skin (lupus band test)

Adapted from Rothfield N: Current approach to SLE and its subsets. DM, October, 1982.

Laboratory studies. A compilation of some of the studies used for the evaluation of LE is listed in Table 16-4. Patients with chronic cutaneous LE but without evidence of systemic disease should have a similar evaluation for documentation because a few of these patients may proceed to develop SLE. A comparison of the laboratory findings in the cutaneous subsets of LE is found in Table 16-5. Changes in values of some of these tests reflect changes in disease activity (Table 16-6).

Antinuclear and anticytoplasmic antibodies. The production of antinuclear and anticytoplasmic antibodies is a fundamental characteristic of LE. Numerous diverse antibodies are produced, and most laboratories have access to facilities that can measure the antibodies listed in Table 16-7. Measurement of these antibodies provides valuable information for diagnosis and prognosis. Quantitative measurement of some of these antibodies such as anti-dsDNA can be made and changes in levels assist in determining disease activity.

TABLE 16-5

COMPARISON OF LABORATORY FINDINGS IN THE CUTANEOUS SUBSETS OF LE[2]

Finding	DLE	SCLE	ALE
ANA titer ($\geq 1:160$)	4%	63%	98%
Anti-dsDNA	Rare	30%	60-80%
ESR greater than 30	Few	59%	90%
LE cell preparation	2%	55%	80%
Low C3 or CH50	Rare	Rare	90%
WBC less than 4,000	7%	19%	17%
Rheumatoid factor latex test positive	15%	19%	37%
Low hemoglobin level	Few	15%	50%
VDRL biologic false-positive	Few	7%	22%
Direct immunofluorescence and the lupus band test			
Lesion	90%	60%	95%
Normal sun-exposed	0	46%	75%
Normal nonexposed	0	26%	50%

TABLE 16-6

LABORATORY STUDIES USED TO DETERMINE DEGREE OF SYSTEMIC ACTIVITY OF LUPUS ERYTHEMATOSUS

Laboratory study	Change of value with increased systemic activity
Lupus band test	Converts to positive
C3, C4, CH50	Concentration decreases
Anti-nDNA antibody	Concentration may increase
LE cell test	Converts to positive
Lymphocyte count	Number decreases
ESR	Value increases

TABLE 16-7

ANTINUCLEAR AND ANTICYTOPLASMIC ANTIBODIES IN SYSTEMIC LUPUS ERYTHEMATOSUS (SLE)

Antigen	Autoantibody	Prevalence	Associations
dsDNA or nDNA	Anti-nDNA	40%-80% varies with disease activity	Highly specific for SLE Indicates poor prognosis High incidence of clinical renal disease High incidence of serum hypocomplementemia Positive LBT*
ssDNA	Anti-ssDNA	40%-80%	Found in most patients with SLE Nonspecific and found in other collagen vascular diseases
A group of small nuclear ribonucleoproteins (RNPs)	Anti-Sm	25%-30%	Highly specific for patients with SLE Patients are at greater risk for development of renal and CNS disease Usually seen in association with anti-nDNA or antinuclear RNP antibodies Associated with positive LBT and hypocomplementemia Indicates potential to develop serious disease
A specific small nuclear RNP	Anti-nuclear RNP	30%-35%	Low incidence of significant renal disease Benign course Increased incidence of Raynaud's phenomenon, arthritis, sclerodactyly, and myositis No correlation with LBT Not specific for SLE
Cytoplasmic RNPs	Anti-Ro (SSA)	25%-30%	Most patients are ANA-negative Increased frequency of photosensitivity, rheumatoid factor, and secondary Sjögren's syndrome Neonatal lupus Subacute cutaneous lupus erythematosus SLE syndrome associated with homozygous C2 and C4 deficiency
Nuclear RNPs	Anti-La (SSB)	10%-15%	Most patients are ANA-negative Almost always associated with Ro

Adapted from Weiss RA, Mogavero HS, Synkowski DR, Provost TT: Diagnostic tests and clinical subsets in systemic lupus erythematosus: update 1983. Ann Allergy **51**:135, 1983.
*LBT, lupus band test.

Measurement of ANA was the first test available for directly measuring antinuclear antibodies in a qualitative and quantitative manner. The test is positive in a high percentage of patients with LE (Table 16-5) and is presently an important screening test.

The ANA test is a nonspecific, very sensitive test that detects many types of antinuclear antibodies. There are no universal standards for performance of ANA tests. The significance of titers varies with different laboratories because of the use of different substrates, but generally titers below 1:16 are considered negative, whereas titers above 1:64 indicate possible SLE. Extremely high titers such as 1:32,000 may be found. Unfortunately, the titer level or change of titer has not been a reliable indicator of disease activity. ANA is detected by indirect immunofluorescence tests. It is performed by applying test serum to an animal tissue section. Antibodies to nuclear antigens attach to the various components of the nucleus. Fluorescein-labeled antihuman immunoglobulins are applied to the preparation and will react with ANA that have attached to the nucleus. The preparation is visualized with a fluorescent microscope. Diverse patterns of nuclear fluorescence (homogeneous, peripheral, speckled, or nucleolar) reflect the binding of antibodies to different nuclear components. Nuclear staining patterns were formerly used as criteria for subsetting,[16] but with the availability of direct measurements for specific autoantibodies, pattern identification has become less important. The test requires interpretation by visual inspection and consequently lacked a high degree of specificity.

Skin biopsy, direct immunofluorescence, and the lupus band test. All patients with suspected LE should have a skin biopsy. The histologic characteristics are listed in Table 16-1.

Direct immunofluorescence of involved skin is a valuable technique that provides additional evidence for the diagnosis of LE. The incidence of positive reactions is listed in Table 16-5. Deposits of IgG, IgM, and complement are found at the dermoepidermal junction and in the walls of the dermal vessels.

The lupus band test (LBT) (Figure 16-12) refers to direct immunofluorescence examination of normal uninvolved skin from either sun-exposed or sun-protected areas.[17] Immunoglobulins and complement are found in uninvolved skin in SCLE, ALE, and some bullous diseases such as pemphigoid.[18] In the absence of bullous disease the test is highly suggestive of either SCLE or ALE. Two studies demonstrate that the LBT can also be used to monitor disease activity.[19,20]

Deposits of immunoglobulin and complement were found in over 90% of patients with active disease and in 33% of those with inactive disease. The finding of such deposits reflected active disease, as did a decrease in serum C3 and C4 levels, elevated anti-dsDNA, the presence of LE cells, lymphopenia, and an elevation of the ESR. In the same patient the band appeared as systemic disease activity began and disappeared with spontaneous remission or improvement caused by prednisone or cytotoxic drugs or both.

The LBT test also has prognostic significance. A 10-year longitudinal study showed that a positive LBT obtained before treatment has important predictive value identifying a subset of SLE patients who develop more aggressive renal disease and have significantly decreased long-term survival.[21] Pretreatment and periodic LBTs were obtained from clinically normal skin from the medial volar forearm. Patients with SLE who were LBT-negative before treatment usually remained negative on repeated testing. LBT-positive patients usually remained positive unless treated with cytotoxic agents or prednisone in doses greater than 40 mg per day. A positive pretreatment LBT was associated with more severe renal disease by both clinical and histologic criteria. A comparison of clinical features in the two groups revealed a 55% prevalence of lupus nephropathy in the LBT-positive group as opposed to 23% in the LBT-negative group. The two groups had similar serum creatinine levels at the time of the initial LBT, but the maximum serum creatinine (mean, 3.0 mg/dl) in the LBT-positive group was significantly higher than the maximum (mean, 1.2 mg/dl) in the LBT-negative group. Of renal biopsies in the LBT-negative group, 9% showed diffuse proliferative glomerulonephritis in contrast to 65% of biopsies in the LBT-positive group. The two groups were compared with regard to outcome; 10-year survival from the time of diagnosis was 95% in the LBT-negative group as opposed to only 54% in the LBT-positive group. No LBT-negative patient died of visceral involvement by SLE. By contrast, 8 of the 11 deaths in the LBT-positive patients were directly related to SLE.

Most hospitals do not have facilities for performing the lupus band test. Cutaneous immunofluorescence laboratories in various parts of the country provide a liquid transport medium and mailing packages; therefore, freezing of specimens is unnecessary. A 3- or 4-mm punch biopsy should be submitted.

Cutaneous Lupus Band Test

A. Erythematous lesion

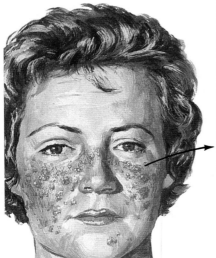

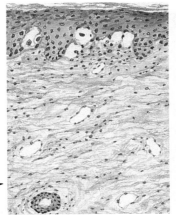

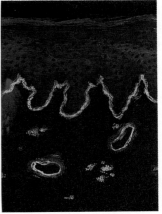

H and E section. Edematous (eosinophilic) subcutaneous tissue with vacuolization of basilar epithelium at dermal-epidermal junction

Immunofluorescence slide:* bandlike granular deposit of gamma globulin and complement at dermal-epidermal junction and in walls of small dermal vessels

B. Normal appearing (nonlesional) skin of lupus patient

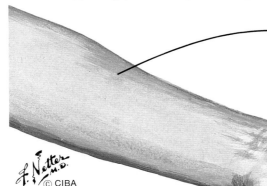

Immunofluorescent bandlike granular deposit may be demonstrated in more than 50% of cases

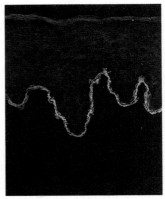

C. Discoid lesion

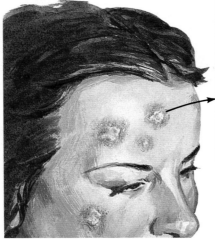

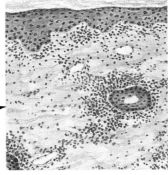

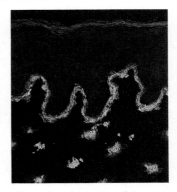

H and E section. Epidermal atrophy, hyalinization of dermis, chronic inflammation around hair follicles

Granular deposits of immune complexes at dermal-epidermal junction and within dermis

*All fluorescence slides stained with fluorescein-labeled rabbit antihuman gamma globulin

Treatment

Sunscreens. Patients should avoid direct exposure to sunlight, particularly during the summer and between the hours of 10 AM and 3 PM. Sunscreens with a sun protection factor of maximum value (currently 15) should be applied if significant sun exposure is anticipated. Encourage patients to apply sunscreens as a routine procedure after morning washing during the summer months.

Topical corticosteroids. Topical corticosteroids are the agents of first choice for all forms of cutaneous LE. Groups I to V topical steroids are required to control discoid LE. They may be applied 3 times a day to all active lesions, including those on the face. Avoid application of potent steroids to the eyelids. Encourage patients to restrict application to the active lesion and to avoid normal surrounding skin. Lesions of SCLE and ALE may be treated with Groups III to V topical steroids applied 3 times a day. Those failing to respond should be advanced to Group II topical steroids. Discontinue treatment when lesions have cleared.

Intralesional corticosteroids. Lesions of discoid LE that are resistant to topical steroids may be well managed with periodic intralesional injections of steroids (e.g., equal parts 1% lidocaine or saline and triamcinolone acetonide [Kenalog] 10 mg/ml). Lesions frequently become inactive after a single injection and may remain in remission for months. Inject with a 27-gauge needle with sufficient solution to blanch the lesion, about 0.1 ml/1 cm lesion.

Antimalarials. Antimalarials are highly effective in the treatment of all forms of cutaneous LE. Fear of retinal toxicity has resulted in much reduced use of these agents during the last 10 years; a timely review article provides recommendations for use and reassurance that toxicity can be avoided.[22] It was discovered that excessive daily dosages influenced retinal damage. The recommended safe and effective dosage for an individual weighing 150 lb is 250 mg of chloroquine (Aralen) once a day or 200 mg of hydroxycholoroquine (Plaquenil) twice a day. Patients can be maintained on this dosage as long as needed, but should have periodic eye evaluations. The ophthalmologist, by serially testing the foveal reflex and the reaction of visual fields to red targets, can detect a state of "premaculopathy." Testing is done before treatment, then every 4 to 6 months during therapy. While the patient is on therapy, premaculopathy is defined as the loss of foveal reflex or the development of paracentral scotomata to red test objects. It is a state of functional loss that is reversible by discontinuation of the drug.

Antimalarials are maintained at the previously recommended dosages until the lesions resolve. They are then reduced to the lowest possible dosage in order to maintain control.

Oral corticosteroids. Occasionally, patients with cutaneous LE will fail to respond to topical steroids and antimalarials. Such patients should discontinue other forms of therapy and begin prednisone, 10 mg 3 times a day, until control is obtained. Oral steroids are then tapered and discontinued; the patient is once more given a trial of conventional therapy.

Figure 16-12 (opposite)
Cutaneous lupus band test. (Copyright 1979, CIBA Pharmaceutical Company, Division of Ciba-Geigy Corporation. Reprinted with permission from Clinical Symposia illustrated by Frank H. Netter, M.D. All rights reserved.)

Dermatomyositis and Polymyositis

Dermatomyositis (DM) is a rare inflammatory disease of skin and muscle of unknown etiology. The term polymyositis is reserved for cases where skin inflammation is absent. Female patients outnumber males by 2:1. Two age groups are affected: children and adults over age 40. Adult DM is associated with malignancy. The clinical picture varies considerably and the following classification of the idiopathic inflammatory myopathies has been suggested.[23]

Group I:	Polymyositis
Group II:	Dermatomyositis
Group III:	DM or polymyositis associated with neoplasia
Group IV:	Childhood dermatomyositis
	Type I: Banker type
	Type II: Brunsting type
Group V:	Polymyositis or DM associated with collagen-vascular disease (overlap syndrome)

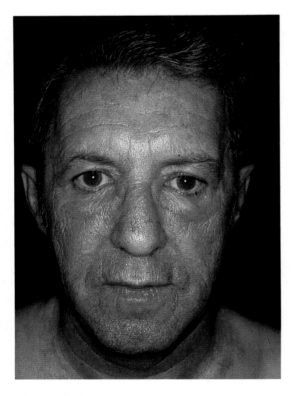

Figure 16-13
Dermatomyositis. Heliotrope (violaceous) discoloration around the eyes and periorbital edema.

Polymyositis

Symmetric painless proximal muscular weakness, especially of the hips and thighs, is characteristic of polymyositis. Neck muscles are commonly involved, leading to weakness in raising the head ("drooped head"). Dysfunction of the pharyngeal muscles may lead to aspiration pneumonia. Weakness progresses over weeks to months; spontaneous remission may occur. Deep tendon reflexes remain normal and atrophy occurs late in the course of the disease. The muscle changes are indistinguishable from those seen in DM.

Dermatomyositis

The associated features of polymyositis may precede, accompany, or follow the skin signs. The course of adult DM may be acute, chronic, recurrent, or cyclic. The various skin manifestations of DM are as follows.

Heliotrope erythema of eyelids. Heliotrope erythema of the eyelids (heliotrope: violet color) is a term used to describe the violaceous discoloration around the eyes (Figure 16-13). Periorbital edema and violet discoloration may be the earliest cutaneous sign or may be a residual finding as diffuse erythema fades. Both upper and lower lids may be involved, but often only the upper lids are.

Gottron's papules. Gottron's papules, a pathognomonic sign for dermatomyositis, are round, 0.2- to 1-cm, smooth, violaceous flat-topped papules that occur over the dorsal interphalangeal joints or along the sides of the fingers. Several lesions appear simultaneously any time during the course of the disease; they tend to remain fixed.

Violaceous scaling patches. A characteristic violet erythema with or without scaling occurs in a localized or diffuse distribution. The localized eruption appears symmetrically over bony prominences such as the knees, elbows, and dorsal interphalangeal joints (Figure 16-14). DM typically involves the knuckles and spares the skin over the phalanges. The distribution is reversed in SLE. The diffuse form begins as a patchy, diffuse dusky-red, or violet erythema of the sun-exposed areas of the face, neck, back, and arms and later may involve the buttocks and legs. Over a period of time the rash becomes confluent and involved areas become minimally raised and slightly scaling. A diffuse deep red erythema (malignant erythema) may appear superimposed on the existing eruption in patients with an evolving malignancy.

Periungual erythema and telangiectasia. Clinically, these are similar to those seen in other connective tissue diseases. The telangiectasia is most prominent on the posterior nail fold and appears as irregular red linear streaks (Figure 16-15). Nailfold capillary microscopy using the ophthalmoscope (see Figure 16-20)[24] reveals a pattern identical to

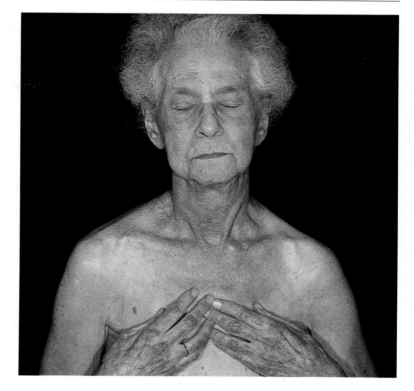

Figure 16-14
Dermatomyositis. Violaceous scaling patches on the face and dorsal interphalangeal joints.

that seen in scleroderma but quite different from that seen in SLE. This technique may therefore be helpful in distinguishing between DM and SLE.

Poikiloderma. Late in the course of the disease, as the erythema fades, a highly characteristic pattern may occur in the same sun-exposed areas occupied by the diffuse erythema. Poikiloderma is a descriptive term for the pattern that consists of finely mottled white and brown pigmentation, telangiectasia, and atrophy. Poikiloderma also occurs as an isolated phenomenon with mycosis fungoides and other rare dermatologic conditions.

Dermatomyositis with neoplasia. There is an increased incidence of malignancy in adult DM. It is reported to be as high as five to seven times that of an age-matched population.[25] Tumors may appear at any site, but the most common sites in order of frequency are the breast, lung, ovary, stomach, colon, uterus, and nasopharynx.[26] Myopathy antedated the diagnosis of cancer in about 60% of cases by a mean interval of about 11 months.[27] In 30% of cases the tumor appeared first and symptoms of DM subsequently appeared, with a mean interval of 16 months. The rash and symptoms of DM may clear after resection of the tumor.

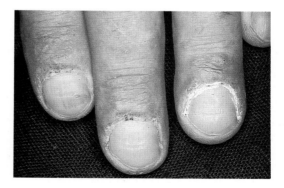

Figure 16-15
Dermatomyositis. Periungual erythema and telangiectasia similar to that seen in other connective tissue diseases.

Childhood dermatomyositis. Childhood DM is a serious illness with a mortality rate of about 25%. A spectrum of inflammatory muscle disease exists. At one end of the spectrum is the lethal form (Banker type), and at the other end the more benign form (Brunsting type). Features of both types are shown in Table 16-8. Signs and symptoms of the more common form (Brunsting type) are similar to the adult form of the disease, except that the course is typically chronic with calcinosis of subcutaneous tissue and periarticular skin, muscle atrophy, and contractures. In some children the disease ends spontaneously. The incidence of cancer is not increased. The rare lethal form of the disease (Banker type) is associated with degenerative vessel changes in the muscles and gastrointestinal tract.

Overlap syndromes. Myositis may occur during the course of other connective tissue diseases such as scleroderma, rheumatoid arthritis, and LE. The most common association is with scleroderma and is termed sclerodermatomyositis. An apparently distinct overlap syndrome, with features of SLE, scleroderma, and polymyositis, is called mixed connective tissue disease (MCTD). Eighty percent of these patients are females, and the peak age of onset is 35 to 40. Clinically, women have swollen hands with tapered fingers, Raynaud's phenomenon, abnormal esophageal motility, myositis, and lymphadenopathy. High titers of antibody (anti-RNP) to an extractable nuclear antigen called ribonucleoprotein (RNP) occur in all such patients but are not unique to MCTD. ANA is present, but anti-Sm is absent.

Diagnosis. Diagnostic measures include biopsy from weak muscles, electromyographic studies, biopsy of involved skin, and measurement of muscle enzymes in serum (creatine phosphokinase [CPK], SGOT, lactate dehydrogenase, aldolase). The level of serum muscle enzymes reflects disease activity; the CPK is usually monitored. Measuring urinary levels of creatine is beneficial; increased levels are an early and sensitive indicator of muscle injury.

Evaluation for possible malignancy. Patients with DM should be evaluated for internal malignancy. A recent review suggests that the discovery of most internal neoplasms resulted from history, physical examination, and routine laboratory studies. A "blind" or nondirected malignancy search was of no value in any of the cases analyzed.[29]

Treatment. The cutaneous eruption may be treated with Group IV and V topical steroids. Exposure to sunlight should be minimized. Rest and good nutrition are important. Oral corticosteroids are the treatment of first choice for most adults who have skin and muscle symptoms. Prednisone (usually 60 mg/day in divided doses) is started, gradually tapered, and changed to an alternate-day schedule after disease activity improves, as indicated by improving clinical signs and decreasing levels of muscle enzymes. Usually the CPK is monitored. Most patients begin to improve after the first month. An immunosuppressive drug such as methotrexate, azathioprine, or cyclophosphamide is substituted for or used in addition to prednisone for patients who fail to improve after 2 months of prednisone. Antimalarials were shown to be effective in treating the cutaneous lesions but not the myositis in a small group of patients with DM.[28] Bed rest is essential for patients with active muscle disease. The signs and symptoms of DM often clear shortly after removal of a malignancy.

TABLE 16-8

TWO TYPES OF DERMATOMYOSITIS IN CHILDREN

Banker type	Brunsting type
Rapid course	Slow course
Weakness, anorexia	Weakness
Dysphagia	No dysphagia
No calcinosis	Calcinosis
Fever, leukocytosis	Afebrile
Intestinal ulceration	No visceral signs
Vascular pathology	Inflammatory myositis
Death	Remission
No steroid response	Steroid response

From Winkelmann RK: Dermatomyositis in childhood. JCE Dermatol **18**(3):13, 1979.

Scleroderma

Scleroderma is a connective tissue disease; the most striking feature is hardening of the skin. Scleroderma may be associated with visceral disease or remain confined to the skin. All forms of scleroderma are more common in females. The degree and extent of involvement are variable, but four syndromes with reasonably constant features can be defined in the spectrum of disease called scleroderma; these are acrosclerosis, CREST syndrome, diffuse systemic sclerosis, and morphea.

Raynaud's phenomenon, a nearly constant feature of scleroderma, precedes the disease or occurs during its course. It does not commonly occur with morphea or localized scleroderma. Raynaud's phenomenon represents an episodic vasoconstriction of the digital arteries and arterioles that is precipitated by cold or stress. It is much more common in women. There are three stages during a single episode: palor (white), vasospasm causes the fingers to turn white, cold and numb; cyanosis (blue), relaxation of vasospasm; and hyperemia (red), relaxation results in reactive hyperemia and the fingers turn red.

Acrosclerosis

This localized form of scleroderma typically begins with either joint pain of the fingers or intermittent edema of the fingers and hands. Over a period of months or years the skin becomes progressively harder and firmly bound. In the last stage (sclerodactyly) the skin of the fingers and hands is thin, shiny, smooth, and tightly bound with the fingers contracted (claw deformity) (Figure 16-16). The fingers narrow or taper distally and the terminal phalanges become shortened as a result of distal bone resorption. Repeated and increasingly severe attacks of Raynaud's phenomenon lead to fingertip ulcerations that leave pitted or star-shaped scars when healed (Figure 16-17). Edema followed by sclerosis may also occur on the face, trunk, and extremities. Facial skin contracts and appears fixed to bone. The nose becomes beak-shaped and the skin around the mouth is drawn into furrows that radiate from the mouth. The disease may progress to visceral involvement with the same features as progressive systemic sclerosis.

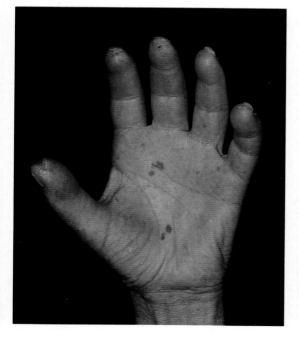

Figure 16-16
Scleroderma (acrosclerosis). The skin is tightly bound down. The fingers are contracted. Telangiectatic mats are evident on the palms. There are fingertip ulcerations.

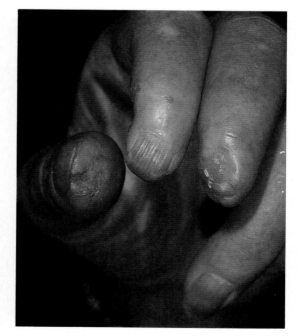

Figure 16-17
Scleroderma (acrosclerosis). Fingertips are narrowed and the fingers are shortened as a result of distal bone resorbtion.

CREST syndrome

A more benign, chronic, and localized variant of scleroderma was labeled the CRST syndrome, which is an acronym for the four clinical features of the disease. The E for esophageal dysfunction was a later addition. The clinical features are calcinosis cutis, Raynaud's phenomenon, esophageal dysfunction, sclerodactyly, and telangiectasia.

In most cases the disease remains localized and progresses slowly for years. Subcutaneous calcinosis occurs most commonly on the palmar aspects of the tips of the fingers. Calcinosis also occurs over the bony prominences of the knees, elbows, spine, and iliac crests. The deposits are firm subcutaneous nodules that may eventually rupture at the surface, discharging fragments of calcium. In response to this foreign material the skin surrounding the calcium becomes painful, red, and sometimes chronically infected. The telangiectasias of the CREST syndrome and scleroderma have a unique morphology. They occur as flat (macular), 0.5-cm rectangular collections of uniform tiny vessels, the so-called telangiectatic mats (Figure 16-18). These mats are most commonly found on the face, palms, and backs of the hands.[30]

Diffuse systemic sclerosis

This most virulent form of scleroderma occurs in the middle-aged and elderly and, like acrosclerosis, begins with skin edema. The hands, face, and limbs may be affected and the disease rapidly progresses to diffuse sclerosis (Figure 16-19). Internal organs are involved in the following order of frequency: gastrointestinal tract, lungs, heart, and kidneys.[31] Esophageal dysfunction is the most common systemic disorder and occurs in one-half the cases. Dilatation and diminished peristalsis of the distal two-thirds of the esophagus lead to dysphagia. Dyspnea occurs with pulmonary fibrosis. Death may occur from renal failure or cardiac disease.

Diagnosis. The clinical features of scleroderma are so characteristic that laboratory studies or skin biopsy are usually unnecessary.

Office nailfold capillary microscopy. A technique has been described for characterizing the telangiectasias seen in the proximal nail fold of the various connective tissue diseases. The scleroderma pattern is distinctive and is also seen in DM. Familiarity with this technique may help differentiate patients with LE and DM from patients who have cutaneous eruptions that appear similar.

Figure 16-18
Scleroderma. Telangiectatic mats.

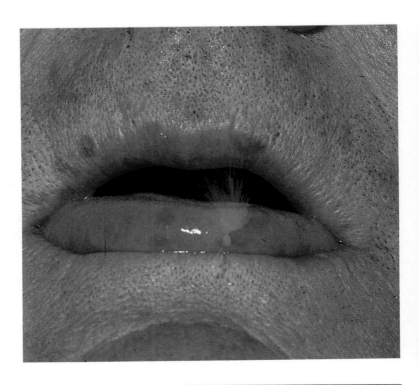

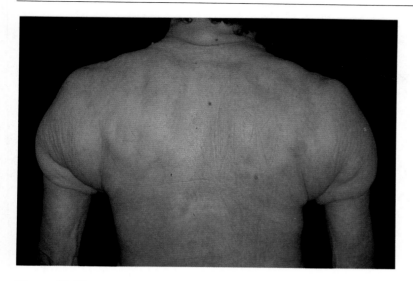

Figure 16-19
Scleroderma. Diffuse systemic sclerosis. Diffuse sclerosis of the limbs.

The technique used by Minkin and Rabhan[7] is as follows:

A drop of mineral oil is placed on each nailfold. The ophthalmoscope is set at +40, resulting in a ×10 magnification. The instrument is placed close to, but not in touch with, the oil. Generally, the capillaries are best seen in the nailfold of the fourth finger. Since the field of observation is smaller than in widefield microscopy, the ophthalmoscope must be moved over the entire nailfold. In normal people, the capillaries are seen as fine regular loops with a small, even space between the afferent and efferent limbs, in a row perpendicular to the nail [Figure 16-20]. The scleroderma pattern, seen in 74% of patients with scleroderma, consists of enlarged and deformed capillaries with dilation of both limbs of the loop, which is often engorged with blood ('sausage loop'). This is associated with marked disorganization of the loop arrangement and many avascular areas (Figure 16-20). The same pattern is seen in 82% of patients with dermatomyositis.

A different pattern is seen in lupus; see the section on lupus.

Treatment. Physical therapy is important in the management of scleroderma. D-penicillamine therapy is effective for both the skin involvement and visceral manifestations of diffuse systemic sclerosis.[32,33]

Figure 16-20
Office nailfold capillary microscopy. (From Minkin W, Rabhan NB: J Am Acad Dermatol 7:190, 1982.)

normal

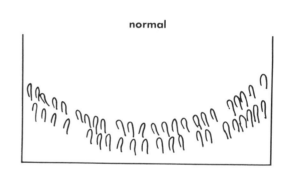

**scleroderma
and dermatomyositis**

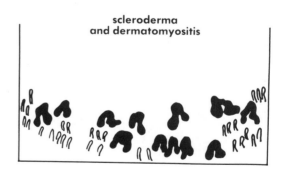

lupus erythematosus

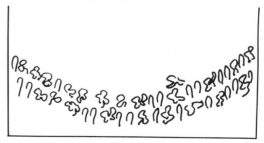

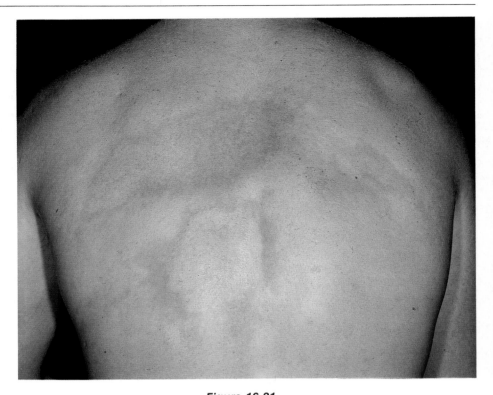

Figure 16-21
Morphea. Early lesions with a violaceous or lilac-colored active inflammatory border.

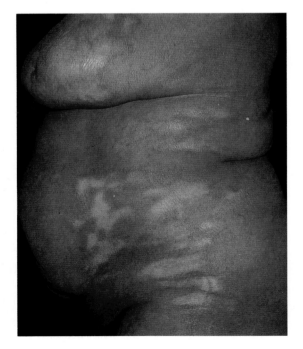

Figure 16-22
Morphea. Thick firm hairless ivory-colored plaques characteristic of long-standing disease.

Morphea

Morphea, or localized scleroderma, is more common in females; it can occur at any age, but is more common after age 30. Like scleroderma, morphea begins spontaneously and involves thickening or sclerosis of the skin. The two diseases differ in appearance, extent of the lesions, and evolution. Scleroderma appears as a bound-down skin thickening with minor skin color change, progresses to involve large contiguous areas of skin, and does not improve with time.

The lesions of morphea begin as one to several circumscribed areas of purplish induration (Figure 16-21). After weeks or months the major portion of the central region of discoloration becomes thickened, firm, hairless, and ivory-colored (Figure 16-22). The smooth, dull, white, waxy surface is elevated, in contrast to the diffusely bound skin of scleroderma. The violaceous or lilac-colored active inflammatory border is a highly characteristic feature of morphea. During the active stage the round-to-oval plaques slowly extend peripherally, but do not increase much in size. Active lesions persist for 1 to 25 years. Inactive lesions leave their mark. Al-

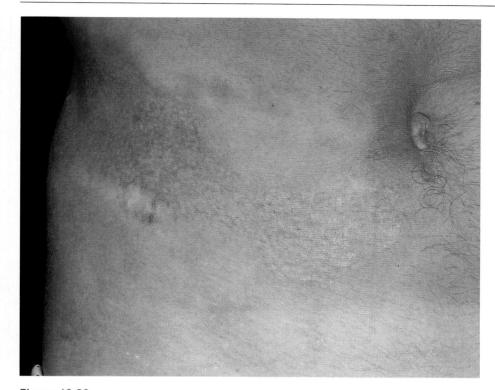

Figure 16-23
Morphea. Inactive disease with atrophy and mottled hyperpigmentation.

though much of the induration and skin thickening disappear, previously involved sites may exhibit atrophy and a mottled brown hyperpigmentation at the border and in the previously thickened plaque area (Figure 16-23). The remainder of the lesion becomes hypopigmented.

Morphea occurs in other patterns. Linear lesions are generally found on the arms or legs. Unlike oval plaque morphea, these lesions may be more firmly anchored and involve deeper structures (Figure 16-24). Multiple small white plaques (guttate morphea) are a rare form of morphea. Most reported cases are probably lichen sclerosis et atrophicus and in fact the two diseases may appear simultaneously in the same patients.[34] The most distinctive form of localized scleroderma is morphea of the frontoparietal face and scalp regions, called "en coup de sabre," so named because it appears that the blade of a sabre has struck a sharp, deep, vertical line on the face (Figure 16-25). The involved site may show all of the features of morphea. In time atrophy of one side of the face may occur, giving the impression that a blade was turned to the side to remove a thickness of skin after landing vertically.

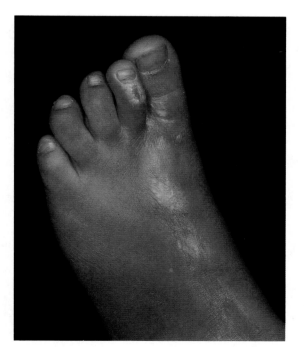

Figure 16-24
Morphea. Linear pattern.

Laboratory diagnosis. Although anti-DNA antibodies have been reported in some children with morphea, no blood studies are characteristically changed in morphea.

Biopsy. The histopathologic features vary with the course of the disease. Early active lesions reveal inflammatory cells in the dermis and subcutaneous tissue. Inflammation is most marked at the violaceous border. The collagen becomes eosinophilic and increases to occupy portions of the subcutaneous fat. Inflammation and sclerosis diminish with time.

Treatment. Inducing atrophy by infiltrating with triamcinolone (10 mg/ml) may be useful in areas where skin thickening has resulted in discomfort or limitation of motion. Thickened tissue offers great resistance to infiltration and scattered pitted areas of atrophy rather than a uniform decrease in plaque thickness may result. Asymptomatic plaques should probably be left alone to resolve spontaneously. Topical steroids and occlusion may induce slight improvement, but are usually worthless.

Hydroxychloroquine sulfate (Plaquenil sulfate, 200 mg) may be considered for cases with multiple lesions that are shown to be in an active inflammatory stage by skin biopsy. The adult dosage is 200 mg of hydroxychloroquine sulfate twice a day. Induration may be markedly reduced or disappear in 2 to 4 months. The medication should be discontinued after lesions improve. The fundi should be examined by an ophthalmologist before antimalarials are started and should be monitored periodically.

Figure 16-25
Morphea "en coup de sabre."

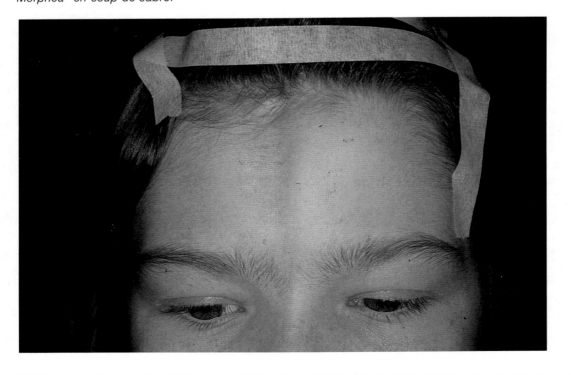

REFERENCES

1. Tan EM, Cohen AS, Fries JF, et al: The 1982 revised criteria for the classification of systemic lupus erythematosus. Arthritis Rheum 25:1271, 1982.
2. Gilliam JN, Sontheimer RD: Distinctive cutaneous subsets in the spectrum of lupus erythematosus. J Am Acad Dermatol 4:471, 1981.
3. O'Loughlin S, Schroeter AL, Jordan RE: Study of lupus erythematosus with particular reference to generalized discoid lupus. Br J Dermatol 99:1, 1978.
4. Uitto J, Santa Cruz DJ, Eisen AZ, et al: Verrucous lesions in patients with discoid lupus erythematosus. Br J Dermatol 98:507, 1978.
5. Sontheimer RD, Thomas JR, Gilliam JN: Subacute cutaneous lupus erythematosus: a cutaneous marker for a distinctive lupus erythematosus subset. Arch Dermatol 115:1409, 1979.
6. Tuffanelli DL, DuBois EL: Cutaneous manifestations of systemic lupus erythematosus. Arch Dermatol 90:377, 1964.
7. Minkin W, Rabhan NB: Office nail fold capillary microscopy using ophthalmoscope. J Am Acad Dermatol 7:190, 1982.
8. O'Loughlin, Schroeter AL, Jordan RE: Chronic urticaria-like lesions in systemic lupus erythematosus. Arch Dermatol 114:879, 1978.
9. Sanchez NP, Winkelmann RK, Schroeter AL, et al: The clinical and histopathologic spectrums of urticarial vasculitis: study of forty cases. J Am Acad Dermatol 7:599, 1982.
10. Christian CL, Sergent JS: Vasculitis syndromes: clinical and experimental models. Am J Med 61:385, 1976.
11. Kallenberg CGM, Wouda AA, The TH: Systemic involvement and immunologic findings in patients presenting with Raynaud's phenomenon. Am J Med 69:675, 1980.
12. Alarcon-Segovia D: Drug induced lupus syndromes. Mayo Clin Proc 44:664, 1969.
13. Rothfield N: Current approach to SLE and its subsets. DM, October, 1982.
14. Alarcon-Segovia D: Drug-induced systemic lupus erythematosus and related syndromes. Clin Rheum Dis 1:573, 1975.
15. Reidenberg MM, Levy M, Drayer DE, et al: Acetylator phenotype in idiopathic systemic lupus erythematosus. Arthritis Rheum 23:569, 1980.
16. Provost TT: Subsets in systemic lupus erythematosus: review article. J Invest Dermatol 72:110, 1979.
17. Burnham TK, Fine G: The immunofluorescent "band" test for lupus erythematosus. III. Employing clinically normal skin. Arch Dermatol 103:24, 1971.
18. Biesecker G, Lavin L, Ziskind M, et al: Cutaneous localization of the membrane attack complex in discoid and systemic lupus erythematosus. N Engl J Med 306:264, 1982.
19. Halberg P, Ullman S, Jorgensen F: The lupus band test as a measure of disease activity in systemic lupus erythematosus. Arch Dermatol 118:572, 1982.
20. Provost TT, Andres G, Maddison PJ, et al: Lupus band test in untreated SLE patients: correlation of immunoglobulin deposition in the skin of the extensor forearm with clinical renal disease and serological abnormalities. J Invest Dermatol 74:407, 1980.
21. Davis BM, Gilliam JN: Prognostic significance of subepidermal immune deposits in uninvolved skin of patients with systemic lupus erythematosus: a 10-year longitudinal study. J Invest Dermatol 83:242, 1984.
22. Olansky AJ: Antimalarials and ophthalmologic safety. J Am Acad Dermatol 6:19, 1982.
23. Pearson CM, Bohan A: The spectrum of dermatomyositis: symposium on rheumatic diseases. Med Clin North Am 61:439, 1977.
24. Herd JK: Nailfold capillary microscopy made easy. Arthritis Rheum 19:1370, 1976.
25. Bohan A, Peter JB: Polymyositis and dermatomyositis. N Engl J Med 292:344, 1975.
26. Barnes BE: Dermatomyositis and malignancy: a review of the literature. Ann Intern Med 84:68, 1976.
27. Masters R: Case records of the Massachusetts General Hospital: case 33-1977. N Engl J Med 297:378, 1977.
28. Woo TY, Callen JP, Voorhees JJ, et al: Cutaneous lesions of dermatomyositis are improved by hydroxychloroquine. J Am Acad Dermatol 10:592, 1984.
29. Callen JP: The value of malignancy evaluation in patients with dermatomyositis. J Am Acad Dermatol 6:253, 1982.
30. Braverman IM: Skin signs of systemic disease. Second edition. Philadelphia, 1981, WB Saunders Co., p 327.
31. Braverman IM: Skin signs of systemic disease. Second edition. Philadelphia, 1981, WB Saunders Co., p 334.
32. Steen VD, Medsger TA, Rodnan GP: D-penicillamine therapy in progressive systemic sclerosis (scleroderma). Ann Intern Med 97:652, 1982.
33. Kang B, Veres-Thorner C, Heredia R, et al: Successful treatment of far-advanced progressive systemic sclerosis by D-penicillamine. J Allergy Clin Immunol 69:297, 1982.
34. Uitto J, Santa Cruz DJ, Bauer EA, et al: Morphea and lichen sclerosis et atrophicus. J Am Acad Dermatol 3:271, 1980.

ADDITIONAL READING

Braverman IM: Skin signs of systemic disease. Second edition. Philadelphia, 1981, W.B. Saunders Co.

Chapter Seventeen

Hypersensitivity Syndromes and Vasculitis

Erythema multiforme
Erythema nodosum
Vasculitis
    Small vessel vasculitis
    Vasculitis of large vessels

Erythema Multiforme

Erythema multiforme (EM) is a relatively common, acute, often recurrent inflammatory disease. Many factors have been implicated in the etiology of EM, including numerous infectious agents, drugs, connective tissue diseases, physical agents, x-ray therapy, pregnancy, and internal malignancies. In about 50% of cases no cause can be found. EM is commonly associated with a preceding herpes simplex or mycoplasma infection such as primary atypical pneumonia. There are some patients who develop EM after each episode of herpes simplex.

Pathogenesis. Recent studies suggest that immune complex formation and subsequent deposition in the cutaneous microvasculature plays a role in the pathogenesis of EM.[1] Deposition of C3, IgM, and fibrinogen around the upper dermal blood vessels, basement membrane zone, and keratinocytes (cytoid bodies) has been found in a majority of patients with EM.[2] Histologically, a mononuclear cell infiltrate is present around the upper dermal blood vessels; in leukocytoclastic vasculitis and other immune complex–mediated cutaneous disease, polymorphonuclear leukocytes are present.

Clinical manifestations. The prodromal symptoms, morphology of the lesions, and intensity of systemic symptoms vary. At one end of the spectrum is the mild form of the disease, with papular eruptions; at the other end is the severe bullous, sometimes fatal Stevens-Johnson syndrome. Milder forms of the disease may be preceded by malaise, fever, or itching and burning at the site where the eruption will occur. The cutaneous eruptions are most distinctive and classification is based on their form.

Target lesions and papules. Target lesions and papules are the most characteristic eruptions. Dusky red round maculopapules appear suddenly in a symmetric pattern on the backs of the hands and feet and the extensor aspect of the forearms and legs (Figure 17-1). The trunk may be involved in more severe cases. Early lesions itch, burn, or are asymptomatic. The diagnosis may not be suspected until the nonspecific early lesions evolve into target lesions during a 24- to 48-hour period (Figures 17-2 to 17-5). The classic "iris" or target lesion results from centrifugal spread of the red maculopapule to a circumference of 1 to 3 cm as the center becomes cyanotic, purpuric, or vesicular. Partially formed targets with annular borders or target lesions on the palms and soles are less distinctive and clinically resemble urticaria. Individual lesions heal in 1 or 2 weeks without scarring but with hypo- or hyperpigmentation while new lesions appear in crops. Bullae and erosions may be present in the oral cavity. The entire episode lasts for approximately 1 month.

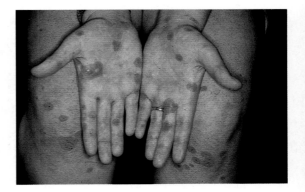

Figure 17-1
Erythema multiforme. Early target lesions demonstrating the typical livid color.

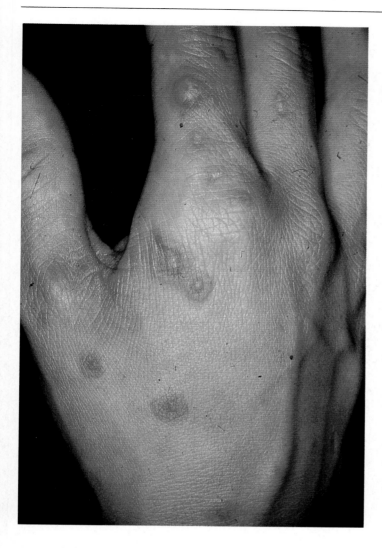

Figure 17-2
*Erythema multiforme. Classic iris
lesions.*

Figure 17-3
*Erythema multiforme. An
episode may be precipitated
by herpes simplex infection.*

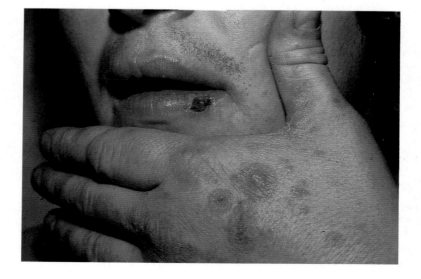

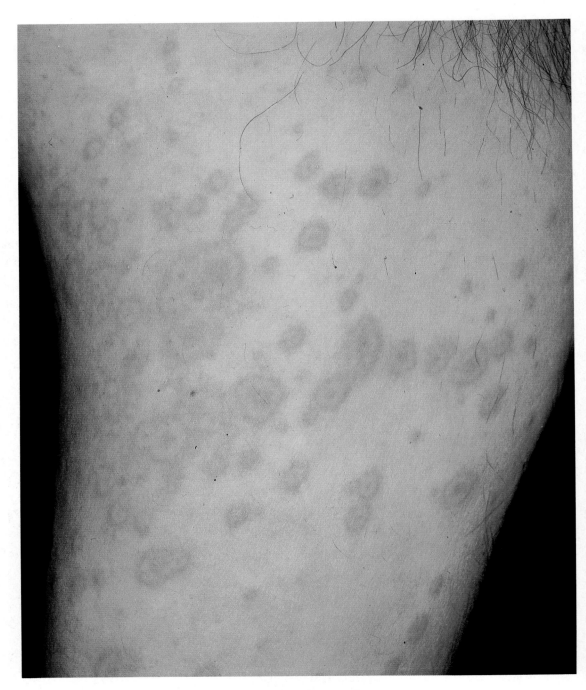

Figure 17-4
Erythema multiforme. A number of target lesions on the upper limb.

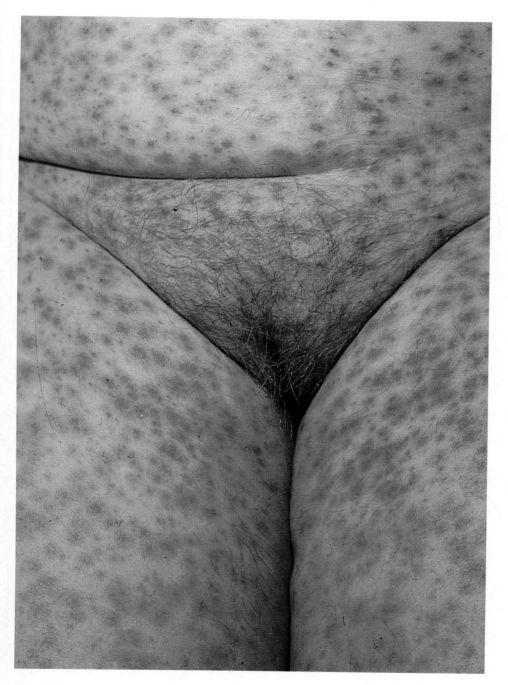

Figure 17-5
*Erythema multiforme. An unusual presentation
with numerous lesions.*

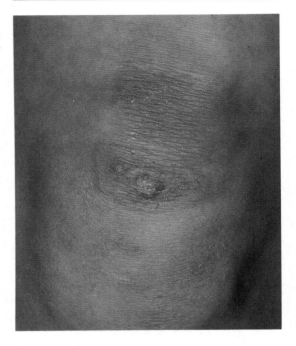

Figure 17-6
Erythema multiforme. Vesiculobullous form. An early lesion on the knee.

Figure 17-7
Erythema multiforme. Vesiculobullous form. Bullae are arising from a portion of an erythematous plaque.

Urticarial plaques. Urticarial plaques may occur without classic target lesions in the same distribution as described above. Unlike hives, all lesions are approximately the same size (1 to 2 cm) and remain unchanged for days.

Vesiculobullous form. This distinctive form of EM begins with 1 to 5 cm red edematous plaques on the extensor surfaces of the extremities; they are found less commonly on the trunk. Lesions may be extensive or confined to a few areas such as the elbows and knees (Figure 17-6). Vesicles or bullae arise from a portion (not the entire surface) of the plaque and may be multiple on a single plaque (Figure 17-7). Lesions are itchy, burning, or painful. They heal in approximately 4 weeks; as with fixed drug eruptions, recurrences may be in the same area. Mucous membrane lesions are more common with this form.

Severe bullous form. Generalized vesiculobullous erythema multiforme of the skin, mouth, eyes, and genitals is called Stevens-Johnson syndrome. The disease occurs most often in children and young adults and affects males more frequently than females. The cutaneous eruption is preceded by symptoms of an upper respiratory infection. Bullae occur suddenly 1 to 14 days after the prodromal symptoms, appearing on the skin, the conjunctivae, the mucous membranes of the nares, the mouth

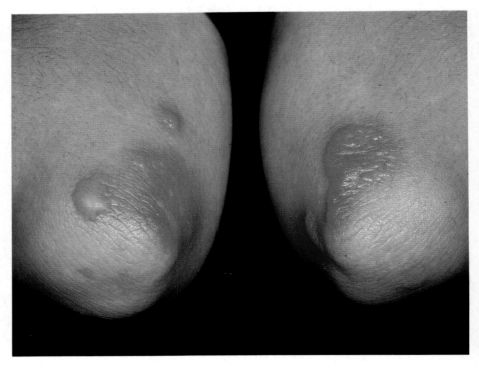

(Figure 17-8), the anorectal junction, the vulvovaginal region, and the urethral meatus. Ulcerative stomatitis leading to hemorrhagic crusting is the most characteristic feature. Corneal ulcerations may lead to blindness. A harsh, hacking cough and patchy changes on chest x-ray indicate pulmonary involvement. Patients with limited disease may be weak and lethargic. The mortality rate approaches 10%. Fever is high during the active stages. New crops of lesions appear, but the disease is self-limited and resolves in approximately 1 month if complications are absent. Oral lesions may continue for months.

Diagnosis. A skin biopsy should be performed if the classic target lesions are not present. Direct immunofluorescence may be helpful in nontypical cases[2] (see Table 15-1). Possible causes should be diligently sought so that recurrences can be avoided.

Treatment. A controversy exists about the use of oral steroids in the treatment of the extensive bullous eruption and Stevens-Johnson syndrome. A recent study in children suggests that treatment with systemic corticosteroids may be associated with delayed recovery and significant side effects.[3] Most physicians presented with a sick child with extensive cutaneous, ocular, and oral lesions elect to treat with oral steroids; most often prednisone (20 mg 2 or 3 times a day) is given for 1 week until new lesions no longer appear. It is then gradually tapered over a 3- or 4-week period.

Other treatment regimens may be as effective. Itching can be controlled with antihistamines. Cutaneous blisters are treated with cool wet Burow's compresses. Topical steroids should not be applied to eroded areas. Papules and plaques may respond to Group II or V topical steroids. Oral symptoms may be relieved by frequent rinsing with lidocaine (Xylocaine Viscous). Patients may tolerate only a liquid or soft diet.

Ocular involvement should be monitored by an ophthalmologist. Significant fluid and electrolyte losses may have to be replaced intravenously. Secondary infection is treated with oral antibiotics.

Figure 17-8
Erythema multiforme. Severe bullous form (Stevens-Johnson syndrome). Bullae are present on the conjunctiva and in the mouth.

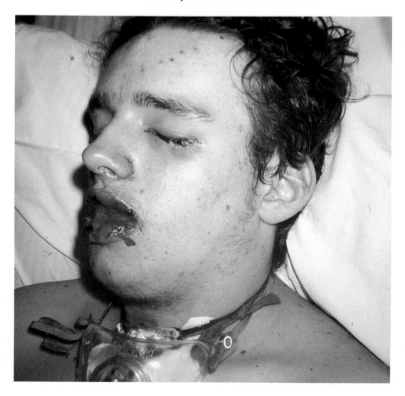

Erythema Nodosum

Erythema nodosum (EN) is a nodular erythematous eruption usually limited to the extensor aspects of the extremities. EN is found in association with a number of different infectious and inflammatory diseases and probably represents a hypersensitivity reaction to an antigen in the septal vessels of the fat lobules.[4] The incidence has decreased in the antibiotic era. EN is seen more frequently in females.

Clinical manifestations and course. Prodromal symptoms of fatigue and malaise or symptoms of an upper respiratory infection precede the eruption by 1 to 3 weeks.

Arthralgia occurs in more than 50% of patients and begins during the eruptive phase or precedes the eruption by 2 to 8 weeks. Symptoms may disappear in a few weeks or persist for 2 years, but they always resolve without destructive joint changes. The rheumatoid factor is negative. Joint symptoms consist of erythema, swelling, and tenderness over the joint, sometimes with effusions (Figure 17-9), morning stiffness and arthralgia, most commonly in the knee, ankles, and wrists, but any joint may be affected; polyarthralgia may last for days.

The eruptive phase begins with flu-like symptoms of fever and generalized aching. The characteristic lesions begin as red, node-like swellings over the shins; as a rule, both legs are affected. Similar lesions may appear on the extensor aspects of the forearms, thighs, and trunk (Figure 17-10). The border is poorly defined and the size varies from 2 to 6 cm. They are oval and their long axis corresponds to that of the limb. During the first week the lesions become tense, hard, and painful; during the second week they become fluctuant, as in an abscess, but never suppurate. The color changes in the second week from bright red to bluish or livid; as absorption progresses, it gradually fades to a yellowish hue resembling a bruise; this disappears in a week or two as the overlying skin desquamates. The individual lesions last about 2 weeks, but new lesions sometimes continue to appear for 3 to 6 weeks. Aching of the legs and ankle swelling may persist for weeks. Recurrences may occur for months or years.

Pulmonary hilar adenopathy may develop as part of the hypersensitivity reaction of EN and is seen in cases of diverse etiology.[5]

Figure 17-9
Erythema nodosum. Erythema, swelling, and tenderness over the joints.

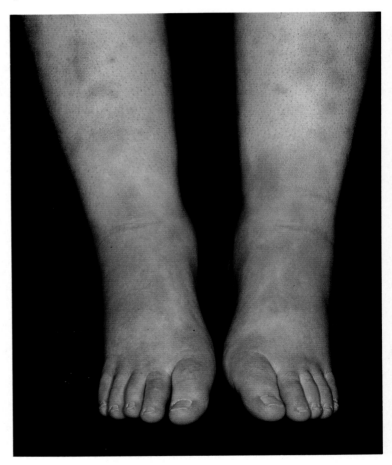

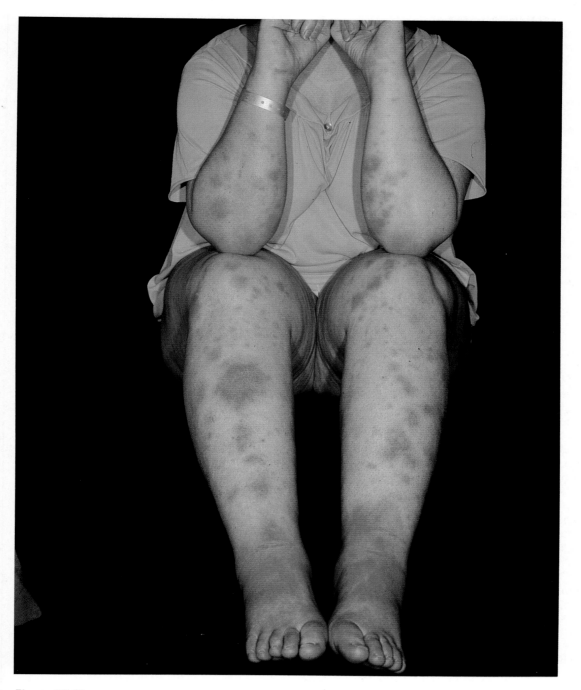

Figure 17-10
Erythema nodosum. Red node-like swelling in the
characteristic distribution.

Pathogenesis and etiology. EN is probably a delayed hypersensitivity reaction to a variety of antigens; it can be elicited by many different diseases. The most common causes today are streptococcal infection and tuberculosis in children and streptococcal infection and sarcoidosis in adults.[6,7]

Coccidioidomycosis (San Joaquin Valley fever) is the most common cause of EN in the west and southwest United States. In approximately 4% of males and 10% of females the primary fungal infection, which may be asymptomatic or involve symptoms of an upper respiratory infection, is followed by the development of EN or erythema multiforme. The lesions appear 3 days to 3 weeks after the termination of the fever caused by the fungal infection.

Histoplasmosis and lymphogranuloma venereum may cause EN. Leprosy is another possible inciting factor. Clinically, erythema nodosum leprosum resembles EN, but its histologic picture is that of leukocytoclastic vasculitis.

Inflammatory bowel diseases such as ulcerative colitis and regional ileitis may trigger EN, usually during active disease with symptoms of abdominal complaints and diarrhea. *Yersinia enterocolitica,* a gram-negative bacillus that causes acute diarrhea and abdominal pain, is a common cause of EN in France and Finland, where the initial cases were reported. Salmonella gastroenteritis has also been implicated.

Sulfonamides, bromides, and oral contraceptives have been reported to cause EN. Several other drugs such as antibiotics, barbiturates, and salicylates are often suspected but seldom proved causes of EN.

EN occurs in up to 20% of cases of sarcoidosis and has also been observed in pregnant women. Many other causes of EN have been reported; most consist of single histories.

Diagnosis. Initial evaluation should include throat culture, antistreptolysin-O titer, chest film, tuberculin purified protein derivative skin test, and sedimentation rate, which is elevated in all patients with EN.

Patients with gastrointestinal symptoms should have a stool culture for *Yersinia enterocolitica.* The bacteria are difficult to isolate in stool culture except in early cases and serologic tests for *Yersinia* are useful in confirming the diagnosis. Notify the laboratory that *Yersinia* infection is possible so that appropriate media and isolation procedures may be used.

Bilateral hilar adenopathy on chest roentgenogram does not establish the diagnosis of sarcoidosis, since hilar adenopathy occurs in EN produced by coccidioidomycosis, histoplasmosis, and streptococcal infections, and as a nonspecific reaction in most cases.

The clinical picture is characteristic in most cases and a biopsy is not required. If histologic confirmation is desired, an excisional rather than a punch biopsy is necessary to sample the subcutaneous fat adequately. Tissue sections show lymphohistiocytic infiltrate, granulomatous inflammation, and fibrosis in the septa of the subcutaneous fat; these are all features of a process called septal panniculitis.

Differential diagnosis. In Weber-Christian panniculitis, localized areas of subcutaneous inflammation tend to occur on the thighs and trunk rather than on the lower legs. Lesions may suppurate and heal with atrophy and localized depressions. Superficial and deep thrombophlebitis and erysipelas must also be differentiated from EN. Panniculitis secondary to pancreatic disease is associated with evidence of pancreatitis. Erythema induratum is characterized by dull red tender nodules on the calves of women; the nodules often ulcerate and heal with scarring.

Treatment. EN in most instances is a self-limited disease and requires only symptomatic relief with salicylates and bed rest. Cases that are recurrent, usually painful, or long lasting require a more vigorous approach.

Potassium iodide may be given in doses of 300 mg orally 3 times each day for 3 to 4 weeks. In different treatment schedules a range of 360 to 900 mg/day is recommended.[8,9] Relief of lesional tenderness, arthralgia, and fever may occur in 24 hours. Most lesions will completely subside within 10 to 14 days. Potassium iodide is not effective in all patients with EN. Patients who receive medication shortly after the initial onset of EN respond more satisfactorily than those with chronic EN. Side effects include nasal catarrh and headache.

Corticosteroids are effective but seldom necessary in self-limited diseases. Recurrence after discontinuation of treatment is common, and underlying infectious disease may be worsened.[10]

Naproxen (Naprosyn, 250 mg twice daily)[11] and indomethacin have been reported to be effective for recurrent unresponsive EN in one case.

Vasculitis

Vasculitis, or angiitis, is defined as inflammation of the vessel wall. The cutaneous vasculitic diseases are classified according to the type of inflammatory cell within the vessel walls (neutrophil, lymphocyte, or histiocyte) and the size and type of blood vessel involved (venule, arteriole, artery, or vein). Some vasculitic diseases are limited to the skin; others involve vessels in many different organs. The clinical presentation varies with the size of the blood vessel involved and the intensity of the inflammation. Numerous cutaneous diseases histologically show some degree of vessel inflammation. Only those diseases with inflammation severe enough to cause necrosis of vessel walls will be discussed here. Necrotizing angiitis is the term given to this group of diseases. These diseases have clinical features that allow one to predict that vessel inflammation and necrosis are taking place and identify the size of vessel involved (Table 17-1).[12]

Small vessel vasculitis

Most of the diseases characterized by necrotizing inflammation of small blood vessels have a number of features in common. Skin lesions reflect various degrees of small vessel necrotizing inflammation; the most common is palpable purpura. There is hypersensitivity to various antigens (drugs, chemicals, microorganisms, and endogenous antigens) with formation of circulating immune complexes deposited in walls of postcapillary venules. The vessel-bound immune complexes activate complement that is chemotactic for polymorphonuclear leukocytes. Leukocytoclastic vasculitis involves postcapillary venules. This is an inflammatory response in the walls of small veins in which leukocytes, by release of lysosomal enzymes, damage vessel walls causing extravasation of erythrocytes. The term leukocytoclastic vasculitis describes the histologic pattern produced when leukocytes fragment (i.e., undergo leukocytoclasis during the inflammatory process, leaving nuclear debris or "dust").

TABLE 17-1

CLINICAL SIGNS OF NECROTIZING VASCULITIS WITH RESPECT TO VESSEL SIZE INVOLVED

Signs	Diseases
SMALL VESSELS (Venules and postcapillary venules)	
Urticaria reflects minimal vessel inflammation and necrosis.	Leukocytoclastic vasculitis
Palpable purpura: exudation and hemorrhage from damaged vessels produce the most characteristic lesion of small-vessel necrotizing vasculitis. The lesion is a red, slightly elevated papule that does not blanch on application of external pressure.	Henoch-Schönlein purpura
	Essential mixed cryoglobulinemia
	Vasculitis associated with connective tissue disease
	Vasculitis associated with malignancies
	Serum sickness and serum sickness–like reactions
	Chronic urticaria (urticarial vasculitis)
Nodules, bullae, or ulcers may be present if vessel wall inflammation and necrosis are intense.	Urticarial prodrome of acute hepatitis type B infection
LARGE VESSELS (Small and medium-sized muscular arteries)	
Necrosis and thrombosis of larger vessels lead to infarction causing subcutaneous nodules, ulceration, and ecchymoses.	Polyarteritis nodosa
	Allergic granulomatosis
	Wegener's granulomatosis
	Giant cell (temporal) arteritis

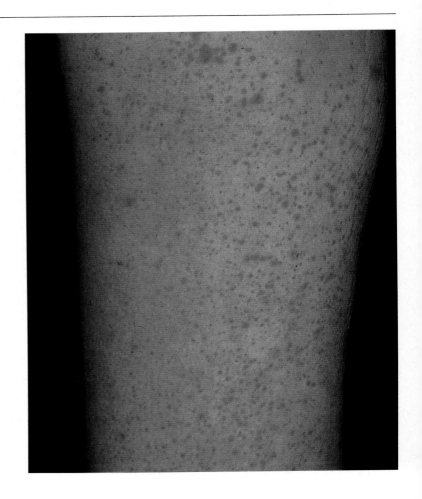

Figure 17-11
Leukocytoclastic vasculitis.
Numerous small hemorrhagic
palpable purpuric lesions are
48 hours old.

Leukocytoclastic vasculitis

Leukocytoclastic vasculitis is the most common form of small-vessel necrotizing vasculitis. The disease may be limited to the skin or involve many different organs, in which case it is called cutaneous-systemic angiitis.[13]

Diagnosis. The characteristic lesions are referred to as palpable purpura. The lesion begins as a localized area of cutaneous hemorrhage that acquires substance and becomes palpable as blood leaks out of damaged venules. Nodules, bullae, and ulcers may arise from these purpuric areas and indicate more severe vessel inflammation and necrosis (Figures 17-11 to 17-14).

A few to numerous discrete purpuric lesions are most commonly seen on the lower extremities, but may occur on any dependent area including the back, if the patient is bedridden, or the arms. Ankle and lower leg edema may occur with lower leg lesions.

Prodromal symptoms include fever, malaise, myalgia, and joint pain. Small lesions itch and are painful; nodules, ulcers, and bullae may be very painful.

Lesions appear in crops and last for 1 to 4 weeks. Recurrences are common and new crops may appear for weeks, months, or years. The disease is usually self-limited and confined to the skin.

Systemic disease. Leukocytoclastic vasculitis has several systemic manifestations; numbers in parentheses indicate approximate percentage of involvement.[14-17]

An analysis of cutaneous leukocytoclastic vasculitis in 82 patients seen by two practicing dermatologists showed that the disease has a better prognosis with less systemic involvement than in those patients seen at medical center clinics.[17]

- Kidneys (50%): Kidney disease is the most common systemic manifestation. Mild vasculitis of the kidneys causes microscopic hematuria and proteinuria. Necrotizing glomerulitis or diffuse glomerulonephritis may lead to chronic renal insufficiency and death.
- Nervous system (40%): Peripheral neuropathy with hypoesthesia or paresthesia is more common than central nervous system (CNS) involvement.

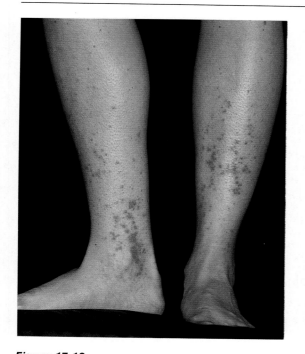

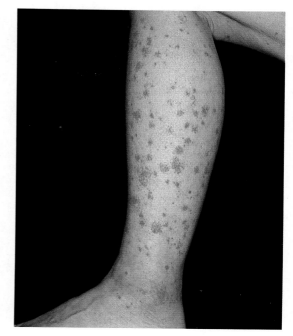

Figure 17-12
Leukocytoclastic vasculitis. Lesions have been present for 4 days and are more hemorrhagic than those illustrated in Figure 17-11.

Figure 17-13
Leukocytoclastic vasculitis. Hemorrhagic areas are more diffuse and the disease is in the process of resolution.

Figure 17-14
Leukocytoclastic vasculitis. An intense eruption with several areas of cutaneous necrosis.

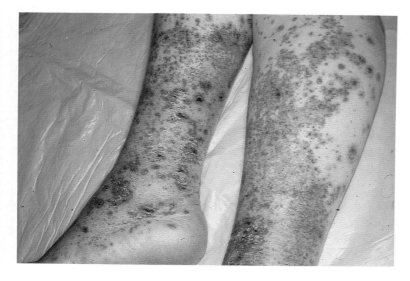

TABLE 17-2

SYNDROMES WITHIN THE BROADER GROUP OF HYPERSENSITIVITY VASCULITIS

Henoch-Schönlein purpura
  Nonthrombocytopenic purpura, joint, gastrointestinal, renal; postinfection or food allergy; tendency to recur several times and resolve; IgA antibody in immune complexes
Essential mixed cryoglobulinemia
  Purpura, arthralgias, anemia, hypergammaglobulinemia, glomerulonephritis; usually IgM rheumatoid factor against IgG; solid evidence for immune complex deposition
Vasculitis associated with connective tissue disease
  Usually rheumatoid arthritis and systemic lupus erythematosus; in rheumatoid arthritis, associated with severe erosive and nodular disease; not caused by corticosteroids; combinations of small venule and small- and medium-sized arteries
Vasculitis associated with malignancies
  Chronic lymphocytic leukemia, lymphoma, Hodgkin's disease, multiple myeloma
Serum sickness and serum sickness–like reactions
  Fever, urticaria, arthralgias, lymphadenopathy 7 to 10 days after primary exposure or 2 to 4 days after secondary exposure (accelerated); heterologous antisera or nonprotein drug (penicillin, sulfa)
Chronic urticaria
  Recurrent episodes or urticaria associated with elevated erythrocyte sedimentation rate, normal or low levels of C1q and C4 and episodic arthralgia; biopsy of urticarial plaque shows necrotizing venulitis
Urticarial prodrome of acute hepatitis type B infection
  Biopsy shows necrotizing venulitis

*Adapted from Haynes, BF: Treatment of the granulomatous vasculitides. Ann Intern Med **89:**671, 1978.

- Gastrointestinal tract (36%): Vasculitis of the bowel causes abdominal pain, nausea, vomiting, diarrhea, and melena.
- Lung (30%): Pulmonary vasculitis may be asymptomatic and be detected only as nodular or diffuse infiltrates on chest film; it may be symptomatic, with cough, shortness of breath, and hemoptysis.
- Joints (30%): Symptoms vary from pain to erythema and swelling.
- Heart (50%): Myocardial angiitis produces arrhythmias and congestive heart failure.

Etiology. In most cases the cause is not determined. Table 17-2[18] lists some reported causes of leukocytoclastic vasculitis.

Evaluation

Clinical studies. Initial clinical studies should include throat culture, antistreptolysin-O titer, urinalysis, stool guaiac test, chest film, complete blood count, antinuclear antibody, hepatitis B surface antigen, cryoglobulin, serum protein electrophoresis, erythrocyte sedimentation rate (ESR), and total hemolytic complement. The ESR is almost always elevated during active vasculitis. A normal ESR in a patient with purpura suggests that immune complex disease is absent. The total hemolytic complement, C3, and C4 may also be low during active disease.

Tests for detecting circulating immune complexes are not routinely available at this time.

Skin biopsy. The clinical presentation is so characteristic that a skin biopsy is generally not necessary. In doubtful cases a punch biopsy should be taken from an early active lesion. Deposition of fibrinoid material, necrosis of vessel walls, and nuclear dust from neutrophil fragmentation will be obscured.

Immunofluorescent studies. These may be done if the diagnosis is not apparent from the clinical presentation and skin biopsy. Biopsy lesions present for less than 24 hours. Vessel wall deposition of immunoglobulin is difficult to demonstrate in older lesions. Experiments have shown that, when histamine is injected intradermally into normal-appearing skin of individuals with active vasculitis, endothelial cell gaps are produced, which permit circulating immune complexes to be trapped in vessel walls.

Dahl[19] suggests the following useful tool to precipitate immune complexes in blood vessel walls for subsequent detection by immunofluorescence. Inject histamine in a 1:1000 dilution intradermally into normal skin in an affected area. Biopsy the site 6 hours later and submit the tissue for direct immunofluorescence examination. IgG, IgM, and C3 have been demonstrated in dermal vessel walls. The presence of IgA, C3, and fibrinogen in blood vessels of a child with vasculitis suggests the diagnosis of Henoch-Schönlein purpura (see Table 15-1).

Treatment. Identify and remove the offending antigen (i.e., drug, chemical, or infection). Short courses of prednisone (40 to 60 mg/day) may be useful for patients with severe symptoms. Cyclophosphamide (50 to 150 mg/day) might be considered either alone or in combination with prednisone for recurrent severe disease.[20] Indomethacin (25 to 50 mg 4 times a day) resulted in complete clearing of lesions in urticarial vasculitis and may be effective in classic leukocytoclastic vasculitis.[21]

Henoch-Schönlein purpura

Henoch-Schönlein purpura (anaphylactoid purpura) is a distinctive syndrome of leukocytoclastic vasculitis seen in children. A streptococcal or viral upper respiratory infection may precede the disease by 1 to 3 weeks. Prodromal symptoms include anorexia and fever. The syndrome is recurrent in 50% of cases, with individual episodes lasting 3 to 6 weeks; these may occur for weeks or months. IgA has been demonstrated in dermal blood vessels. The clinical features[22-24] are as follows.

Nonthrombocytopenic purpura is most common on the extremities. The lesions evolve from urticarial papules into the classic palpable purpura. Localized edema of the feet, hands, scalp, and periorbital regions occurs more frequently in the very young.

Abdominal symptoms were reported in 66% of patients under the age of 16. They included abdominal pain and colic, nausea, vomiting, and diarrhea, which may be accompanied by signs of gastrointestinal bleeding.

Joint pain occurs without signs of inflammatory joint disease. Several joints were involved in approximately 30% of patients.

Kidney disease is found; 25% to 50% of patients may develop hematuria and proteinuria that in a few cases persist after the other symptoms have passed. Some degree of chronic nephritis occurs in 25% of those with renal disease.

Essential mixed cryoglobulinemia

Cryoglobulinemia may be found in a number of disorders. However, a distinctive syndrome has been described for which there is no identifiable underlying disease.[25] The features are purpura with leukocytoclastic small vessel vasculitis with immune complexes made up of IgM rheumatoid factor directed against IgG molecules, mixed cryoglobulinemia with hepatitis B antigen, present in most cases, arthralgia, and glomerulonephritis. The prognosis is poor.

Vasculitis associated with connective tissue disease

Typical small-vessel leukocytoclastic vasculitis may occur with any of the connective tissue disorders, but most commonly it appears with systemic lupus erythematosus and rheumatoid arthritis. Patients with rheumatoid arthritis may develop large vessel vasculitis similar to that seen with polyarteritis nodosa.

Vasculitis associated with malignancy

Small-vessel vasculitis may be seen in association with certain malignancies; these are usually lymphoid or reticuloendothelial neoplasms such as chronic lymphocytic leukemia, lymphoma, Hodgkin's disease, and multiple myeloma.

Urticaria

A significant number of patients with chronic urticaria have been shown to have histologic and immunopathologic findings of small-vessel necrotizing vasculitis.[26] Vasculitis has also been demonstrated in the urticarial plaques in some patients with serum sickness and hepatitis type B infection.[27] These are discussed in Chapter 6.

Vasculitis of large vessels
Polyarteritis nodosa

The term nodosa means a node or swelling. Polyarteritis nodosa is a rare disease occurring most commonly after age 50. There may be a history of chronic infection, drug ingestion, or acute streptococcal infection. Necrotizing vasculitis occurs in various stages along segments of arteries and at bifurcation points, resulting in clinical signs of ischemia and infarction. Aneurysmal dilatation at bifurcation points is detected in visceral organs by angiography and as subcutaneous, sometimes pulsating, nodules in the skin. Multiple organ systems may be involved[28]; the most common are kidney (glomerulosclerosis, cortical infarction) and cardiovascular (coronary arteritis, particularly in children, myocardial infarction, hypertension), gastrointestinal (infarction of bowel segments), and neurologic (asymmetric polyneuritis) systems.

Cutaneous signs are found in approximately 25% of cases.[29] Subcutaneous nodules (less than 2 cm) recur in groups or crops, sometimes along the course of an artery; they are most commonly found on the lower leg. There is small, relatively superficial, punched-out ulceration in the center of a brownish tinted area overlying nodules. Ecchymosis occurs after infarction of vessel walls in a segment or bifurcation.

Without treatment most cases lead to death in less than 2 years.

A benign chronically relapsing cutaneous periarteritis nodosa has been described, which lacks multisystem involvement but has similar cutaneous lesions.[30] Patients with cutaneous disease without clinical or laboratory evidence of systemic disease will have a benign course and will remain free of systemic disease.

Allergic granulomatosis

Allergic granulomatosis (Churg-Strauss syndrome) is characterized clinically by the triad of asthma, peripheral eosinophilia (greater than 1500/mm³), and fever. Vessels are grossly affected, as in polyarteritis nodosa, but histologically show granulomatous inflammation in addition to leukocyte invasion. Multisystem visceral and cutaneous disease similar to polyarteritis nodosa follows the initial triad of signs and symptoms.

Wegener's granulomatosis

This is a rare, fatal necrotizing granulomatous vasculitis occurring after age 40 and characterized by the triad of ulceration and granulomas of the upper and lower respiratory tract, leading to nasal, tracheal, bronchial and laryngeal ulceration, and multiple nodular cavitary infiltrates of the lung parenchyma. Focal and segmental glomerulitis sometimes develop into necrotizing glomerulonephritis. Other multisystem visceral and cutaneous signs are similar to those of the other syndromes of large vessel systemic vasculitis. Most patients die of renal failure if not treated. The disease responds well to cyclophosphamide.

Giant-cell (temporal) arteritis

Giant-cell (temporal) arteritis (Figure 17-15), a necrotizing granulomatous vasculitis of branches of the carotid artery (superficial temporal and occipital and branches of the internal carotid artery), occurs after age 50. The syndrome in the prodromal phase produces fever, a high ESR, stiffness, aching, and muscle pain.

In the active phase there is unilateral headache, erythema, and pain over the artery, loss of arterial pulses, tender nodules along the course of the artery, loss of vision, pain while eating, and sometimes massive skin ulceration of the scalp. In the chronic phase patient recovers from the active phase, but symptoms similar to the prodromal phase continue.

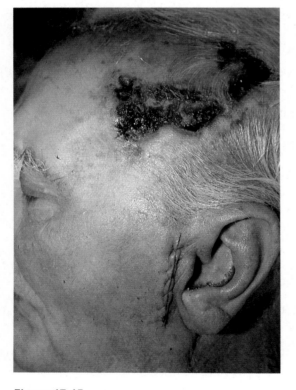

Figure 17-15
Temporal arteritis. There is massive ulceration of the temporal and scalp region. The temporal artery has been biopsied.

REFERENCES

1. Buchkell LL, Mackel SE, Jordan RE: Erythema multiforme: direct immunofluorescence studies and detection of circulating immune complexes. J Invest Dermatol **74**:372, 1980.
2. Finan MC, Schroeter AL: Cutaneous immunofluorescence study of erythema multiforme: correlation with light microscopic patterns and etiologic agents. J Am Acad Dermatol **10**:497, 1984.
3. Rasmussen JE: Erythema multiforme in children: response to treatment with systemic corticosteroids. Br J Dermatol **95**:181, 1976.
4. Hannuksela M: Erythema nodosum migrans. Acta Derm Venereol **53**:313, 1973.
5. Braverman IM: Hypersensitivity syndromes. In Skin signs of systemic disease. Second edition. Philadelphia, 1981, WB Saunders Co.
6. Simila S, Pietila J: The changing etiology of erythema nodosum in children. Acta Tuberculosea Pneumologica Scand **46**:159, 1965.
7. MacPherson P: A survey of erythema nodosum in a rural community between 1954 and 1968. Tubercle **51**:324, 1970.
8. Horio T, Imamura S, Danno K, et al: Potassium iodide in the treatment of erythema nodosum and nodular vasculitis. Arch Dermatol **117**:29, 1981.
9. Whiting DA, Schultz EJ: Treatment of erythema nodosum and nodular vasculitis with potassium iodide. Br J Dermatol **94**:75, 1976.
10. Soderstron RM, Krull EA: Erythema nodosum: a review. Cutis **21**:806, 1978.
11. Lehman CW: Control of chronic erythema nodosum with naproxen. Cutis **26**:66, 1980.
12. Soter NA: Clinical presentations and mechanisms of necrotizing angiitis, of the skin, J Invest Dermatol **67**:354, 1976.
13. Braverman IM: Skin signs of systemic disease. Second edition. Philadelphia, 1981, WB Saunders Co.
14. Ramsay C, Fry L: Allergic vasculitis. Clinical and histological features and incidence of renal involvement. Br J Dermatol **81**:96, 1969.
15. Winkelman RK, Ditto WB: Cutaneous and visceral syndromes of necrotizing or "allergic" angiitis: a study of thirty-eight cases. Medicine **43**:59, 1964.
16. Lopez LR, Schocket AL, Stanford RE, et al: Gastrointestinal involvement in leukocytoclastic vasculitis and polyarteritis nodosa. J Rheumatol **7**:677, 1980.
17. Ekenstram EA, Callen JP: Cutaneous leukocytoclastic vasculitis. Arch Dermatol **120**:484, 1984.
18. Fauci AS: Hypersensitivity vasculitis. The spectrum of vasculitis: clinical, pathologic, immunologic, and therapeutic considerations. Ann Intern Med **89**(part 1):660, 1978.
19. Dahl MV: Clinical immunodermatology. Chicago, 1981, Year Book Medical Publishers, Inc.
20. Sams WM, Thorne EG, Small P, et al: Leukocytoclastic vasculitis: review article. Arch Dermatol **112**:219, 1976.
21. Millns JL, Randle HW, Solley GO, et al: The therapeutic response of urticarial vasculitis to indomethacin, J Am Acad Dermatol **3**:349, 1980.
22. Allen DM, Diamond LK, Howell DA: Anaphylactoid purpura in children (Schölein-Henoch syndrome). Am J Dis Child **99**:833, 1960.
23. Ansell BM: Henoch-Schönlein purpura with particular reference to prognosis of the renal lesion, Br J Dermatol **82**:211, 1970.
24. Emery H, Later W, Schaller JG: Henoch-Schoenlein vasculitis. Arthritis Rheum **20**:385, 1977.
25. Meltzer M, Franklin EC, Elias K, et al: Cryoglobulinemia: A clinical and laboratory study. II. Cryoglobulins with rheumatoid factor activity. Am J Med **40**:837, 1966.
26. Monroe EW, Schulz CT, Maize JC, et al: Vasculitis in chronic urticaria: an immunopathologic study. J Invest Dermatol **76**:103, 1981.
27. Sergent JS, Lockshin MD, Christian CL, et al: Vasculitis with hepatitis B antigenemia: long term observations in nine patients. Medicine **55**:1, 1976.
28. Cohen RD, Conn DL, Ilstrup DM: Clinical features, prognosis, and response to treatment in polyarteritis. Mayo Clin Proc **55**:146, 1980.
29. Ketron LW, Burnstein JC: Cutaneous manifestations of periarteritis nodosa. Arch Dermatol Syph **40**:929, 1939.
30. Diaz-Perez JL, Schroeter AL, Winkelmann RK: Cutaneous periarteritis nodosa. Arch Dermatol **116**:56, 1980.

Chapter Eighteen

Light-Related Diseases and Disorders of Pigmentation

Photobiology

Sunlight has profound effects on the skin and is associated with a variety of diseases (Table 18-1). Ultraviolet light causes most photobiologic skin reactions and diseases. The accepted unit for measuring the wavelength of light is the nanometer (nm). The solar radiation reaching the earth is a continuous spectrum consisting of wavelengths of electromagnetic energy above 290 nm. By convention, ultraviolet light is divided into UVA (320 to 400 nm; long wave, black light), UVB (290 to 320 nm; middle wave, sunburn), and UVC (100 to 290 nm; short wave, germicidal).

UVA penetrates window glass, interacts with topical and systemic chemicals and medication, causes immediate and delayed tanning, and contributes little to erythema and burning.

UVB is absorbed by window glass. Prior exposure to UVA enhances the sunburn reaction from UVB. UVB is the principal cause of erythema and burning and produces tanning more efficiently than UVA.

UVC is almost completely absorbed by the ozone layer of the earth's atmosphere.

Suntan and Sunburn

Light-induced skin changes depend on genetic factors and the intensity and duration of exposure. Tanning follows moderate and intense sun exposure and occurs in two stages. The first stage, immediate pigment darkening (IPD), is caused primarily by UVA. The skin becomes brown while exposed, but fades rapidly after exposure. IPD is caused by a photochemical change in existing melanin, not by an increase in melanin. A lasting tan requires the synthesis of new melanin; a more lasting tan becomes visible within 72 hours.

The sunburn reaction occurs in stages. With sufficient exposure, erythema appears within minutes (immediate erythema), fades, and then reappears and persists for days (delayed erythema). Vascular permeability of varying degrees results in edema and blisters. Desquamation occurs within a week. Sunburn is best treated with cool wet water compresses. Topical anesthetic preparations containing lidocaine provide some relief. Benzocaine incorporated in some sunburn preparations is a sensitizer and should be avoided. A 4- to 6-day course of prednisone (20 mg twice a day for adults) may abort a potentially intense reaction. Protection with sunscreens can, if used properly, prevent burning in even the fair-skinned individual.

TABLE 18-1

CLASSIFICATION OF ABNORMAL REACTIONS TO SOLAR RADIATION

Normal individuals
Sunburn reaction
Immediate pigment darkening or
tanning reaction
Delayed tanning (melanogenesis)
Degenerative and neoplastic
Actinic damage
Actinic keratosis
Basal cell carcinoma
Squamous cell carcinoma
Malignant melanoma
Idiopathic
Polymorphous light eruptions
Hydroa aestivale
Hydroa vacciniforme
Photosensitivity
Phototoxicity
Photoallergy

Photoaggravated diseases
Acne
Darier's disease
Dermatomyositis
Discoid lupus erythematosus
Hailey-Hailey disease
Herpes simplex labialis
Lichen planus actinicus
Lymphogranuloma venereum
Pemphigus foliaceus
Psoriasis
Rosacea
Metabolic
Erythropoietic porphyria
Erythropoietic protoporphyria
Porphyria cutanea tarda
Variegate porphyria

Sun Protection

The value of protecting the skin from excess sun exposure has been appreciated only recently. The increasing frequency of skin malignancy in sun-exposed areas and the awareness that skin wrinkling is greatly accelerated by ultraviolet light have stimulated efforts to better understand the photobiologic properties of sunlight. People enjoy sun exposure, but they should be informed of how to effectively limit sun exposure without interfering with their lifestyle.

Methods of sun protection. Natural protection is provided by the stratum corneum and the skin pigment melanin. People vary widely in their natural ability to tan or burn. A sun-reactive skin typing system has been devised to classify individuals according to their ability to tan or burn. These categories (Table 18-2) are useful guides for recommending sunscreening agents and devising programs for sun protection.

TABLE 18-2

SKIN TYPES AND RECOMMENDED SUNSCREEN PROTECTION FACTORS

Skin type	Sensitivity to UV*	Sunburn and tanning history	Recommended sun protection factor†
I	Very sensitive	Always burns easily; never tans	10 or more
II	Very sensitive	Always burns easily; tans minimally	10 or more
III	Sensitive	Burns moderately; tans gradually and uniformly (light brown)	8 to 10
IV	Moderately sensitive	Burns minimally; always tans well (moderate brown)	6 to 8
V	Minimally sensitive	Rarely burns, tans profusely (dark brown)	4
VI	Insensitive	Never burns; deeply pigmented (black)	None indicated

From Pathak, MA: Sunscreens. J Am Acad Dermatol **7**:285, 1982.
*Based on first 30 to 45 minutes of sun exposure after winter season or no sun exposure.
†Based on outdoor field studies.

TABLE 18-3

SUN PROTECTION FACTORS OF SOME BRAND NAME SUNSCREENS UNDER INDOOR AND OUTDOOR CONDITIONS*

Trade name	Ingredients	Type of sunscreen	Sun protection factor (SPF)		Resistance to	
			Indoor solar simulator	Outdoor sunlight	Sweating	Water immersion
PABA sunscreens						
PreSun 15	5% PABA in 50%-70% ethyl alcohol	Clear lotion	15	15	Excellent	Poor
Pabanol		Clear lotion	15	6-8	Fair	Poor
Sunbrella		Clear lotion	15	6	Fair	Poor
PABA-ester combination sunscreens						
SuperShade 15	7% octyldimethyl PABA + 3% oxybenzone	Milky lotion	15-18	6-9	Excellent	Good
Total Eclipse 15	2.5% glyceryl PABA + 2.5% octyldimethyl PABA + 2.5% oxybenzone	Milky lotion	15-18	9-12	Excellent	Good
MMM What-A-Tan!	3.0% octyldimethyl PABA + 2.5% benzophenone-3	Milky lotion	15-20	10	Excellent	Good
PreSun 15	5% PABA + padimate 0 + 3% oxybenzone	Milky lotion	15-20	8-10	Excellent	Good
Clinique 19	Phenylbenzimidazole-5-sulfonic acid + 2.5% octyldimethyl PABA	Milky lotion	15-19	7-8	Good	Fair
Sundown 15	7% padimate 0 + 5% octylsalicylate + 4% oxybenzone	Milky lotion	15-20	10-11	Excellent	Good

PABA ester sunscreens

Block Out	3.3% isoamyl-*p*-*N,N*-dimethylaminobenzoate (padimate A)	Lotion/gel	6-8	6	Good	Fair
Pabafilm	3.3% isoamyl-*p*-*N,N*-dimethylaminobenzoate (padimate A)	Lotion/gel	6-8	4-6	Good	Fair
Sundown	3.3% isoamyl-*p*-*N,N*-dimethylaminobenzoate (padimate A)	Lotion	8-10	4-6	Good	Fair
Original Eclipse	3.5% padimate A + 3.0% octyldimethyl PABA	Lotion	8-10	4-6	Fair	Fair
Aztec	5.0% homomenthyl salicylate + 2.5% amyl-*p*-dimethyl aminobenzoate	Lotion	6-8	4	Fair	Poor
Sea & Ski	3.3% octyldimethyl PABA	Cream	7-8	4	Fair	Poor

Non-PABA sunscreens

Piz Buin-8*	5% ethyl-hexyl-*p*-methoxycinnamate +	Cream	15-20	10-12	Excellent	Good
Ti. Screen	3% 2-hydroxy-4-methoxybenzophenone + 4% 2-phenyl-benzimidazole sulfonic acid	Cream	16-22	10-12	Excellent	Good
Piz Buin-8*	5% ethyl-hexyl-*p*-methoxycinnamate+	Milky lotion	20-22	10-12	Excellent	Good
Ti. Screen	3% 2-hydroxy-4-methoxybenzophenone	Milky lotion	16-20	10-12	Excellent	Good
Piz Buin-4*	4.5% ethyl-hexyl-*p*-methoxycinnamate	Milky lotion	10-12	4-6	Fair	Fair
Uval	10% 2-hydroxy-4-methoxybenzophenone-5-sulfonic acid	Milky lotion	10-12	4	Poor	Poor
Coppertone	8% homomenthylsalicylate	Lotion	3.5-4	2	Poor	Poor

Physical sunscreens

A-Fil	Titanium dioxide + zinc oxide + talc, kaolin, iron oxide or red veterinary petrolatum	Cream	6-8	4-6	Good	Fair
RV Paque		Cream	6-8	3-4	Good	Fair
Shadow		Cream	4-6	2-4	Good	Fair
Reflecta		Cream	6-8	4-6	Good	Fair
Covermark		Cream	6-8	4-6	Good	Fair
Clinique		Cream	6-8	4-6	Good	Fair

From Pathak, MA: Sunscreens. J Am Acad Dermatol **7**:285, 1982.
*Not available in the United States.

Recommend the following to minimize sun exposure:

1. Avoid sun exposure between 11 AM and 3 PM.
2. Start with short exposures of 15 to 20 minutes in the morning or late afternoon.
3. Wear protective clothing and a hat.
4. Use sunscreens of appropriate strength based on skin type.

Every effort should be made to avoid sunburn. People who take short winter vacations in the South are particularly apt to burn. Total sun exposure during a lifetime is greatest on the face, back of the neck, bald head, ears, forearms, backs of the hands, and exposed lower legs. The effects of sunlight can readily be appreciated by comparing the lateral (sun-exposed) to the medial (sun-protected) surfaces of the forearm in older individuals. Sunburns are particularly harmful and great emphasis should be placed on preventing burns. Patients frequently relate how permanent freckling occurred on the upper back after one severe burn.

Sunscreens. Sunscreens are topical agents that protect the skin from ultraviolet light. Chemical sunscreens such as para-aminobenzoic acid (PABA) selectively absorb ultraviolet radiation in the spectral range of 290 to 320 nm, whereas those containing more than one chemical may protect in the 290- to 360-nm range. Sunscreens are incorporated into cosmetically acceptable lotion and cream bases. Physical sunscreens contain particles of substances, such as titanium dioxide, that scatter both ultraviolet and visible radiation.

The effectiveness of sunscreens is expressed as the sun protection factor, or SPF. The SPF is defined as the ratio of the least amount of UVB energy (minimal erythema dose, or MED) required to produce a minimal erythema reaction through a sunscreen product film to the amount of energy required to produce the same erythema without any sunscreen application.[1] An individual who wears a sunscreen with an SPF of 8 will require 8 times longer than usual to develop erythema.

The SPF for commercially available products is derived from tests with laboratory light sources and therefore is not a true measure of the sunscreen's ability to protect. SPF values determined for a number of products by use of natural sunlight were found to be lower than those derived in the laboratory. These values, along with other characteristics of a number of commercially available sunscreen products, are listed in Table 18-3.

Experimental evidence has shown that sunscreens prevent actinic skin damage and sun-related tumors, such as squamous cell carcinoma.[2]

Adverse reactions to sunscreens include contact dermatitis and staining of clothing. Patients who develop contact dermatitis to a sunscreen containing a chemical such as PABA should change to a product that contains a different class of chemical, such as one containing a benzophenone.

Sunscreens do not promote tanning. People vary greatly in their ability to burn. Those who want some tan should choose a product with an SPF of 2 to 8 and increase exposure times conservatively.

Polymorphous Light Eruption

Polymorphous light eruption (PLE) is the most common light-induced skin disease seen by the practitioner. There are several different morphologic subtypes. Not only is the clinical picture variable, but symptoms may change over the years.

There are several morphologic subtypes, but individual patients tend to develop the same type each year. Lesions usually heal without scarring. The eruption appears first on limited areas, but becomes more extensive during subsequent summers. Most people with PLE will have exacerbations each summer for many years; a few will have temporary remissions. The disease may begin at any age. The amount of light exposure needed to elicit an eruption varies greatly from one patient to another. Patients can tolerate a certain minimum exposure time, such as 30 minutes, after which the eruption appears. Light sensitivity decreases with repeated sun exposure; this phenomenon is referred to as hardening. The eruption may cease to appear after days or weeks of repeated sun exposure. Those exposed to sunlight year around rarely develop PLE. Most patients show symptoms 2 hours after exposure.

The most common initial symptoms are burning, itching, and erythema. The eruption usually lasts for 2 to 3 days, but in some cases it does not clear until the end of summer. Many patients experience malaise, chills, headache, and nausea starting about 4 hours after exposure but lasting only 1 or 2 hours. The most commonly involved areas are the vee of the chest (the area exposed by open-necked shirts), the backs of the hands, extensor aspects of the forearms, and the lower legs in women. Women are affected more often than men. Reports vary concerning the wavelength of light responsible for inducing lesions. Most reports in the United States claim that UVB causes PLE, but in a large series from Germany lesions could be reproduced only with UVA.[3]

Clinical types. There are a number of clinical types of PLE.[3] The *papular type* is the most common form (Figure 18-1). The *plaque type* is the second most common pattern. Plaques may be superficial or urticarial. They may coalesce to form larger plaques and at times are eczematous (Figures 18-2 and 18-3). The *papular vesicular* type is less common. It occurs primarily on the vee area of the chest

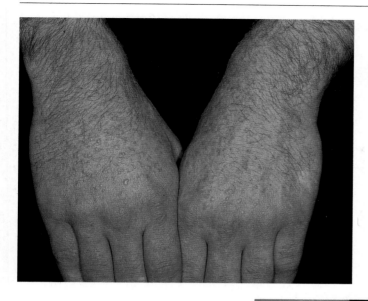

Figure 18-1
Polymorphous light eruption. Papular type.

Figure 18-2
Polymorphous light eruption. Plaque type.

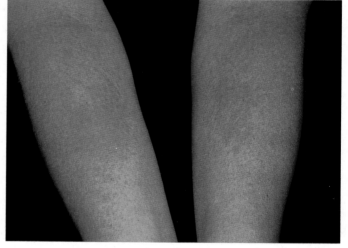

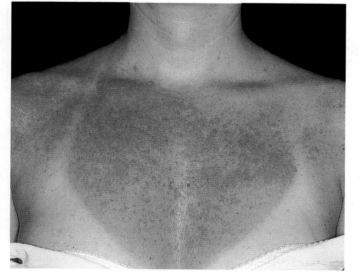

Figure 18-3
Polymorphous light eruption. Plaque type.

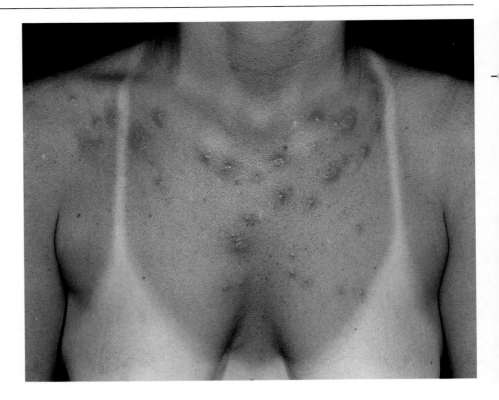

and usually begins with urticarial plaques from which groups of vesicles arise. Unlike other vesicular eruptions, the vesicles break and healing occurs quickly (Figure 18-4).

Erythema multiforme—type lesions and distribution are similar to classic erythema multiforme, with lesions most frequent on the backs of the hands and extensor forearms. The rare *hemorrhagic* type is characterized by hemorrhagic papules or purpura.

Differential diagnosis. The papular form resembles atopic dermatitis. PLE is less pruritic and occurs in a sun-exposed distribution, not in crease areas as in atopic dermatitis.

The plaque-like lesions and histology of systemic and discoid lupus erythematosus may be identical to PLE. The characteristic direct and indirect immunofluorescence patterns of lupus erythematosus will clarify the diagnosis.

Treatment. Many patients improve with repeated exposure to sunlight; this is the so-called hardening phenomenon. Protective clothing should be worn over involved areas. Sun exposure during times of maximum intensity (between 11 AM and 3 PM) should be avoided. Sunscreens with maximum sun-protecting factors, such as PreSun 15, should be used. Group II to V topical steroids will reduce pruritus and hasten resolution.

Trisoralen and natural sunlight[4] treatment is simple and effective for patients who do not improve with the above routine measures and who have significant eruptions each summer. Give 5 mg of 4, 5′, 8-trimethylpsoralen (Trisoralen) for every 20 to 25 pounds of body weight, the average dosage being five to six tablets, followed by sunlight 2 or more hours later. Start in the early spring with 15 minutes of sunlight the first day and increase the exposure by several minutes each day. Apply topical steroids if the disease is activated by treatment. Maximum protection will be reached 3 weeks after a 1-week course of treatment and a single course will offer a minimum of 6 weeks of protection. The course is repeated each month during the spring and summer months. Protective glasses such as NoIR should be worn for the remainder of the day after taking Trisoralen.

PUVA therapy is the "indoor method"; it utilizes another psoralen, 8-methoxypsoralen, and artificial UVA light exposure. However, it is much more expensive. See the discussion on treatment of psoriasis for details.

Antimalarials may be effective and should be considered for patients resistant to all other modes of treatment.[5] Antimalarials need only be used during the summer months; therefore, the total dosage taken will be small. Although the risk of eye damage is slight, ophthalmologic examinations should be obtained periodically to monitor for antimalarial toxicity.

Hydroa Aestivale and Hydroa Vacciniforme

Hydroa aestivale (summer prurigo of Hutchinson) and hydroa vacciniforme are rare but very distinctive light-induced eruptions. They may represent a type of PLE peculiar to children. The onset is before puberty and males are affected more frequently. Moderate itching occurs before and during the eruption. The lesions of hydroa aestivale consist of papules with weeping and crusting. The eruption is most prominent on the face, ears, and backs of the hands, but involvement of non-sun-exposed areas, especially the buttocks, is not uncommon. The rash fades, but may persit through the winter months. There is evidence for genetic transmission. UVB light reproduced the lesions in many cases.

Hydroa vacciniforme (Figure 18-5) is similar to hydroa aestivale, except that tense umbilicated vesicles resembling smallpox appear on the face, ears, chest, and backs of the hands; after breaking and forming a crust, they may heal with scarring. Both diseases usually clear after puberty. Sunscreens, sun avoidance, Group V topical steroids, and wet compresses are measures to control these diseases.

Figure 18-5
Hydroa vacciniforme. Umbilicated vesicles resembling smallpox in a sun-exposed distribution in a young boy.

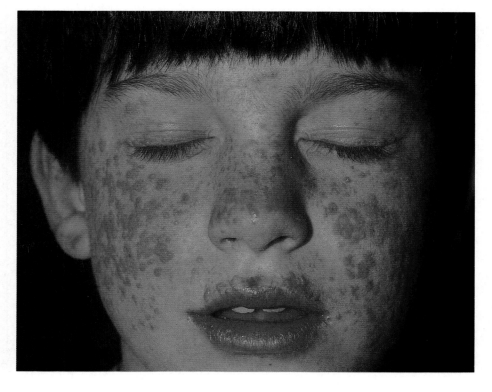

Hepatic Porphyrias

Porphyria refers to a group of diseases caused by enzymatic defects in the heme biosynthetic pathway. Each type of porphyria is associated with a specific enzymatic defect that may result in the accumulation of porphyrin metabolites in blood, urine, feces, and various tissues such as skin and liver. Certain porphyrin metabolites accumulate in the skin and are autooxidized, becoming capable of absorbing light in wavelengths between 400 and 410 nm. That energy is transferred to oxygen, which generates peroxides and causes the blisters seen in porphyria cutanea tarda and variegate porphyria. The porphyrias are classified into two groups, erythropoietic and hepatic, on the basis of the source of the excess porphyrin and the clinical features. The erythropoietic porphyrias are very rare and will not be discussed.

Porphyria cutanea tarda

Porphyria cutanea tarda (PCT) is the most common type of porphyria. An acquired form is precipitated by certain drugs (e.g., alcohol and estrogens);[6] there is also an inherited form. Since most people who consume alcohol or take estrogens do not develop prophyria, it is likely that genetic factors are important in the pathogenesis of nonfamilial cases. This genetic predisposition may explain why some patients on chronic hemodialysis develop PCT.[7,8]

The clinical features in order of frequency are blistering and milia in sun-exposed areas, increased skin fragility, facial hypertrichosis, hyperpigmentation, sclerodermoid changes, and dystrophic calcification with ulceration[9] (Figures 18-6 and 18-7). Serum iron and liver function tests are abnormal in about 60% of cases. The diagnosis is confirmed by demonstrating an elevated urine uroporphyrin level.

Phlebotomy is the treatment of choice. Chloroquine in very low doses may also be used.

Variegate porphyria

Variegate porphyria is an autosomal dominant disorder, most common in white South Africans, that has the same cutaneous signs as PCT, in addition to episodes of acute abdominal pain and neuropsychiatric symptoms such as depression and seizures. Acute attacks are precipitated by drugs such as barbiturates, sulfonamides, alcohol, and estrogens. High levels of fecal protoporphyrins are found during acute attacks.

Treatment consists of avoiding precipitating factors.

Figure 18-6
Porphyria cutanea tarda. There is increased facial hair around the eyes. Chronic sun exposure has resulted in blistering, erosions, and atrophic scars on the backs of the hands.

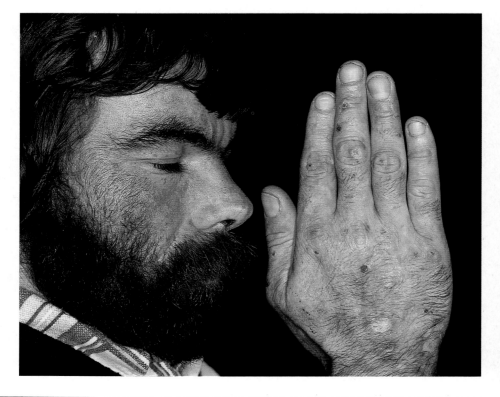

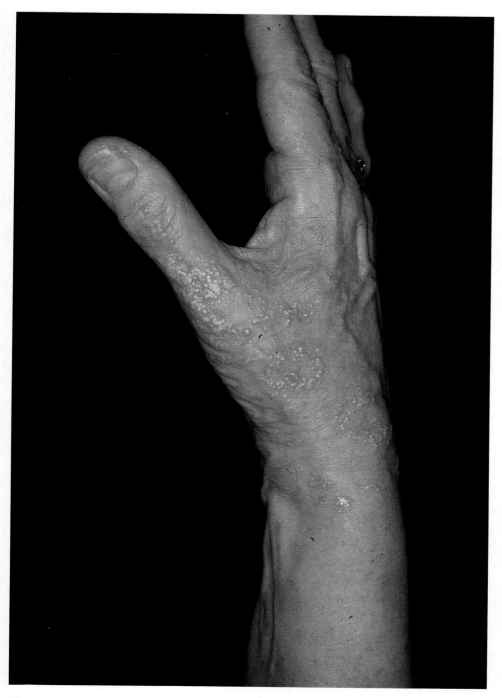

Figure 18-7
*Porphyria cutanea tarda. White milia form during
the healing process.*

Phototoxic Reactions

Phototoxic reactions are nonallergic cutaneous responses induced by a variety of topical and systemic agents. The frequency of these eruptions has decreased as physicians aware of the photosensitive potential of certain drugs have chosen alternatives. Phototoxicity occurs when a photosensitizer is absorbed into the skin either topically or systemically in appropriate concentrations and is exposed to adequate amounts of specific wavelengths of light, usually UVA. Theoretically, if sufficient quantities of chemical and light are delivered, the reaction should occur in all exposed individuals. In fact the response varies. A minimal clinical response consists of an almost imperceptible erythema followed by prolonged hyperpigmentation.

An example is berlock dermatitis caused by the psoralen compounds in oil of bergamot, formerly used in some perfumes. A maximal response consists of tingling of the exposed skin and erythema occurring shortly after exposure, followed within 24 hours by burning edema and vesiculation. This is followed by a bullous reaction lasting for days (Figure 18-8). Desquamation occurs, and residual hyperpigmentation may persist for 1 year or more (Figure 18-9). Intense reactions follow exposure to celery by salad makers, to wild parsnip (Figures 18-10 and 18-11) in meadows, and to ingestion of drugs such as chlorothiazides and demeclocycline.

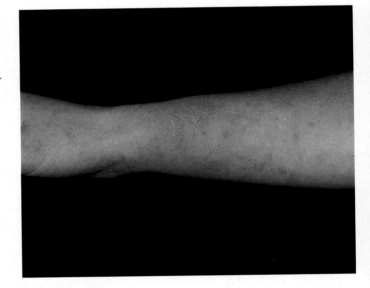

Figure 18-8
Phototoxic eruption. Diffuse erythema and vesiculation occurred 24 hours after preparing celery in a commercial processing plant.

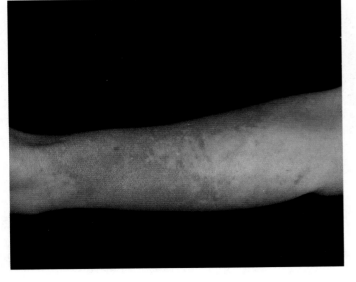

Figure 18-9
Phototoxic eruption. The patient pictured in Figure 18-8 developed diffuse hyperpigmentation in the previously inflamed areas 2 weeks after the acute episode.

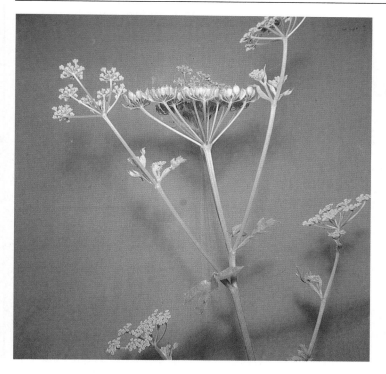

Figure 18-10
The wild parsnip. A cause of phototoxic eruptions.

Figure 18-11
Phototoxic reaction. Streaks of vesicles occurred after the patient laid in a field of wild parsnips.

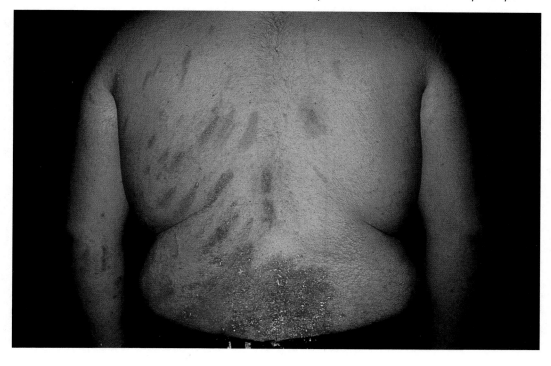

TABLE 18-4

AGENTS CAUSING PHOTOTOXIC REACTIONS

Internal drugs
    Benoxaprofen (Oraflex)*
    Chlorpromazine
    Chlorothiazides
    Demeclocycline (Declomycin)
    8-methoxypsoralens
    Trimethylpsoralen
    Nalidixic acid (NegGram)
    Many others reported, but rare
Topical agents
    Coal tar derivatives
    Perfumes

Plants containing psoralen compounds
    (phytophotodermatitis)
    Celery
    Gas plant (burning bush, dittany)
    Meadow grass (agrimony)
    Parsnip (wild parsnip)
    Persian limes
    Many others reported, but rare

*No longer available.

The distribution of phototoxic reactions is sharply limited to areas of sun exposure. Topical exposure to solutions or plants produces bizarre patterns of inflammation, such as streaks from brushing against a plant or haphazard lines from celery juice. Systemic exposure results in a generalized intense erythema in sun-exposed skin. The characteristic areas are the forehead, nose, malar eminences, cheeks, upper ears, lateral and posterior neck, vee of the chest, extensor surfaces of the forearms, backs of the hands, and prominences of the pretibial and calf areas. Photoonycholysis, which is sep-aration of the nails from the nail beds, may occur with drugs such as tetracycline, demeclocycline, and benoxaprofen.[10,11] The upper eyelids, nasolabial folds, and submental areas are typically spared.

Management consists of eliminating the suspected compound or drug. Many drugs not listed in Table 18-4 can, on rare occasions, cause a phototoxic reaction. When simple elimination fails to establish the offending agent, phototesting by physicians experienced with such procedures should be performed.

TABLE 18-5

DISORDERS OF PIGMENTATION

Hypopigmentation	Hyperpigmentation
Acquired	Circumscribed brown
Chemical-induced	Café-au-lait spots
Halo nevus	Diabetic dermopathy
Idiopathic guttate hypomelanosis	Erythema ab igne
Pityriasis alba	Fixed drug eruption
Postinflammatory hypopigmentation	Freckles
Tinea versicolor	Lentigo in children
Vitiligo	Peutz-Jeghers syndrome
Congenital	Lentigo in adults
Albinism, partial (piebaldism)	Melasma
Albinism, total	Phytophotodermatitis
Nevus anemicus	Diffuse brown
Tuberous sclerosis	Addison's disease
	Biliary cirrhosis
	Hemochromatosis
	Malignant melanoma (metastatic)

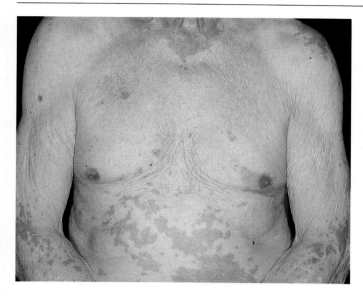

Figure 18-12
Vitiligo. There is almost total loss of pigment. Benoquin, a potent depigmenting agent, could be used for cosmetic purposes to remove the remaining pigment.

Photoallergy

Photoallergic reactions are now rare and are primarily of historic interest. Ultraviolet light initiates a reaction between skin protein and a chemical or drug to form an antigen. A delayed hypersensitivity reaction follows and the clinical presentation is, like poison ivy, eczematous inflammation. Some patients without additional drug exposure continue to flare for years when exposed to sunlight; this is termed a persistent light reaction.

Disorders of Hypopigmentation

Diseases with hypopigmentation or hyperpigmentation are listed in Table 18-5. The most common and distinctive are described below.

Vitiligo

Vitiligo is an acquired loss of pigmentation characterized histologically by absence of melanocytes. It is an autosomal dominant trait of variable penetrance and affects both sexes equally. Approximately 1% of the population is affected; 50% of cases begin before age 20. The pigment loss may be localized or generalized.[12]

The hypopigmented macules have a well-defined border. The loss of pigmentation may be inapparent in fair-skinned individuals, but disfiguring in blacks. Examination with the Wood's light will accentuate the hypopigmented areas and is useful for examining light-complected patients. The white macules often have a hyperpigmented border; this is most apparent in fair-skinned individuals.

Initially, the disease is limited; it then progresses slowly over a period of years (Figure 18-12). Com-

monly involved sites include the backs of the hands (Figure 18-13), the face, and body folds, including axillae and genitalia (Figure 18-14). White areas are common around body openings such as eyes, nostrils, mouth, nipples, and umbilicus. Vitiligo occurs at sites of trauma, such as around the elbows and in previously sunburned skin. Many patients with vitili-

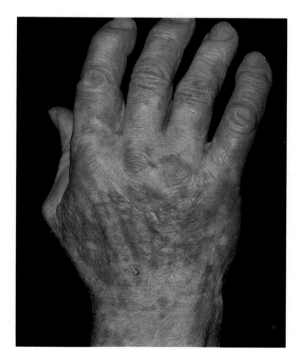

Figure 18-13
Vitiligo of the backs of the hands, a commonly involved site.

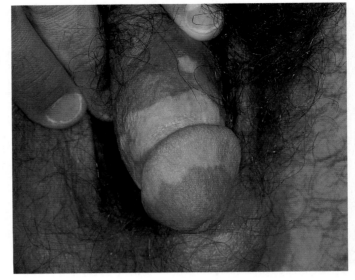

Figure 18-14
Vitiligo of the penis, a commonly involved site.

go will develop halo nevi. Most patients with vitiligo have no other associated findings; however, vitiligo has been reported to be associated with alopecia areata, hyperthyroidism, Addison's disease, pernicious anemia, diabetes mellitus, and melanoma.[13] Vitiligo is part of the Vogt-Koyanagi syndrome of vitiligo, uveitis, and deafness.

Treatment. Vitiligo in fair-skinned individuals is usually not a significant cosmetic problem. The condition becomes more apparent in the summer months when tanning accentuates normal skin. Tanning may be prevented with sunscreens having an SPF of 15.

However, vitiligo is a significant cosmetic problem in people with dark complexions and repigmentation with psoralens may be worthwhile. Patients must be selected carefully for this program and

should be informed of the following facts. Vitiligo of the backs of the hands, palms, and soles almost never responds;[14] repigmentation may not be complete and the partially treated areas may appear more bizarre than they did initially. The response is slow and treatment may have to be continued for months or years. Patients who accept these limitations can obtain good results in many instances.

The following program is to be used with natural sunlight.[15] Patients treated with artificial light in the dermatologist's office with PUVA will have an individualized program.

For adults and children over 12, the dosage is 20 mg of 8-methoxypsoralen (Oxsoralen) or 10 mg of trisoralen (Trioxsalen). The dose should be taken 2 to 4 hours before measured periods of sun exposure. Maximum solar radiation is received between

TABLE 18-6

TREATMENT OF VITILIGO WITH PSORALENS; SUGGESTED SUN EXPOSURE GUIDE

	Basic skin color	
	Light	**Medium**
Initial exposure	15 min	20 min
Second exposure	20 min	25 min
Third exposure	25 min	30 min
Fourth exposure	30 min	35 min
Subsequent exposure	Gradually increase exposure based on erythema and tenderness	

11 AM and 3 PM. The patient should be treated only twice each week during the first 2 weeks to determine the degree of sun sensitivity. Treatments may be more frequent after this initial period. A persistent faint erythema is the desired result. The beginning of repigmentation requires 10 to 50 treatments and appears as round perifollicular brown macules that enlarge and coalesce. The schedule in Table 18-6 is suitable for most patients. Sunglasses, such as NoIR, should be worn during the day of treatment. For cosmetic purposes, lesions may be temporarily dyed brown with Neo-Dyoderm or Vita-dye.

Idiopathic guttate hypomelanosis

Idiopathic guttate hypomelanosis (white spots on the arms and legs) is characterized by small white spots with a sharply demarcated border.[16,17] They are located on the exposed areas of hands, forearms, and lower legs in middle-aged and elderly people (Figure 18-15). Patients have signs of early aging and sun exposure, including keratosis, lentigines, and xerosis in the same areas. The condition is asymptomatic. There is no treatment.

Pityriasis alba

Pityriasis alba is a common finding that is probably more usual in patients with the atopic diathesis (see the chapter on atopic dermatitis). The condition appears in most instances before puberty. The face, neck, and arms are the most common sites. The lesions begin as a nonspecific erythema and gradually become scaly and hypopigmented. The hypopigmentation is transient and results from mild dermal inflammation and the ultraviolet screening effect of the scaly skin. The condition gradually improves after puberty. Treatment consists of lubrication. Mild inflammation responds to Group VI topical steroids, but the degree of pigmentation is not affected by any treatment.

The condition is often confused with vitiligo and tinea versicolor. Vitiligo does not scale. The potassium hydroxide preparation is positive in tinea versicolor.

Nevus anemicus

Nevus anemicus is a rare lesion most frequently observed on the chest or back of females. The lesions consist of a well-defined white macule with an irregular border, often surrounded by smaller white macules (Figure 18-16). Histologically, the skin appears normal; the pale color has been attributed to local blood vessel sensitivity to catecholamines.[18] The lesion is most often confused with tinea versicolor or vitiligo. The white macule lacks the scale of tinea and during Wood's light examination does not become as prominent as in vitiligo.

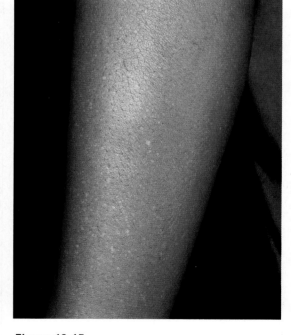

Figure 18-15
Idiopathic guttate hypomelanosis. White spots on the arms and lower legs occur in the middle-aged and the elderly.

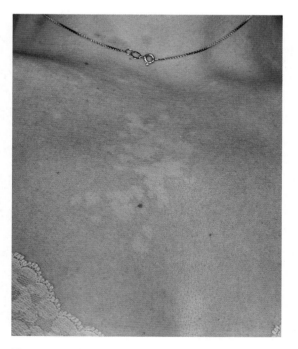

Figure 18-16
Nevus anemicus.

Figure 18-17
Tuberous sclerosis. Ash leaf–shaped hypopigmented macules.

Tuberous sclerosis

Hypopigmented macules (oval, ash leaf–shaped or stippled) that are concentrated on the arms, legs, and trunk are the earliest visible sign of tuberous sclerosis[19-20] (Figure 18-17). (See also the chapter on skin signs of internal disease.) They are present in 40% to 90% of patients with the disease and number from 1 to 32 in affected individuals.

Disorders of Hyperpigmentation

Freckles

Freckles or ephelides are small red or light brown macules that are promoted by sun exposure and fade during the winter months. They are usually confined to the face, arms, and back. The number varies from a few spots on the face to hundreds of confluent macules on the face and arms. They occur as an autosomal dominant trait and are most often found in fair-complected individuals. The use of sunscreens prevents the appearance of new freckles and helps prevent the darkening that typically accompanies sun exposure.

Lentigo in children

A lentigo is a small (0.5- to 2-cm) tan, brown, or black oval-to-round macule that is darker than a freckle and is not affected by sunlight. Freckles darken with sun exposure. Lentigines may increase in number during childhood and adult life or fade at any time. The Peutz-Jeghers syndrome consists of mucocutaneous pigmentation consisting of many blue-brown lentigines, less than 0.5 cm in diameter, on the buccal mucosa and other areas of the glabrous skin, accompanied by generalized intestinal polyposis.[21,22]

Lentigo in adults

Lentigo, or liver spot, occurs in sun exposed areas of the face, arms, and hands (Figure 18-18). The lesions vary in size from 0.2 to 2.0 cm and become more numerous with advancing age. To rule out lentigo maligna melanoma, a biopsy should be taken from any lentigo that develops a highly irregular border, localized increase in pigmentation, or localized thickening. Hydroquinone preparations are occasionally useful for bleaching these lesions (see treatment of melasma).

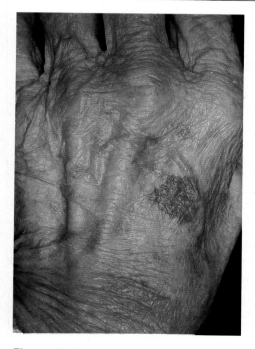

Figure 18-18
Lentigo (liver spots). A brown macule that appears in chronically sun exposed areas.

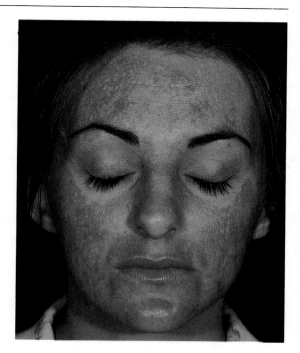

Figure 18-19
Melasma (mask of pregnancy). Diffuse brown hyperpigmentation may occur during pregnancy or while taking oral contraceptives.

Melasma

Melasma (chloasma or mask of pregnancy) is an acquired brown hyperpigmentation involving the face and neck in genetically predisposed women. The pigmentation develops slowly without signs of inflammation and may be faint or dark. The forehead, malar eminences, upper lip, and chin are most frequently affected (Figure 18-19). Melasma occurs during the second or third trimester of pregnancy, gradually fades after delivery, and darkens with subsequent pregnancies. Melasma is also seen in some women taking oral contraceptives.[23]

Treatment. Sun exposure must be minimized. Sunscreens with the highest sun protection factor should be used. Depigmentation may be accomplished with the use of bleaching creams containing hydroquinone.[24,25] This agent is available in 2% concentrations without prescription (Eldoquin, Eldopaque, Porcelana, and Solaquin) and by prescription in 3% (Melanex) and 4% (Eldoquin-Forte, Eldopaque-Forte, and Solaquin Forte) concentrations. Hydroquinone is a potential sensitizer and

skin sensitivity should be tested before use by applying a small amount to the cheek or arm once each day for 2 days (open patch testing). The development of intense erythema or vesiculation indicates an allergic reaction and precludes further use. Sun protection is essential during and after use of bleaching agents. Products such as Eldopaque have a tinted sunblocking cream base. Patients who object to a tinted preparation may use products that contain benzophenone and PABA ester sunscreens such as Saloquin Forte or Solaquin. These preparations must be used for months and in many cases will result in gradual depigmentation. Sun protection must be accomplished both during and after treatment.

The monobenzyl ether of hydroquinone (Benoquin) is a potent depigmenting agent and is used only for final depigmentation in disseminated vitiligo. Hydroquinones will also bleach freckles and lentigenes, but not café-au-lait spots or pigmented nevi.

Café-au-lait spots

Café-au-lait spots are uniformly pale brown macules found on any cutaneous surface, which vary in size from 0.5 to 20 cm (Figures 18-20 and 25-11). (See also the section on neurofibromatosis in the chapter on cutaneous manifestations of internal disease.) They may be present at birth, are estimated to be present in 10% to 20% of normal children, and increase in number and size with age. Six or more spots greater than 1.5 cm in diameter are presumptive evidence of neurofibromatosis (von Recklinghausen's disease) in young children over 5 years of age. In children under 5 years, five or more café-au-lait spots greater than 0.5 cm in diameter suggest the diagnosis of neurofibromatosis. Café-au-lait spots are present in 90% to 100% of patients with von Recklinghausen's disease. Smaller spots 1 to 4 cm in diameter in the axillae (axillary freckling or Crowe's sign) are a rare but diagnostic sign of neurofibromatosis. There is an increased incidence of café-au-lait spots in tuberous sclerosis. Similar lesions, but with a more irregular border (shaped like the coast of Maine), are seen in polyostotic fibrous dysplasia (Albright's syndrome). The smooth regular border of the café-au-lait macules of neurofibromatosis have been compared to the coast of California.

Macromelanosomes, or larger than normal pigment granules, have been detected with the electron microscope in the café-au-lait spots of some patients with neurofibromatosis, but their absence does not rule out the diagnosis. Café-au-lait spots cannot be lightened by hydroquinone bleaching agents.

Diabetic dermopathy

Asymptomatic, round, atrophic hyperpigmented areas on the shins (shin spots) are the most common cutaneous manifestation of diabetes. Lesions may also appear on the forearms, the anterior surface of the lower thighs, and the sides of the feet. Men are affected twice as often as women and the incidence is greatest in patients with diabetic neuropathy. They may be initiated by trauma. Lesions begin as round-to-oval, flat-topped, red, scaly papules that may become eroded. The lesions eventually clear or heal with epidermal atrophy or hyperpigmentation.

Figure 18-20
Café-au-lait spots. Irregular brown macules that are found in 10% to 20% of normal children. Number and size are increased in neurofibromatosis. (See Fig. 25-11.)

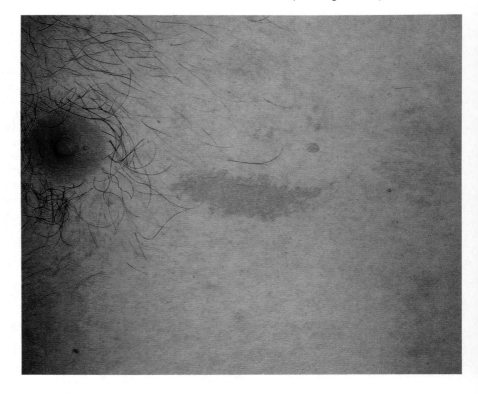

Erythema ab igne

Chronic exposure to heat from a wood stove, fireplace, electric blanket, electric heater, hot water bottle, or hot compress may cause a distinctive cutaneous eruption with a reticular pattern. The eruption initially appears as reticular erythema, but brown hyperpigmentation develops with repeated exposure (Figure 18-21). The pigmentation may fade in time or be permanent. The eruption must be differentiated from livido reticularis, which occurs with diseases such as leukocytoclastic vasculitis. Livido reticularis is a reddish-purple reticular pigmentation probably caused by restricted blood flow through the horizontal venous plexus. The color persists, but brown hyperpigmentation does not occur.

Figure 18-21
Erythema ab igne. Reticular brown hyperpigmentation that develops in areas chronically exposed to heat. A heating pad used for several months produced the eruption depicted here.

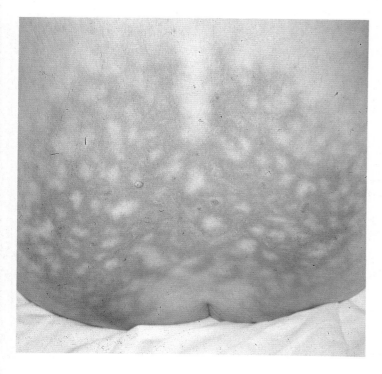

REFERENCES

1. Pathak MA: Sunscreens: topical and systemic approaches for protection of human skin against harmful effects of solar radiation. J Am Acad Dermatol 7:285, 1982.
2. Wulf HC, Poulsen T, Brodthagen H, Klaus HJ: Sunscreens for delay of ultraviolet induction of skin tumors. J Am Acad Dermatol 7:194, 1982.
3. Holzle E, Plewig G, Hofmann C, Elke RM: Polymorphous light eruption: experimental reproduction of skin lesions. J Am Acad Dermatol 7:111, 1982.
4. Jillson OT: Treatment of polymorphous light eruption with Trisoralen ® and natural sunlight. Cutis 29:592, 1981.
5. Epstein JH: Polymorphous light eruption. J Am Acad Dermatol 3:329, 1980.
6. Thiers BH: The porphyrias. J Am Acad Dermatol 5: 621, 1981.
7. Poh-Fitzpatrick M, Bellet N, DeLeo VA, et al: Porphyria cutanea tarda in two patients treated with hemodialysis for chronic renal failure. N Engl J Med 299:292, 1978.
8. Garcia Parilla J, Ortega R, Pena ML, et al: Porphyria cutanea tarda during maintenance hemodialysis. Br Med J 280:1358, 1980.
9. Grossman M, Bickers DR, Poh-Fitzpatrick MB, et al: Porphyria cutanea tarda: clinical features and laboratory findings in 40 patients. Am J Med 67:277, 1979.
10. Greist MC, Norins AL: Benoxaprofen: a new arthritis medication that causes phototoxicity. J Am Acad Dermatol 7:689, 1982.
11. McCormack L, Elgart ML, Turner ML: Benoxaprofen-induced photo-onycholysis. J Am Acad Dermatol 7: 678, 1982.
12. Lerner AB, Norland JJ: Vitiligo: the loss of pigment in skin, hair and eyes. J Dermatol 5:1, 1978.
13. Betterle C, Del Prete GF, Peserico A, et al: Autoantibodies in vitiligo. Arch Dermatol 112:1328, 1976.
14. Mosher DB, Fitzpatrick TB, Ortonne JP: Abnormalities of pigmentation. In Dermatology in General Medicine. New York, 1979, McGraw-Hill Book Co.
15. Trisoralen, ® package insert. Bryan, Ohio, Elder Pharmaceuticals, Inc.
16. Savall R, Ferrandiz C, Ferrer I, et al: Idiopathic guttate hypomelanosis. Br J Dermatol 103:635, 1980.
17. Cummings K, Cottel WI: Idiopathic guttate hypomelanosis. Arch Dermatol 93:184, 1966.
18. Greaves MW, Birkett D, Johnson C: Nevus anemicus: a unique catecholamine-dependent nevus. Arch Dermatol 102:172, 1970.
19. Hurwitz S, Braverman IM: White spots in tuberous sclerosis. J Pediatr 77:587, 1970.
20. Fitzpatrick TB, Szabó G, Hori Y, et al: White leaf-shaped macules: earliest visible sign of tuberous sclerosis. Arch Dermatol 98:1, 1968.
21. Reid JD: Intestinal carcinoma in the Peutz-Jeghers syndrome. JAMA 229:833, 1974.
22. Papaioannon A, Critselis A: Malignant changes in the Peutz-Jeghers syndrome. N Engl J Med 289:694, 1973.
23. Sanchez NP, Pathak MA, Sato S, et al: Melasma: a clinical, light microscopic, ultrastructural, immunofluorescence study. J Am Acad Dermatol 4:698, 1981.
24. Pathak MA, Fitzpatrick TB, Parrish JA, et al: Treatment of melasma with hydroquinone (abstract). J Invest Dermatol 76:324, 1981.
25. Kligman AM, Willis I: A new formula for depigmenting human skin. Arch Dermatol 111:40, 1975.

ADDITIONAL READINGS

Fitzpatrick TB, et al: Biology and diseases of dermal pigmentation. New York, 1981, Columbia University Press.
Ortonne J-P, Mosher DB: Vitiligo and other hypomelanoses of hair and skin (Topics in Dermatology Series). New York, 1983, Plenum Publishing Corp.

Seborrheic Keratosis

Seborrheic keratoses are common growths that originate in the epidermis. They are of unknown origin and without malignant potential. One must be familiar with all of the characteristics and variants of this lesion to differentiate it from others and prevent unnecessary destructive procedures. Seborrheic keratosis can be easily and quickly removed and, if correctly executed, will heal with little or no scarring. Most people will develop at least one seborrheic keratosis at some point in their lives.

Many seborrheic keratoses occur in sun-exposed areas. The number varies from less than 20 in most individuals to numerous lesions on the face or trunk. They are sharply circumscribed and vary from 0.2 to more than 3 cm in diameter. They appear to be stuck to the skin surface and, in fact, occur totally within the epidermis (Figure 19-1). The surface characteristics vary with the age of the lesion and location. Those on the extremities are often subtle, flat, or minimally raised and are slightly scaly with accentuated skin lines (Figures 19-2 and 19-3). Lesions on the face (Figures 19-4 and 19-5) and trunk (Figures 19-6 and 19-7) vary considerably in appearance, but the characteristics common to all lesions are the well-circumscribed border, the stuck-on appearance, and the variable tan-brown-black color. The border may be round and smooth or irregular and notched, resembling a malignant melanoma (Figure 19-8).

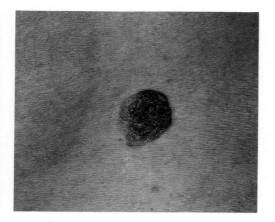

Figure 19-1
Seborrheic keratosis. The most common presentation. A brown-black nodule with an irregular surface that crumbles when picked.

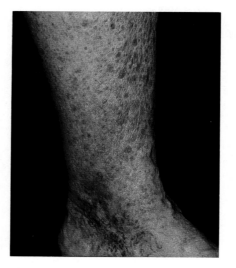

Figure 19-2
Seborrheic keratosis. Lesions on the distal extremities are flatter and do not accumulate dense surface keratin.

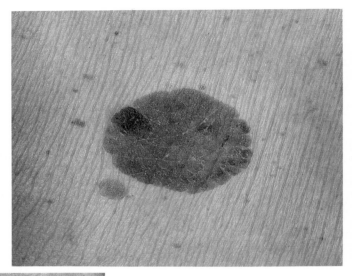

Figure 19-3
Seborrheic keratosis. A typical distal extremity lesion that is broad, flat, and comparatively smooth-surfaced.

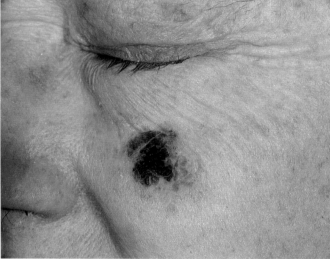

Figure 19-4
Seborrheic keratosis. Lesions may become darkly pigmented if the surface keratin is retained for long periods.

Figure 19-5
Seborrheic keratosis. Very large lesions may form along the hairline and temple.

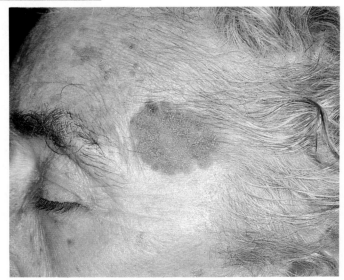

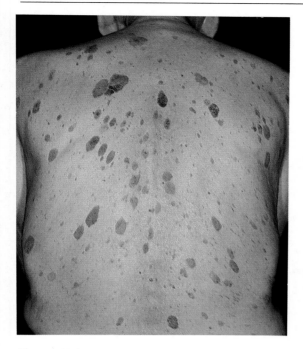

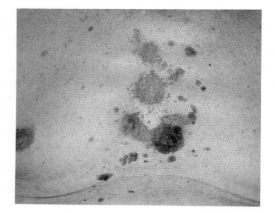

Figure 19-6
Seborrheic keratosis. Lesions are very common on the back; an individual may have numerous lesions on the sun-exposed back and none on the buttocks.

Figure 19-7
Seborrheic keratosis. The presternal area is a common site. Different levels of keratin retention are depicted in this photograph.

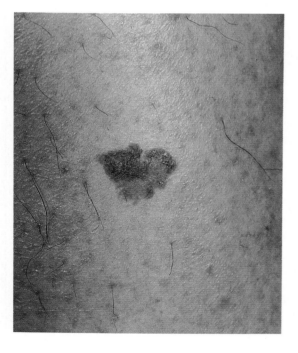

Figure 19-8
Seborrheic keratosis mimicking malignant melanoma. There is variation in pigmentation and the border is irregular and notched, but the surface is regular with dense keratin.

The surface characteristics show considerable variation. Smooth, dome-shaped tumors have 1-mm white or black pearls of keratin embedded in their surface; these are called horn pearls (Figures 19-9 and 19-10). Broader and flatter lesions may have a verrucous surface (Figure 19-11). The most common lesions are oval-to-round flattened domes with a granular or irregular surface that crumbles when picked (Figure 19-1). Although generally asymptomatic, they can be a source of itching, especially in the elderly who have a tendency to unconsciously manipulate these protruding growths. Irritation can also be initiated by chafing from clothing or from maceration in intertriginous areas such as under the breasts. When inflamed, the lesions become slightly swollen and develop an irregular red flare in the surrounding skin. Itching and erythema can then appear spontaneously in other seborrheic keratoses that have not been manipulated (Figure 19-12). The only treatment is to apply topical steroids or to remove all inflamed lesions. With continued inflammation, the seborrheic keratosis loses most of its normal characteristics and becomes a bright red, oozing mass with a friable surface. This irritated seborrheic keratosis itches intensely (Figure 19-13).

Sign of Leser-Trélat. The sudden appearance of numerous seborrheic keratoses has been reported as a sign of internal malignancy.[1,2] However, this is a rare occurrence and patients with numerous seborrheic keratoses need not be evaluated for malignancy unless the lesions erupt abruptly.

Treatment. Lesions are removed for cosmetic purposes or to eliminate a source of irritation. Since these growths appear entirely within the epidermis, scalpel excision is unnecessary. They are easily removed with cryosurgery or curettage. Lesions to be curetted are first anesthetized with lidocaine introduced with a needle or jet injector (Dermo-jet). The jet injector should be fired directly into the center of the lesion to provide instantaneous and almost painless anesthesia. This technique is particularly useful when several lesions are to be removed at one time. With multiple strokes, a small curette is smoothly drawn through the lesion. (See Figure 26-8, page 551.) Seborrheic keratosis on the face or other areas with inappreciable underlying support can be softened before curettage with the electric needle. Monsel's solution controls bleeding and the site remains exposed to heal. Some lesions are tenaciously fixed to the skin and resist curettage; others are on sites difficult to curette, like the eyelid. These can be dissected with curved blunt-tipped scissors.

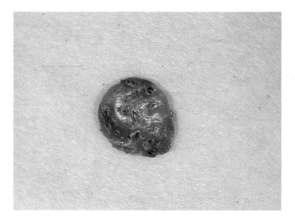

Figure 19-9
Seborrheic keratosis. Smooth dome-shaped tumor with tiny round black areas on the surface (horn pearls).

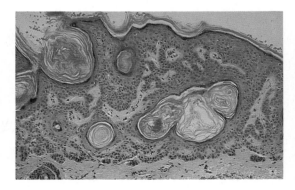

Figure 19-10
Seborrheic keratosis. Histology of tumor in Figure 19-9. There is benign epidermal thickening. Tiny keratin-filled cysts open onto the surface. Brown pigmentation is most evident in the basal layer.

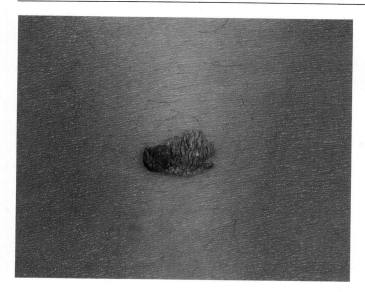

Figure 19-11
Seborrheic keratosis with a verrucous surface resembling a filiform wart. (See Fig. 12-2, p. 241.)

Figure 19-12
Irritated seborrheic keratosis. A single lesion developed an erythematous border; subsequently, inflammation occurred at the base of many other seborrheic keratoses.

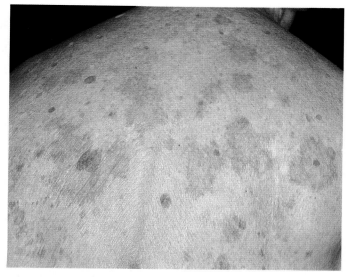

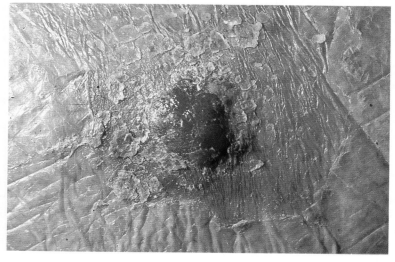

Figure 19-13
Irritated seborrheic keratosis. A bright red oozing mass simulating a pyogenic granuloma.

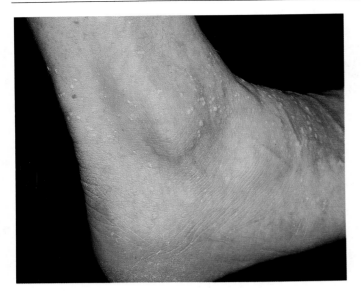

Figure 19-14
Stucco keratosis. Multiple small scaling lesions in a typical location.

Figure 19-15
Stucco keratosis. Many white dry scaly lesions on the forearm and back of the hand. Note also the several brown seborrheic keratoses on the back of the hand.

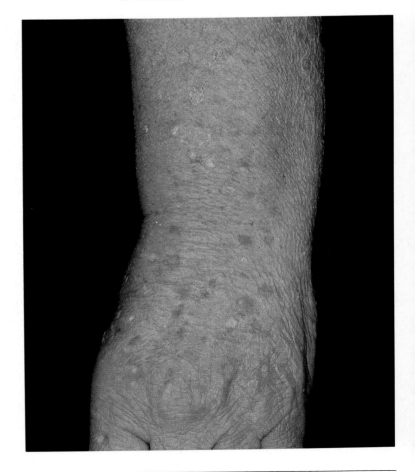

Stucco Keratosis

In the elderly, stucco keratoses, sometimes referred to as barnacles, are common, nearly inconspicuous lesions occurring on the lower legs (Figure 19-14), especially around the Achilles tendon area, the dorsum of the foot, and the forearms (Figure 19-15).[3] The 1- to 10-mm, round, very dry, stuck-on lesions are considered by patients to be simply a manifestation of dry skin. The dry surface scale is easily picked intact from the skin without bleeding, but recurs shortly thereafter. They can be removed with curettage or cryosurgery.

Dermatosis Papulosa Nigra

Young and middle-age blacks may develop multiple brown-black, 2- to 3-mm smooth, dome-shaped papules on the face. They probably represent a type of seborrheic keratosis. Patients who desire removal should be informed that white hypopigmented scarring may result. Determine the patient's response by curetting or freezing one or two lesions and permitting complete healing.

Cutaneous Horn

Cutaneous horn refers to a hard conical projection composed of keratin and resembling an animal horn. It occurs on the face, ears, and hands (Figure 19-16) and may become very long. Warts, seborrheic keratosis, actinic keratosis, and squamous cell carcinoma may all retain keratin and produce horns. Treatment is performed by local scissor excision or blunt dissection.

Figure 19-16
*Cutaneous horn. **A,** A hard conical projection composed of keratin. **B,** After blunt dissection this lesion was histologically confirmed as a wart.*

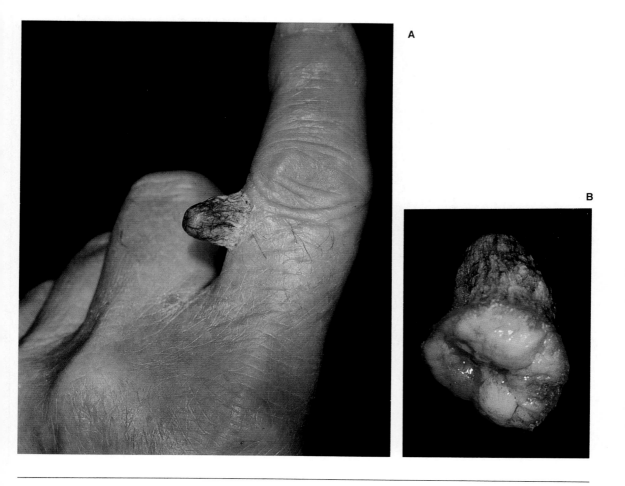

A

B

Figure 19-17
Acquired digital fibrokeratoma. A rare lesion resembling a cutaneous horn, the base of which is surrounded by a collarette of elevated skin.

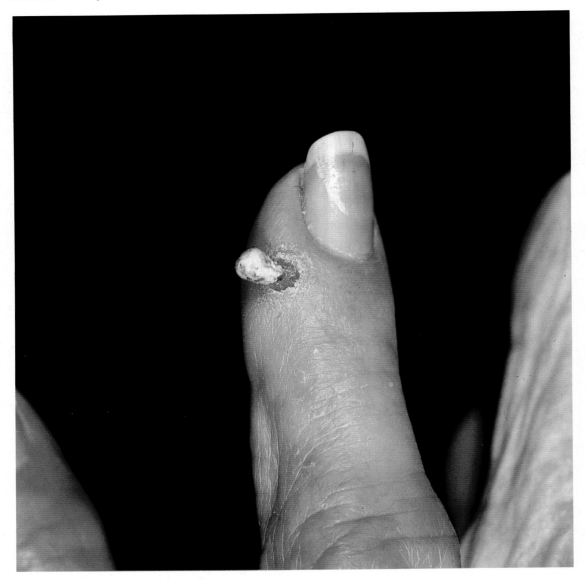

Acquired Digital Fibrokeratoma

This is a rare lesion that resembles a cutaneous horn or supernumerary digit and occurs around the finger joints. A short projection of collagen and capillaries is covered by epithelium and occasionally by retained keratin (Figure 19-17). The projection may be surrounded by a collarette of elevated skin. Treatment is performed by simple scissor dissection and bleeding is terminated by Monsel's solution.

Skin Tags (Acrochordons)

Skin tags are a common tumor of the neck, axillae, and groin that occur more commonly in females. They can begin in the second decade as a tiny, brown, oval excrescence attached by a short broad-to-narrow stalk (Figure 19-18). With time, the tumor can increase to 1 cm as the stalk becomes long and narrow (Figure 19-19). Patients complain that they are bothersome when wearing clothing or jewelry. One study suggests that skin tags may be a means for identifying patients at increased risk for colonic polyps.[4] The stalks are easily removed by scissor excision or with a light touch of the electrocautery.

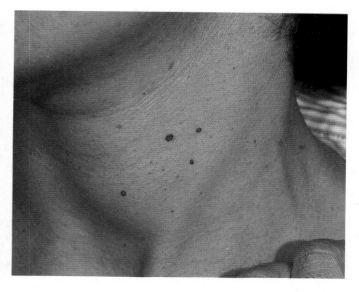

Figure 19-18
Skin tags. Multiple round black oval excrescences attached by a short broad-to-narrow stock.

Figure 19-19
Skin tag. A polypoid mass on a long narrow stock. Some nevi have an identical appearance.

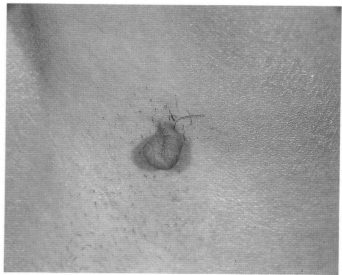

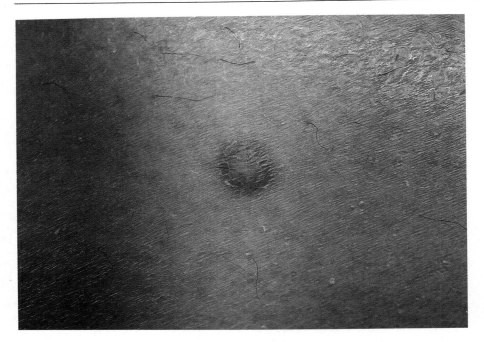

Figure 19-20
Dermatofibroma. A typical lesion on the lower legs that is slightly elevated, round, and hypopigmented, with a scaling surface.

Dermatofibroma

Dermatofibromas are common, benign, asymptomatic to slightly itchy lesions occurring more frequently in females. They vary from 1 to 10 and can be found anywhere on the extremities and trunk, but are most likely to occur on the anterior surface of the lower legs. Dermatofibromas may not be tumors; rather they may represent a fibrous reaction to trauma or an insect bite. They appear as 3- to 10-mm, slightly raised, pink-brown, sometimes scaly, hard growths that retract beneath the skin surface during attempts to compress and elevate them with the thumb and index finger (Figures 19-20 and 19-21).

Treatment. Some patients object to the color of the lesion and therefore request excision. These lesions are most commonly found on the lower legs, where elliptical excisions closed with sutures may result in a wide, unsightly scar. An alternative is to shave the brown surface with a #15 surgical blade and allow the wound to granulate and reepithelialize. The healed area remains hard because a portion of the fibrous tissue has remained. The brown color may reappear in some lesions. Conservative cryosurgery may also eliminate the color and part of the tumor.

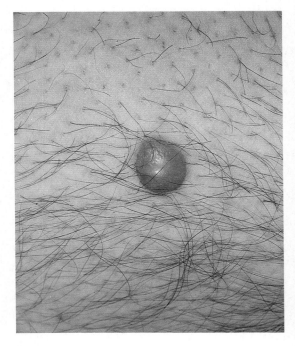

Figure 19-21
Dermatofibroma. This lesion is elevated, very firm, and lacks the typical brown hyperpigmentation of most dermatofibromas.

Hypertrophic Scars and Keloid

Injury in a predisposed individual can result in an abnormally large scar. A hypertrophic scar is inappropriately large, but remains confined to the wound site; a keloid extends beyond the margins of injury (Figure 19-22). There are histologic differences between hypertrophic scars and keloids. Keloids are often symptomatic and complaints arise about tenderness, pain and hyperesthesia, particularly in the early stages of development. Keloids are most common on the shoulders and chest, but may occur on any skin surface. Blacks are more susceptible and sometimes develop facial keloids. Some patients with cystic acne of the back and chest form numerous keloidal scars (Figure 19-23).

Treatment. Several techniques can be used for treating keloids. Inducing atrophy with an intralesional injection of triamcinolone (Kenalog) 10 mg/ml is adequate for most small lesions; a 27-gauge needle is used. To distribute the suspension evenly, inject while continually advancing the needle. Particles of steroid that have not been properly dispersed will remain visible as white flecks in the scar tissue. Inject with firm pressure until the lesion blanches. Early keloids have softer proliferating connective tissue and are more inclined to improve with intralesional injections than are older inactive lesions. Inject every 4 weeks until a significant response is noted. Subsequently, decrease the frequency and concentration of injections to avoid over compensation and telangiectasia.

Other techniques include radiation therapy, excision,[5] and a combination of freezing and intralesional steroid injection.[6] Large keloids may be excised, followed by intralesional steroid injection of the closed surgical wound. Injections are repeated for several months at 4-week intervals.

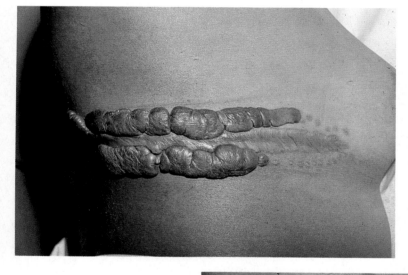

Figure 19-22
Keloid. A mass of keloids arising from suture marks in a black patient.

Figure 19-23
Keloid. Numerous confluent keloids arising from a patient with cystic acne.

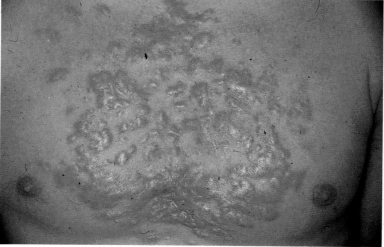

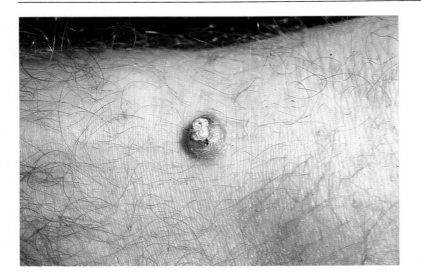

Figure 19-24
Keratoacanthoma. An early dome-shaped tumor with a central keratin plug.

Keratoacanthoma

Keratoacanthoma is a relatively common, benign, epithelial tumor that previously was considered to be a variant of squamous cell carcinoma. After careful observation of the growth characteristics and histology, keratoacanthoma was recognized as a distinct entity.

Keratoacanthoma begins as a smooth, dome-shaped, red papule that resembles molluscum contagiosum (Figure 19-24). In a few weeks the tumor may rapidly expand to 1 or 2 cm and develop a central keratin-filled crater, frequently covered with crust (Figure 19-25). The growth retains its smooth surface unlike a squamous cell carcinoma. Untreated, growth stops and the tumor remains unchanged for an indefinite period of time. In the majority of cases it then regresses, frequently healing with scarring. Keratoacanthoma occurs most commonly as a solitary growth on exposed areas of the face and dorsum of the hand, but may occur on any site. On occasion, multiple keratoacanthomas appear or a single lesion extends over several centimeters. These rare variants are resistant to treatment and are unlikely to undergo spontaneous remission.

Treatment. There is no advantage in waiting for spontaneous regression to occur, since most keratoacanthomas ultimately heal with scarring. There are many ways of managing keratoacanthomas: conventional excision, electrodesiccation and curettage,[7] intralesional injections of 5-fluorouracil,[8,9]

Figure 19-25
Keratoacanthoma. Classic presentation of a fully developed tumor. A round smooth dome-shaped mass with a central keratin-filled crater.

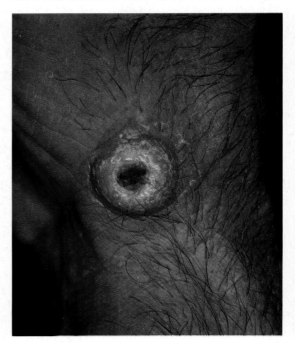

cryosurgery, or radiotherapy.[10] All produce acceptable results. I prefer blunt dissection[11] because it is simple and fast, has a high rate of cure, and results in good cosmetic appearances (see the chapter on skin surgery). Excellent results have been reported with 5-fluorouracil injections.[8,9] The tumor is injected with 0.1 to 0.2 ml of a solution of 50 mg/ml of 5-fluorouracil (available as fluorouracil injection 500 mg/10 ml ampul). Injections are given at weekly intervals until the lesion clears. Reported time for healing varies from 1 to 9 weeks.

Epidermal Nevus

The term nevus means a congenital defect of the skin characterized by the localized excess of one or more types of cells in a normal cell site. Histologically, the cells are identical to or closely resemble normal cells. Epidermal nevus should be a general term to designate an excess of one type of epidermally derived cells (e.g., squamous cell or sebocyte). However, the term is commonly reserved for congenital growths in which the predominant cell is the keratinocyte. Such localized lesions are designated nevus verrucosus and lesions with linear distribution are designated nevus unius lateris.

These well-circumscribed growths are present at birth or appear in infancy or childhood. They are round, oval or oblong, elevated, flat-topped, yellow-tan to dark brown with a uniformly warty or velvety surface (Figure 19-26). They appear more commonly on the limbs than on the scalp. Considering their unusual appearance and occasional itching, they are generally inconsequential. Occasionally, the growths are very large and disfiguring. The very rare epidermal nevus syndrome consists of extensive epidermal nevi associated with skeletal, cardiovascular, and central nervous system disorders.[12] Treatment may be attempted with cryosurgery or dermabrasion, but recurrences are common, and surgical excision produces the most predictable results.

Figure 19-26
Epidermal nevus. A congenital lesion, which is often linear, and has a dark brown, warty or velvety surface.

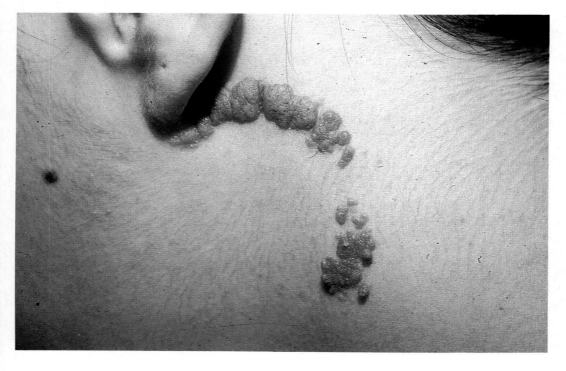

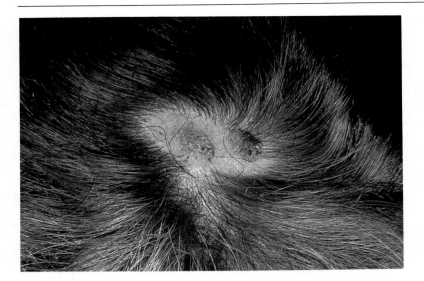

Figure 19-27
*Nevus sebaceous. A typical lesion on the scalp
of a postpubertal male.*

Nevus Sebaceous

Nevus sebaceous is a distinctive growth of the scalp, face, and neck, which sustains age-related modifications in morphology.[13] The nevus occurs singly and is asymptomatic. Two-thirds of cases are present at birth; the others develop in infancy or early childhood. Males and females are equally affected.

Lesions are oval to linear, varying from 0.5 × 1.0 cm to 7 × 9 cm. Most lesions occur on the scalp (Figure 19-27); less frequently they are found on the forehead and cheeks. The lesions in infants and younger children are smooth, waxy, hairless thickenings. During puberty there is a massive development of sebaceous glands with epidermal hyperplasia within the lesion (Figure 19-28). At this stage they change clinically by developing a verrucous surface covered with numerous closely aggregated yellow to dark brown papules. When this transformation becomes noticeable, parents become worried and seek medical attention.

In about 20% of cases there is a third phase of evolution that involves the development of secondary neoplasia in the mass of the nevus. A number of benign and malignant "nevoid tumors" may occur, the most common of which is the basal cell carcinoma.[14]

Treatment. Plastic surgical excision is the treatment of choice. Attempts at local destruction with electrocautery or cryosurgery may lead to recurrence.

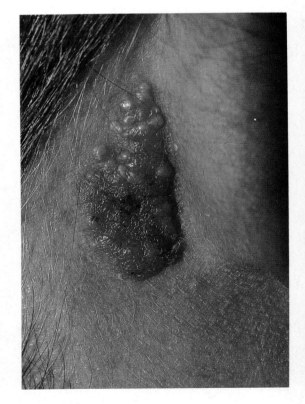

Figure 19-28
*Nevus sebaceous. A white globular surface
indicative of sebaceous gland hyperplasia that
occurs after puberty.*

Chondrodermatitis Nodularis Chronica Helicis

This uncommon disorder occurs on the lateral surface of the helix and occasionally on the anti-helix, a site rarely occupied by other growths. One (occasionally more) firm 2- to 6-mm nodule appears spontaneously. It subsequently develops a central scale lacking the keratinous plug of a keratoacanthoma (Figure 19-29). Removal of the scale reveals a small central erosion. Unlike the full distended margins of a squamous or basal cell carcinoma, the sides of this mass slope down from the center. The small mass is dull red to white and painful. During the active stage the base may become red and swollen; pain is constant. Pressure of any type becomes intolerable. As the mass attains its maximum size it becomes lighter in color, but remains symptomatic. The cause of this disorder is unknown, but chronic sun exposure may be a factor. Men over the age of 40 make up 90% of the patients.

Histologically, the dermis shows collagen degeneration with granulation tissue, edema, and inflammation.

Treatment. Excision with blunt-tipped curved scissors produces immediate relief. Cut down to and expose the cartilage. In an attempt to eradicate all foci of inflammation, gently electrodesiccate the base (see Figures 26-6 and 26-7). Bleeding is controlled with Monsel's solution. The wound will granulate and heal with a minimum defect. Recurrences are common if all sites of inflammation have not been eradicated. Patients refusing surgery may be treated with intralesional triamcinolone (10 mg/ml) once every 2 to 3 weeks until clear. Some degree of pain will persist throughout the treatment period.

Figure 19-29
Chondrodermatitis nodularis chronica helicis. A painful firm nodule with scaling in the center occupying a commonly observed site on the lateral surface of the helix.

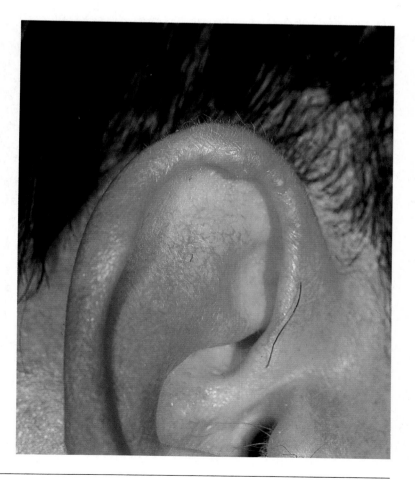

Epidermal Cyst

The common epidermal or sebaceous cyst occurs primarily on the face, back, or base of the ears, chest, and back. The cyst wall is lined with stratified squamous epithelium that produces keratin. The round, protruding, smooth-surfaced mass is movable and varies in size from a few millimeters to several centimeters. The cyst communicates with the surface through a narrow channel, with the surface opening presenting as a small, round, sometimes imperceptible, keratin-filled orifice—a blackhead (Figure 19-30). Epidermal cysts may originate from comedones; such lesions are superficial with a large black keratinous plug on the surface. They are referred to as giant comedones and are commonly found on the back (Figure 19-31). Cysts may either remain small for a period of years or progressively develop. Spontaneous rupture of the wall results in discharge of the soft yellow keratin into the dermis.

A tremendous inflammatory response ensues and the sterile purulent material either points and drains through the surface or is slowly reabsorbed. If the wall is destroyed during the inflammatory process, the cyst will not recur.

Treatment. Like boils, fluctuant inflamed cysts must be drained and evacuated. Small cysts are removed by making a linear incision with a #11 blade over the surface and, if possible, through the orifice. The soft keratinous material is expressed through the orifice and the remaining material is dislodged with a #1 curette. After total evacuation, firm pressure generally forces the cyst wall through the incision where it can be grasped with the forceps and separated with scissors from connective tissue. To absorb blood and serum, the wound is compressed for several minutes. If necessary, the wound edges may be supported with Steri-strips. Excision is the procedure of choice for large cysts.

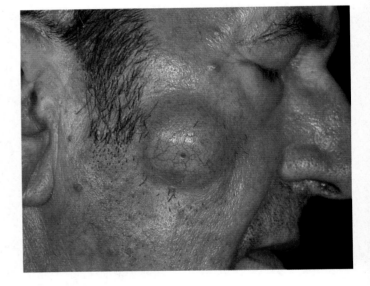

Figure 19-30
Epidermal cyst. The keratin-filled orifice (blackhead) communicating with the surface is not usually as prominent as illustrated here.

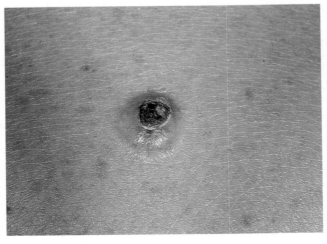

Figure 19-31
Giant comedon. A superficial epidermal cyst commonly found on the back.

Pilar Cyst

The pilar cyst occurs most commonly in the scalp and, like epidermal cysts, is freely movable. They are frequently multiple and may become large masses (Figure 19-32). The epithelial-lined wall produces keratin of a different quality than that of the epidermal cyst, but rupture of the wall creates the same intense reaction. The cyst contains concentric layers of dry keratin that over time may become macerated, soft, and cheesy.

Treatment. Except for the largest structures, pilar cysts can be satisfactorily removed through a linear excision, avoiding suture closure. The following procedure should be used. Cut the hair over the cyst and make a 5- to 15-mm linear incision. With firm pressure, express the contents and dislodge remaining fragments with a #1 curette. Firmly press the curette against the inner wall of the cyst and move it back and forth to dislodge the cyst from its surroundings. The wall is firm and has a smooth, glazed surface easily separated from connective tissue. Hold the cut edge of the cyst with forceps and, applying continuous pressure to the sides of the wound, separate the cyst from the supporting connective tissue with a blunt dissecting instrument such as a Schamberg or blunt-tipped scissors. The cyst will literally pop out of the wound. To control bleeding, apply firm pressure for 5 minutes. Dressings or bandages are unnecessary and the scalp may be gently shampooed several hours later.

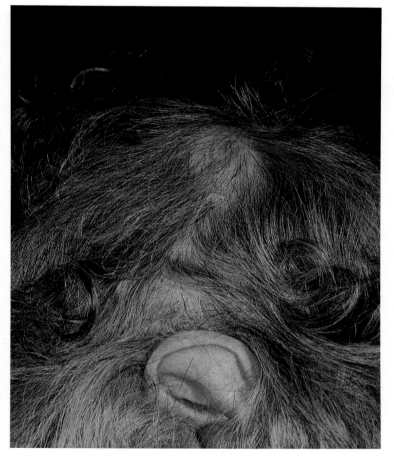

Figure 19-32
Pilar cyst. A freely movable cystic mass found on the scalp. Communication with the surface is rarely observed.

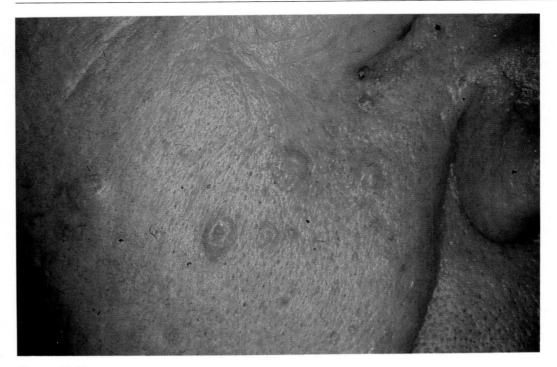

Figure 19-33
Senile sebaceous hyperplasia (cheek). Note central umbilication.

Figure 19-34
Senile sebaceous hyperplasia (lower lids). A common site in the elderly.

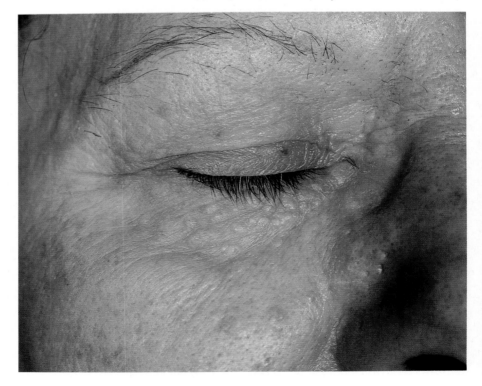

Senile Sebaceous Hyperplasia

Senile sebaceous hyperplasia consists of small tumors composed of enlarged sebaceous glands. They begin as pale yellow slightly elevated papules; with time, they become yellow, dome-shaped, and umbilicated. Senile sebaceous hyperplasia with telangiectasia may be mistaken for a basal cell carcinoma. The lesions occur after age 30 and gradually become more numerous. They are commonly found on the forehead, cheeks (Figure 19-33), lower lid (Figure 19-34), and nose. Treatment consists of removal of the elevated portion of the papule. A pitted scar will result if the entire structure is removed with a curette. The superficial portion of the lesion may be removed by shave excision or destroyed with cryosurgery or electrosurgery.

Syringoma

Syringomas are sweat duct tumors composed of firm flesh-colored papules that occur on the lower lids (Figure 19-35) and, less commonly, on the forehead, chest, and abdomen of women. The lesions appear at puberty and slowly become more numerous. The tumors have no malignant potential. They may be removed for cosmetic purposes by electrosurgery or cryosurgery. Lesions on the lower lid may be destroyed by trichloroacetic acid.

Figure 19-35
Syringoma on the lower lid of a young woman.

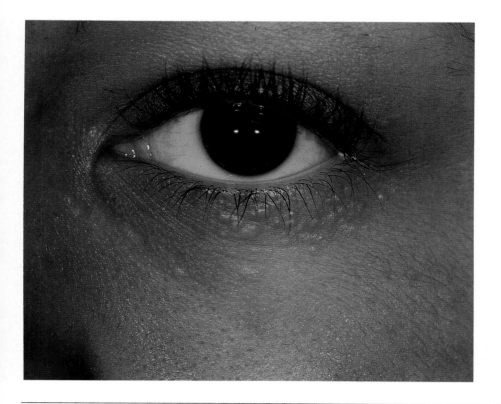

REFERENCES

1. Venencie PY, Perry HO: Sign of Leser-Trélat: report of two cases and review of the literature. J Am Acad Dermatol **10**:83, 1984.

2. Greer KE, Hawkins H, Hess C: Leser-Trélat associated with acute leukemia. Arch Dermatol **114**:1552, 1978.

3. Schnitzler L, Verret JL, Schubert B, et al: Stucco keratosis: histologic and ultrastructural study in 3 patients. Ann Dermatol Venereol **104**:489, 1977.

4. Leavitt J, Klein I, Kendricks F, et al: Skin tags: a cutaneous marker for colonic polyps. Ann Intern Med **98**:928, 1983

5. Pollack SV, Goslen B: The surgical treatment of keloids. J Dermatol Surg Oncol **8**:1045, 1982.

6. Ceilley RI, Babin RW: The combined use of cryosurgery and intralesional injections of suspensions of fluorinated adrenocorticosteroids for reducing keloids and hypertropic scars. J Dermatol Surg Oncol **5**:54, 1979.

7. Reymann F: Treatment of keratoacanthomas with curettage. Dermatologica **155**:90, 1977.

8. Eubanks SW, Gentry RH, Patterson JW, May DL: Treatment of multiple keratoacanthomas with intralesional fluorouracil. J Am Acad Dermatol **7**:126, 1982.

9. Goette DK, Odom RB: Successful treatment of keratoacanthoma with intralesional fluorouracil. J Am Acad Dermatol **2**:212, 1980.

10. Farina AT, Leider M, Newall J, et al: Radiotherapy for aggressive and destructive keratoacanthomas. J Dermatol Surg Oncol **3**:177, 1977.

11. Habif TP: Extirpation of keratoacanthomas by blunt dissection. J Dermatol Surg Oncol **6**:652, 1980.

12. Solomon LM: Epidermal nevus syndrome. Mod Prob Paediatr **17**:27, 1975.

13. Mehregan A, Pinkus H: Life history of organoid nevi: special reference to nevus sebaceus of Jadassohn. Arch Dermatol **91**:574, 1965.

14. Nagy R, Vasily DB: Pseudomelanoma in nevus sebaceus of Jadassohn. Arch Dermatol **115**:1004, 1979.

15. Wade TR: Chondrodermatitis nodularis chronica helicis. A review with emphasis on steroid therapy. Cutis **24**:406, 1979.

Chapter Twenty

Premalignant and Malignant Skin Tumors

Basal Cell Carcinoma

Basal cell carcinoma (BCC) is the most common malignant cutaneous neoplasm found in human beings. Fair skin and the degree of sun exposure are important risk factors. BCC is commonly found on the face and rarely on the backs of the hands, although both sites receive approximately the same quantity of solar radiation. BCC is rare in blacks. The tumor may occur at any age, but the incidence of BCC increases markedly after age 40. However, the incidence in younger people is rising, possibly as a result of increased sun exposure. Unfortunately, there was formerly a tendency to regard BCC as nonmalignant because the tumor rarely metastasizes. BCC advances by direct extension and destroys normal tissue. Left untreated or inadequately treated, the cancer can penetrate subcutaneous tissue into the bone and subsequently into the brain. Metastasis is rare, but possible.[1]

Pathophysiology and histology

The cells of a BCC resemble those of the basal layer of the epidermis. They are basophilic, have a large nucleus, and appear to form a basal layer by forming an orderly line around the periphery of tumor nests in the dermis, a feature referred to as palisading (Figure 20-1). Tumors with large nests of tumor cells (e.g., nodular BCC) are the least aggressive, whereas tumors with numerous small nests, each containing a few basal cells in a fibrous stroma (e.g., morpheaform BCC), may be more dangerous. The superficial BCC, the least aggressive of all BCCs, is observed more commonly on the extremities and back and contains buds of atypical basal cells extending from the basal layer of the epidermis (Figure 20-2).

BCC grows by direct extension and appears to require the surrounding stroma to support its growth. This may explain why the cells are not capable of metastasizing through blood vessels or lymphatics. The course of BCC is unpredictable. It can remain small for years with little tendency to grow, particularly in the elderly, or it may grow rapidly.

Clinical types

BCC occurs in many different clinical forms that vary in appearance and potential for aggressiveness.

Nodular BCC. Nodular BCC is the most common form. The lesions begins as a pearly white, dome-shaped papule resembling a molluscum contagiosum or dermal nevus (Figure 20-3). The mass extends peripherally, and telangiectatic vessels become prominent and easily recognizable through the thin epidermis. The growth pattern is irregular, forming an oval mass whereby the surface may become multilobular (Figure 20-4). The center frequently ulcerates and bleeds and subsequently accumulates crust and scale (Figures 20-5 and 20-6). Ulcerated BCCs were formerly designated "rodent ulcers."

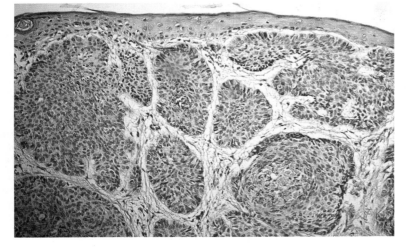

Figure 20-1
Nodular basal cell carcinoma. Nests of atypical basal cells are found in the dermis.

Figure 20-2
Superficial basal cell carcinoma. Buds of atypical basal cells extending from the basal layer of the epidermis.

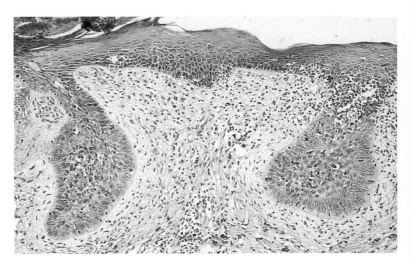

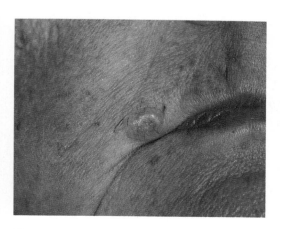

Figure 20-3
Nodular basal cell carcinoma. A pearly white, dome-shaped mass with prominent telangiectatic vessels that resembles a dermal nevus.

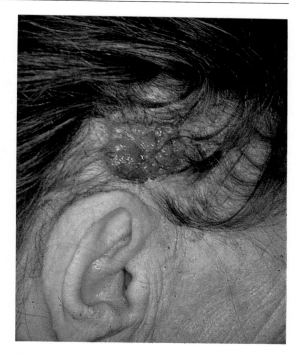

Figure 20-4
Nodular basal cell carcinoma. A relatively large mass with a multilobular surface.

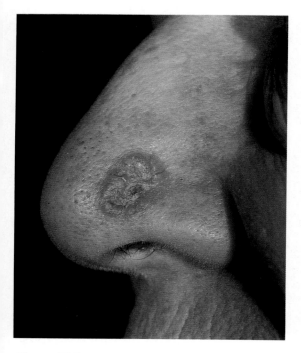

Figure 20-5
Nodular basal cell carcinoma. The center has ulcerated and is covered with a crust.

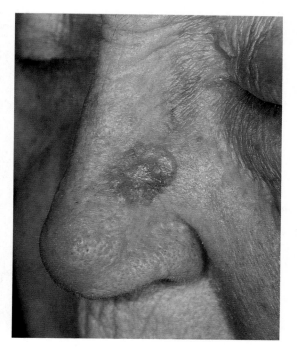

Figure 20-6
Nodular basal cell carcinoma (rodent ulcer). Degeneration and ulceration in the center.

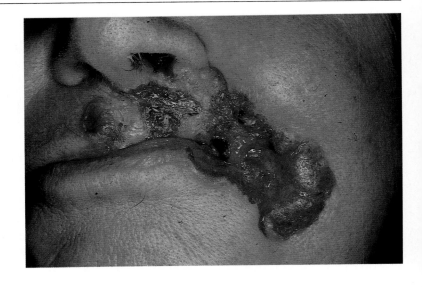

Figure 20-7
Nodular basal cell carcinoma. Tumor grew for 8 years before the patient requested help.

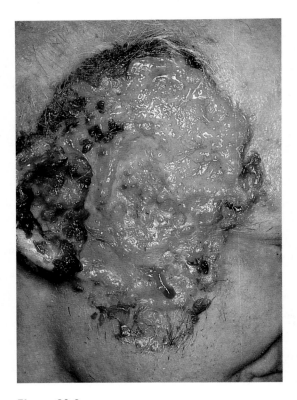

Figure 20-8
Basal cell carcinoma. Recurrence over a broad area after multiple surgical procedures.

Ulcerated areas heal with scarring and the patient often assumes that the condition is improving. This cycle of growth, ulceration, and healing continues as the mass extends peripherally and deeper; masses of enormous size may be attained (Figures 20-7 and 20-8). The tissue mass of a nodular BCC has a distinctive consistency that can be observed during curettage or while taking a biopsy. The tissue mass has poor cohesive forces and collapses or breaks down when manipulated with a curette. This is an important diagnostic feature that supports the clinical impression during the biopsy.

Pigmented BCC. Nodular BCC may contain melanin that imparts a brown, black, or bluish color through all or part of the lesion. Clinically, the lesion resembles a melanoma, but close inspection reveals the characteristically elevated, pearly white, translucent border and the biopsy confirms the diagnosis (Figure 20-9).

Cystic BCC. This variant of nodular BCC appears as a smooth round cystic mass. The cystic BCC behaves like the nodular BCC (Figure 20-10).

Sclerosing or morpheaform BCC. Morpheaform BCC is an insidious tumor possessing innocuous surface characteristics that can mask its potential for deep, wide extension. The tumor is waxy, firm, flat to slightly raised and either pale white or yellowish and resembles localized scleroderma; therefore, the designation morpheaform (Figure 20-11). The borders are indistinct and blend with normal skin. The tissue is rigid and difficult or impossible to remove with a curette. Localization of this tumor by inspection or biopsy is impossible. Treatment consists of wide excision or preferably Mohs' chemosurgery.

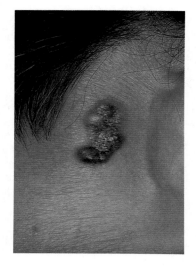

Figure 20-9
Pigmented basal cell carcinoma. A dark mass that resembles a melanoma. The tumor has all of the features of a nodular basal cell carcinoma.

Figure 20-10
Cystic basal cell carcinoma that has invaded the lower lid.

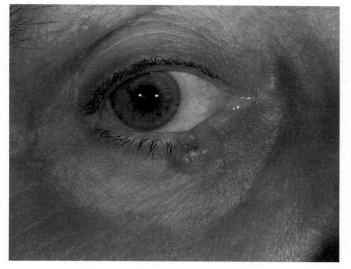

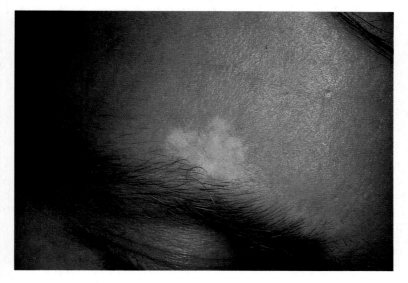

Figure 20-11
Sclerosing basal cell carcinoma. A firm yellow mass; the surface has a waxy consistency. Borders are ill-defined.

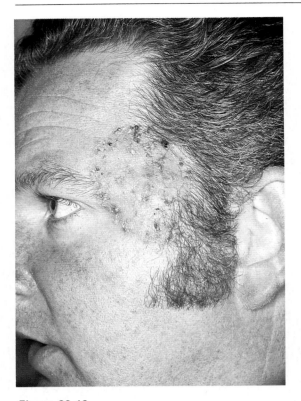

Figure 20-12
Superficial basal cell carcinoma. A large round flat plaque with a scaling border. Diagnosis of tinea was made initially.

Superficial BCC. The least aggressive BCC is the superficial BCC. This tumor occurs most frequently on the trunk and extremities, but may occur on the face (Figure 20-12). There may be one or more lesions. The tumor spreads peripherally, sometimes for several centimeters and invades after a considerable period of time. The circumscribed, round-to-oval, red, scaling plaque resembles a plaque of eczema, psoriasis, or Bowen's disease (Figure 20-13). However, careful inspection of the border reveals its thin, raised, pearly white nature (Figure 20-14). The characteristic features can also be observed by eliminating the redness with finger pressure.

Nevoid BCC syndrome. This rare, autosomal dominant disease possesses the following features: widespread BCC appearing at birth or early childhood, numerous small pits on the palms and soles, odontogenic cysts of the jaws, bifid ribs, and osseous, endocrine, central nervous system, and connective tissue abnormalities.[2] The tumors may become aggressive after puberty.

Management

There are several factors to consider before choosing the best treatment modality. The most important are cell type, tumor size, and location. In general, electrodesiccation and curettage afford excellent results for small (less than 10 mm) nodular BCCs located on the forehead and cheeks. Larger forehead and cheek nodular BCCs with well-defined margins should be excised and closed; electrosurgery for large tumors results in large unsightly scars. The margins of sclerosing BCCs cannot be determined by inspection, and either excision or Mohs' chemosurgery should be performed. Superficial BCCs of any size can be adequately removed by electrosurgery.

Tumors around the nose, eye, and ear require management by experts such as a dermatologic surgeon capable of performing Mohs' chemosurgery. BCCs of the nose and inner canthi are particularly dangerous. The skin rests close to bone and cartilage and tumor cells initially invade and proceed to migrate undetected along periosteum or perichondrium. Healing occurs over inadequately treated tumors and deep invasion and lateral extension can remain undetected, resulting in a tumor of massive proportions. Extension to the eye and brain is possible. Patients treated for BCC should be followed periodically for 5 or more years. Patients with one BCC often develop another.

The following section outlines various treatment modalities. Specific techniques are described in the chapter describing skin surgery.

Electrosurgery. This is most beneficial for small to medium-size nodular and superficial BCCs.[3-5] Electrosurgery is not appropriate for morpheaform BCC because margins cannot be clinically defined. However, it is particularly useful for ear lesions where mobilization of skin for closure after excision is difficult. Curettage requires firm dermis on all sides and below the tumor to enable the curette to distinguish between dermis and soft tumor. If the tumor encroaches on the fat, the curette cannot distinguish between fat and soft tumor and an alternate procedure must be used. Wounds created by electrosurgery ooze serum and accumulate crust during a 2- to 6-week healing period.

Excision surgery. Excisional surgery is preferred for large tumors or those with poorly defined margins on the cheeks, forehead, trunk, and legs. The cosmetic result is good and healing requires less time than with electrosurgery. Excision with primary closure is technically difficult on the ears and nose. The advantage of feeling the tumor is lost and adequate margins must be taken.

Cryosurgery. Cryosurgery is utilized for small to large BCCs of the nodular and superficial type. It is not indicated for deeply invasive tumors unless

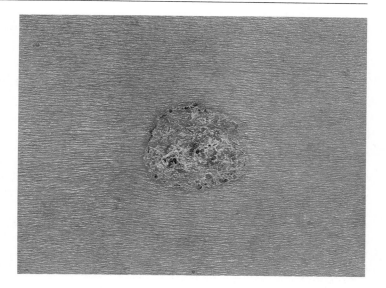

Figure 20-13
*Superficial basal cell carcinoma.
Surface has eroded in several areas
and formed a crust.*

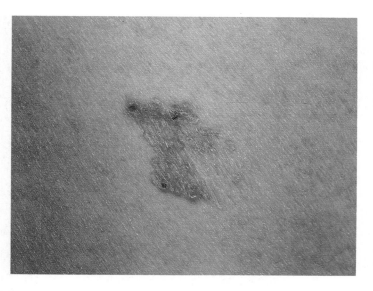

Figure 20-14
*Superficial basal cell carcinoma.
A slightly raised pearly translucent
plaque on the chest.*

thermocouples are used to measure depth of freeze.

Mohs' chemosurgery. Mohs' chemosurgery can be used for all types and sizes of BCCs. Chemosurgery is unnecessarily destructive for smaller lesions or lesions with well-defined clinical margins such as nodular or superficial multicentric BCCs.

Mohs' chemosurgery is the treatment of choice for most sclerosing BCCs and other BCCs with poorly defined clinical margins, tumors in areas of potentially high recurrence such as the nose or eyelid, very large primary tumors, and large recurrent BCCs.

Radiation. Radiation is useful for elderly patients who can not tolerate minor surgical procedures. In areas such as those around the eyelids and lips in which preservation of normal surrounding tissue is of prime consideration, radiation therapy may produce the best cosmetic result.[6] The treatment requires a number of outpatient visits that may be difficult for debilitated patients.

5-Fluorouracil. 5-Fluorouracil (5-FU) should not be used for the treatment of any BCC with the exception of some occurring in the rare nevoid BCC syndrome.[7] 5-FU can destroy surface tumor without affecting deeper cells.

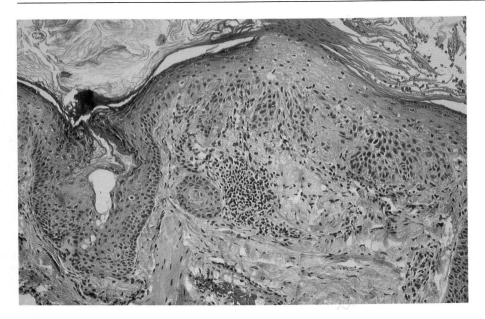

Figure 20-15
Actinic keratosis. Keratin and crust are present on the surface. Atypical epithelial cells are confined to the epidermis and do not involve the follicular structure.

Actinic Keratosis

Actinic keratoses are common, sun-induced, premalignant lesions that increase with age. Light-complexioned individuals are more susceptible than those with dark-complexions. Years of sun exposure are required to induce sufficient damage to cause lesions. After several years a small percentage of lesions may degenerate into squamous cell carcinomas. Squamous cell carcinomas that evolve from actinic keratosis may be aggressive.[8] Histologically, an actinic keratosis consists of atypical squamous cells confined to the epidermis (Figure 20-15). Penetration through the dermoepidermal junction and into the dermis indicates the development of a squamous cell carcinoma.

Actinic keratoses begin as an area of increased vascularity, with the skin surface becoming slightly rough. Very gradually an adherent yellow crust forms, the removal of which may cause bleeding (Figures 20-16 and 20-17). The extent of disease varies from a single lesion to involvement of the entire forehead, balding scalp, or temples. Induration, inflammation, and oozing suggest degeneration into malignancy. Keratin may accumulate, forming a cutaneous horn particularly on the superior aspects of the pinna (Figure 20-18). All patients with actinic keratosis should be examined carefully for BCC.

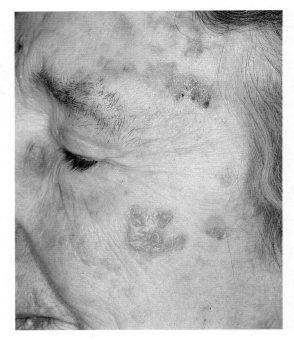

Figure 20-16
Actinic keratosis. Early lesions are present on the forehead. A more advanced lesion with yellow adherent scale is seen on the cheek.

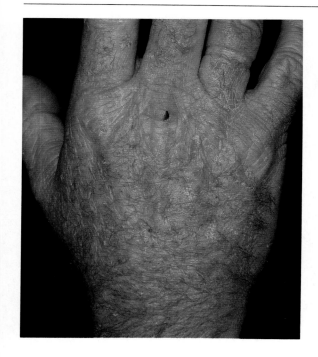

Figure 20-17
Actinic keratosis. Several oval to round red indurated lesions with adherent scale.

Figure 20-18
Actinic keratosis. Three actinic keratoses are forming cutaneous horns.

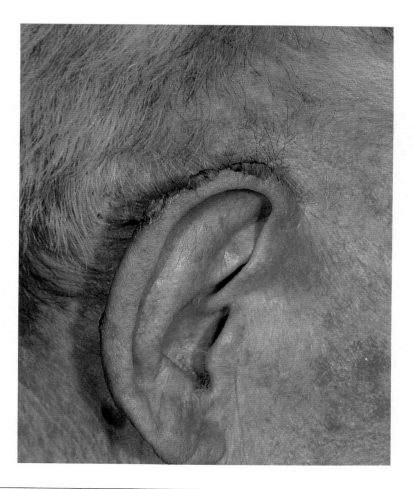

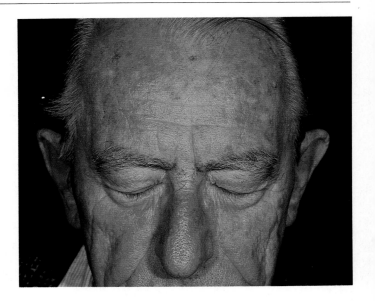

Figure 20-19
Actinic keratosis. Diffuse involvement of the forehead. Lesions are superficial. Lesions on the cheek were not clinically apparent.

Management

Sunscreens. Patients should make every effort to prevent further sun damage. This does not mean hibernating for a lifetime. Sunscreens are best applied in the morning on days when significant sun exposure is anticipated. Apply sunscreens to the face, lower lips, ears, back of the neck, backs of the hands, and forearms. Hats should cover bald heads. The physician should explain that, although sunscreens are used, additional lesions may occur.

Surgical removal. Individual indurated lesions or those with thick crusts should be removed with minor surgical procedures. It is unnecessary to biopsy lesions less than 0.5 cm. Larger lesions or those occurring around or on the vermilion border of the lips should be examined. Cryosurgery or electrodesiccation and curettage will easily remove small lesions. The cosmetic results may be superior with conservative cryosurgery.

Topical chemotherapy with 5-fluorouracil. 5-FU is an effective topical treatment for many cases of actinic keratosis.[9] The agent is incorporated into rapidly dividing cells, resulting in cell death. Normal cells are less affected and clinically appear unaffected. Inflammation is induced during this process. Thick, indurated lesions become most

---

TABLE 20-1

GUIDELINES FOR CHOICE OF 5-FU CONCENTRATION AND DURATION OF THERAPY ACCORDING TO SITE

Site	5-FU* (%)	Early signs of inflammation (days)	Duration of treatment (weeks)
Face, lips	1-2	3-5	3
Scalp	5	4-7	4
Neck	5	4-7	4
Arms, hands	5	10-14	6-8
Back	5	10-14	4-6
Chest	5	10-14	4-6

From Goette, KD: Topical chemotherapy with 5-fluorouracil. J Am Acad Dermatol **4**:633, 1981.
*Topical preparations include Efudex 2% and 5% solutions (10 ml) and 5% cream (25 gm); Fluoroplex 1% solution (30 ml) and 1% cream (30 gm).

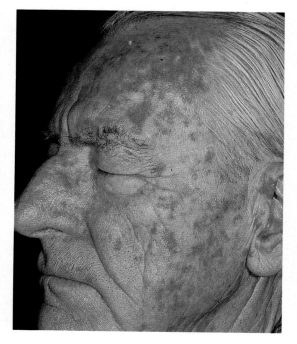

Figure 20-20
*Actinic keratosis. Treatment with topical 5-FU.
Maximum intensity of inflammation was reached 3
weeks after starting treatment. The medication
has inflamed the cheek lesions that were not
clinically apparent before treatment.*

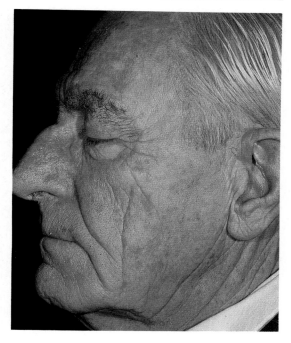

Figure 20-21
*Actinic keratosis. Five weeks after starting topical
5-FU. Residual erythema was present in
previously inflamed areas. All skin surfaces are
smooth.*

inflamed and may best be managed by surgically removing them before instituting topical chemotherapy. The available preparations of 5-fluorouracil are given in Table 20-1.

Patients should be cautioned about the various stages of inflammation encountered during treatment. Emphasize that a considerable degree of discomfort may be experienced for 1 week or more during periods of intense inflammation. Pharmaceutical companies that supply 5-FU also provide patient information sheets with color photographs of the various stages of inflammation.

Treatment technique and expected results.
Sparingly apply the preparation twice each day and massage thoroughly (Figures 20-19, 20-22, and 20-24.) Some authors suggest using topical steroids during the entire treatment period to suppress inflammation and decrease patient discomfort. This technique, however, may increase the difficulty of determining the conclusion of therapy.

In the early inflammatory phase erythema first appears in treated areas at predictable intervals (Table 20-1). In the severe inflammatory phase (Figure 20-20) erythema, edema, burning, stinging and oozing reach maximum intensity at different in-

tervals depending on the site treated and the thickness of the lesions. In the lesion disintegration phase (Figures 20-23 and 20-25), erosion or ulceration, intense inflammation, discomfort, pain, crusting, eschar formation, and evidence of reepithelialization occur. The approximate duration until this point is reached is listed in Table 20-1. Treatment is stopped at this phase.

Treatment is discontinued and cool compresses are applied for 20 minutes as needed for comfort. Group V topical steroids may be applied to red areas to suppress inflammation and pruritus. Do not apply topical steroids to eroded or ulcerated areas. Appearance of a purulent exudate suggests infection and oral antistaphylococcal antibiotics should be started. In the healng phase (Figure 20-21) residual erythema and hyperpigmentation persist for several weeks.

Patients should remain free of lesions for months and possibly years, but recurrences can be anticipated.[10] Very frequently, unsupervised patients inadequately treat their own newly evolving lesions with the result of surface healing and unaffected deeper abnormal cells. Medication should be discarded when treatment has terminated.

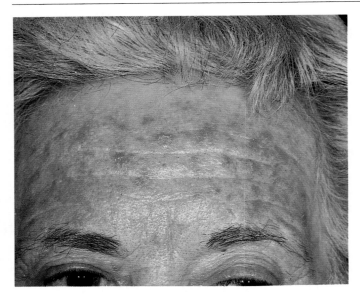

Figure 20-22
Actinic keratosis before treatment with topical 5-FU. Lesions are more advanced than those depicted in Figure 20-19.

Figure 20-23
Actinic keratosis. Three weeks after starting topical 5-FU. Lesion disintegration phase with ulceration and crusting.

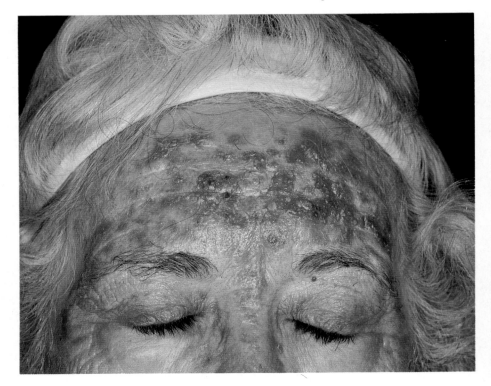

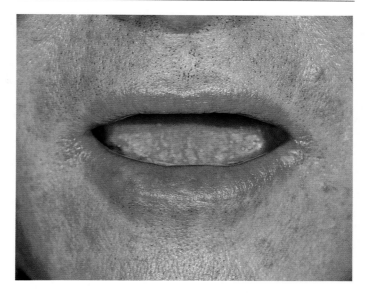

Figure 20-24
*Actinic cheilitis. Before treatment with topical
5-FU. The lower lip is white and smooth. The
non-sun-exposed upper lip is normal.*

Figure 20-25
*Actinic cheilitis. Two weeks after starting topical
5-FU. The entire lower lip is ulcerated.*

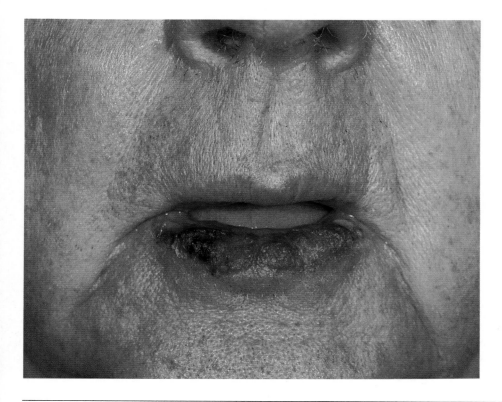

TABLE 20-2

LESIONS FROM WHICH SQUAMOUS CELL CARCINOMA ORIGINATES

Actinic keratosis	Leukoplakia
Cutaneous horn	Lichen sclerosis et atrophicus (vulva)
Bowen's disease	Sites of chronic infection
Erythroplasia of Queyrat	Chronic sinus tracts
Chemical exposure	Osteomyelitis
Arsenic (internal)	Thermal burn scars (Marjolin's ulcer)
Tar (external), except therapeutic tars	Radiation-damaged skin

Squamous Cell Carcinoma

Squamous cell carcinoma (SCC) is a tumor arising in the epithelium. It is a disease common to the middle-aged and the elderly. Like basal cell carcinomas, SCCs are most common in sun-exposed areas; however, distribution is different. SCC's are common on the scalp, backs of the hands, lower lip, and ear. Marjolin's ulcers are SCCs that arise in areas of chronic injury (burn, chronic stasis ulcers, open fracture, crush injury). SCC also occurs from epidermal diseases of unknown origin such as Bowen's disease (Table 20-2).

Pathophysiology. Atypical squamous cells originate in the epidermis and proliferate for an indefinite period. A flat, scaly lesion becomes an indurated SCC when cells penetrate the epidermal basement membrane and proliferate in the dermis.

Clinical manifestations. SCCs that arise in actinically damaged skin were previously thought to have a minimal potential for metastasis. A recent large study showed that such lesions may be aggressive. Their ability to metastasize is related to the size, degree of differentiation, and depth of invasion.[11] SCCs originating on the lip (Figure 20-26) or from apparently normal skin are aggressive and have an affinity to metastasize to the regional lymph nodes and beyond. SCC arising from actinic keratosis may have a thick adherent scale. The tumor is soft and freely movable and may have a red inflamed base. These lesions are most frequently observed on the bald scalp, forehead (Figure 20-27), and backs of the hands (Figure 20-28). Cutaneous horns may begin as actinic keratosis and degenerate into SCC.

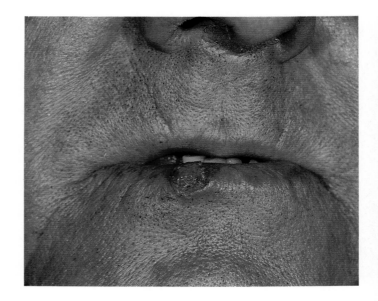

Figure 20-26
Squamous cell carcinoma. The sun-exposed lower lip is a common site for squamous cell carcinoma.

Those SCCs beginning in actinically damaged skin, but not from actinic keratosis, appear as firm, movable, elevated masses with a sharply defined border and little surface scale (Figure 20-29). Small squamous cell carcinomas evolving from actinic keratosis are treated by electrodesiccation and curettage. Larger tumors or those on or near the vermilion border of the lips are best excised. Larger tumors or those around the nose and eyes require special consideration; see the section on treatment of basal cell carcinoma located in these specific areas. Regional lymph nodes should be clinically examined.

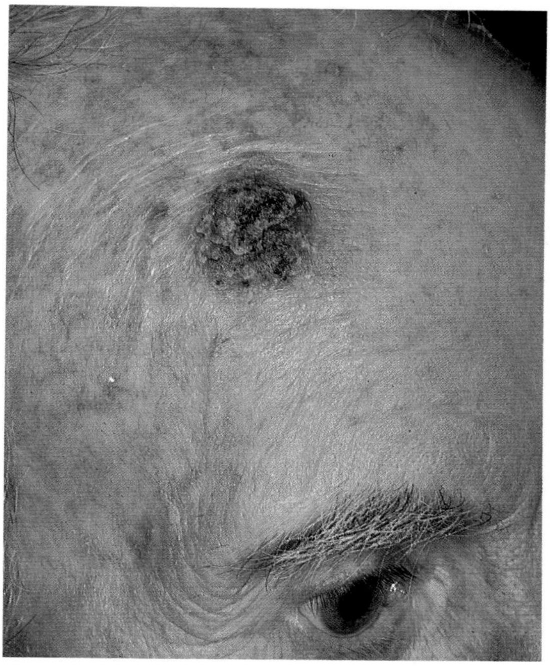

Figure 20-27
Squamous cell carcinoma. Malignant degeneration occurred in an actinic keratosis that had been present for years.

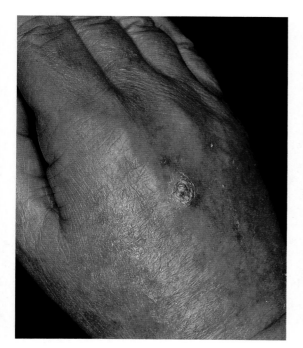

Figure 20-28
Squamous cell carcinoma. Malignant degeneration of an actinic keratosis.

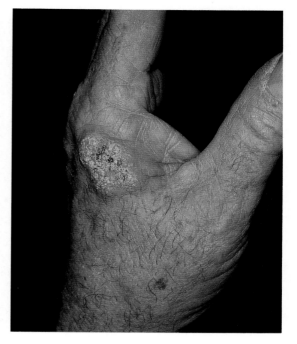

Figure 20-29
Squamous cell carcinoma. The mass grew rapidly and there was no history of a preexisting actinic keratosis.

Bowen's Disease

Bowen's disease, also referred to as squamous cell carcinoma in situ, appears on any part of the body as a slightly elevated, red, scaling plaque with well-defined borders (Figures 20-30 and 20-31). Bowen's disease may closely resemble psoriasis (Figure 20-32), chronic eczema, or superficial basal cell carcinoma. The plaque grows very slowly by lateral extension and may eventually, after several months or years, invade the dermis, producing induration and ulceration. When confined to the epidermis, the atypical cells, in contrast to actinic keratosis, involve epidermal appendages, particularly the hair follicle (Figure 20-33). Atypical cells are also found at the periphery of lesions in clinically uninvolved skin. Atypical cells in the epidermal lining of the hair follicle, while still confined to the epidermis, are deeper and more difficult to reach by treatment modalities such as topical 5-FU or electrosurgery, which permit access only to superficial areas. The cause of this disease is unknown, but several patients with this rare disease were formerly treated with arsenic. Association of Bowen's disease with internal malignancy has been suggested by some studies, but refuted by others.[12,13]

Small lesions may be successfully treated with electrodesiccation and curettage or cryosurgery. Larger lesions are treated with 5-FU cream applied twice a day for 4 to 8 weeks. Treatment is discontinued when erosion and superficial necrosis occur. A large area surrounding the lesion should be treated to destroy the clinically inapparent disease. Some authors suggest plastic occlusion to enhance penetration to the hair follicle.[14] Close followup of patients after treatment is required because recurrences are relatively common.

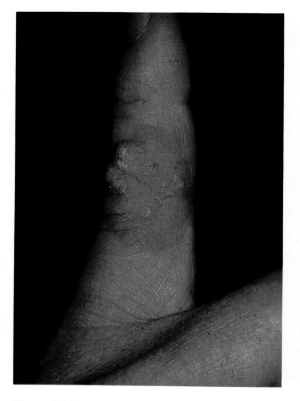

Figure 20-30
Bowen's disease. The red plaque is well defined with scale and some crust on the surface.

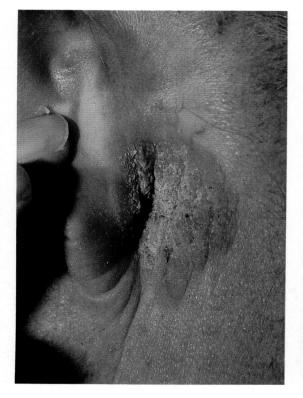

Figure 20-31
Bowen's disease. The plaque is more indurated than the lesion depicted in Figure 20-30. Scale and crust cover much of the surface.

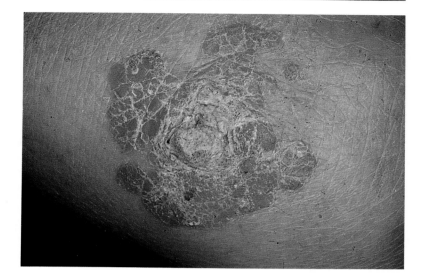

Figure 20-32
Bowen's disease. The well-defined borders and silvery scale impart a psoriasiform quality to this lesion.

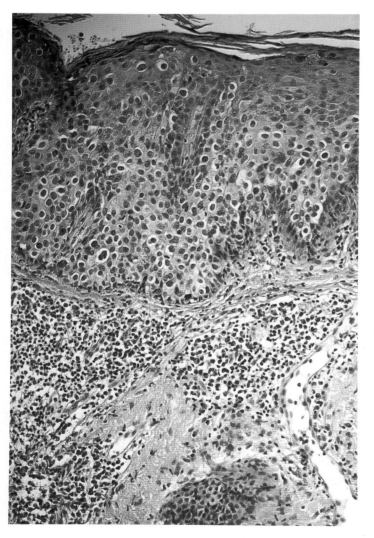

Figure 20-33
Bowen's disease. Atypical cells are present throughout the entire thickness of the epidermis. The dermoepidermal junction remains distinct and intact.

Erythroplasia of Queyrat

Clinically and histologically, erythroplasia of Queyrat of the penis resembles Bowen's disease and is probably the same entity. It appears exclusively under the foreskin of the uncircumcised penis and is a moist, slightly raised, well-defined, red, smooth or velvety plaque (Figure 20-34). Like Bowen's disease of the skin, it grows slowly and has the potential for degeneration into squamous cell carcinoma. Similar lesions may occur on the vulva. 5-FU cream is the treatment of choice and recurrences are unlikely because the hair follicles that serve as foci for recurrence are absent on the penile mucosa.[15]

Bowenoid Papulosis

Wade et al[16] described an apparently new condition, Bowenoid papulosis of the genitalia (vulva and circumcised penis), which histologically resembles Bowen's disease. It occurs in individuals between the ages of 15 to 30 for periods of 2 months to 10 years. Many patients have a history of genital infection with viral warts or herpes simplex. Asymptomatic, discrete, slightly scaly, skin-colored to violaceous papules averaging 4 mm and plaques are located on the vulva, shaft and, less frequently, glans. They appear to remain indolent, but their biologic potential is unknown. Treat for 3 to 5 weeks with 5% 5-FU cream until inflamed or remove with electrodesiccation and curettage or cryosurgery.

Figure 20-34
Erythroplasia of Queyrat. A moist, glistening, slightly raised plaque. Similar lesions may occur on the vulva.

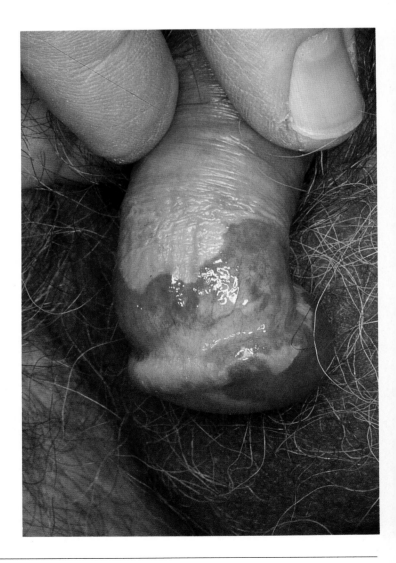

Leukoplakia

The term leukoplakia is used to designate a white patch on the vermilion border of the lips, oral mucosa, or vulva that, histologically, exhibits changes varying from mild scaling and epidermal thickening to carcinoma in situ. Clinically, the patches are white, slightly elevated, usually well-defined plaques that show little tendency to extend peripherally. A small percentage of lesions may eventually degenerate into squamous cell carcinoma. The differential diagnosis includes candidiasis, lichen planus, habitual cheek biting, and white sponge nevus. Small lesions may be biopsied and simply followed if the histology is benign. Excise, electrodesiccate, or freeze with liquid nitrogen plaques that histologically exhibit atypical features.

Leukoplakia of the vulva and the lip can be successfully treated with 5-FU. Lip lesions are treated twice daily with applications of 1% 5-FU solution until erythema and erosions become marked, about 10 to 21 days. Discomfort is intense and can be relieved with cool compresses or topical lidocaine gel. Cigarette or pipe smoking, the probable cause in many cases, must be terminated.

Marjolin's Ulcer

Squamous cell carcinomas that occur at sites of chronic inflammation (Marjolin's ulcers) are more aggressive than those that develop from actinic keratosis or Bowen's disease.[17] They occur in unstable burn or radiation scars, stasis ulcers, and chronic sinus tracts of osteomyelitis. Their appearance is masked by inflamed hypertrophic tissue.

Verrucous Carcinoma

Verrucous carcinoma is a term encompassing three rare entities: epithelioma cuniculatum (plantar surface of the foot), giant condylomata of Buschke-Lowenstein (perineum), and oral florid papillomatosis. Histologically, the tumor displays epidermal thickening with local invasion minus cellular atypia. With few exceptions, metastasis is rare. In their early stages all tumors may be mistaken for warts (Figure 20-35). However, tumors are unresponsive to locally destructive procedures and slowly over months or years increase in size, become indurated, and deeply penetrate the dermis. Conservative local excision or Mohs' chemosurgery is the treatment of choice.[18]

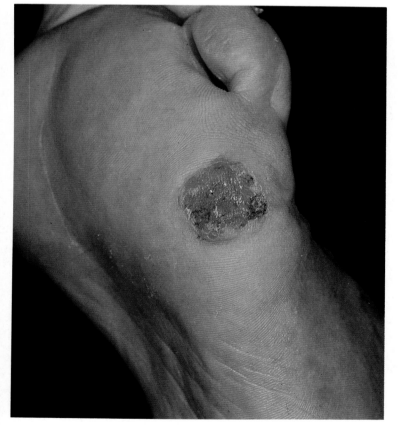

Figure 20-35
*Verrucous carcinoma
(epithelioma cuniculatum).
A lesion present for months,
which was suspected of being
a plantar wart.*

Arsenical Keratoses and Other Arsenic-Related Skin Diseases

Pentavalent, inorganic arsenic dispensed years ago for psoriasis and other diseases may cause a number of problems. Arsenical keratoses are discrete, round, wart-like or pointed keratotic lesions appearing 20 or more years after long-term arsenic ingestion (Figure 20-36). Arsenical keratoses may degenerate into squamous cell carcinoma. Lesions are most common on the palms and soles, but may occur elsewhere. Bowen's disease, multiple basal cell carcinomas, and changes in pigmentation characterized by small, round, white macules ("rain drops on a hyperpigmented background") are additional findings in patients with chronic arsenic ingestion. No treatment is necessary for arsenical keratosis unless signs of degeneration occur.

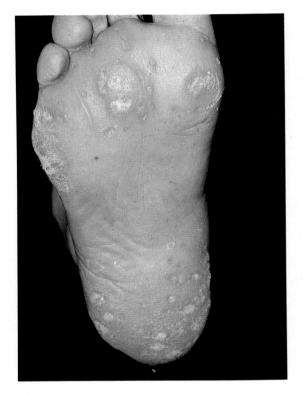

Figure 20-36
Arsenical keratoses. Discrete, wart-like keratotic lesions occur on the palms and soles.

Mycosis Fungoides

Mycosis fungoides (MF) is a rare T-cell lymphoma[19] that probably originates in the skin and occurs in the fifth and sixth decades. The name is misleading because the disease is not of fungal origin. The course is unpredictable, sometimes resulting in death in less than 1 year and sometimes lasting for several decades. There are three phases in the evolution of the disease; when the third or tumor phase has begun, survival time is less than 3 years.[20]

The early manifestations are those of a persistent, nonspecific, itchy, eczematous eruption. This premycotic phase persists for months or years. The rash resembles asteatotic eczema or atopic dermatitis with the exception that the involved areas tend to remain fixed in location and size and the margins are sharply delineated. Spontaneous remissions do occur. Parapsoriasis en plaque and poikiloderma atrophicans vasculare have characteristic features that allow one to predict with a greater degree of certainty that the evolution of typical MF may occur.

Poikiloderma atrophicans vasculare occurs on the abdomen, buttock, and thigh as plaques with telangiectasia, fine wrinkly atrophy, and mottled pigmentation (Figure 20-37). The form of parapsoriasis that evolves into MF has the morphologic features of poikiloderma, but the plaques may be smaller and more widespread. Histologic examination of these early lesions reveals a superficial perivascular infiltrate composed of small lymphocytes. A scant number of lymphocytes may be found in the epidermis.

Gradually, the second or plaque stage is entered when dusky red-to-brown, sometimes scaly plaques develop and itching becomes more persistent and intense. The plaques vary in shape with round, oval, arciform, or serpiginous patterns, occasionally with central clearing. The extent of involvement varies from a few isolated areas to involvement of a major portion of the skin (Figure 20-38). Itching may be intolerable. Histologically, the plaques exhibit a superficial, deep, perivascular lymphocytic infiltrate with collections of lymphocytes (Pautrier's microabscesses) within a thickened epidermis. The infiltrate becomes mixed (lymphocytes, eosinophils, and plasma cells) as the plaque stage progresses. Some of the lymphocytes are atypical, retaining a large, hyperconvoluted or cerebriform nucleus ("mycosis cell") (see Figure 20-41). The plaque stage persists for an indefinite period. Plaques either regress, remain stationary, or evolve into nodules and tumors.

Tumors develop from preexisting plaques or originate from red or normal skin (Figure 20-39). Itching may decrease in intensity. Tumors vary in size, some becoming huge or mushroom-shaped; there-

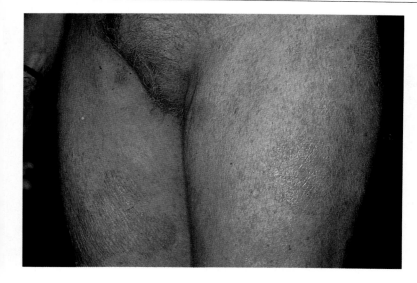

Figure 20-37
Mycosis fungoides
(poikiloderma vasculare
atrophicans). Red-brown
hyperpigmented plaques
with an atrophic, wrinkled
surface tend to remain fixed
in location.

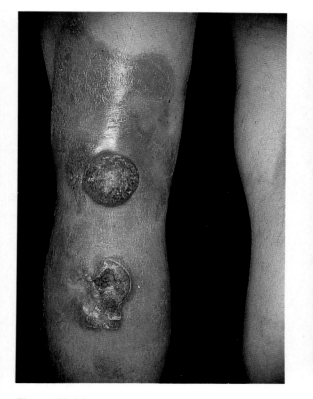

Figure 20-38
Mycosis fungoides. Plaque and tumor stage.

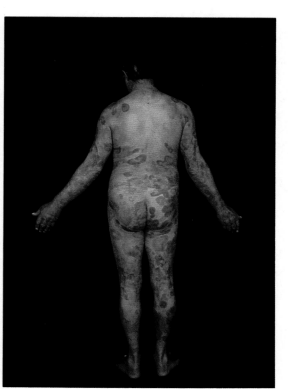

Figure 20-39
Mycosis fungoides. Tumor stage.

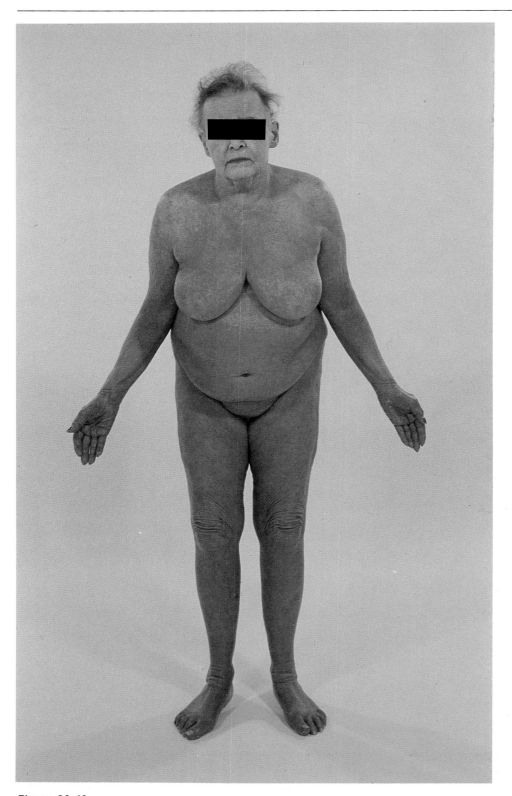

Figure 20-40
*Sézary syndrome. Generalized erythroderma with
scaling and thickening of the palms and soles.*

fore, the term mycosis, in use for 150 years. Necrosis and ulceration of plaques and tumors are common.

In the early stages the disease remains confined to the skin. Superficial lymphadenopathy may be detected in the plaque stage and deep lymphadenopathy with visceral metastasis, such as to spleen, lungs, or gastrointestinal tract, may occur during the tumor stage.[21]

A closely related disease called the Sézary syndrome is regarded by many observers as the leukemic form of MF[22] (Figure 20-40). Sézary syndrome is characterized by erythroderma with pruritus, scaling, and thickening of the palms and soles. Skin biopsy may reveal features resembling those found in the early stages of classic MF. Circulating cells with hyperconvoluted nuclei (Sézary cells) appear to be identical to those found in the skin infiltrates of MF[23] (Figure 20-41).

The following are the most commonly used treatments for the early stages of MF: topical nitrogen mustard,[24] total body surface electron beam therapy,[25] PUVA (oral psoralens with long-wave ultraviolet light),[26] and topical BCNU [1,3-bis(2-chloroethyl)-1-nitrosourea].[27] Systemic chemotherapy is indicated for the tumor or visceral stages. All of these treatment modalities may be initially successful in inducing remissions, but none appear to prolong survival.

The etiology of this unusual disease is unknown. One theory states that, in predisposed individuals, chronic occupational exposure to industrial or environmental allergens results in persistent antigenic stimulation.[28] This stimulation incites a chronic, inflammatory response in the skin, leading to a breakdown of immune surveillance eventually resulting in malignancy.

Figure 20-41
Sézary cells. Nuclei are hyperconvoluted.

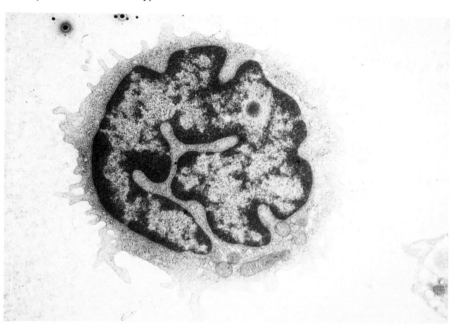

Paget's Disease of the Breast

Paget's disease of the breast, a unilateral disease of the breast, results from invasion of the epidermis of the nipple, areola, and surrounding skin by malignant cells originating from an underlying ductal carcinoma.[29] The disease begins insidiously in one breast with a small area of erythema on the nipple, which drains serous fluid and forms crust. The inflammation is attributed to trauma, and partial healing comforts the patient. Patients equate lumps rather than inflammatory changes with cancer and consequently fail to seek treatment, and the disease continues. Malignant cells migrate through the epidermis and the disease becomes initially apparent on the areola and, at a much later date (a year or more), on the surrounding skin (Figure 20-42). The process appears eczematous, but the plaque is indurated and has sharp margins that remain relatively fixed in location for weeks. Clinically and histologically, the process is very similar to Bowen's disease; however, Bowen's disease of the nipple is rare. Ulceration is a late finding.

An underlying carcinoma of the breast may be palpated. Treatment after biopsy is surgical. A crucial point to note is that Paget's disease of the breast is a unilateral disease, whereas eczematous inflammation of the nipples is common and nearly invariably bilateral. Paget's disease of the male nipple is extremely rare and is more aggressive than disease in females.[30]

Figure 20-42
Paget's disease of the breast. A red scaling plaque drains serous fluid and forms crust. The lesion appears eczematous but, unlike eczema, is unilateral.

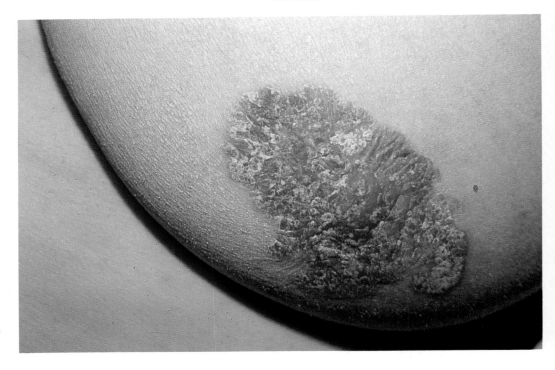

Extramammary Paget's Disease

Paget's disease of the anogenital region is a rare disease occurring in elderly men and women. The disease may be associated with an underlying adenocarcinoma or carcinoma of the rectum. As with Paget's disease of the breast, the epidermis is infiltrated with malignant cells that migrate laterally. Biopsy often reveals cells that are exterior to the clinically apparent areas, a fact explaining the high rate of recurrence after excision. The disease in females appears as a white-to-red, scaling or macerated, infiltrated plaque, most frequently observed on the labia majora (Figure 20-43). Persistent itching and burning are common. The clinical presentation closely resembles lichen sclerosis et atrophicus, lichen simplex chronicus, leukoplakia, or chronic yeast infection. Surgery is the treatment of choice. Recurrent Paget's disease of the vulva has been treated successfully with topical bleomycin.[31]

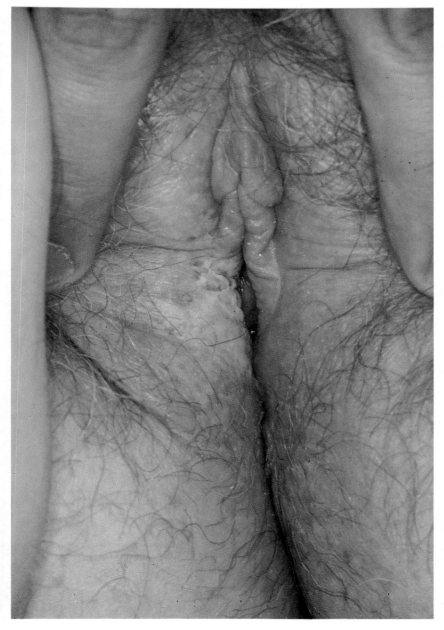

Figure 20-43
Extramammary Paget's disease. A white plaque with ill-defined borders on the labia.

Cutaneous Metastasis

The incidence of cutaneous metastasis in patients with malignancy is approximately 1% or 2%. In a series of papers Brownstein and Helwig described several aspects of cutaneous metastasis.[32-34] They determined the incidence and relative importance of the sex of the patient, location of the metastatic growth, morphology of the metastatic lesion, and histologic features of the metastatic lesions in identifying the site of the primary tumor. The incidence of some of these features is summarized in Tables 20-3 and 20-4 and illustrated in Figure 20-44. The most helpful information for localizing the primary tumor is the sex of the patient and the location of the skin tumor.

TABLE 20-3

METASTATIC TUMORS OF THE SKIN: SITE OF PRIMARY TUMOR BY SEX OF PATIENT

Primary tumor	Men		Women	
	No.	%	No.	%
Lung	117	24	9	4
Large intestine	90	19	22	9
Melanoma	62	13	13	5
Oral cavity (squamous cell carcinoma)	57	12	2	1
Kidney	29	6	1	0
Stomach	28	6	1	0
Esophagus	15	3	0	0
Sarcoma*	15	3	4	2
Pancreas	12	2	3	2
Breast	9	2	168	169
Urinary bladder	8	2	2	1
Salivary glands (adenocarcinoma)	8	2	0	0
Prostate	5	1	—	—
Skin (squamous cell carcinoma)	5	1	0	0
Thyroid	4	1	0	0
Penis (squamous cell carcinoma)	3	1	—	—
Liver	3	1	0	0
Gallbladder	2	0	1	0
Testicle	2	0	—	—
Small intestine	2	0	1	0
Ovary	—	—	10	4
Uterine cervix	—	—	4	2
Miscellaneous	6	1	1	0
TOTAL	482	100	242	99†

From Brownstein MH, Helwig EB: Metastatic tumors of the skin. Cancer **29**:1298, 1972.
*Includes leiomyosarcoma, rhabdomyosarcoma, fibrosarcoma, chondrosarcoma, Ewing's sarcoma, osteogenic sarcoma, and undifferentiated sarcomas.
†Percentages do not add to 100 because of rounding.

TABLE 20-4

METASTATIC TUMORS OF THE SKIN: PRIMARY TUMORS BY SITE OF
CUTANEOUS METASTASIS IN MEN

Primary tumor	Scalp	Face	Neck	Upper extremities	Chest	Abdomen	Back	Pelvis	Lower extremities	Multiple sites	Total
Lung	12	6	10	6	39	16	17	2	3	6	117
Large intestine	1	1	2	4	4	40	3	33	1	1	90
Melanoma	1	4	3	10	15	4	10	3	11	1	62
Oral cavity	0	12	41	1	1	0	0	0	1	1	57
Kidney	5	6	1	4	3	4	3	1	2	0	29
Stomach	1	1	2	1	4	16	1	0	0	2	28
Esophagus	0	3	4	0	3	1	3	1	0	0	15
Sarcoma	1	3	2	0	3	2	2	1	0	1	15
Other	1	5	10	3	15	23	2	4	1	5	69
TOTAL	22	41	75	29	87	106	41	45	19	17	482

From Brownstein MH, Helwig EB: Metastatic tumors of the skin. Cancer **29**:1298, 1972.

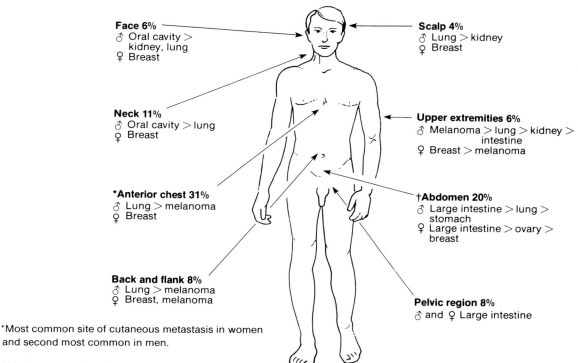

Face 6%
♂ Oral cavity >
   kidney, lung
♀ Breast

Scalp 4%
♂ Lung > kidney
♀ Breast

Neck 11%
♂ Oral cavity > lung
♀ Breast

Upper extremities 6%
♂ Melanoma > lung > kidney >
   intestine
♀ Breast > melanoma

*Anterior chest 31%
♂ Lung > melanoma
♀ Breast

†Abdomen 20%
♂ Large intestine > lung >
   stomach
♀ Large intestine > ovary >
   breast

Back and flank 8%
♂ Lung > melanoma
♀ Breast, melanoma

Pelvic region 8%
♂ and ♀ Large intestine

*Most common site of cutaneous metastasis in women and second most common in men.

†Most common site of cutaneous metastasis in men and second most common in women.

Figure 20-44
Patterns of cutaneous metastasis. 724 patients. Percentages are of total number of cases. (Adapted from Brownstein MN, Helwig EB: Arch Dermatol **105**:862, 1972.)

Morphology of metastatic lesions. The most common representation of cutaneous metastasis is an aggregate of discrete, firm, nontender, skin-colored nodules that appear suddenly, grow rapidly, attain a certain size (often 2 cm), and remain stationary (Figure 20-45). Accurate clinical diagnosis is rare; the lesions are most frequently diagnosed as cysts or benign fibrous tumors. In several instances the clinical picture is that of a vascular tumor such as a pyogenic granuloma, hemangioma, or Kaposi's sarcoma (Figure 20-46).

The second most common pattern of cutaneous metastasis is inflammation with erythema, edema, warmth (Figures 20-47 and 20-48), and tenderness. The primary tumor is usually in the breast, and malignant cells spread to the subepidermal lymphatic vessels where they create obstruction. The initial diagnosis is frequently a bacterial infection such as erysipelas or cellulitis. The patient is, however, afebrile and appears healthy.

The third and least common pattern simulates a cicatricial condition and resembles discoid lupus erythematosus or morphea. Asymptomatic sclerodermoid plaques, sometimes associated with hair loss, are most frequently located on the scalp and are caused by metastasis from breast cancer.

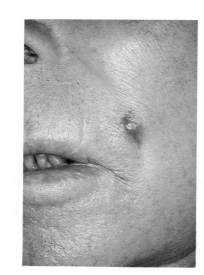

Figure 20-45
Metastatic carcinoma of the prostate. Clinical diagnosis was basal cell carcinoma.

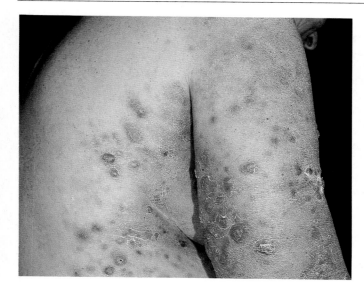

Figure 20-46
Metastatic carcinoma of the breast. Nodules appear vascular and resemble Kaposi's sarcoma.

Figure 20-47
Inflammatory cutaneous metastasis with erythema, edema, and crusting.

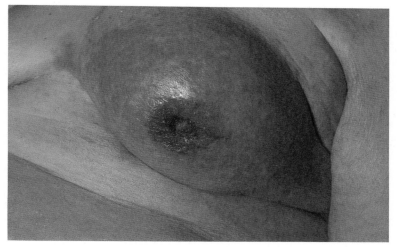

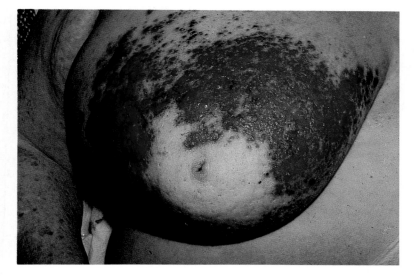

Figure 20-48
Inflammatory cutaneous metastasis. Erosion and crusting resemble infected eczema.

Histology of cutaneous metastasis. In general the histologic features[32-34] of the primary and metastatic tumor are similar, but the metastatic tumors are often less differentiated. Frequently, biopsy specimens are not interpreted as originating from a distant site. Adenocarcinoma metastatic to the skin is most often secondary to cancer of the large intestine, lung, or breast. Squamous cell carcinoma metastatic to the skin generally originates from the oral cavity, lung, or esophagus. Undifferentiated lesions usually originate from the breast or lungs.

Mode of spread. Tumors that invade veins, such as carcinoma of the kidney and lung, frequently occur as cutaneous metastasis in diverse skin sites distant from the primary tumor. Cancers that invade lymphatics, such as carcinoma of the breast and squamous cell carcinoma of the oral cavity, appear late in the course of the disease and may invade skin overlying the primary tumor.

REFERENCES

1. Domarus HV, Steven PJ: Metastatic basal cell carcinoma. J Am Acad Dermatol 10:1043, 1984.
2. Totten JR: The multiple nevoid basal cell carcinoma syndrome. Cancer 46:1456, 1980.
3. Kopf AW, Bart RS, Schrager D, et al: Curettage-electrodesiccation treatment of basal cell carcinomas. Arch Dermatol 113:439, 1977.
4. Whelan CS, Deckers PJ: Electrocoagulation for skin cancer: an old oncologic tool revisited. Cancer 47:2280, 1981.
5. Salasche SJ: Curettage and electrodesiccation in the treatment of midfacial basal cell epithelioma. J Am Acad Dermatol 8:496, 1983.
6. Albright SD: Treatment of skin cancer using multiple modalities. J Am Acad Dermatol 7:143, 1982.
7. Labandter HP, Ryan RF: 5 fluorouracil in management of Gorlin's syndrome. N Engl J Med 298:913, 1978.
8. Moller R, Reymann F, Hou-Jensen K: Metastases in dermatological patients with squamous cell carcinoma. Arch Dermatol 115:703, 1979.
9. Goette DK: Topical chemotherapy with 5-fluorouracil: a review. J Am Acad Dermatol 4:633, 1981.
10. Simmonds WL: Management of actinic keratosis with topical 5-fluorouracil. Cutis 18:298, 1976.
11. Immerman SC, Scanlon EF, Christ M, et al: Recurrent squamous cell carcinoma of the skin. Cancer 51:1537, 1983.
12. Callen JP, Headington J: Bowen's and non-Bowen's squamous intraepidermal neoplasia of the skin: relationship to internal malignancy. Arch Dermatol 116:422, 1980.
13. Andersen S LaC, Nielsen A, Reymann F: Relationship between Bowen disease and internal malignant tumors. Arch Dermatol 108:367, 1973.
14. Sturm HM: Bowen's disease and 5-fluorouracil. J Am Acad Dermatol 1:513, 1979.
15. Goette DK, Elgart M, DeVillez RL, et al: Erythroplasia of Queyrat: treatment with topically applied 5-fluorouracil. JAMA 232:934, 1975.
16. Wade TR, Kopf AW, Ackerman AB: Bowenoid papulosis of the genitalia. Arch Dermatol 115:306, 1979.
17. Barr LH, Menard JW: Marjolin's ulcer. Cancer 52:173, 1983.
18. Mora RG: Microscopically controlled surgery (Mohs' chemosurgery) for treatment of verrucous squamous cell carcinoma of the foot (epithelioma cuniculatum). J Am Acad Dermatol 8:354, 1983.
19. Kung PC, Berger CL, Goldstein G, et al: Cutaneous T cell lymphoma: characterization by monoclonal antibodies. Blood 57:261, 1981.
20. Epstein EH Jr, Levin DL, Croft JD Jr, et al: Mycosis fungoides: survival, prognostic features, response to therapy, and autopsy findings. Medicine 15:61, 1972.
21. Long JC, Mihm MC: Mycosis fungoides with extracutaneous dissemination: a distinct clinicopathologic entity. Cancer 34:1745, 1974.
22. Miller RA, Coleman CN, Fawcett HD, et al: Sezary syndrome: a model for migration of T lymphocytes to skin. N Engl J Med 303:89, 1980.
23. Edelson RL: Cutaneous T cell lymphoma: mycosis fungoides, Sezary syndrome, and other variants. J Am Acad Dermatol 2:89, 1980.
24. Halprin KM, Comerford M, Presser SE, et al: Ultraviolet light treatment delays contact sensitization to nitrogen mustard. Br J Dermatol 105:71, 1981.
25. Niscle LZ, Safai B, Kim JH: Effectiveness of once-weekly total skin electron beam therapy in mycosis fungoides and Sezary syndrome. Cancer 47:870, 1981.
26. Molin L, Thomsen K, Volden G, et al: Photochemotherapy (PUVA) in pretumor stage of mycosis fungoides: report from the Scandinavian Mycosis Fungoides Study Group. Acta Derm Venereol 61:47, 1980.
27. Zackheim HS, Epstein EH Jr: Treatment of mycosis fungoides with topical nitrosourea compounds: further studies. Arch Dermatol 111:1564, 1975.
28. Thiers BH: Controversies in mycosis fungoides. J Am Acad Dermatol 7:1, 1982.
29. Paone JF, Baker RR: Pathogenesis and treatment of Paget's disease of the breast. Cancer 48:825, 1981.
30. Satiani B, Powell RW, Mathews WH: Paget's disease of the male breast. Arch Surg 112:587, 1977.
31. Watring WG, Roberts JA, Lagasse LD, et al: Treatment of recurrent Paget's disease of the vulva with topical bleomycin. Cancer 41:10, 1978.
32. Brownstein MH, Helwig EB: Metastatic tumors of the skin. Cancer 29:1298, 1972.
33. Brownstein MH, Helwig EB: Patterns of cutaneous metastasis. Arch Dermatol 105:862, 1972.
34. Brownstein MH, Helwig EB: Spread of tumors to the skin. Arch Dermatol 107:80, 1973.

Chapter Twenty-One

Nevi and Malignant Melanoma

Melanocytic nevi
    Common forms
    Special forms
    Management
Malignant melanoma
    Dysplastic nevi
    Benign lesions that resemble melanoma
    Management

Melanocytic Nevi

Nevi, or moles, are benign tumors composed of nevus cells derived from melanocytes. Moles are so common that they appear on virtually every person. They are present in 1% of newborns and increase in incidence throughout infancy and childhood, reaching a peak at puberty. Size and pigmentation may increase at puberty and during pregnancy. A few may continue to appear throughout life. These tumors exist in a variety of characteristic forms that must be recognized to distinguish them from malignant melanocytic tumors, or melanomas. Except for certain types, such as large congenital nevi and dysplastic nevi, most nevi have a very low malignancy potential.

There are many myths concerning moles, such as that hairs should not be plucked and that moles should not be removed or disturbed. These myths should be clarified. The well-publicized increase in the incidence of melanoma has stimulated the lay person's interest and concern regarding pigmented lesions.

Nevi may occur anywhere on the cutaneous surface. There is a strong correlation between sun exposure and number of nevi. Acquired nevi on the buttock or female breast are unusual.

Nevi vary in size, shape, surface characteristics, and color. The important fact to remember is that each nevus tends to remain uniform, retaining a uniform color and shape. Although various shades of brown and black may be present in a single lesion, the colors are distributed over the surface in a uniform pattern.

Melanomas consist of malignant pigment cells that grow and extend with little constraint through the epidermis and into the dermis. Such unrestricted growth produces a lesion with a haphazard or disorganized appearance, which varies in shape, color, and surface characteristics. The characteristics of uniformity cannot always be relied on to differentiate benign from malignant lesions. Very early melanomas may appear quite uniform, having a round or oval shape with a homogeneous brown color. Careful inspection of such lesions with a powerful hand lens may reveal irregularities in the border or minute areas of regression.

Common forms

Nevi may be classified as acquired or congenital, but a clinical classification based on appearance and conventional nomenclature will be used here.

During childhood, nevi begin as flat junction nevi; they evolve into compound nevi and later become dermal nevi in adulthood. However, this evolution does not occur consistently. The subdivision into three types of nevi is based on the location of the nevus cells in the skin (Table 21-1). Nevi with cells confined to the dermoepidermal junction area tend to be flat, whereas those with cells confined to the dermis are usually elevated.

Junction nevi. Junction nevi are flat (macular) or slightly elevated. They are light brown to brown-black, with uniform pigmentation that may be slightly irregular with a reticular black pattern (Figures 21-1 to 21-3). The surface is smooth and flat-to-slightly-elevated, and the border is round or oval and symmetric. Most lesions are hairless. The size varies from 0.1 to 0.6 cm; some are larger. Junction nevi may change into compound nevi after childhood but remain as junction nevi on palms, soles, and genitalia. Junction nevi are rare at birth and generally develop after age 2. Degeneration into melanoma is very rare.

TABLE 21-1

CHARACTERISTICS OF NEVI

	Surface	Color	Histology
Junction nevus	Flat, slightly elevated, smooth	Brown, black	Nevus cells at dermoepidermal junction
Compound nevus	Slightly elevated, dome-shaped, smooth, verrucoid (warty)	Flesh, brown, "halo nevus"	Nevus cells at dermoepidermal junction and upper dermis
Dermal nevus	Dome-shaped, smooth, verrucoid (warty), pedunculated (on a stalk), sessile (broad base)	Brown, black, becomes lighter with age; white or translucent with telangiectatic vessels, "halo nevus"	Nevus cells in dermis, sometimes among fat cells

---

Shapes

Slightly elevated

Dome

Flat

Polypoid

Warty

Pedunculated

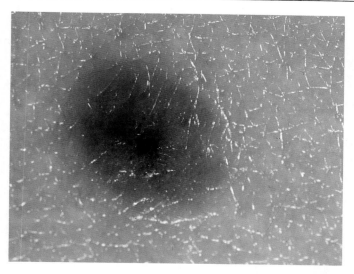

Figure 21-1
Junction nevus. The lesion is flat; pigmentation is darker in the center.

Figure 21-2
Junction nevus. The border is smooth; speckled black pigment is uniformly distributed over the surface.

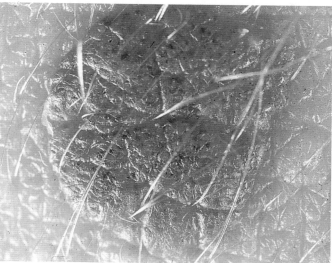

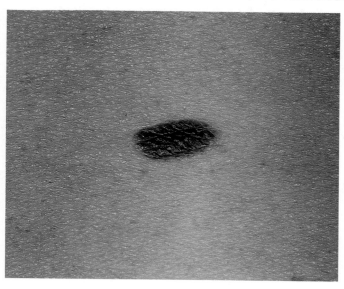

Figure 21-3
Junction nevus. The color and shape of this black lesion are uniform.

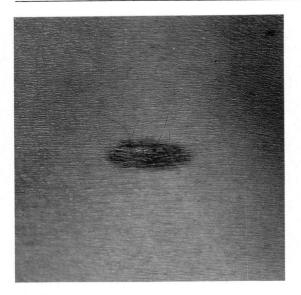

Figure 21-4
Compound nevus. The center is elevated and the surrounding area is flat, retaining the features of a junction nevus.

Compound nevi. Compound nevi are slightly elevated and flesh colored or brown. They are elevated, smooth, or warty and become more elevated with increasing age. They are uniformly round, oval, and symmetric. Hair may be present (Figure 21-4). A white halo may appear at the periphery and the lesion is then referred to as a halo nevus.

Dermal nevi. Dermal nevi are brown or black but may become lighter or flesh colored with age. Lesions vary in size from a few millimeters to a centimeter. The variety of shapes reflects the evolutionary process in which moles extend outward with age and nevus cells degenerate and become replaced by fat and fibrous tissue.

Dome-shaped lesions are the most common (Figures 21-5 and 21-6). They generally appear on the face and are symmetric with a smooth surface. They may be white or translucent with telangiectatic vessels on the surface mimicking basal cell carcinoma. The structure may be warty (Figure 21-7) or polypoid (Figure 21-8). Pedunculated lesions with a narrow stalk are located on the trunk, neck, axilla, and groin. They may appear as a soft, flabby, wrinkled sack (Figure 21-9). Elevated nevi are exposed and are prone to trauma from clothing and so forth; this may result in bleeding and inflammation, influencing patients to perceive them as malignant. White borders may appear, creating a halo nevus. Degeneration to melanoma is very rare, but dermal nevi may resemble nodular melanoma; therefore knowledge of duration is important.

Figure 21-5
Dermal nevus. Dome shaped.

B

A

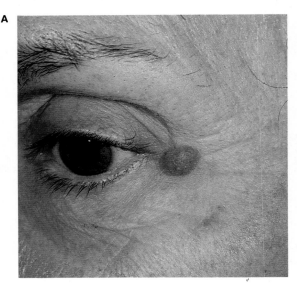

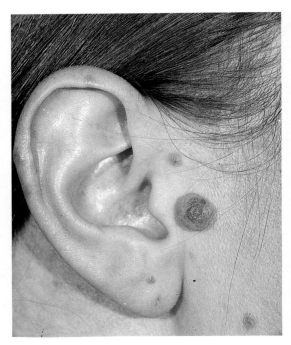

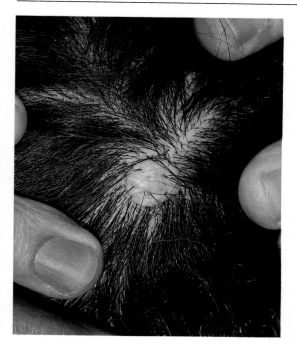

Figure 21-6
Dermal nevus. Flesh colored and dome shaped.

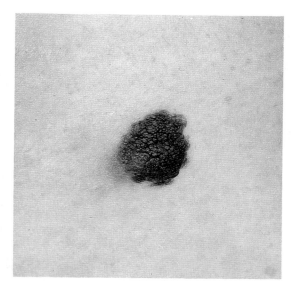

Figure 21-7
Dermal nevus. Warty (verrucous) surface.

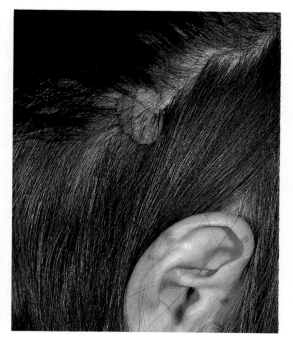

Figure 21-8
Dermal nevus. Polypoid.

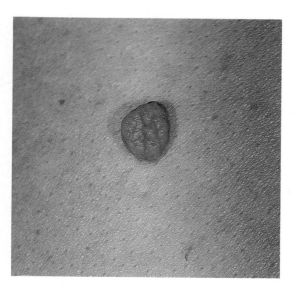

Figure 21-9
Dermal nevus. Papillomatous with a soft, flabby, wrinkled surface.

Special forms

Special forms include congenital nevus, halo nevus, nevus spilus, Becker's nevus, benign juvenile melanoma (Spitz nevus), and blue nevus. These will be discussed below.

Congenital nevi. Congenital nevi (birthmarks) are present at birth and vary in size from a few millimeters to several centimeters covering wide areas of the trunk, an extremity, or the face. Not all pigmented lesions present at birth are congenital nevi; café-au-lait spots may also be present at birth. The largest lesions are referred to as giant hairy nevi. Giant congenital nevi on the trunk are referred to as bathing trunk nevi (Figure 21-10).

Congenital nevi may contain hair; if present, it is usually coarse. They are uniformly pigmented, with various shades of brown or black predominating (Figure 21-11), but red or pink may be a minor or sometimes predominant color (Figure 21-12). Most are flat at birth, but become thicker during childhood and the surface becomes verrucous and sometimes nodular.

The risk of developing melanoma in very large lesions is significant.[1,2] Malignant transformation may occur early in childhood; therefore, large thick lesions should be removed as soon as possible.[3] The risk of developing malignancy may be related to the number of melanocytes and consequently to the size and thickness; however, melanomas have developed in small congenital nevi. The risk of malignant degeneration for smaller congenital nevi is unknown. A report showed histologic features of congenital nevi in 8.1% of melanoma specimens studied.[4] Because of the possibility of malignant degeneration of congenital nevi, some experts recommend that all congenital nevi be considered for prophylactic excision.[5]

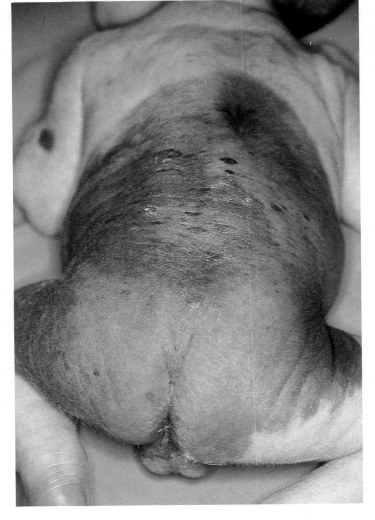

Figure 21-10
Giant congenital nevus (bathing trunk nevus).

Halo nevi. A compound or dermal nevus that develops a white border is called a halo nevus. The depigmented halo is symmetric and round or oval with a sharply demarcated border (Figure 21-13). There are no melanocytes in the halo area and histologically chronic inflammatory cells may be present. Most are located on the trunk; they are absent on palms and soles. Halo nevi develop spontaneously, most commonly during adolescence. They may occur as an isolated phenomenon or several nevi may spontaneously develop halos. Halos may repigment with time or the nevus may disappear. Repigmentation does not follow removal of nevus. The incidence of vitiligo may be increased in patients with halo nevi.[6] A halo rarely develops around malignant melanoma; the halo in such instances is usually not symmetric (Figure 21-22, *E*). Removal of a halo nevus is unnecessary unless the nevus has atypical features. Parental concern over this impressive change is often reason for a conservative excision.

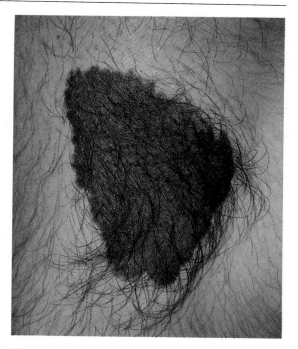

Figure 21-11
Congenital hairy nevus. The border is irregular and appears notched, but that characteristic is maintained in a uniform manner around the entire border.

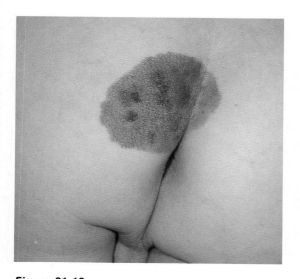

Figure 21-12
Congenital nevus. Pigmentation is variable and nonuniform but a biopsy showed all such areas were benign.

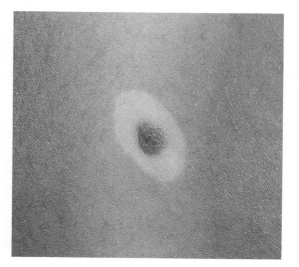

Figure 21-13
Halo nevus. A sharply defined white halo surrounds this compound nevus.

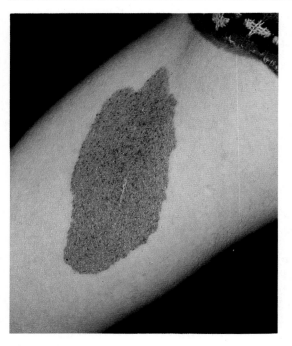

Nevus spilus. Nevus spilus is a hairless, oval, or irregularly shaped brown lesion that is dotted with darker brown-to-black spots.[7,8] The brown area is usually flat and the black dots may be slightly elevated and contain typical nevus cells (Figures 21-14 to 21-16). There is considerable variation in size, ranging from 1 to 20 cm; they may appear at any age. The anatomic position or time of onset is not related to sun exposure. Degeneration into melanoma is not documented.

Becker's nevus. Becker's nevus is not a nevocellular nevus because it lacks nevus cells. The lesion is a developmental anomaly consisting of either a brown macule (Figure 21-17), a patch of hair, or both (Figure 21-18). Nonhairy lesions may develop hair at a later date. The lesions appear in adolescent men on the shoulder, submammary area, and upper and lower back.[9] Becker's nevus varies in size and may enlarge to cover the entire upper arm or shoulder. The border is irregular and sharply demacated. Malignancy has never been reported.

Figure 21-14
Nevus spilus. A large brown macular lesion resembling a café-au-lait spot. Tiny black papules are uniformly distributed over the surface.

Figure 21-15
Nevus spilus. The macular pigmentation is less prominent than in the lesion illustrated in Figure 21-14.

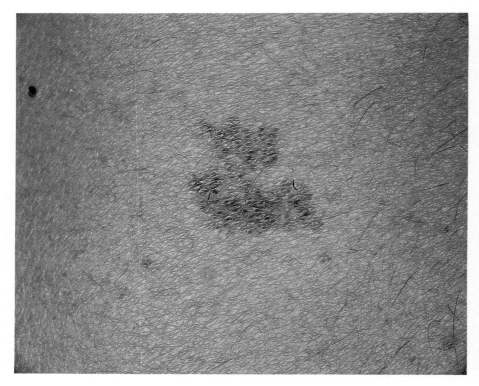

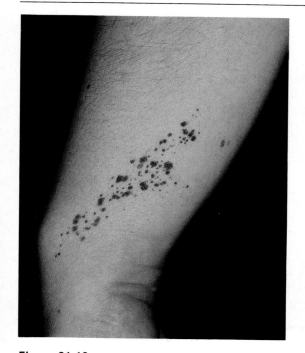

Figure 21-16
Nevus spilus. The macular pigmentation is almost entirely absent. The multiple papules containing nevus cells predominate. Compare this to Figure 21-14.

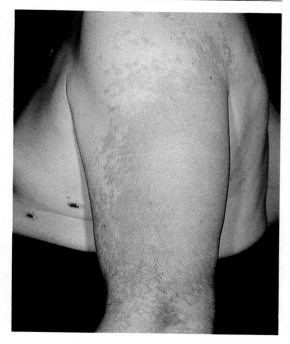

Figure 21-17
Becker's nevus. A huge brown macule. Only a small area of this lesion contains hair.

Figure 21-18
Becker's nevus. A typical lesion with macular pigmentation and hair.

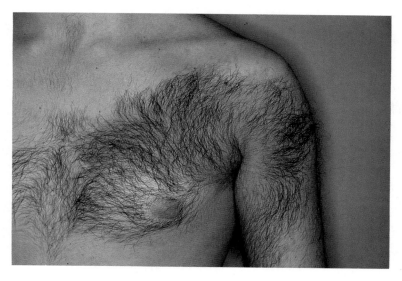

Benign juvenile melanoma. Benign juvenile melanoma (Spitz nevus)[10] is most common in children, but does appear in adults. The term melanoma was used because the clinical and histologic appearance is similar to melanoma. The tumors are hairless, red or reddish-brown, dome-shaped papules or nodules with a smooth (Figure 21-19) or warty surface; they vary in size from 0.3 to 1.5 cm. The color results from increased vascularity, and bleeding sometimes follows trauma. Benign juvenile melanoma are usually solitary, but may be multiple. They appear suddenly and, unlike slowly evolving common moles, patients can sometimes date their onset. The benign juvenile melanoma should be removed for microscopic examination. Histologic differentiation from melanoma is sometimes difficult.

Blue nevus. The blue nevus is a slightly elevated round regular nevus that is usually less than 0.5 cm and contains large amounts of pigment located in the dermis (Figure 21-20). The brown pigment absorbs the longer wavelengths of light and scatters blue light (Tyndall effect). The blue nevus appears in childhood and is most common on the extremities and dorsum of hands. A rare variant, the cellular blue nevus, is larger (usually greater than 1.0 cm), nodular, and frequently located on the buttock. Malignant degeneration of these larger blue nevi into melanomas has been reported.[11]

Figure 21-19
Benign juvenile melanoma (Spitz nevus). A reddish dome-shaped nodule that generally appears in children.

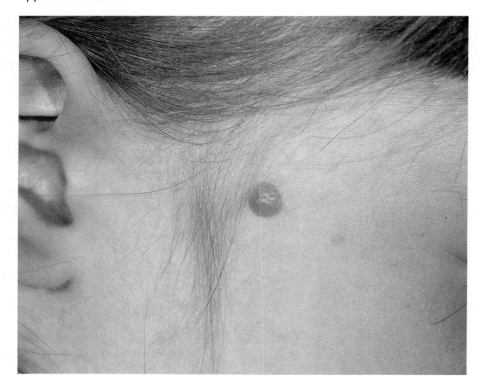

Management

Any pigmented lesion suspected of being malignant should be biopsied or referred for a second opinion. Suspected lesions should be completely removed by excisional biopsy down to and including subcutaneous tissue. (See chapter on cutaneous surgery for techniques.) Patients frequently request removal of nevi for cosmetic purposes. These may be removed either by shave excision or by simple excision and closure with sutures. Most common nevi are small and consequently shave excision is adequate. Some nevus cells remain with shave excision and therefore some repigmentation is possible. Residual pigmentation may be removed at a later time with electrocautery or cryosurgery.

It is good practice to biopsy all pigmented lesions; therefore total removal by electrocautery should be avoided. An unusual histologic picture resembling melanoma may follow partial removal of nevi.[12] In this case the pathologists should always be notified that the submitted tissue was acquired from a previously treated area.

The incidence of melanomas in small congenital nevi is unknown. Some experts suggest that small congenital nevi be considered for prophylactic excision.[5] Large congenital nevi (bathing trunk nevi) are at definite risk for development of melanoma in childhood and are managed by the plastic surgeon.[3]

If parents are concerned, the mole part of a halo nevus may be removed by shave or excision. Nevus spilus is flat and would necessitate excision and closure if the patient desired removal. Becker's nevus is usually too large to remove and is best left untouched. The hair may be shaved or permanently removed. Benign juvenile melanoma should be excised and examined. Blue nevi are deep dermal structures and must be surgically excised if removal is desired.

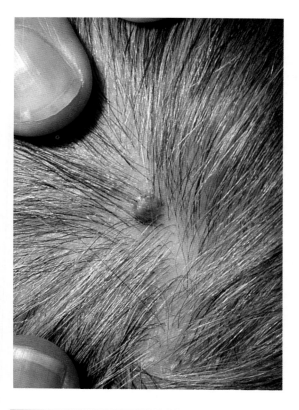

Figure 21-20
Blue nevus. Most lesions are small and round.

Malignant Melanoma

Malignant melanoma is a tumor arising from cells of the melanocytic system. This entity has been recognized for years, but until recently no criteria for its early diagnosis had been established. The incidence of melanoma is increasing and may be reaching epidemic proportions. Alterations of the upper atmosphere by pollutants such as fluorocarbons, resulting in increased UVB radiation, and increased recreational sun exposure may be the two most important factors responsible for the disproportionate rise in the incidence of melanoma.

Malignant melanoma is one of the most dangerous tumors. It has the ability to metastasize to any organ, including the brain and heart. Therefore it is imperative that all physicians be familiar with the features of early preinvasive melanoma and include a complete skin examination as part of routine physical examinations. Referral or excisional biopsy is indicated for suspected lesions. The previous practice of waiting and watching for a change may result in a death. Criteria for the early diagnosis of malignant melanoma have been established and can be appreciated by all physicians and patients.

Signs of malignant transformation. The goal is to recognize melanomas at the earliest stage. Changes in shape and color are important early signs and should always arouse suspicion. Ulceration and bleeding are late signs; hope of cure diminishes greatly if the diagnosis has not been made before such changes. The specific signs that appear during the evolution of each type of melanoma are listed and illustrated on the following pages. A list of all possible changes at all stages of development is presented in Table 21-2.

TABLE 21-2

SIGNS SUGGESTING MALIGNANCY IN PIGMENTED LESIONS

Sign	Implication
Change in color	
Sudden darkening: brown, black	Increased number of tumor cells, the density of which varies within the lesion, creating irregular pigmentation
Spread of color into previously normal skin	Tumor cells migrating through epidermis at various speeds and in different directions (horizontal growth phase)
Red	Vasodilatation and inflammation
White	Areas of regression or inflammation
Blue	Pigment deep in dermis, sign of increasing depth of tumor
Change in characteristics of border	
Irregular outline	Malignant cells migrating horizontally at different rates
Satellite pigmentation	Cells migrating beyond confines of primary tumor
Development of depigmented halo	Destruction of melanocytes by possible immunologic reaction and inflammation
Changes in surface characteristics	
Scaliness	
Erosion	
Oozing	
Crusting	
Bleeding	
Ulceration	
Elevation	
Loss of normal skin lines	
Development of symptoms	
Pruritus	
Tenderness	
Pain	

Characteristics of benign moles. Benign moles have a more uniform tan, brown, or black color. The border is regular and the lesion is roughly symmetric; if the lesion could be folded in half the two halves would superimpose. Most acquired benign moles are 6 mm or less in diameter. Most occurred early in life and the only notable change is a slight uniform elevation during pregnancy or with age.

Clinical classification. Melanoma either begins de novo or develops from a preexisting lesion such as a congenital or dysplastic nevus. A classification into several different types was devised after observing that the microscopic anatomy at the periphery of the elevated tumor mass was variable and showed characteristic patterns that could be correlated with distinctive clinical presentations.[13-15] The proposed types are superficial spreading melanoma (SSM), lentigo maligna melanoma (LMM), nodular melanoma (NM), and acral-lentiginous melanoma (ALM).

Some melanomas do not conform to this clinical-pathologic classification and may be labeled exclusively malignant melanoma. Malignant melanoma may be a single entity that has various clinical and histologic forms varying with the degree of differentiation of the tumor cell. The potential for a melanocyte to degenerate and become neoplastic is probably influenced by a number of factors, including degree of skin pigmentation, heredity, immunologic status, quantity of solar radiation, sex of the individual, and position on the body.

Growth characteristics. Once a melanocyte becomes neoplastic, constraints on its localization are removed and it may leave its assigned position at the basal layer of the epidermis. A well-differentiated malignant melanocyte retains its affinity for the epidermis and may slowly grow horizontally, only to be restrained or eliminated in some areas by a still competent immunologic system. Years of slow growth and regression by a number of such cells on the face produce the LMM. A more immature group of cells would be more aggressive and extend and regress at a faster rate, stimulating new vessel formation and inflammation. Such biologic behavior could be expected to produce the SSM. Melanomas in which the cells are extending laterally are considered to be in the horizontal (radial) growth phase.[16] This phase may endure for months or years. A poorly differentiated cell knows no bounds, has no affinity for the epidermis, and grows both horizontally and vertically, producing a mass or NM. Melanomas in which cells have begun to grow vertically into the dermis and form a mass are considered to be in the vertical growth phase.[16]

The validity of classification by type has yet to be settled. The classification, however, enables one to understand the growth and evolution of malignant melanoma and is therefore an aid in making an early diagnosis. The various types of melanomas have specific characteristics.[17,18]

Superficial spreading melanoma. The SSM (Figure 21-21) is most common in middle age, from the fourth to fifth decade. It develops anywhere on the body, but most frequently on the upper back of both sexes and on the legs of women. SSM begins in a nonspecific manner and then changes shape by radial spread and regression. The random migration of cells, along with the process of regression, results in lesions with an endless variety of shapes and sizes. The shape is bizarre if left untreated for a period of years. The hallmark of SSM is the haphazard combination of many colors, but it may be uniformly brown or black. Colors may become more diverse as time proceeds. A dull red color is frequently observed; this may occupy a small area or dominate the lesion. The precursor radial growth phase may last for months or more than 10 years. Nodules appear when the lesion is approximately 2.5 cm in diameter.[19]

Nodular melanoma. The NM (Figure 21-22) occurs most often in the fifth or sixth decade. It is more frequent in males than females with a ratio of 2:1. It is found anywhere on the body. NM has no radial growth phase.

NM is most commonly dark brown, red-brown, red-black, or occasionally amelanotic (flesh-colored). This is the type most frequently misdiagnosed because it resembles a blood blister, hemangioma, or a flesh-colored dermal nevus. NM is dome-shaped, polypoid, or plaque-like.

Lentigo maligna melanoma. The age of presentation of LMM (Figure 21-23) is usually the sixth or seventh decade. Most are located on the face, but 10% are on other exposed sites, such as arms and legs.

The radial growth phase is called lentigo maligna or Hutchinson's freckle. The radial growth phase may last for 10 years, and a vertical growth phase may never develop.

Years of migration and regression produce lesions with a shape more varied and bizarre than SSM. The color is more uniform than SSM color, but red and white may later occur. Tumors generally are in the center of the lesion away from the border. LMM may ulcerate or undergo changes similar to other lesions when they enter the tumor stage. Nodules are usually single and generally appear when the lesion has reached 5 to 7 cm, but may occur in much smaller lesions.

Text continued on p. 472.

SUPERFICIAL SPREADING MELANOMA

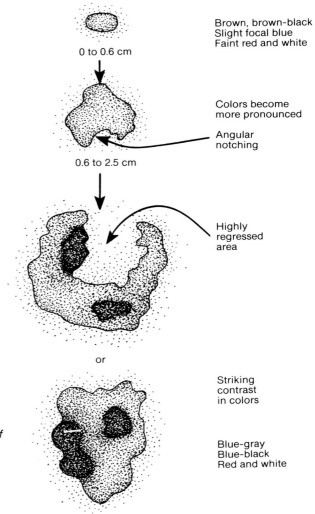

**Initial phase
(months to years)**
1. Flat, not palpable
2. Color variation slight
3. Indistinguishable from other early melanomas

0 to 0.6 cm

Brown, brown-black
Slight focal blue
Faint red and white

**Radial growth phase
(months to 10 years)**
1. Border irregular
2. Areas of regression appear with angular notching
3. Thick areas appear at about 2.5 cm—herald onset of vertical phase

0.6 to 2.5 cm

Colors become more pronounced

Angular notching

**Vertical growth phase
(months to years)**
1. Numerous patterns, depending on degree of growth and regression
2. Tumors palpable
Plaquelike elevation at border
Nodules in center
3. Areas of ulceration and scaling

Highly regressed area

or

Striking contrast in colors

Blue-gray
Blue-black
Red and white

Figure 21-21
Supeficial spreading melanomas in all stages of development. The small early lesions have irregular borders, irregular pigmentation, and small white areas indicating regression. The largest tumors show an accentuation of all of these features. Centimeters indicate size of original lesion.

A

B
1.3 cm

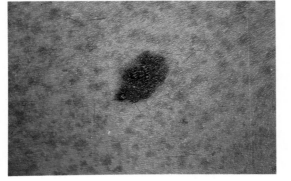

C
1.5 cm

1.3 cm

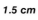

1.5 cm

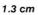

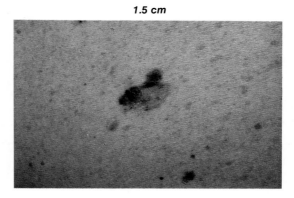

1.5 cm

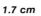

F

G

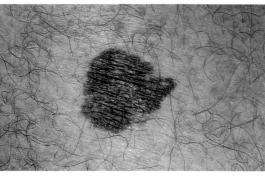

1.7 cm

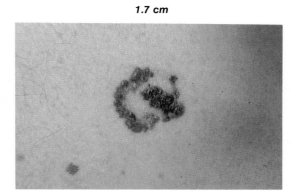

1.7 cm

H

I

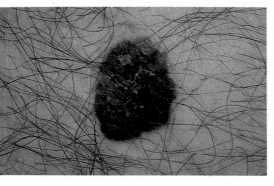

2 cm

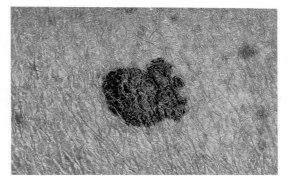

3 cm

J

K

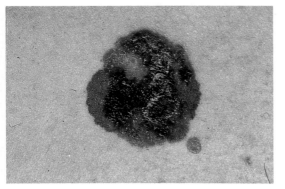

2.8 cm

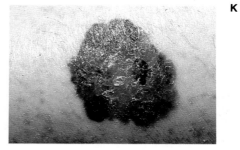

NODULAR MELANOMAS

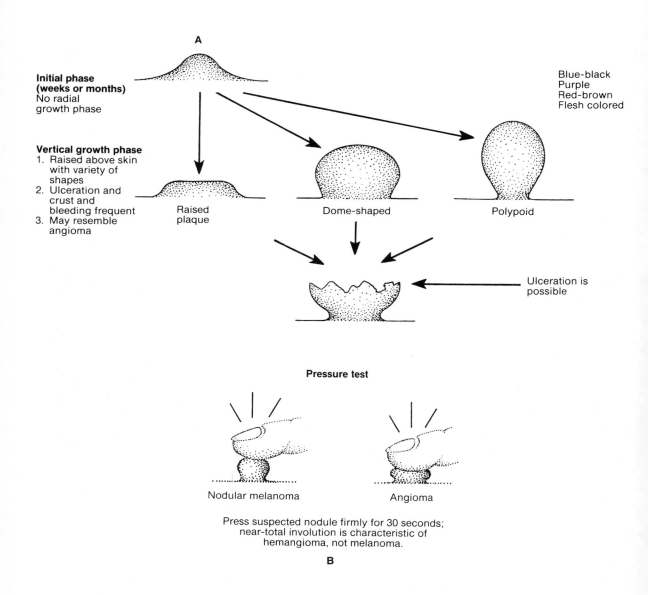

A

**Initial phase
(weeks or months)**
No radial
growth phase

Blue-black
Purple
Red-brown
Flesh colored

Vertical growth phase
1. Raised above skin
   with variety of
   shapes
2. Ulceration and
   crust and
   bleeding frequent
3. May resemble
   angioma

Raised
plaque

Dome-shaped

Polypoid

Ulceration is
possible

Pressure test

Nodular melanoma

Angioma

Press suspected nodule firmly for 30 seconds;
near-total involution is characteristic of
hemangioma, not melanoma.

B

Figure 21-22
*There are raised plaque, dome-shaped, and
polypoid lesions. Some appear to be originating
from nevi. A halo has developed around one of
the plaque-shaped melanomas.*

C
1.8 cm

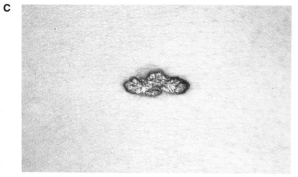

D
1.2 cm

2 cm

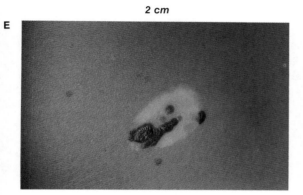

2.4 cm

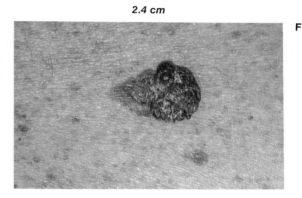

E

F

2 cm

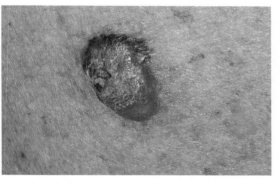

G

2.5 cm

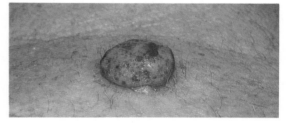

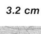

H

3 cm

3.2 cm

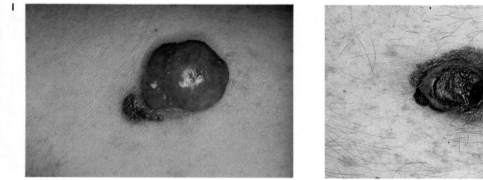

I

J

LENTIGO MALIGNA-MELANOMA

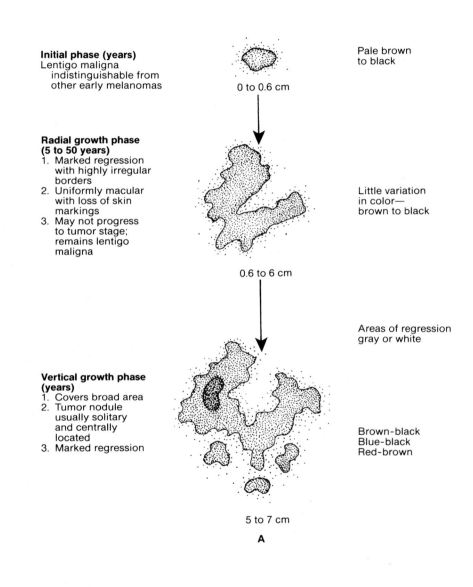

Initial phase (years)
Lentigo maligna
  indistinguishable from
  other early melanomas

0 to 0.6 cm

Pale brown
to black

**Radial growth phase
(5 to 50 years)**
1. Marked regression
   with highly irregular
   borders
2. Uniformly macular
   with loss of skin
   markings
3. May not progress
   to tumor stage;
   remains lentigo
   maligna

0.6 to 6 cm

Little variation
in color—
brown to black

Areas of regression
gray or white

**Vertical growth phase
(years)**
1. Covers broad area
2. Tumor nodule
   usually solitary
   and centrally
   located
3. Marked regression

Brown-black
Blue-black
Red-brown

5 to 7 cm

A

Figure 21-23
*The lesions grow slowly and regress for several
years, forming highly irregular borders. The color
remains brown or black until the tumor stage is
reached.*

B

2 cm

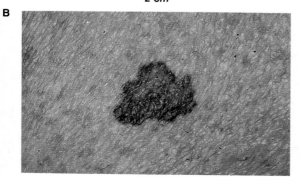

C

2.5 cm

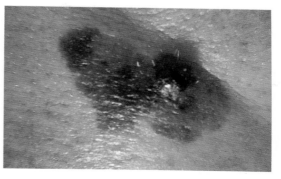

D

2.5 cm

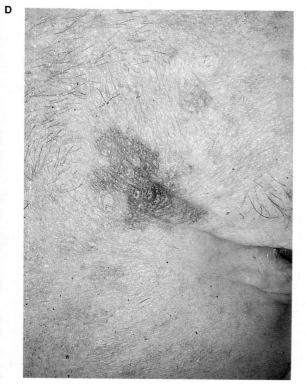

E

5 cm

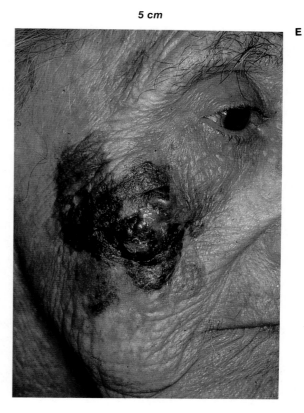

Acral-lentiginous melanoma. ALM (Figure 21-24) appears on the palms, soles, and terminal phalanges. It is similar in clinical presentation to LMM; it has the same colors and tendency to remain flat. ALM is most frequent in blacks and orientals. Small areas of elevation may be associated with deep invasion; it is very aggressive and metastasizes early.[20-22] The sudden appearance of a pigmented band originating at the proximal nail fold (Hutchinson's sign) is suggestive of acral-lentiginous melanoma.

Dysplastic nevi

It is well established that malignant melanoma may develop de novo and evolve into one of the four patterns described or it may develop from a preexisting pigmented lesion such as a congenital nevus. A new precursor lesion, the dysplastic nevus (DN) with a reported incidence of 2% to 8% (Figures 21-25 and 21-26), has recently been described; as data accumulate, it may be established as the single most important precursor lesion of melanoma.

DN was initially recognized as a precursor to melanoma in patients with familial cutaneous melanoma, in which the tendency to develop melanoma is genetically transmitted. This syndrome was named the "B-K mole syndrome"[23] from two of the probands, and the precursor nevi were designated as B-K moles and later referred to as dysplastic nevi.[24] Dysplastic nevi have since been observed in 8% of patients with nonfamilial (sporadic) melanoma and their transformation into SSM has been photographically documented. Dysplastic nevi are found on the skin of 90% of patients with hereditary melanomas, and over 50% of melanomas in this group are associated histologically and probably evolve from dysplastic nevi.[25-27] The lifetime risk of developing cutaneous melanoma among the white population in the United States is about 0.6%, or 1 in 150. The overall lifetime risk among patients with DN is estimated at 10%. The lifetime risk of melanoma approaches 100% for those people with DN from families with two or more first-degree relatives having cutaneous melanoma.[28]

These unusual nevi differ in a number of important ways from typical acquired pigmented nevi or moles; see Table 21-3.

The following recommendations for management of patients with DN are from the National Institutes of Health Consensus Development Conference statement, October 24-26, 1983.[29]

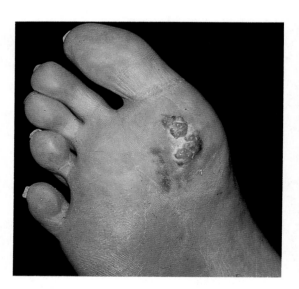

Figure 21-24
Acral-lentiginous melanoma.

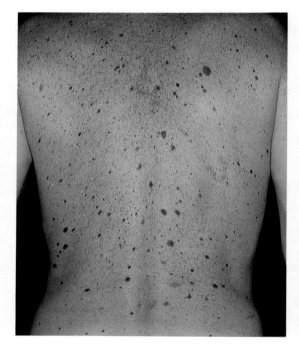

Figure 21-25
Dysplastic nevi. There are numerous large nevi present. Superficial spreading melanomas have been removed from the upper back and the midline on the left side (note scars).

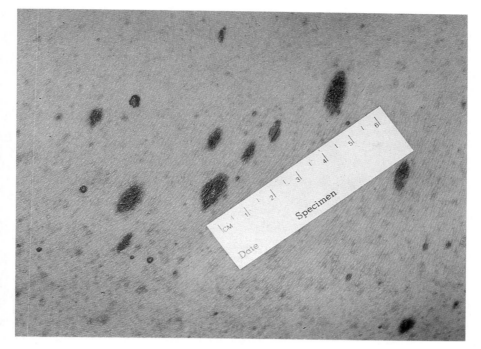

Figure 21-26
Dysplastic nevi. A closeup view of the lower right back of the patient depicted in Figure 21-25. Nevi are larger than 1 cm and irregularly pigmented.

TABLE 21-3

DIFFERENCES BETWEEN DYSPLASTIC AND COMMON NEVI

Characteristics	Dysplastic nevi	Common nevi
Distribution	Back most common, upper and lower limbs, sun-protected areas, female breasts, scalp, buttock, groin	Usually sun-exposed areas; anywhere on body surface
Number	Less than 10 to greater than 100	10 to 40
Age at onset	Appear as normal nevi at age 2 to 6; increase in number and size at puberty; new nevi appear throughout life	Appear at age 2 to 6; grow vertically in uniform manner throughout life; several may appear at puberty
Size	Usually greater than 5 mm and commonly greater than 10 mm	Usually less than 6 mm
Shape and contour	Irregular border; flat (macular) areas	Round, symmetric, uniformly macular or papular
Color	Variable within a single lesion; brown, black, red, pink	Uniform tan, brown, black; darken during pregnancy or at adolescence; become lighter with age

Derived from Greene MH, Clark WH Jr, Tucker MA, et al: Acquired precursors of cutaneous malignant melanoma. The familial dysplastic nevus syndrome. N Engl J Med **312:**91, 1985.

Classification. Classify patients into one of two groups:

1. DN with a family history of melanoma.
2. DN without a family history of melanoma.

Classification requires an accurate family history and evaluation of first-degree relatives.

Diagnosis
1. Physical examination: examine the entire integument including scalp and eyes.
2. Excisional biopsy: biopsy at least one or more atypical appearing DN.

Familial screening
1. If family history suggests melanoma, examine all first-degree relatives.
2. If a melanoma is found in any of these family members, all blood relatives should be examined to determine the extent of the risk of melanoma in the kindred.

Treatment and follow-up
1. Excision of any DN with any feature of early melanoma.
2. Follow-up with examination every 3 to 6 months for patients with DN and any family history of melanoma.

Benign lesions that resemble melanoma

Typical nevi or other lesions such as seborrheic keratosis may have features that suggest melanoma. These lesions should be biopsied (Figures 21-27 to 21-33).

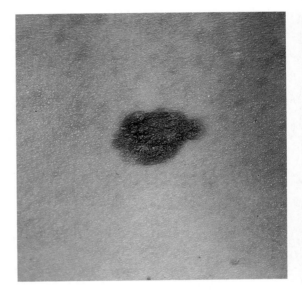

Figure 21-27
Nevus with an irregular border and a variety of colors resembling superficial spreading melanoma.

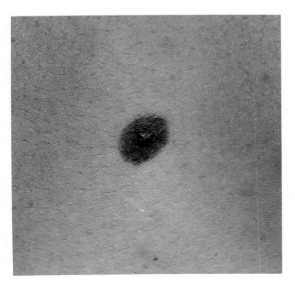

Figure 21-28
Nevus with a dark nodule in the center resembling nodular melanoma.

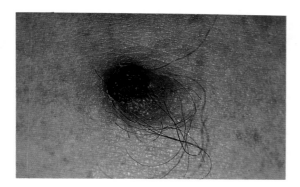

Figure 21-29
Nevus with recent hemorrhage suggesting malignant degeneration.

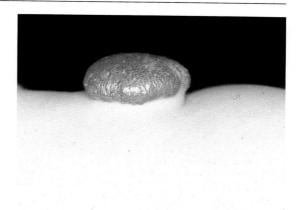

Figure 21-30
Hemangioma (nodular shaped) resembling nodular melanoma.

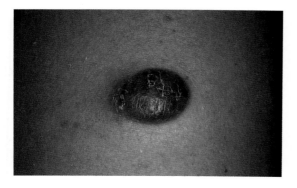

Figure 21-31
Traumatized hemangioma suggesting malignant degeneration.

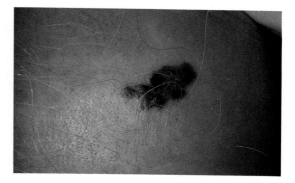

Figure 21-32
Seborrheic keratosis with an irregular border simulating a superficial spreading melanoma.

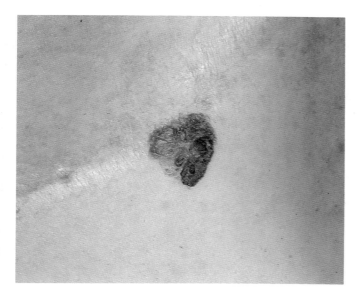

Figure 21-33
Seborrheic keratosis with an irregular elevated surface simulating the plaque type of nodular malignant melanoma.

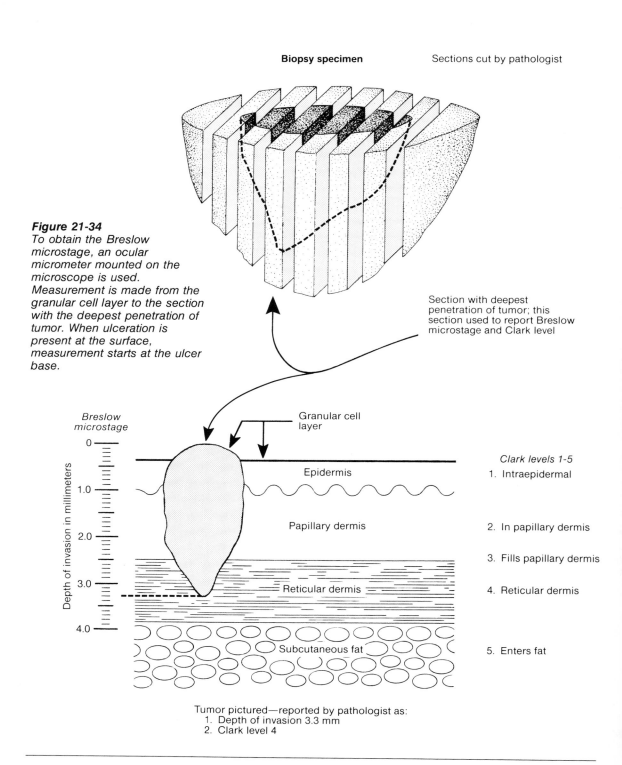

Biopsy specimen   Sections cut by pathologist

Figure 21-34
To obtain the Breslow microstage, an ocular micrometer mounted on the microscope is used. Measurement is made from the granular cell layer to the section with the deepest penetration of tumor. When ulceration is present at the surface, measurement starts at the ulcer base.

Section with deepest penetration of tumor; this section used to report Breslow microstage and Clark level

Breslow microstage

Granular cell layer

Depth of invasion in millimeters

0
1.0
2.0
3.0
4.0

Clark levels 1-5

Epidermis   1. Intraepidermal

Papillary dermis   2. In papillary dermis

3. Fills papillary dermis

Reticular dermis   4. Reticular dermis

Subcutaneous fat   5. Enters fat

Tumor pictured—reported by pathologist as:
    1. Depth of invasion 3.3 mm
    2. Clark level 4

Management

Biopsy. The prognosis and extent of surgery to be performed is based on tumor type, thickness, and level of invasion. The pathologist can report this information if provided with an excisional biopsy of the entire lesion deep enough to include subcutaneous fat. If total excision is impractical, an incisional biopsy should be taken from what is considered to be the deepest part of the tumor. The deepest portion is generally the area with the highest surface elevation. Punch biopsy may not be sufficient because it yields such a small piece of tissue that the problem may go undetected.

Pathology report. The pathology report (Figure 21-34) should include the following.

Tumor type. This is reported as superficial spreading, nodular, lentigo maligna, acral-lentiginous melanoma, or unclassifiable. The degree of ulceration, inflammation, cell differentiation, and mitotic activity is reported.

Tumor thickness (Breslow microstage). The tumor is step sectioned. The section with the deepest level of penetration of tumor is used to measure thickness. An ocular micrometer is placed on the microscope. The pathologist measures, in millimeters, the thickness of the tumor from the granular cell layer to the deepest part of the tumor. If the granular layer is absent, the measurement is taken from the highest part of the ulcerated surface. The report is given as Breslow level, followed by the depth reported in millimeters.[30,31]

Tumor thickness (Clark level). Clark was the first to propose that the depth of penetration of melanoma should be reported in a specific manner using a specified convention.[32] He proposed that tumor depth should be reported by anatomic site (i.e., epidermis, depth in dermis, etc.). Pathologists continue to report depth of invasion by Clark levels but prognosis and extent of surgery are based on the depth of invasion measured in millimeters.

Clinical staging. Clinical staging refers to the extent of disease determined by physical examination. Stage I consists of local disease. Stage II is enlarged regional lymph nodes determined by palpation. In stage III, there is clinical evidence of disseminated disease through, for instance, positive liver scan or chest roentgenogram.

Prognosis. Many factors affect prognosis,[33-36] including clinical stage, location, and size.

Clinical stage I. A series of studies have demonstrated that, for clinical stage I disease, the specific location and the primary tumor thickness are the variables whose values most accurately predict rates of recurrence and death even if regional lymph nodes also contain metastases (Table 21-4).

Locations where the prognosis is worse than for tumors of comparable thickness elsewhere are called high-risk subsites. These are the BANS area (the upper back, posterolateral upper arm, posterolateral neck, posterior scalp, and hands and feet.

Melanomas less than 0.85 mm thick in any location and melanomas from 0.85 to 1.69 mm thick on the face, anterior neck, extremities excluding the posterolateral upper arm, and lower trunk rarely metastasize. However, melanomas larger than 3.60 mm on the trunk or 2.75 mm on the hands and feet nearly always result in death.

TABLE 21-4

PROBABILITY OF DEATH (%) FROM MELANOMA IN THE FIRST 7½ YEARS AFTER DIAGNOSIS OF CLINICAL STAGE I MELANOMA*

Thickness range (mm)	NonBANS† extremities excluding hands and feet	NonBANS head and neck	NonBANS trunk	Hands and feet	BANS
<0.85	0	0	0	0	2
0.85-1.69	0	0	3	0	22
1.70-3.64	14	36	23	40	42
≥3.65	17	35	78	100	67

Reprinted from Day CL Jr, Mihm MC Jr, Lew RA, et al: Cutaneous malignant melanoma: prognostic guidelines for physicians and patients. Ca-A Cancer Journal for Clinicians **32**(2) © 1982, American Cancer Society.

*A 7½ year death rate from melanoma determined by life table analysis of 598 clinical stage I patients from the Massachusetts General Hospital and New York University Medical Center.

†BANS = Upper back, posterolateral arm, posterior and lateral neck, and posterior scalp.

Clinical stage II. Approximately 30% of clinical stage II patients live 5 years and 10-year survivors are uncommon.

Clinical stage III. Patients with distant metastases surgically resected and judged to be clinically free of disease have a median survival time of 16 months versus 5 months for patient with unresectable distant metastases.

Surgical management of clinical stage I melanoma. Clinical stage I melanoma is managed surgically. The surgeon must decide on the resection margins and whether to perform a regional node dissection.

Resection margins. Traditionally, surgeons have excised melanomas with a border of normal skin at least 5 cm from the edge of the tumor, giving a specimen over 10 cm in diameter. The necessity of performing such a radical procedure has been questioned. Smaller resection margins have been proposed as a reasonable compromise until data from prospective trials become available.[37-39] For melanomas less than 0.85 mm thick, the proposed margin would be 1.5 cm of clinically normal skin surrounding the lesion. For melanomas 0.85 mm thick or greater, the suggested margin is 3 cm or less of clinically normal skin around the lesion. Smaller margins may be indicated to preserve vital structures.[39]

Elective regional node dissection. The criteria for performing an elective regional node dissection have not been established at this time; there is a great deal of conflicting information.[40-42] The available data suggest that patients with clinical stage I disease who are most likely to benefit from elective regional node dissection are those with melanomas from 0.85 to 1.69 mm on the BANS areas and those with melanomas from 1.70 to 3.64 mm thick on any area. Some surgeons perform regional node dissections for tumors thicker than 3.64 mm.

REFERENCES

1. Kaplan EN: The risk of malignancy in large congenital nevi. Plast Reconstr Surg **53**:421, 1974.
2. Kopf AW, Bart RS, Hennessey P: Congenital nevocytic nevi and malignant melanomas. J Am Acad Dermatol **1**:123, 1979.
3. Lanier VC, Pickrell KL, Georgiade NG: Congenital giant nevi: clinical and pathological considerations. Plast Reconstr Surg **58**:48, 1976.
4. Rhodes AR, Sober AJ, Day CL, et al: The malignant potential of small congenital nevocellular nevi: an estimate of association based on a histologic study of 234 primary melanomas. J Am Acad Dermatol **6**:230, 1982.
5. Rhodes AR: Small congenital nevi (reply). J Am Acad Dermatol **7**:687, 1982.
6. Bleehen SS, Ebling FJ: Disorders of skin color. In A Rook, DS Wilkinson, FJ Ebling, editors. Textbook of dermatology, third edition. Oxford, 1979, Blackwell Scientific Publications.
7. Stewart DM, Altman J, Mehregan AH: Speckled lentiginous nevus. Arch Dermatol **114**:895, 1978.
8. Cohen HJ, Minkin W, Frank SB: Nevus spilus. Arch Dermatol **102**:433, 1970.
9. Bart RS, Kopf A: Extensive melanosis and hypertrichosis (Becker's nevus). J Dermatol Surg Oncol **3**:379, 1977.
10. Paniago-Pereira C, Maize JC, Ackerman AB: Nevus of large spindle and/or epithelioid cells (Spitz's nevus). Arch Dermatol **114**:1811, 1978.
11. Merkow LP, Burt RC, Hayeslip DW, et al: A cellular and malignant blue nevus. Cancer **24**:886, 1969.
12. Connors RC, Ackerman AB: Histologic pseudomalignancies of the skin. Arch Dermatol **112**:1767, 1976.
13. Mihm MC Jr, Fitzpatrick TB, Brown MM, et al: Early detection of primary cutaneous malignant melanoma: a color atlas. N Engl J Med **289**:989, 1973.
14. Mihm MC, Clark WH, Reed RJ: The clinical diagnosis of malignant melanoma. Semin Oncol **2**:105, 1975.
15. Kopf AW, Bart RS, Rodríguez-Sains RS, et al: Clinical diagnosis of cutaneous malignant melanoma. In Malignant melanoma. New York, 1979, Masson Publishing USA Inc.
16. Clark WH Jr, Ainsworth AM, Bernardino EA: The developmental biology of primary human malignant melanomas. Semin Oncol **2**:83, 1975.
17. Sober AJ, Fitzpatrick TB, Mihm MC: Primary melanoma of the skin: recognition and management. J Am Acad Dermatol **2**:179, 1980.
18. Sober AJ, Fitzpatrick TB, Mihm MC, et al: Malignant melanoma of the skin, and benign neoplasms and hyperplasias of melanocytes in the skin. In Dermatology in general medicine. New York, 1979, McGraw-Hill Book Co.
19. McGovern VJ, Mihm MC Jr, Bailly C, et al: The classification of malignant melanoma and its histologic reporting. Cancer **32**:1446, 1973.
20. Feibleman CE, Stoll H, Maize JC: Melanomas of the palm, sole, and nail bed: clinicopathologic study. Cancer **46**:2492, 1980.
21. Paladugu RR, Winberg CD, Yonemoto RH: Acral lentiginous melanoma: a clinicopathologic study of 36 patients. Cancer **52**:161, 1983.
22. Patterson RH, Helwig EB: Subungual malignant melanoma: a clinicopathologic study. Cancer **46**:2074, 1980.
23. Clark WH Jr, Reimer RR, Greene M, et al: Origin of familial malignant melanomas from heritable melanocytic lesions: "the B-K mole syndrome." Arch Dermatol **114**:732, 1978.
24. Pellegrini AE: The dysplastic nevus syndrome: what is it? Am J Dermatopathol **4**:453, 1982.
25. Reimer RR, Clark WH Jr, Greene MH, et al: Precursor lesions in familial melanoma: a new genetic preneoplastic syndrome. JAMA **239**:744, 1978.
26. Elder DE, Goldman LI, Goldman SC, et al: Dysplastic nevus syndrome: a phenotypic association of sporadic cutaneous melanoma. Cancer **46**:1787, 1980.
27. Happle R, Traupe H, Vakilzadeh F, et al: Arguments in favor of a polygenic inheritance of precursor nevi. J Am Acad Dermatol **6**:540, 1982.
28. Greene MH, Clark WH Jr, Tucker MA, et al: Melanoma risk in familial dysplastic nevus syndrome (abstract). J Invest Dermatol **82**:424, 1984.

29. Precursors to malignant melanoma. National Institutes of Health Consensus Development Conference Statement, Oct 24-26, 1983. J Am Acad Dermatol **10**:683, 1984.

30. Breslow A: Prognosis in stage I cutaneous melanoma: tumor thickness as a guide to treatment. In Pathology of malignant melanoma. New York, 1981, Masson Publishing USA Inc.

31. Breslow A, Cascinelli N, van der Esch EP, et al: Stage I melanoma of the limbs: assessment of prognosis by levels of invasion and maximum thickness. Tumori **64**:373, 1978.

32. Suffin SC, Waisman J, Clark WH, et al: Comparison of the classification by microscopic level (stage) of malignant melanoma by three independent groups of pathologists. Cancer **40**:3112, 1977.

33. Day CL Jr, Mihm MC Jr, Sober AJ, et al: Prognostic factors for melanoma patients with lesions 0.76-1.69 mm in thickness: an appraisal of "thin" level IV lesions. Ann Surg **195**:30, 1982.

34. Day CL Jr, Mihm MC Jr, Lew RA, et al: Prognostic factors for patients with clinical stage I melanoma of intermediate thickness (1.51-3.99 mm): a conceptual model for tumor growth and metastasis. Ann Surg **195**:35, 1982.

35. Day CL Jr, Lew RA, Mihm MC Jr, et al: A multivariate analysis of prognostic factors for melanoma patients with lesions 3.65 mm in thickness: the importance of revealing alternate Cox models. Ann Surg **195**:44, 1982.

36. Day CL Jr, Mihm MC Jr, Lew RA, et al: Cutaneous malignant melanoma: prognostic guidelines for physicians and patients. CA **32**:113, 1982.

37. Day CL Jr, Mihm MC Jr, Sober AJ, et al: Narrower margins for clinical stage I malignant melanoma. N Engl J Med **306**:479, 1982.

38. Kirkwood JM, Ariyan S, Nordlund JJ: Malignant melanoma margins. N Engl J Med **307**:439, 1982.

39. Day CL Jr, Lew RA: Malignant melanoma prognostic factors. 3. Surgical margins. J Dermatol Surg Oncol **9**:797, 1983.

40. Veronesi U, Adamus J, Bandiera DC, et al: Inefficacy of immediate node dissection in stage I melanoma of the limbs. N Engl J Med **297**:627, 1977.

41. Balch CM, Murad TM, Soong SJ, et al: Tumor thickness as a guide to surgical management of clinical stage I melanoma patients. Cancer **43**:883, 1979.

42. Petrelli NJ: Opinion: lymph node dissection for stage I melanoma: the unresolved dilemma. CA **32**:314, 1982.

ADDITIONAL READINGS

Ackerman AB, editor: Malignant melanoma and other melanocytic neoplasms. Am J Dermatopathol **6**(suppl), summer 1984. Also available in hard cover: New York, 1984, Masson Publishing USA, Inc.

Ackerman AB, editor: Pathology of malignant melanoma. New York, 1981, Masson Publishing USA, Inc.

Balch CM, Milton GW, editors: Cutaneous melanoma, clinical management and treatment results worldwide. Philadelphia, 1985, JB Lippincott Co.

Kopf AW, Bart RS, Rodriguez-Sains RS, et al: Malignant melanoma. New York, 1979, Masson Publishing USA, Inc.

Chapter Twenty-Two

Vascular Tumors and Malformations

Nevus flammeus (port wine stains)
Salmon patches
Strawberry hemangioma
Cavernous hemangioma
Cherry angioma
Angiokeratomas
Venous lake
Lymphangioma circumscriptum
Spider angioma
Hereditary hemorrhagic telangiectasia
Pyogenic granuloma
Kaposi's sarcoma

A number of different congenital vascular malformations occur in the skin. Vascular structures may be abnormal in size, present in abnormal numbers, or both. Several of these lesions have been referred to previously as capillary hemangiomas. That term has been abandoned in favor of the more specific terms discussed. Most represent developmental malformations and do not appear to be genetically determined.

Nevus Flammeus (Port Wine Stains)

In most cases this distinctive lesion is a developmental anomaly that is not genetically transmitted. Nevus flammeus is a significant cosmetic problem that, unlike some other congenital vascular malformations, does not fade with age. These nevi are usually unilateral; they frequently occur on the face, but also appear elsewhere (Figure 22-1). They may be a few millimeters in diameter or cover an entire limb (Figure 22-2). Size remains stable throughout life. Nevus flammeus appears at birth as flat, irregular, red-to-purple patches. Initially, the lesion is smooth, but later it may become papular, simulating a cobble-stone surface. The entire depth of the dermis contains numerous dilated vessels.

Nevus flammeus may be a component of neurocutaneous syndromes (Table 22-1) (e.g., Sturge-Weber syndrome, which is nevus flammeus of the trigeminal area, or Klippel-Trenaunay-Weber syndrome). When it occurs over the midline of the back, it may be associated with an underlying spinal cord arteriovenous malformation.[1]

In the past, treatment has been unsatisfactory, but significant improvement can now be obtained with the argon laser.[2-4] The argon laser's visible blue-green light is absorbed selectively by the red pigment, hemoglobin, transforming the radiant energy into heat, which in turn coagulates blood vessels up to 0.5 mm in diameter. Therefore, the color and size of the blood vessels in nevus flammeus are ideal for treatment with the argon laser. Dispersion of energy in deeper tissues results in some scarring.

Individuals are treated as outpatients; patients 12 and under are not usually treated, since cooperation during the procedure is necessary. Studies show that the patients who benefit most from the therapy are those who are 37 or older with lesions with a definite purple color and who, on histologic examination, show large, ectatic vessels filled with red blood cells.[4]

The cosmetic appearance of some patients with port wine stain can be significantly improved by using a tinted waterproof makeup such as Dermablend (Dermablend Corrective Cosmetics, Farmingdale, NJ) or Covermark, manufactured by Lydia O'Leary, Moonachie, NJ (Figures 22-3 and 22-4). A cosmetic kit for matching skin tone is available directly from Lydia O'Leary. Contact the company as to availability. Experienced people are located in several areas of the country to help with application techniques and color selection. Dermablend is available in nine primary shades. Covermark is available in 10 different shades. A setting powder and cleanser are used with these cosmetics. Both are waterproof. Dermablend is nationally distributed and is available at department stores and independent pharmacies.

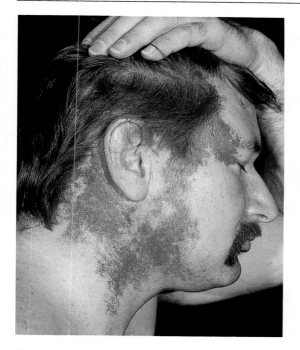

Figure 22-1
Nevus flammeus. An extensive lesion with a
relatively smooth surface.

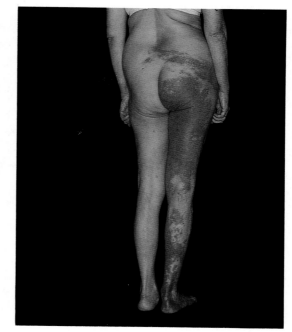

Figure 22-2
Nevus flammeus covering the entire lower limb.
The affected limb is 2 inches longer than the
normal side.

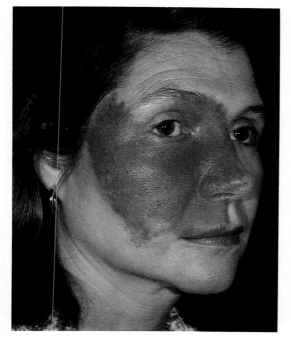

Figure 22-3
Nevus flammeus with a papular surface.

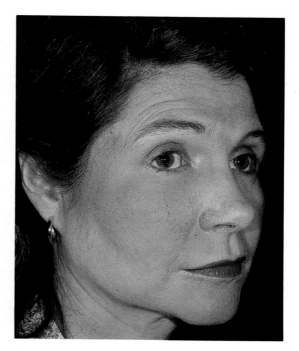

Figure 22-4
Same patient as in Figure 22-3 after applying
Covermark makeup.

TABLE 22-1

NEUROCUTANEOUS SYNDROMES WITH VASCULAR ABNORMALITIES*

	Cobb syndrome	Sturge-Weber syndrome	Osler-Weber-Rendu syndrome
Synonym	Cutaneomeningo-spinal angiomatosis	Encephalotrigeminal angiomatosis	Hereditary hemorrhagic telangiectasia
Inheritance	Not familial	Dominant partial trisomy or not familial	Autosomal dominant
Sex distribution	More in males	Equal	Equal
Age of onset	Childhood or adolescence	Two-thirds with hemangioma at birth	Childhood
Skin lesion	Port wine stain or angiokeratomas in dermatomal distribution corresponding within segment or two of area of spinal cord involvement†	1. Ipsilateral capillary angioma or port wine stain in distribution of superior and middle branches of the trigeminal nerve†; associated cavernous changes may occur 2. No consistent relationship between extent of skin lesion and degree of meningeal involvement	Telangiectasia (skin and mucous membranes)†
CNS findings	1. Arteriovenous or venous angioma of the spinal cord† 2. Neurologic signs of cord compression or anoxia	1. Angioma of meninges† 2. Intracranial gyriform calcifications 3. Mental retardation (60%)† 4. Epilepsy (usually focal)† 5. Hemiparesis contralateral to skin lesions† 6. Visual impairment (50% have one or more of various eye abnormalities)†	Angiomas in the brain or spinal cord with signs of localized tumor
Associated findings	1. Angioma of vertebrae 2. Renal angioma 3. Kyphoscoliosis	1. Renal angioma 2. Coarctation of aorta 3. High arched palate 4. Abnormally developed ears	1. Pulmonary arteriovenous anastomoses 2. Hemorrhage from lesions in mouth, GI tract, GU tract and associated anemia
Diagnostic aids	1. Lateral spine x-ray 2. Myelography 3. Selective spinal angiography	1. EEG 2. Skull x-ray 3. Cerebral angiography	None
Treatment	Surgical removal of spinal cord angioma if possible	1. Anticonvulsants 2. Surgical removal of intracranial lesion if possible 3. Cosmetic procedures for skin lesions	Cautery of bleeding lesions

From Jessen T, Thompson S, Smith EB: Arch Dermatol **113**:1582, 1977. Copyright 1977, American Medical
*CNS, central nervous system; GI, gastrointestinal; GU, genitourinary; EEG, electroencephalogram.
†Major component of the syndrome.

Fabry-Anderson syndrome	Ataxia telangiectasia	von Hippel-Lindau disease
Angiokeratoma corporis diffusum	Cephalo-oculocutaneous telangiectasia syndrome	Angiomatosis retinae et cerebelli syndrome
Recessive trait (X chromosome)	Autosomal recessive	Autosomal dominant
Males tend to full syndrome: 1. Angiokeratomas 2. Extremity pain 3. High blood pressure 4. Cardiomegaly 5. Albuminuria 6. Hypohidrosis	Equal	Equal
Childhood	Childhood	Adult
1. Small clustered angiokeratomas (symmetric, mucosal, increased over bony prominences) 2. Palmar mottling	1. Telangiectasia (increased in sun-exposed areas)† 2. Inelasticity	1. Port wine stains in some; most with no cutaneous lesions 2. Café-au-lait spots
1. Cerebral vascular accidents 2. Neuronal glycolipid deposition (peripheral neuritis)	1. Progressive cerebellar ataxia (voluntary movements)† 2. Ocular telangiectasia (spread from canthal fold)† 3. Peculiar eye movements (nystagmus, poor control)† 4. Retarded 5. Slow dysarthric speech 6. Decreased tendon reflexes	1. Cerebellar hemangioblastoma and cyst† 2. Spinal hemangioblastoma (rarely) 3. Retinal hemangiomas (tangle of vessels away from disk)†
1. Stooped posture 2. Slender limbs, thin, weak muscles 3. Dilated, tortuous conjunctival and retinal vessels 4. Varicose veins and stasis edema 5. Scant facial hair 6. Hypogonadism	1. Sinopulmonary infections† 2. Hypoplastic or absent thymus 3. Small spleen 4. Retarded growth 5. Malignancies (reticulum cell sarcoma, Hodgkin's disease, lymphosarcoma, gastric carcinoma)	1. Phecochromocytoma 2. Pancreatic cysts 3. Hepatic angiomas 4. Renal hypernephromas (20%) 5. Polycythema (erythropoietic substance from tumor)
1. Urinary glycolipids (ceramide trihexoside) 2. Slit lamp 3. Biopsy, renal or marrow (lipid deposits)	1. Diminished or absent IgA 2. Increased serum alpha-fetoprotein	1. Hemogram (polycythemia) 2. Urinalysis, excretory urograms 3. Skull x-ray, angiogram 4. Myelogram
Symptomatic	1. Control infections 2. Plasma infusions (IgA) 3. Thymus transplant 4. Transfer factor	Supportive

Association.

Salmon Patches

Salmon patches are actually variants of nevus flammeus; they are present in approximately 40% to 70% of newborns at birth. They are red, irregular, macular patches resulting from dilatation of dermal capillaries. The most common site is on the nape of the neck (Figure 22-5), where the lesion is referred to as a stork bite. They are often inconspicuous and covered by hair. Those patches occurring on the glabella and upper eyelids are sometimes mistaken for pressure or forceps marks. Salmon patches on the face fade within a year, but those on the nape may persist for life.

Strawberry Hemangioma

Strawberry hemangioma occurs at birth or evolves in the first few months of life. It consists of a collection of dilated vessels in the dermis surrounded by masses of proliferating endothelial cells. The proliferating endothelial cells may be responsible for the unique growth characteristics of this lesion. The lesion begins as a nodular mass or as a flat, ill-defined telangiectatic macule that is mistaken for a bruise. Strawberry hemangiomas grow rapidly for weeks or months, forming a nodular, protuberant, compressible mass of a few millimeters to several centimeters that is sharply delineated (Figure 22-6). Vital structures can be compressed and rapidly growing areas may ulcerate; however, most have a benign course. An inactive phase lasting several months is followed by involution in over 90% of cases.[5] The mass shrinks and fades during the scarring process. Involution usually has begun in most cases by age 3; hemangiomas present after ages 7 to 9 will infrequently undergo further regression.

Management. Lesions that are relatively small and indolent should remain untouched to involute spontaneously. In most cases the result is very satisfactory. Small areas of bleeding and ulceration are treated with cool wet compresses. Rapidly growing lesions, or those that have the potential for interfering with vital structures such as the eyes or auditory canals, should be treated with prednisone (2 to 4 mg/kg) given in divided doses twice a day.[6,7] Most lesions stabilize and markedly regress in 2 to 4 weeks. Prednisone may then be given in a single early morning dose, tapered on an alternate-day schedule for a few weeks, and then discontinued. A second course of treatment is given for recurrences. Lesions not regressing by late childhood may be evaluated for surgical excision.

Cavernous Hemangioma

Cavernous hemangioma is a collection of dilated vessels deep in the dermis and subcutaneous tissue, which is present at birth. The clinical appearance is a pale, skin-colored, red or blue, ill-defined, rounded mass (Figure 22-7). Like strawberry hemangioma, the lesion enlarges for several months, becomes stationary for an indefinite period, and then undergoes spontaneous resolution. Cavernous hemangiomas are managed like strawberry hemangiomas.

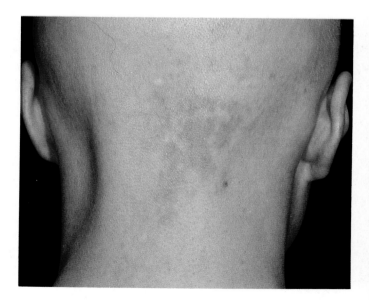

Figure 22-5
Salmon patch (stork bite). A variant of nevus flammeus found in many individuals on the nape of the neck.

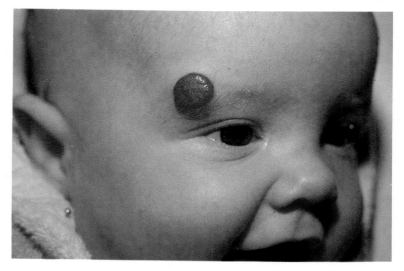

Figure 22-6
Strawberry hemangioma. A nodular protuberant mass that undergoes spontaneous involution in over 90% of the cases.

Figure 22-7
Cavernous hemangioma. A blue, thick, rounded mass. This lesion has a strawberry hemangioma on the surface.

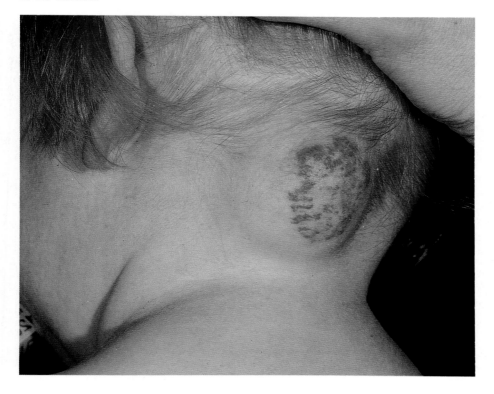

Cherry Angioma

The most common vascular malformation is the benign cherry or senile angioma. These 0.5- to 5-mm smooth, firm, deep red papules occur in virtually everyone after age 30 and numerically increase with age. Patients recognize them as new growths, prompting concerns about malignancy. They are most common on the trunk (Figure 22-8) and vary in number from a few to hundreds. Trauma produces slight bleeding. The papules are easily removed by scissor excision or electrodesiccation and curettage.

Angiokeratomas

Angiokeratoma is a lesion characterized by dilatation of the superficial dermal blood vessels and hyperkeratosis of the overlying epidermis. The term is applied to six different vascular malformations. The most common are angiokeratomas of the scrotum (Fordyce spots) (Figure 22-9) or vulva, characterized by multiple 2- to 3-mm red-to-purple papules, which occasionally bleed with trauma. If desired, removal is performed by simple scissor excision or electrodesiccation and curettage.

The other forms are rare. They consist of red-brown-black hyperkeratotic plaques varying in size and distribution. Numerous cutaneous angiokeratomas are part of the Fabray-Anderson syndrome (Table 22-1).

Venous Lake

Venous lake is a dark blue, slightly elevated 0.2- to 1-cm lesion composed of a dilated, blood-filled vascular channel. These lesions are common on sun-exposed surfaces of the vermilion border of the lip (Figure 22-10), face, and forearms. They occasionally bleed after trauma and can be removed by electrodesiccation.

Lymphangioma Circumscriptum

This uncommon but distinctive malformation, located in the upper dermis, consists of dilated lymph channels that communicate with deeper lymph channels. The appearance of the lesion has been compared to a mass of frog eggs ("frog spawn") and consists of a group of straw-colored, fluid-filled vesicles on a dull red or brown base (Figure 22-11). Some lesions contain a mixture of vascular and lymph channels. Most can be destroyed by electrosurgery, but recurrences may occur from residual communications with deep lymph channels.

Figure 22-8
Cherry angioma. Multiple small red papules commonly occur on the trunk.

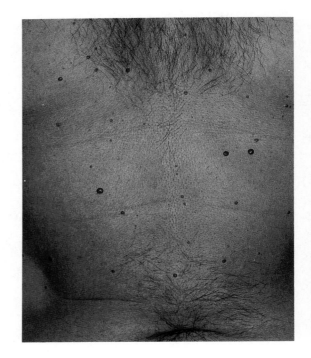

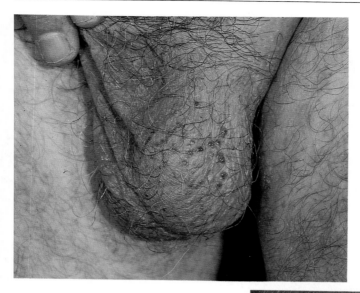

Figure 22-9
Angiokeratomas (Fordyce). Multiple red to purple papules consisting of multiple small blood vessels.

Figure 22-10
Venous lake. A dilated blood-filled channel typically seen on the lower lip.

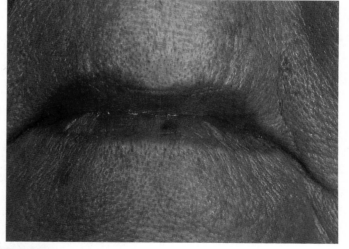

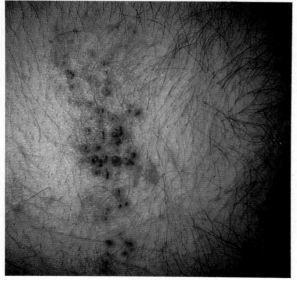

Figure 22-11
Lymphangioma circumscriptum. Dilated lymph channels. Appearance has been compared to a mass of frogs eggs ("frog spawn").

Spider Angioma

Spider angioma forms as an arteriole (spider body), becomes more prominent near the surface of the skin, and radiates capillaries (spider legs) (Figure 22-12). They occur in many normal individuals and frequently appear in children. Once formed, they tend to be permanent. Bleeding rarely occurs. Spider angiomas are most common on the exposed surfaces of the face and arms. They increase in number with liver diseases and during pregnancy and are probably stimulated by higher than normal estrogen concentrations. Spider angioma is to be distinguished from the flat patches of tiny vessels of uniform size (telangiectatic mats) seen in scleroderma.

Anesthesia is unnecessary in the following procedure for treatment. Force the blood out of the spider by pressing firmly on the lesion; with continuous pressure, move the finger slightly to one side to expose the central arteriole and then gently electrodesiccate the central arteriole. If the arteriole has been destroyed, the radiating capillaries cannot fill. Remaining radiating capillaries are destroyed by drawing the electrocautery in short strokes over the capillary. Incompletely destroyed lesions may recur. Vigorous desiccation may cause a pitted scar.

Figure 22-12
Spider angioma. A common lesion consisting of a central arteriole and several radiating capillaries.

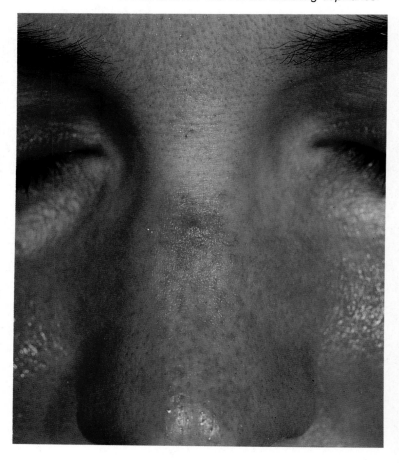

Hereditary Hemorrhagic Telangiectasia

Hereditary hemorrhagic telangiectasia (HHT) is an autosomal dominantly inherited malformation of blood vessels.[8] The characteristic lesion begins as a tiny flat telangiectasia with a few vessels radiating from a single point. Rarely, there is a large central arteriole as seen in spider angioma. Engorged lesions are fragile and bleed easily with the slightest trauma. Few to numerous lesions occur primarily on the lips, tongue (Figure 22-13), nasal mucosa, forearms, hands and fingers, and throughout the gastrointestinal tract, but any skin area or internal organ may be involved. HHT is the most common cause of pulmonary arteriovenous anastomoses.[9] Although lesions may be prominent during childhood, they are most often so small and subtle that stretching of the lip is required to accentuate them. By the third or fourth decade, telangiectasias become more apparent and the diagnosis is easily made. Recurrent bleeding from nasal or gastrointestinal telangiectasia can be fatal in a small number of cases. Bleeding points are treated by electrocautery. Most patients have a normal life expectancy.

Figure 22-13
Hereditary hemorrhagic telangiectasia. Several lesions are present on the lip and tongue.

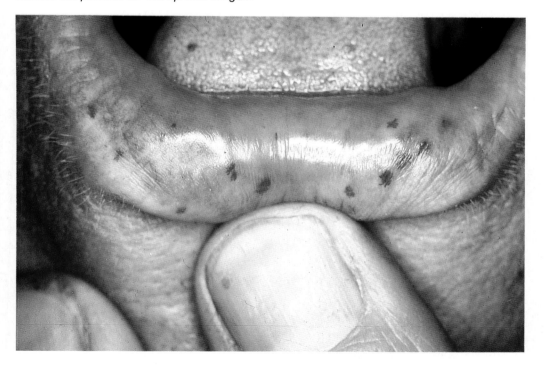

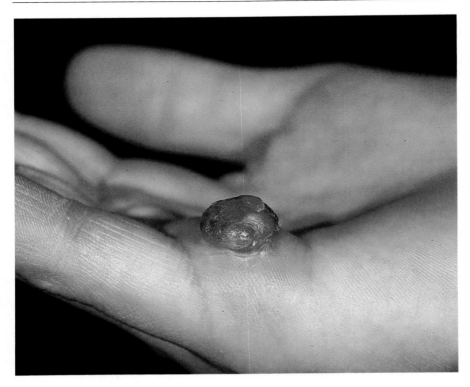

Figure 22-14
Pyogenic granuloma. A dome-shaped tumor with a moist fragile surface. The lesion may bleed profusely with the slightest trauma.

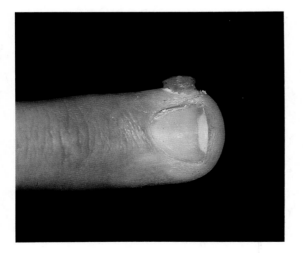

Figure 22-15
Side view of a pyogenic granuloma demonstrating the white collarette of scale often observed at the base.

Pyogenic Granuloma

Pyogenic granuloma is a small (less than 1 cm), rapidly growing, yellow-to-bright red, dome-shaped (Figure 22-14) fragile protrusion that has a glistening, moist-to-scaly surface. The base of the lesion is often surrounded by a collarette of scale (Figure 22-15). Pyogenic granulomas are most commonly seen in the head and neck region and on the extremities, especially the fingers. The slightest trauma causes bleeding that is difficult to control. The dermis is composed of a mass of capillaries. The name pyogenic suggests an infectious origin, but the lesion is probably caused by trauma.

Treatment consists of firm and thorough curettage of the base and border followed by electrodesiccation. Pyogenic granuloma will recur if the minutest piece of abnormal tissue remains.

Kaposi's Sarcoma

Kaposi's sarcoma is a rare vascular neoplasm generally appearing on the feet or lower legs. It begins as violaceous macules and papules (Figure 22-16) and very slowly progresses to form plaques with multiple red-purple nodules (Figure 22-17). Kaposi's sarcoma is relatively common in certain parts of Africa. Until recently, it was rarely seen in the United States and Europe, occurring exclusively in elderly men of Jewish, Greek, or Italian descent. Progression of this disease in the elderly is slow and, although lymph node and visceral involvement can occur, most of these patients die from unrelated causes.

A rapidly progressive form of Kaposi's sarcoma appears in a substantial fraction of the homosexual population with the acquired immunodeficiency syndrome. Lesions tend to be smaller (often 1 cm or less in diameter), less violaceous, raised, and nodular.[10] Some have a pityriasis rosea–like pattern of oval violaceous macules and plaques on the neck, trunk, and arms. Lesions tend to be widespread and not limited to the lower extremities. Many patients have tumor involvement of internal organs, for example, the gastrointestinal tract.[11]

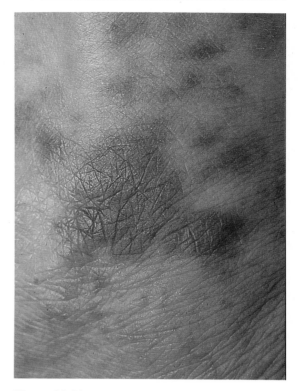

Figure 22-16
Kaposi's sarcoma. Early lesion consisting of violaceous macules and plaques.

Figure 22-17
Kaposi's sarcoma. Purple nodules are most commonly seen on the lower legs.

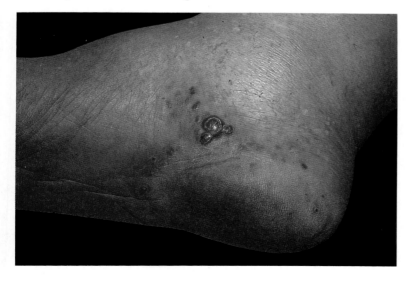

REFERENCES

1. Jessen T, Thompson S, Smith EB: Cobb syndrome. Arch Dermatol 113:1587, 1977.
2. Ohmori S, Haung C-K: Recent progress in treatment of port wine staining by argon laser: some observations on prognostic value of relative spectroeflectance (RSR) and histologic classification of lesions. Br J Plast Surg 34:249, 1981.
3. Cosman B: Experience in argon laser therapy of port-wine stains. Plastic Reconstr Surg 65:119, 1980.
4. Noe JM, Barsky SH, Geer DE, et al: Port wine stains and the response to argon laser therapy: successful treatment and the predictive role of color, age and biopsy. Plastic Reconstr Surg 65:130, 1980.
5. Illingworth RS: Thoughts on the treatment of vascular nevi. Arch Dis Child 51:138, 1976.
6. Edgerton MT: The treatment of hemangiomas: with special reference to the role of steroid therapy. Ann Surg 183:517, 1976.
7. Brown SH, Neerhout RC, Ronkalsrud GW: Prednisone therapy in the management of large hemangiomas in infants and children. Surgery 71:168, 1972.
8. Braverman IM: Skin signs of systemic disease. Philadelphia, 1981, WB Saunders Co.
9. Hodgson CH, Burchell HB, Good CA, et al: Hereditary hemorrhagic telangiectasia and pulmonary arteriovenous fistula. N Engl J Med 261:625, 1959.
10. Gottlieb GJ, Ackerman AB: Kaposi's sarcoma: an extensively disseminated form in young homosexual men. Hum Pathol 13:882, 1982.
11. Friedman-Kien AE: Disseminated Kaposi's sarcoma in homosexual men. Ann Intern Med 96:693, 1982.

Chapter Twenty-Three

Hair Diseases

Anatomy and physiology
Evaluation of hair loss
Generalized hair loss
Localized hair loss

Physicians are frequently confronted with hair-related problems. Most complaints are from patients with early onset pattern baldness. The physician must be able to recognize this normal, inherited hair loss pattern so that detailed and expensive evaluations can be avoided. Other patients have complaints about abnormal hair growth; these diseases must be recognized and not dismissed as balding. The signs of hair loss or excess growth are at times subtle. The signs usually seen with cutaneous disease, such as inflammation, may be absent. A systematic approach to evaluation is essential.

Anatomy and Physiology

The hair follicle is formed in the embryo by a club-shaped epidermal downgrowth, the primary epithelial germ that is invaginated from below by a capillary-containing dermal structure called the papilla of the hair follicle. The central cells of the downgrowth form the hair matrix, the cells of which make the hair shaft and surrounding structures. The mitotic rate of the hair matrix is greater than that of any other organ. Hair growth is greatly influenced by any stress or disease process that can alter mitotic activity. The growing shaft is surrounded by several concentric layers (see Figure 1-2). The outermost layer is called the outer root sheath. It is static and continuous with the epidermis. The inner root sheath (Henle's layer, Huxley's layer, and cuticle) protects and molds the growing hair, but disintegrates before reaching the surface. The hair shaft that emerges has three layers, an outer cuticle, a cortex, and sometimes an inner medulla, all of which are composed of dead protein. The cortex cells in the growing hair shaft rapidly synthesize and accumulate proteins while in the lower regions of the hair follicle. Systemic diseases and drugs may interfere with the metabolism of these cells and reduce the hair shaft diameter.

Growth cycle. Humans have a mosaic growth pattern; hair growth and loss are not cyclic or seasonal, as in some mammals, but occur at random so that hair loss is continuous (Figure 23-1). Each hair follicle undergoes repeated cycles of growth, rest, and shedding. The duration of the cycle varies with body location and can be modified by stress and disease. There are three stages in the hair growth cycle. These are catagen (transitional phase), telogen (resting phase), and anagen (growing phase).

Catagen. Approximately 3% of scalp hairs are in this 2- to 3-week transitional phase at any one time. Cell division in the hair matrix stops and the resting or catagen stage begins. The outer root sheath degenerates and retracts around the widened lower portion of the hair shaft. The lower follicle shrinks away from the connective tissue papilla and ascends to the level of the insertion of the papillary muscle.

Telogen. All activity ceases and the structure rests during the telogen phase. The telogen phase in the scalp lasts for about 100 days.[1] About 12% of scalp hair is in the telogen phase at any one time. The telogen phase is much longer in the eyebrows, arms, and legs. The inactive dead hair or club hair has a solid, hard, dry, white node at its proximal end; the white color results from lack of pigment. The club hair is firmly held in place; it is not ejected until a new anagen hair grows up and forces it out. About 25 to 100 telogen hairs are shed each day; possibly twice this number are lost on the days the hair is shampooed.

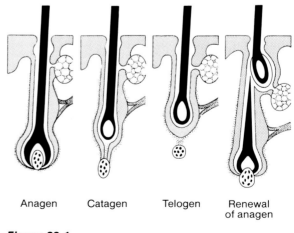

Anagen   Catagen   Telogen   Renewal of anagen

Figure 23-1
Phases in the life cycle of a hair.

TABLE 23-1

SYSTEMATIC APPROACH TO HAIR LOSS

History
  Sudden versus gradual loss
  Presence of systemic disease or high fever
  Recent psychologic or physical stress
  Medication or chemical exposure
Examination
  Localized versus generalized
  Scarring versus nonscarring
  Inflammatory versus noninflammatory
  Density—normal or decreased
  Presence of follicular plugging
Skin disease in other areas

Diagnostic procedures
  Hair pluck
    Telogen effluvium versus anagen
      effluvium
    Possible trichotillomania
  Potassium hydroxide examination for
    fungi
  Scalp biopsy
    Scarring alopecia
    Trichotillomania
  Hormone studies

TABLE 23-2

HAIR LOSS

Generalized*	Localized†
Telogen effluvium	Androgenic alopecia
Acute blood loss	Male-pattern
Childbirth	Female-pattern
Crash diets (inadequate protein)	Hirsutism
Drugs	Alopecia areata
Coumarins	Trichotillomania
Heparin	Traction alopecia
Propranolol	Scarring alopecia
Vitamin A	Developmental defects: aplasia cutis
High fever	Physical injury: burns, pressure
Hypo- and hyperthyroidism	Infection
Physical stress, e.g., surgery	Fungal: kerion
Physiologic, e.g., neonate	Bacterial: folliculitis, furuncle
Psychologic stress	Viral: herpes zoster
Severe illness, e.g., systemic lupus	Neoplasms
erythematosus	Metastatic carcinoma
Anagen effluvium	Sclerosing basal cell carcinoma
Cancer chemotherapeutic agent	Others
Poisoning	Lupus erythematosus
Thallium (rat poison)	Lichen planus
Arsenic	Cicatricial pemphigoid
Radiation therapy	Scleroderma
Generalized patchy	
Secondary syphilis-"moth eaten" alopecia	

*Diffuse uniform loss, but many hairs left randomly distributed in area of loss.
†Most or all hair missing from involved area.

TABLE 23-3

FEATURES DIFFERENTIATING TELOGEN EFFLUVIUM AND ANAGEN EFFLUVIUM

Clinical presentation	Telogen	Anagen
Onset of shedding after insult	2-4 months	1-4 weeks
Percent hair lost	20-50	80-90
Type hair lost	Normal club (white bulb)	Anagen hair (pigmented bulb)
Hair shaft	Normal	Narrowed or fractured

Anagen. The anagen phase begins with resumption of mitotic activity in the hair bulb and dermal papilla. The follicle grows down and meets the dermal papilla, recapitulating the embryonic events of development of the hair follicle. A new hair shaft forms and forces the tightly held club hair out. During anagen, hair grows at an average rate of 0.35 mm/day or 1 cm in 28 days;[2] this rate diminishes with age. Scalp hair remains in an active growing phase for an average of 2 to 6 years on the scalp. The active growing phase is much shorter and the resting stage is longer for arm, leg, eyelash, and eyebrow hairs and explains why these hairs remain short. About 85% of scalp hair is in an active growing phase at any one time.

Types of hair. There are three types of hair. Lanugo hairs are the fine hairs found on the fetus; similar fine hairs (peach fuzz) found on the adult are called vellus hairs. The coarse pigmented hairs of the scalp, beard, and axillary and pubic areas are called terminal hairs and are influenced by the androgen concentration. Hair on the rest of the body is independent of androgens.

Evaluation of Hair Loss

The causes of hair loss (alopecia) are numerous. A classification will be used, which is based primarily on distribution (i.e., localized versus generalized). A systematic approach for evaluation of hair loss is outlined in Table 23-1. Traditionally, the alopecias have been divided into scarring or nonscarring, but the presence of scarring is sometimes difficult to appreciate and some diseases cause scarring at one time and not at another. Scarring when present is a helpful sign; it should always be searched for.

Generalized hair loss

Diffuse hair loss (Table 23-2) usually occurs without inflammation or scarring. The loss affects hairs throughout the scalp in a more or less uniform pattern. The hair pluck test is important for differential diagnosis.

Telogen effluvium. A number of events have been documented that prematurely terminate anagen and cause an abnormally high number of normal hairs to enter the resting or telogen phase (Table 23-3). The follicle is not diseased, but has had its biologic clock reset and undergoes a normal involutional process. Usually no more than 50% of the patient's hair is affected. Scarring and inflammation are absent. Resting hairs on the scalp are retained for about 100 days before they are forced out by a new hair. Therefore, telogen hair loss should occur about 3 months after the event that terminated normal hair growth.

Kligman[3] explained this process and identified the various precipitating events (Table 23-2). The most common causes are briefly discussed. High fever from any cause may result in a sudden diffuse loss of club hairs 2 to 3 months later. Hair loss begins abruptly and lasts about 4 weeks. Telogen counts (see below) vary from 30% to 60%. Full recovery can be expected. Diffuse but primarily frontotemporal hair loss occurs in a significant number of women 1 to 4 months after childbirth. The loss can be quite significant, but complete recovery occurs in less than 1 year. Both severe emotional and physical traumas have been documented to cause diffuse hair loss. Hair loss has been reported as occurring 2 weeks after severe psychologic or physical trauma, but since this is too short a time for the induction of the telogen phase, the loss must have occurred by another mechanism, such as loss from alopecia areata.

Anagen effluvium. Anagen effluvium (Tables 23-2 and 23-3) is the abrupt loss of hair from follicles that continue in their growing phase. The insult causes a change in the rate of hair growth, but does not convert the follicle to a different growth phase, as occurs in telogen effluvium. An abrupt insult to the metabolic and follicular reproductive apparatus must be delivered to create such an event.

Cancer chemotherapeutic agents, thallium salts (rat poison), and radiation therapy are capable of such an insult.[4,5] The rapidly dividing cells of the matrix and cortex are affected. High concentrations of anti-metabolites or radiation bring all metabolic processes to an abrupt halt and the entire hair and hair root are shed intact. Insults of less intensity slow the mitotic rate of the bulb and cortex cells, causing bulb deformity and narrowing of the lower hair shaft. Narrow weakened hair shafts are easily broken and shed without bulbs. Since 90% of scalp hair is in the anagen phase, a large number of hairs can be affected. Patients with 10% to 20% of their hair remaining after an insult almost certainly have had an anagen effluvium.

Hair pluck evaluation. The most accurate technique for establishing the anagen-telogen ratio is to abruptly extract hairs from the scalp with a rubber-tipped needle holder.[6] Make the instrument by placing rubber-tubing needle protectors from prepackaged injectable drugs over the jaws of a small needle-holder. Firmly grasp about 50 hairs at the same height and rotate the needle-holder one turn to ensure a firm hold on the hairs. Apply slight tension on the hairs, then with a quick positive upward motion extract the hairs. The pain is intense but of short duration.

Cut the excess hair 1 cm from the roots, float the hairs onto a wet microscope slide or Petri dish, and examine with the ×10 lens (Figure 23-2). Baden[7] reported a simple technique for staining plucked anagen hairs that allows them to be easily distinguished from plucked telogen hairs. Anagen Hair Dye (4-dimethylaminocinnamaldehyde [DACA], ob-tained from Dermatologic Lab and Supply, Inc., Council Bluffs, Iowa) reacts with citrulline, an amino acid found only in the internal root sheath. The stain is dropped on the root ends of a hair pluck preparation, and the hairs are moved gently from side to side for 15 to 20 seconds to allow penetration of the dye.

Telogen hairs have small unpigmented ovoid bulbs and do not contain an internal root sheath; therefore, they do not stain with DACA. Anagen hairs have larger, elongated, pigmented (if hair is pigmented) bulbs shaped like the end of a broom, surrounded by a narrow internal root sheath. DACA stains the root sheath a bright red color.

In some diseases hair fragments without bulbs are obtained during a hair pluck. Processes that interfere with cell division cause the shaft to be poorly formed and therefore apt to break under tension. Alopecia areata, antimetabolite therapy, and small doses of ionizing radiation will interrupt the mitotic activity in the cells along the hair shaft that normally contribute cells to the growing hair follicle.

Localized hair loss (Table 23-2)

Androgenic alopecia in males. Baldness in males is not a disease, but rather a physiologic reaction induced by androgens in genetically predisposed men. The pattern of inheritance is unknown. There are two populations of scalp follicles: androgen-sensitive follicles on the top and androgen-independent follicles on the sides and back of the scalp. In genetically predisposed individuals and under the influence of androgens, terminal hair follicles are transformed into vellus-like follicles and the terminal hair is shed and replaced by fine light vellus hair. Triangular frontotemporal recession occurs normally in most males and females after puberty. The first signs of balding are increased fronto-temporal recession accompanied by midfrontal recession. Hair loss in a round area on the vertex follows and the density of hair decreases, sometimes rapidly, over the top of the scalp.

Patients who begin balding at an early age are most distressed and are tempted to consult "experts" at hair clinics. These clinics offer a variety of topical preparations, all of which have absolutely no value. Warn patients who seek your advice for hair loss not to become involved in these long-term and expensive programs. Selected patients may be referred for hair transplants, plastic surgical rotation flaps, or wigs.

Adrenal androgenic female-pattern alopecia. Chronic, progressive, diffuse hair loss in women in their twenties and thirties is a frequently encountered complaint. These women, who usually have a normal menstrual cycle and lack any abnormalities evident on physical examination, have been classified as having "male-pattern baldness,"

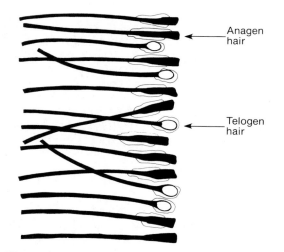

Figure 23-2
Hair pluck preparation showing anagen and telogen hairs.

Anagen hair

Telogen hair

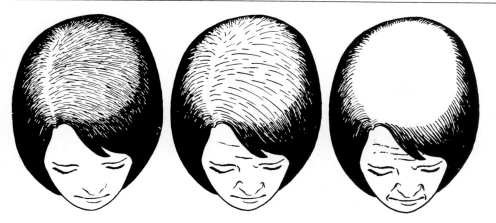

Figure 23-3
*The evolution of the female type of androgenic alopecia. (From Ludwig E: Br J Dermatol **97:**247, 1977.)*

a genetic trait, and dismissed without further evaluation. Recent studies have shown that many of these women have increased levels of the serum adrenal androgen dehydroepiandrosterone-sulfate (DHEAS) and a distinct pattern of central scalp alopecia, which has been called adrenal androgenic female-pattern alopecia.

With male-pattern baldness, there is a gradual regression of the hair on the central scalp and gradual frontotemporal recession, as well as a gradual decrease in hair-shaft diameter in the areas of hair loss. In contrast, most women with diffuse alopecia experience a gradual loss of hair on the central scalp, with retention of the normal hairline without frontotemporal recession. There is a variety of anagen hair diameters. With advancing age, the central thinning becomes more pronounced; contrary to male-pattern baldness, a fringe of hair along the frontal hairline persists (Figure 23-3).[8] In exceptional cases a course similar to that in men is seen, with deep frontotemporal recession.

Laboratory findings. The laboratory investigation of female patients with diffuse alopecia with both female and male patterns is outlined in Table 23-4. Laboratory evaluation for androgenic alopecia should initially include determination of the serum

TABLE 23-4

LABORATORY VALUES FOR EVALUATION OF DIFFUSE FEMALE ALOPECIA*

	Female-pattern alopecia	Female-pattern alopecia with hirsutism	Male-pattern alopecia (frontotemporal recession)
DHEAS*	Normal or elevated	Normal or elevated	Elevated
T	Normal	Normal or elevated	Elevated
TeBG	Normal	Decreased or normal	Decreased or normal
T/TeBG	Normal	Elevated	Elevated
Prolactin†			

Adapted from Kasick JM, Bergfeld WF, Steck WD, et al: Adrenal androgenic female-pattern alopecia: sex hormones and the balding woman. Cleve Clin Q **50:**111, 1983.
*DHEAS, dehydroepiandrosterone-sulfate, T, total serum testosterone; TeBG, testosterone-estradiol binding globulin; T/TeBG, androgenic index.
†If elevated, suspect pituitary disease, e.g., pituitary prolactin-secreting adenoma.

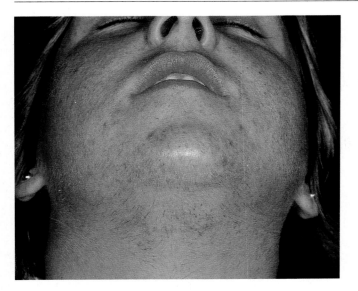

Figure 23-4
*Hirsutism. Growth of terminal hair on the chin and
neck of a young woman.*

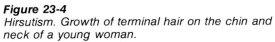

Figure 23-5
Hirsutism. A prominent escutcheon in a woman.

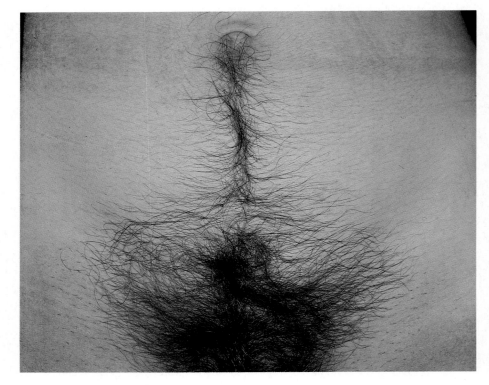

TABLE 23-5

SIGNS OF VIRILIZATION

Acne and increased sebum production	Increased muscle mass
Clitoral hypertrophy	Infrequent or absent menses
Decrease in breast size	Heightened libido
Deepening of the voice	Hirsutism
Frontotemporal balding	Malodorous perspiration

TABLE 23-6

CAUSES OF HIRSUTISM

Without virilization	With virilization
Racial: variations of normal	Ovarian tumors
Pregnancy	Adrenal disease
Menopause	Congenital adrenal hyperplasia
Idiopathic: androgen elevation of	Adrenal tumors
unknown cause	
Drugs	
Androgens	
Diazoxide	
Glucocorticoids	
Minoxidil	
Oral contraceptives (progestational	
components)	
Phenytoin	

DHEAS and total serum testosterone (T) levels, testosterone-estradiol binding globulin (TeBG) for the T/TeBG ratio, and serum prolactin levels.[9]

Treatment. Several reports have indicated that spironolactone is a highly effective and safe drug for the treatment of hirsutism. One small study showed that some women with adrenal androgenic alopecia had an increased growth of scalp hair with a decrease in the amount of daily hair loss when treated with 25 to 50 mg of spironolactone taken twice daily for periods ranging from 3 to 12 months. Some had a reduction of serum DHEAS.[9]

Hirsutism. Hirsutism in women is defined as the growth of terminal hair in the male distribution on the face, body, and pubic area accompanied by frontotemporal scalp hair recession (Figures 23-4 and 23-5). These areas contain androgen-sensitive hair. Hirsutism by itself or associated with other signs of virilization (Table 23-5) may be a sign of an endocrine disorder.

A classification of hirsutism is listed in Table 23-6. Most women have some terminal hair in the so-called male sexual pattern. Normal variations are great and women of certain ethnic groups, such as women of eastern Mediterranean descent may have dense facial and body hair with a male escutcheon. Such individuals would be recognized as perfectly normal in their countries of origin and can be reassured. Women who develop hirsutism well after puberty, especially if accompanied by signs of virilization such as infrequent or absent menses, require further evaluation. Hormones capable of causing virilization may originate from ovarian or adrenal disease. Braunstein has designed an approach for establishing the etiology of hirsutism.[10]

Braunstein method for evaluation of hirsutism. In the Braunstein method for evaluating hirsutism (Figure 23-6) the presence or absence of virilization is first established. Serum testosterone and serum DHEAS (abbreviated in Figure 23-6 as DHEA-sulfate or D-S) levels are obtained. Additional tests are ordered as indicated in the flow sheet.[10]

Treatment of hirsutism. After ovarian and adrenal diseases have been investigated and treated appropriately if present, hirsutism may be dealt with in a variety of ways.

Cosmetic approach. Excess facial hair may be plucked, shaved, bleached, wax stripped, or removed by chemical depilatories or electrolysis. Shaving does not increase the thickness or rate of growth.

Glucocorticoids. Glucocorticoids suppress adrenal and ovarian androgen production. Administer dexamethasone (0.5 to 0.75 mg orally) at night. Nighttime administration will reduce the early morning peak of adrenocorticotropic hormone secretion and generally does not cause the typical side effects of glucocorticoid excess or prolonged adrenal suppression. About 30% to 50% of patients will note improvement on this program.[10]

Oral contraceptives. The estrogen component of oral contraceptives decreases the ovarian and adrenal androgen production and stimulates the liver to produce increased quantities of testosterone-estradiol-binding globulin. The circulating globulin binds and decreases the concentration of active serum androgens. The same criteria for choosing an oral contraceptive are used for hirsutism and acne. Effective preparations are those with high

Figure 23-6 (opposite)
Flow sheet for the evaluation of a patient with hirsutism with or without associated virilization. DHEA-sulfate (D-S), dehydroepiandrosterone sulfate; LH, luteinizing hormone; FSH, follicle stimulating hormone. (From Braunstein GD: Female reproductive disorders. In Hershman JM, editor. Management of endocrine disorders. Philadelphia, 1980, Lea & Febiger.)

concentrations of estrogen and a progestin with low androgen activity. Agents containing 100 μg of mestranol and 2 mg of norethindrone (Ortho-Novum 2 mg; Norinyl 2 mg) meet this criteria. If the high dose of estrogen is not tolerated, preparations containing 80 μg of mestranol and 1 mg of norethindrone (Norinyl-1 + 80 21- or 28-day; Ortho-Novum 1/80-21 or -28) may be substituted. Approximately 50% of patients treated with oral contraceptives for 6 months or more will improve.[10]

Cimetidine. Cimetidine blocks androgen action at the hair follicle and would be expected to be effective whether the source of the excess androgen is ovarian or adrenal. One study showed that 300 mg of cimetidine 5 times daily for 3 months significantly reduced the rate of hair growth in severely hirsute women.[11]

Spironolactone. Spironolactone inhibits enzymes required for synthesis of androgens in gonadal and adrenal cells and acts by competitive in-

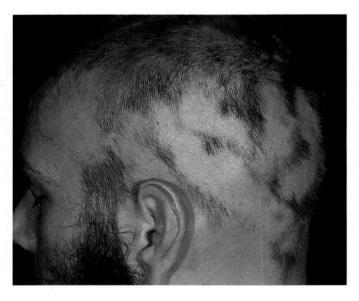

Figure 23-7
Alopecia areata. Multiple round and oval patches of hair loss.

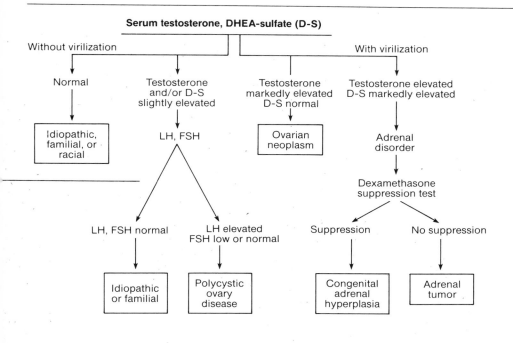

Serum testosterone, DHEA-sulfate (D-S)

Without virilization — With virilization

Without virilization:

Normal → Idiopathic, familial, or racial

Testosterone and/or D-S slightly elevated → LH, FSH

LH, FSH normal → Idiopathic or familial

LH elevated FSH low or normal → Polycystic ovary disease

With virilization:

Testosterone markedly elevated D-S normal → Ovarian neoplasm

Testosterone elevated D-S markedly elevated → Adrenal disorder → Dexamethasone suppression test

Suppression → Congenital adrenal hyperplasia

No suppression → Adrenal tumor

hibition at the hair follicle. Administration of 200 mg of spironolactone per day resulted in definite improvement with marked reduction in the quantity and notable improvement in the quality of facial hair in one study. Improvement was noted in 2 months and was maximal at 6 months.[12]

Alopecia areata. Alopecia areata is a common asymptomatic disease characterized by the rapid onset of total hair loss in a sharply defined, usually round, area. Most patients are under 40 and have no other associated findings. A wide spectrum of involvement is seen. The majority of patients report the sudden occurrence of one or several 1 to 4 cm areas of hair loss on the scalp that can be easily concealed by covering with adjacent hair (Figure 23-7). The skin is smooth and white or may have short stubs of hair. The hair shaft in alopecia areata is poorly formed and breaks off at the surface. A short (3 mm) broken hair that tapers toward a small but normal club bulb may be extracted from the periphery of the bald patch. This hair is shaped like an exclamation point and is referred to as an exclamation point hair.

Regrowth begins in 1 to 3 months and may be followed by loss in the same or other areas. The prognosis for total permanent regrowth in cases with limited involvement is excellent. The new hair is usually of the same color and texture, but may be fine and white (Figure 23-8). Occasionally the white color remains. The eyelashes, beard, and rarely other parts of the body may be involved. Total hair

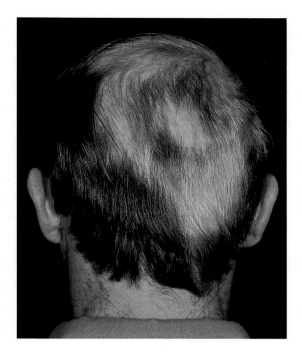

Figure 23-8
Alopecia areata. The hair has regrown white.

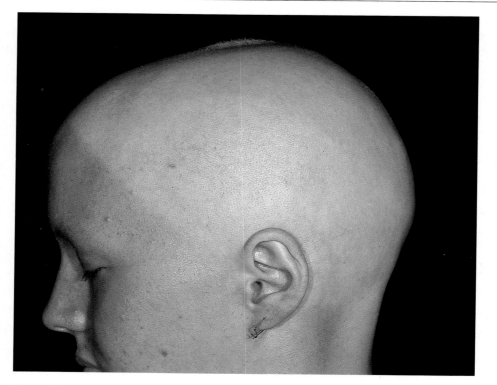

Figure 23-9
Alopecia totalis. The hair has regrown for short periods. The prognosis for normal regrowth is poor.

loss of the scalp (alopecia totalis) (Figure 23-9), seen most frequently in young people, may be accompanied by cycles of growth and loss, but the prognosis for long-term regrowth is poor. Total body hair loss (alopecia universalis) is very rare. Nail pitting and longitudinal striations may be seen in one or all nails in some patients with alopecia areata (Figure 24-8, page 509).

The diagnosis is made by observation. A biopsy is rarely necessary. The dermis contains a lymphocytic infiltrate around a small follicle that despite all the inflammation has managed to remain in the anagen phase. The etiology is unknown. Stress is frequently cited and some patients date the onset of hair loss from a traumatic event.[13] Alopecia areata may be associated with thyroid disease, pernicious anemia,[14,15] Addison's disease, vitiligo,[16] lupus erythematosus, ulcerative colitis,[17] and Down's syndrome. Circulating autoantibodies and follicular deposits of C3 and IgG have been reported.[18] The significance of these findings is unknown.

Treatment

Observation. The majority of patients with a few small areas of hair loss can be assured that the prognosis for regrowth is excellent. If there is great anxiety or if bald areas cannot be concealed, then intralesional injections should be considered.

Intralesional injection. Hair growth can be stimulated in a majority of cases with an intradermal injection of triamcinolone acetonide (Kenalog) (2.5 to 10 mg/ml).[19,20] The suspension is delivered uniformly throughout the bald area by simultaneously injecting and advancing the needle. Inject just enough of the suspension to momentarily blanch the skin. Injections may be repeated at 4-week intervals. Atrophy, especially with the 10 mg/ml dosage, is the major side effect. The results in most cases are gratifying, but there is no evidence that intralesional steroid injections alter the course of disease and the hair may once again be shed. This treatment should be reserved for patients with a few small areas of hair loss.

Systemic steroids. Oral and intramuscular steroids will predictably restore hair growth, but one can forsee with the same degree of certainty that the hair will be lost when treatment is stopped.[21] Except in the most unusual circumstances systemic steroids should be avoided.

Anthralin. Anthralin in a petrolatum base (Anthra-Derm ointment 1%, 0.5%, 0.25%, or 0.1%; see

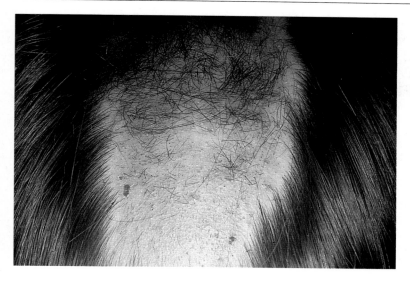

Figure 23-10
*Trichotillomania. Several short
hairs are randomly distributed
in the involved site.*

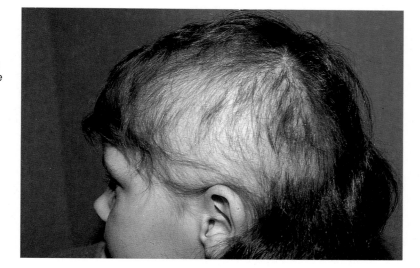

Figure 23-11
*Trichotillomania. Hair has been
manually extracted from a wide
area of the scalp. There is
no inflammation or scarring.*

Table 8-2) applied once daily in concentrations high enough to induce a visible dermatitis of marked erythema and mild itching has been reported to induce hair growth.[22] The mechanism of action is unknown, but the treatment is safe and may be considered for refractory cases.

Dinitrochlorobenzene (DNCB). Hair growth may be stimulated by inducing a contact allergy at the sites of hair loss. DNCB will induce sensitivity in most individuals and has been used as a therapeutic agent in many trials. Its use has been curtailed because of its potential carcinogenicity. Other contact allergens are being investigated.[24]

Minoxidil (topical solution). Minoxidil, a potent direct peripheral vasodilator used to control severe hypertension, is being evaluated in several centers for treatment-resistant alopecia areata.[25]

Trichotillomania. Trichotillomania is the act of manually removing hair by manipulation. This conscious or subconscious habitual act or tic is most commonly performed by young children and adolescents during inactive periods in the classroom, while watching television, or in bed while waiting to fall asleep. Hair is twisted around the finger and pulled or rubbed until extracted or broken. The favorite site is the easily reached frontoparietal region of the scalp, but any scalp area or eyebrows and eyelashes may be attacked. The affected area has an irregular angulated border and the density of hair is greatly reduced, but the site is never bald as in alopecia areata. Several short broken hairs are randomly distributed in the involved site. Hair that grows beyond 0.5 to 1 cm can be grasped by small fingers and is extracted (Figures 23-10 and 23-11).

Diagnosis. First ask the patient if he or she manipulates the hair. Parents or teachers may be aware of the habit. A potassium hydroxide and Wood's light examination may have to be performed to rule out noninflammatory tinea capitis. Areas of alopecia areata are completely devoid of hair. In questionable cases a hair pluck can be performed and will show 100% of the hairs in the active growing or anagen phase. Skin biopsy will show absence of hairs in follicles, but is rarely necessary.

Treatment. Most patients are psychologically stable and require only a discussion of the problem with an understanding physician or parent. Patients with extensive involvement or who persist should have a psychiatric evaluation.

Traction (cosmetic) alopecia. Prolonged tension created by certain hair styles such as braids or ponytails, hair rollers, and hot hair straightening combs, may result in temporary and rarely permanent hair loss in an area corresponding exactly to the stressed hair. The scalp appears normal or shows evidence of inflammation and sometimes scarring. Temporary or permanent occipital alopecia secondary to pressure ischemia may occur on the scalp of patients left on their backs in the same position during surgery.

Scarring alopecia. A great number of diseases cause scarring, and if they happen to occur in the scalp, hair follicles may be destroyed, resulting in scarring or cicatricial alopecia. Many can be recognized by their characteristic presentation.

Discoid lupus erythematosus. Discoid lupus erythematosus in the scalp is characterized by localized erythematous areas of hair loss that show prominent follicular plugging. With time, plugged follicles disappear and the skin becomes smooth, atrophic, and scarred. Biopsy and immunofluorescence will help establish the diagnosis.

Lichen planus. Lichen planus in the scalp appears as violaceous papules or as an area of alopecia with follicular plugging. If scarring occurs, the follicular plugs are lost and at this stage the diagnosis cannot be made with certainty by biopsy. This type of scarring alopecia without evidence of lichen planus in other areas has been called pseudopelade.

Aplasia cutis congenita. A small blister or eroded area, usually in the midline of the scalp, may be present at birth. It represents a congenital absence of a portion or a full thickness of skin. In most cases the area heals spontaneously. Larger areas of aplasia may be associated with other developmental defects.

REFERENCES

1. Rook A, Dawber R: Diseases of the hair and scalp. Oxford 1982, Blackwell Scientific Publications.
2. Munro DD: Hair growth measurement using intradermal sulphur 35 L-cystine. Arch Dermatol **93**:119, 1966.
3. Kligman AM: Pathologic dynamics of human hair loss. I. Telogen effluvium. Arch Dermatol **83**:175, 1961.
4. Webster JR, Huff S, Gecht MC: Thallotoxicosis. Arch Dermatol **78**:278, 1958.
5. Levantine A, Almeyda J: Drug induced alopecia, Br J Dermatol **89**:549, 1973.
6. Maguire HC Jr, Kligman AM: Hair plucking as a diagnostic test. J Invest Dermatol **43**:77, 1964.
7. Baden HP, Kubilus J, Baden L: A stain for plucked anagen hairs. J Am Acad Dermatol **1**:121, 1979.
8. Ludwig E: Classification of the types of androgenic alopecia (common baldness) occurring in the female sex. Br J Dermatol **97**:247, 1977.
9. Kasick JM, Bergfeld WF, Steck WD, et al: Adrenal androgenic female-pattern alopecia: sex hormones and the balding woman. Cleve Clin Q **50**:111, Summer 1983.
10. Braunstein GD: Female reproductive disorders. In Hershman JM, editor. Management of endocrine disorders. Philadelphia, 1980, Lea & Febiger.
11. Vigersky RA, Mehlman I, Glass AR, et al: Treatment of hirsute women with cimetidine. N Engl J Med **303**:1042, 1980.
12. Cumming DC, Yang JC, Rebar RW, et al: Treatment of hirsutism with spironolactone. JAMA **247**:1295, 1982.
13. Greenberg SI: Alopecia areata: a psychiatric surgery. Arch Dermatol **72**:454, 1955.
14. Muller SA, Winkelman RK: Alopecia areata. Arch Dermatol **88**:290, 1963.
15. Friedmann PS: Alopecia areata and autoimmunity. Br J Dermatol **105**:153, 1981.
16. Anderson I: Alopecia areata: a clinical study. Br Med J **2**:1250, 1950.
17. Allen HB, Moschella SL: Ulcerative colitis associated with skin and hair changes. Cutis **14**:85, 1974.
18. Bystryn J, Orentreich N, Stengel F: Direct immunofluorescence studies in alopecia areata and male pattern alopecia. J Invest Dermatol **73**:317, 1979.
19. Abell E, Munroe DD: Intralesional treatment of alopecia areata with triamcinolone acetonide by jet injector. Br J Dermatol **88**:55, 1973.
20. Porter D, Burton JL: A comparison of intralesional triamcinolone hexacetonide and triamcinolone acetonide in alopecia areata. Br J Dermatol **85**:272, 1971.
21. Winter RJ, Kern F, Blizzard RM: Prednisone therapy for alopecia areata: a follow-up report. Arch Dermatol **112**:1549, 1976.
22. Schmoeckel C, Weissmann I, Plewig G, et al: Treatment of alopecia areata by anthralin-induced dermatitis. Arch Dermatol **115**:1254, 1979.
23. Swanson NA, Mitchell AJ, Leahy MS, et al: Topical treatment of alopecia areata: contact allergen vs primary irritant therapy. Arch Dermatol **117**:384, 1981.
24. Case PC, Mitchell AJ, Swanson NA, et al: Topical therapy of alopecia areata with squaric acid dibutylester. J Am Acad Dermatol **10**:447, 1984.
25. Weiss VC, West DP, Fu TS, et al: Alopecia areata treated with topical Minoxidil. Arch Dermatol **120**:457, 1984.

Chapter Twenty-Four

Nail Diseases

Anatomy and Physiology

The nail unit consists of several components (Figure 24-1). The nail plate is hard translucent dead keratin. The nail fold includes the skin surrounding the lateral and proximal aspects of the nail plate. The proximal nail fold overlies the matrix. Its keratin layer extends onto the proximal nail plate to form the cuticle. Capillary loops at the tip of the nail fold are normally small and inapparent, but they become distinct in diseases such as systemic lupus erythematosus and scleroderma. The proximal nail-fold epithelium covers the proximal nail plate for a few millimeters, then makes a 180 degree turn and curves back into direct contact with the nail plate. It makes another 180 degree turn and becomes continuous with the nail matrix. The matrix epithelium synthesizes the nail plate. The lunula (white half-moon), which is visible through the nail plate, is the distal aspect of the nail matrix. It is continuous with the nail bed. The nail bed extends from the distal nail matrix to the hyponychium. It consists of parallel longitudinal ridges with small blood vessels at their base (Figure 24-2). Bleeding induced by trauma or vessel disease, such as lupus, occurs in the depths of these grooves, producing the splinter hemorrhage pattern viewed through the nail plate. The hyponychium is a short segment of skin lacking nail cover; it begins at the distal nail bed and terminates at the distal groove.

Nails grow continuously, but their growth rate decreases with both age and poor circulation. Fingernails, which grow faster than toenails, grow at the rate of 0.5 to 1.29 mm per week. It takes approximately 5.5 months for a fingernail to grow from the matrix to the free edge and approximately 12 to 18 months for a toenail to be replaced. A reduction in the rate of matrix cell division like that which occurs during certain systemic diseases (e.g., scarlet fever) causes thinning of the nail plate (Beau's lines).

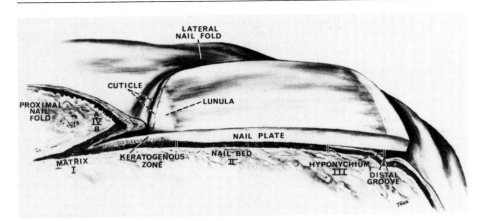

Figure 24-1
Diagrammatic drawing of an adult fingertip,
showing nail structures through a longitudinal
midline plane. (From Zaias N, Ackerman BA:
Arch Dermatol **107**:193, 1973. Copyright 1973,
American Medical Association.)

Figure 24-2
Dermal topography underlying nail unit.
The nail bed consists of parallel
longitudinal ridges with small blood
vessels at their base. Anatomic
pathology of splinter hemorrhages is
obvious. (From Zaias N, Ackerman BA:
Arch Dermatol **107**:193, 1973. Copyright
1973, American Medical Association.)

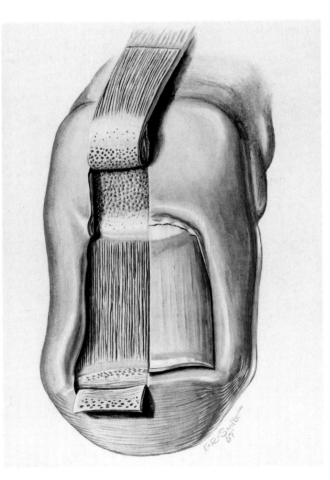

Normal Variations

The shape and opacity of the nail vary considerably among individuals. Aging may increase or decrease nail thickness. Longitudinal ridging is common in aging, but this variant is occasionally observed among the young. Beading occurs at all ages, but is more common in the elderly (Figure 24-3). The beads cover part or most of the plate surface and are arranged longitudinally. A pigmented band or bands occur in over 90% of blacks (Figure 24-4). The sudden appearance of such a band in whites may result from a melanoma and necessitates further investigation.

Figure 24-3
Longitudinal ridging and beading. A variant of normal most commonly seen in the elderly.

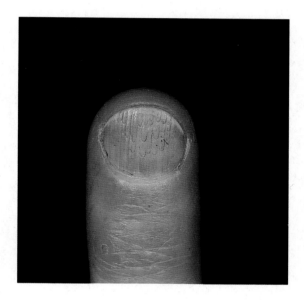

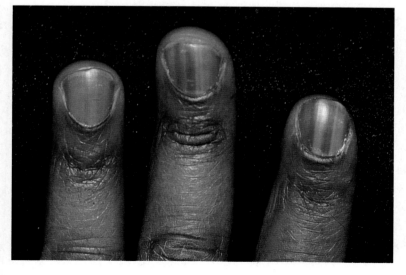

Figure 24-4
Pigmented bands occur as a normal finding in over 90% of blacks.

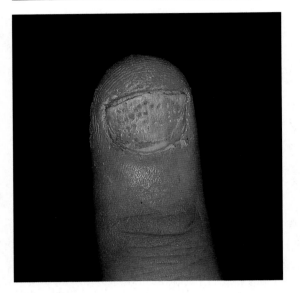

Figure 24-5
Psoriasis. Pitting is the most common nail change found in psoriasis.

Figure 24-6
Psoriasis. Onycholysis, subungual debris, and nail plate distortion are shown. These changes are often misinterpreted as being fungal in origin.

Nail Disorders Associated with Skin Disease

Psoriasis. The incidence of nail involvement in psoriasis varies from 10% to 50%. Nail involvement usually occurs simultaneously with skin disease, but may occur as an isolated finding. Pitting, onycholysis, discoloration, subungual thickening, and nail plate alterations take place. Pitting, or sharply defined ice-pick–like depressions in the nail plate, are the most common finding (Figure 24-5). The number, distribution pattern, and depth vary. Pitting is observed in normal nails and in patients with alopecia areata, but in general psoriatic pits are deeper. Pits form as the nail substance is shed, which is a process analagous to the shedding of psoriatic skin scale.

Separation of the nail from the nail bed, or onycholysis, is common; unlike traumatic onycholysis, it is frequently accompanied by yellow discoloration. Separation begins at the distal groove and may involve several nails. Psoriasis of the hyponychium results in the accumulation of yellow scaly debris, which elevates the nail plate. The debris is commonly mistaken for nail fungus infection. Severe psoriasis of the matrix and nail bed results in grossly malformed nails and nail bed splinter hemorrhages are common (Figure 24-6).

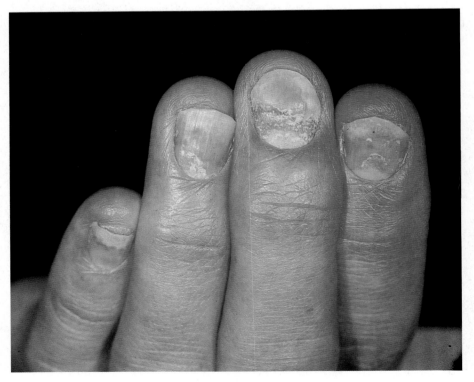

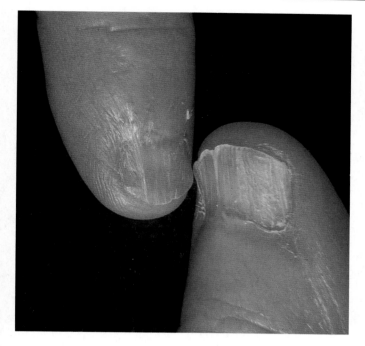

Figure 24-7
Lichen planus. Inflammation of the matrix results in adhesion of the proximal nail fold to the scarred matrix, a pterygium.

Treatment is unsatisfactory. Intralesional injections into the matrix with triamcinolone acetonide (2.5 to 5 mg/ml) delivered with a 30-gauge needle produce the most satisfactory results.[1] The painful procedure is repeated every 3 or 4 weeks. There is little merit in treating psoriatic nails with psoralen UVA (PUVA) or topical 5-fluorouracil (5-FU).

Lichen planus. Nail involvement may accompany any form of lichen planus (LP). The matrix, nail bed, and nail folds may be involved in producing a variety of changes, few of which are characteristic. Minimal inflammation of the matrix induces longitudinal grooving and ridging, which is the most common finding for lichen planus of the nail. Scarring may follow LP of the nail matrix. A pterygium, caused by adhesion of a depressed proximal nail fold to the scarred matrix, may occur after intense matrix inflammation (Figure 24-7). The nail plate distal to this focus is either absent or thinned out.

Matrix lesions may respond to intralesional triamcinolone acetonide (2.5 to 5 mg/ml) delivered with a 30-gauge needle every 3 to 4 weeks. Severe cases will respond to prednisone (20 to 30 mg/day). This may require a long course of treatment in which the risks may outnumber the advantages.

Alopecia areata. Many patients with alopecia areata have shallow pitting or surface stipling in a uniform or grid-like pattern (Figure 24-8).

Darier's disease. A number of nail changes are reported with Darier's disease (keratosis follicularis),[2] but white longitudinal streaks are the most common and the most characteristic.

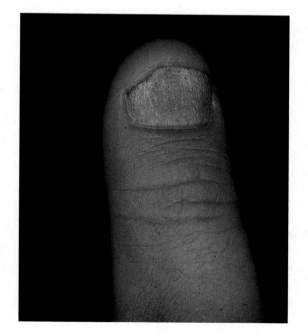

Figure 24-8
Alopecia areata. Shallow pitting occurs in some patients with alopecia areata.

Acquired Disorders

Infections

Acute paronychia. The rapid onset of painful bright red swelling of the proximal and lateral nail fold may occur spontaneously or follow trauma or manipulation. Superficial infections are characterized by an accumulation of purulent material behind the cuticle (Figure 24-9). The small abscess is drained by inserting the pointed end of a comedo extractor or a similar instrument between the proximal nail fold and the nail plate. Pain is abruptly relieved. A diffuse painful swelling suggests deeper infection and cases not responding to antistaphylococcal antibiotics may require deep incision. Acute paronychia rarely evolves into chronic paronychia.

Chronic paronychia. Chronic paronychia evolves slowly and begins with tenderness and mild swelling around the proximal and lateral nail folds (Figure 24-10). Bakers, dishwashers, and dentists, for example, whose hands are repeatedly exposed to moisture, are at greatest risk. Manipulation of the cuticle will accelerate the process. Typically, many or all fingers are involved simultaneously. The cuticle separates from the nail plate, leaving the space between the proximal nail fold and the nail plate exposed to infection. Many organisms, both pathogens and contaminants, thrive in this warm moist intertriginous space. The skin around the nail becomes pale red, tender, or painful and swollen. Occasionally a small quantity of pus can be expressed from under the proximal nail fold. A culture of this material may grow candida or gram-positive and gram-negative organisms. The nail plate is not infected and maintains its integrity, although its surface becomes brown and rippled. There is no subungual thickening such as that present in some fungal infections. The process is chronic and responds very slowly to treatment. Psoriasis of the fingers shows a similar form, with a possible secondary-yeast infection.

Treatment. Every attempt must be made to keep the hands dry. Avoid using medicines with an ointment base; they are too occlusive and interfere with the necessary drying process. Patients should refrain from washing dishes and from washing their own hair. Rubber or plastic gloves are of some value, but moisture accumulates in them with prolonged use.

Oral antibiotics do not penetrate this distal site in sufficient concentration. Furthermore, the variety of organisms is too numerous for response by any single oral agent. The most effective treatment is to place one or two drops of 3% thymol in 70% ethanol, which must be compounded by a pharmacist, at the proximal nail fold and wait for this liquid to flow by capillary action into the space created by the absent cuticle. Slight elevation of the proximal nail fold with a flat toothpick will facilitate penetration. This should be repeated 2 to 3 times each day for months until the cuticle is reformed. Patients with long-standing inflammation may never reform the cuticle.

Pseudomonas infection. Repeated exposure to soap and water causes maceration of the hyponychium and softening of the nail plate. Separation of the nail plate (onycholysis) exposes a damp macerated space between nail plate and nail bed, which is a fertile site for the growth of pseudomonas. The nail plate assumes a green-black color[3] (Figure 24-11). There is little discomfort or inflammation. This presentation may be confused with subungual hematoma (see Figure 24-20), but the absence of pain with pseudomonas infection serves to establish the diagnosis. Zaias[4] recommends applying a few drops of a 1 part Chlorox–4 parts water mixture under the nail 3 times a day. Vinegar (5% acetic acid) applied under the nail twice daily is also very effective treatment.

Herpetic whitlow. Dentists and nurses are at risk of acquiring herpes simplex infection of the fingertip. The appearance and course of the disease resemble that at other body sites with the exception of extreme pain from the swollen fingertips (see Figure 12-33).

Tinea of the nails. Tinea of the nails[5] is also called tinea unguium. Dermatophytes are responsible for most finger and toenail infections, but the so-called nonpathogenic fungi (contaminants), and candida in the rare syndrome of chronic mucocutaneous candidiasis, can also infect the nail plate. Nail infection may occur simultaneously with hand or foot tinea or occur as an isolated phenomenon. The disease is very common in adults, but may also occur in children.

Trauma predisposes to infection. There is a tendency to label as a fungus infection any process involving the nail plate, but many other cutaneous diseases can change the structure of the nail; differential diagnosis is discussed at the end of this section.

There are four distinctive patterns of nail infection described by Zaias.[5] Several patterns of infection may occur simultaneously in the nail plate. *Trichophyton rubrum* and *T mentagrophytes* invade nail plate more frequently than *T violaceum* and *T tonsurans. Aspergillus, Cephalosporium, Fusarium,* and *Scopulariopsis,* generally considered contaminants or nonpathogens, have been isolated from infected nails. They may be found in any pattern of nail infection, especially distal subungual onychomycosis and white superficial onychomycosis. The contaminants do not respond to griseofulvin. The technique for preparation of the nail for potassium hydroxide wet mount is described in the chapter pertaining to fungal infections.

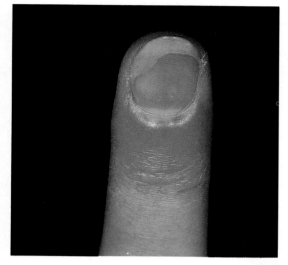

Figure 24-9
Acute paronychia. Erythema and purulent material occur at the proximal nail fold.

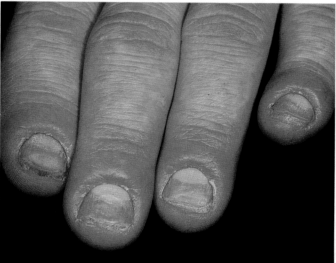

Figure 24-10
Chronic paronychia. Erythema and swelling of the nail folds. The cuticle is absent. Chronic inflammation has caused horizontal ridging of the nails.

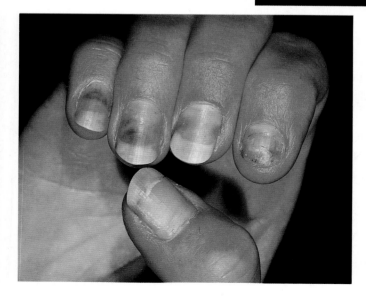

Figure 24-11
Pseudomonas *colonized the space between the nail and nail plate after onycholysis had occurred, imparting a green color to the nail plate.*

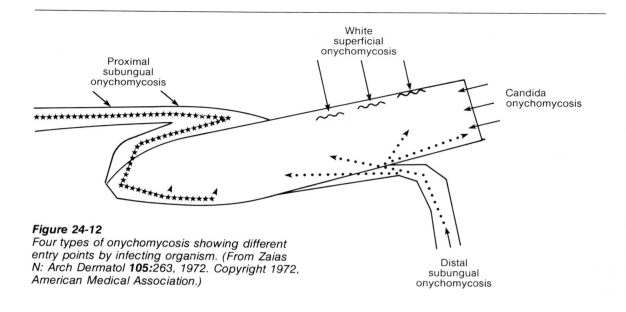

Figure 24-12
*Four types of onychomycosis showing different entry points by infecting organism. (From Zaias N: Arch Dermatol **105:**263, 1972. Copyright 1972, American Medical Association.)*

Patterns of infection. The four patterns of nail infection are described below and illustrated in Figure 24-12.

Distal subungual onychomycosis. In distal subungual onychomycosis (Figure 24-13), the most common pattern of nail invasion, the distal nail plate turns yellow or white as an accumulation of hyperkeratotic debris causes the nail to rise and separate from the underlying bed. Fungus grows in the substance of the plate, causing it to crumble and fragment. A large mass composed of thick nail plate and underlying debris may cause discomfort with footwear.

White superficial onychomycosis. This is caused by surface invasion of the nail plate. This condition is frequently a result of *T mentagrophytes.* The surface of the nail is soft, dry, and powdery and can easily be scraped away. The nail plate is not thickened and remains adherent to the nail bed.

Proximal subungual onychomycosis. This condition results from an infection within the substance of the nail plate, but the surface remains intact. Transverse white bands begin at the proximal nail plate and are carried distally with outward growth of the nail plate (Figure 24-13). *T. rubrum* is the most common cause.

Candida onychomycosis. Nail plate infection caused by *Candida albicans* is seen almost exclusively in chronic mucocutaneous candidiasis. It generally involves all of the fingernails (Figure 24-14). The nail plate thickens and turns yellow-brown.

There are many other patterns of infection. Linear yellow or dark brown streaks appear at the distal end and grow proximally. In others, some or all of the nail plate may appear yellow; in these areas, the nail can be separated from the underlying bed.

Differential diagnosis. Psoriasis is most commonly confused with onychomycosis, and the two diseases may coexist. Moreover, psoriatic nail disease may develop as an isolated phenomenon without other cutaneous signs. The single distinguishing feature of psoriasis, pitting of the nail plate surface, is not a feature of fungal infection. Leukonychia, which are white spots or bands that appear proximally and proceed out with the nail, are probably caused by minor trauma and may be confused with proximal subungual onychomycosis. Eczema or habitual picking of the proximal nail fold will induce the nail plate to be wavy and ridged, but its substance remains intact and hard. Numerous less common nail diseases may be confused with tinea unguium.

Treatment

Oral therapy. Treating tinea of the nails can be discouraging.[6] Topical creams and lotion do not penetrate nail plate and are of little value except in controlling inflammation at the nailfolds. Expensive, long-term oral therapy, if effective, is often followed by reinfection when the pills are discontinued. Oral therapy has the highest success rate with fingernail and nail infections in young individuals. See the treatment section in the chapter on fungal infection for dosages and duration of treatment with griseofulvin and ketoconazole.

Mechanical reduction of infected nail plate. A nail clipper with plier handles may be used to remove substantial amounts of hard, thick debris. One should insert the pointed tip of the instrument as far

Figure 24-13
Distal subungual onychomycosis of the large toe and proximal subungual onychomycosis of the second toe.

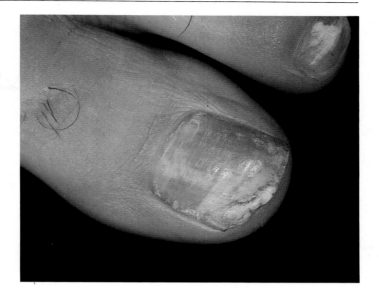

Figure 24-14
Candida onychomycosis in a patient with chronic mucocutaneous candidiasis. All of the fingernails are infected.

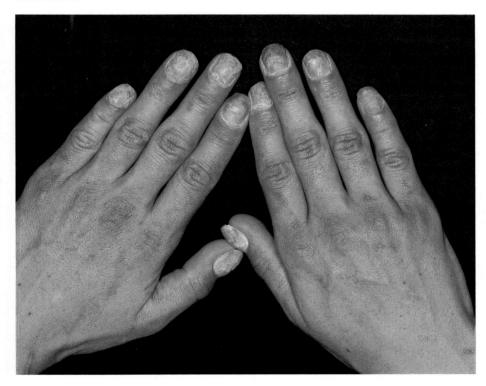

down as possible between diseased nail and nail bed. Adherent thick nail plate can be reduced by sanding or cutting the surface layers with the clippers. Removal of the infected nail may accelerate resolution of the infection.

Surgical removal. Painful or extremely infected nails (usually the nail of the first toe) can be removed by a simple surgical procedure. Local anesthesia is induced with 2% lidocaine by digital block. Hemostasis is maintained by a rubber-band tourniquet placed at the proximal end of the finger or toe. The nail is freed by simultaneously pushing and-opening flat, blunt-tipped scissors between the nail and nail bed and subsequently extracting with a forceps. The proximal nail fold is inspected carefully for any remaining nail fragment. The rubber band is removed and a bulky dressing is applied for 48 hours to control bleeding. Antifungal creams are later applied twice a day.

Nonsurgical avulsion of nail dystrophies. By use of the method of Farber and South,[7] symptomatic dystrophic nails may be painlessly removed with a urea compound. The technique has its most important application in removing hypertrophic mycotic nails and can be used to treat other hypertrophic conditions of the nail plate, such as psoriatic nails. The procedure also facilitates subsequent treatment with topical antifungal agents. The technique will remove only grossly diseased or dystrophic nails, not normal nails. Urea ointment is not commercially available and must be compounded by a pharmacist.

The urea formulation found most effective is urea, 40%, 120 gm; white beeswax, or soft parafin, 5%, 15 gm; anydrous lanolin, 20%, 60 gm; white petrolatum, 25%, 75 gm; and silica gel, type H, 10%, 30 gm. Urea powder and silica gel are blended in after the other ingredients have been combined and melted at 85° C. The mixture has a 4-month shelf life.

Cloth adhesive tape is used to cover the normal skin surrounding the affected nail plate, which has been pretreated with tincture of benzoin. The urea compound is generously applied directly to the nail surface and covered with a piece of plastic or Saranwrap. This in turn is covered with a finger cut from a plastic glove and held in place with adhesive tape (Figure 24-15). Patients are instructed to keep the area completely dry with the aid of plastic gloves or booties. The patients return to the physician in 7 to 10 days. At that time the treated nails are removed, when possible, either by lifting the entire nail plate from the nail bed or by cutting the abnormal portions with a nail cutter. This is followed by light curettage until clinically normal nail is reached at all margins (Figure 24-16).

Onycholysis. Onycholysis, the painless separation of the nail from the nail bed, is common. Sepa-

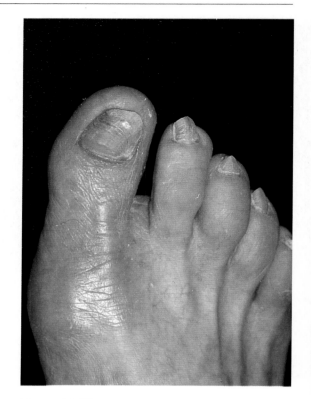

Figure 24-15
Infected nail before application of urea formulation.

ration usually begins at the distal groove and progresses, irregularly, proximally, causing part or most of the plate to become separated (Figure 24-17). The nonadherent portion of the nail is opaque with a white, yellow, or green tinge. The causes for onycholysis include psoriasis, trauma, *Candida,* or *Pseudomonas* infections, ingested drugs,[8] and allergic contact dermatitis, for instance, to nail hardener.

When other signs of skin disease are lacking, onycholysis is most frequently seen in women with long fingernails. With normal activity the extended nail inadvertently strikes objects and acts as a lever arm to pry the nail from the nail bed. Photoonycholysis may occur with tetracycline antibiotics and benoxaprofen (Oraflex).* Treatment is simple. All of the separated nail is removed and the fingers are kept dry. Removing the separated nail eliminates the lever arm and dryness discourages infection. Do not cover the cut nails; occlusion promotes maceration. Discourage any form of manipulation.

*Benoxaprofen is no longer available.

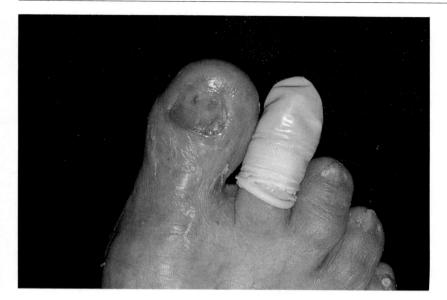

Figure 24-16
Infected nail of the large toe depicted in Figure 24-15 has been dissolved by the urea formulation.

Figure 24-17
Onycholysis. Separation of the nail plate starts at the distal groove. Minor trauma to long fingernails is the most common cause.

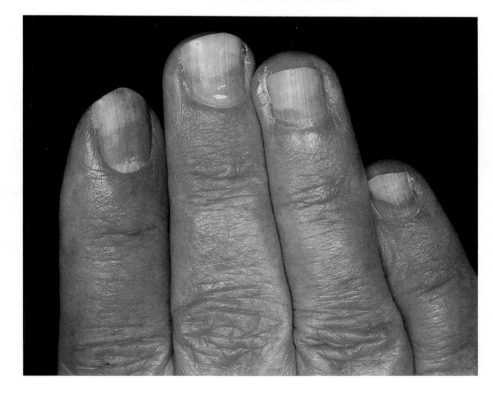

Trauma

Nail and cuticle biting. Nail biting is a nervous habit that usually begins in childhood and lasts for years. One or all nails may be chewed as far as the lunula. The nail plate is chiseled and bitten from the nail bed by the teeth. Nail growth occurs during periods of physical activity, but periods of physical inactivity seem to promote zealous nail biting. Thin strips of skin on the lateral and proximal nail fold may also be stripped (Figure 24-18). Patients are aware of their habit, but seem powerless to control it. Painting the nail plate with a distasteful preparation such as Nailicure (Purepac) or Sally Hansen Nail Biter may help discourage the habit.

Nail plate excoriation. Digging or excoriating the nail plate is much less common than biting. This destructive practice may result in gross deformity of the nail plate.

Hang nail. Triangular strips of skin may separate from the lateral nail folds, particularly during the winter months. Attempts at removal may cause pain and extension of the tear into the dermis. Separated skin should be cut before extension occurs. Constant lubrication of the fingertips with skin creams and avoidance of repeated hand immersion in water are beneficial.

Ingrown toenail. Ingrown toenail is common; the large toe is most frequently affected. The nail

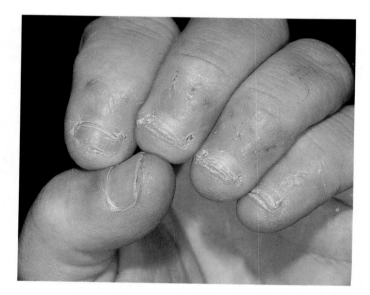

Figure 24-18
Nail and cuticle biting.

Figure 24-19
Ingrown toenail. Swelling and inflammation occur at the lateral nail fold.

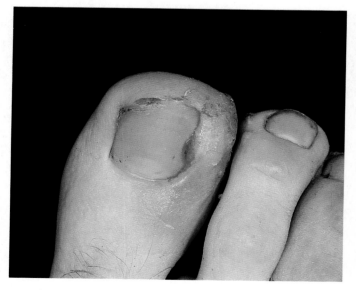

pierces the lateral nailfold and enters the dermis, where it acts as a foreign body. The first signs are pain and swelling. The area of penetration becomes purulent and edematous as exuberant granulation tissue grows alongside the penetrating nail (Figure 24-19). Ingrown nails occur from lateral pressure of poorly fitting shoes, improper or excessive trimming of the lateral nail plate, or after trauma.

Treatment. Ingrown toenail is a mechanical problem. Infiltrate the lateral nail fold with 1% or 2% lidocaine. Insert nail-splitting scissors under the ingrown nail parallel to the lateral nail fold. Insert the tip toward the matrix until resistance is met, then cut and remove the wedge-shaped nail. With a curette, remove all granulation tissue and control bleeding with Monsel's solution. For a few days the inflamed site is treated with a cool Burow's wet compress until the swelling and inflammation have subsided. Shoes should be worn that allow the toes to fall naturally without compression. The new nail is forced up and over the lateral nail fold by inserting cotton under the lateral nail margin and allowing it to remain in place for weeks. Patients with recurrent ingrown nails may require the use of phenol for permanent destruction of the lateral portions of the nail matrix.[9]

Subungual hematoma. Subungual hematoma (Figure 24-20) may result from trauma to the nail plate, which causes immediate bleeding and pain. The quantity of blood may be sufficient to cause separation and loss of the nail plate. The old method of puncturing the nail with a red-hot paper clip tip remains the quickest and most effective method of draining the blood. Trauma to the proximal nail fold causes hemorrhage that may not be apparent for days. The nail plate may emerge from the nail fold with blood stains that remain until the nail grows out.

Nail hypertrophy. Gross thickening of the nail plate may occur with tight-fitting shoes or other forms of chronic trauma. The nail plate is brown and very thick and points to one side. Shoes compress the nail plate against the toe and cause pain. The substance of the nail plate may be reduced with sandpaper or a file, or the nail matrix can be permanently destroyed with phenol.[9]

White spots or bands. White spots (leukonychia punctata) in the nail plate are a common finding, which possibly result from cuticle manipulation or other mild forms of trauma (Figure 24-21). The spots or bands appear at the lunula or appear spontaneously in the nail plate and subsequently disappear or grow out with the nail.[10]

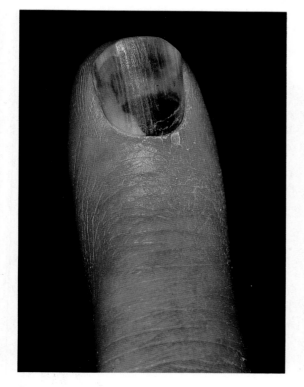

Figure 24-20
Subungual hematoma. A proteus or pseudomonas infection might be suspected if there were no history of trauma.

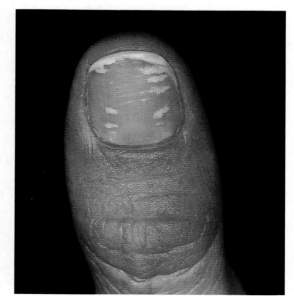

Figure 24-21
White spots (leukonychia punctata). A common finding often mistaken for a fungal infection.

Distal plate splitting. A change that may resemble or be analogous to the scaling of dry skin is the splitting into layers or peeling of the distal nail plate. This occurrence, usually found in women, may result from repeated water immersion.

Habit-tic-deformity. Habit-tic-deformity is a common finding caused by biting or picking a section of the proximal nail fold of the thumb with the index fingernail. The resulting defect consists of a longitudinal band of horizontal grooves that often have a yellow discoloration. The band extends from the proximal nail fold to the tip of the nail (Figure 24-22). This should not be confused with the nail rippling that occurs with chronic paronychia or chronic eczematous inflammation of the proximal nail fold. The ripples of chronic inflammation appear as rounded waves (Figure 24-23), in contrast to the closely spaced sharp grooves produced by continuous manipulation.

The method of formation is demonstrated for the patient. Some patients are not aware of their habit and others who admit to nail picking do not realize that they have created the defect. Patients who can discontinue manipulation will grow relatively normal nails; there are those, however, who find it impossible to stop.

Median nail dystrophy. Median nail dystrophy is a distinctive nail plate change of unknown origin. A longitudinal split appears in the center of the nail plate. Several fine cracks project from the line laterally, giving the appearance of a fir tree. The thumb is most often affected (Figure 24-24). There is no treatment, and after a few months or years, the nail can be expected to return to normal. Recurrences are possible.

Pincer nails (curvature). Inward folding of the lateral edges of the nail results in a tube- or pincer-shaped nail. The nail bed is drawn up into the tube and may become painful. The toenails are more commonly involved. Shoe compression has been considered responsible, but the etiology is uncertain. If pain is significant, surgical removal of the nail or reconstruction of the nail unit is required.

Figure 24-22
Habit-tic deformity. A common finding on the thumbs caused by picking the proximal nail fold with the index finger.

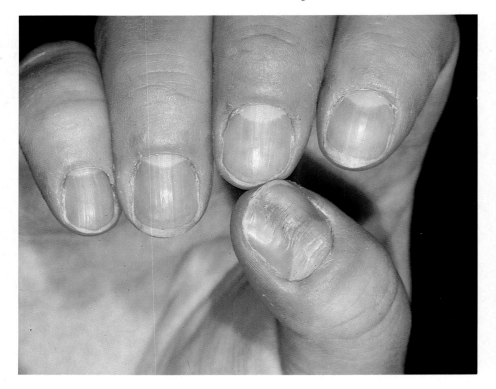

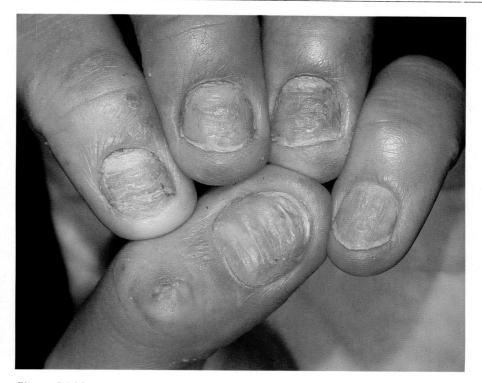

Figure 24-23
Nail rippling caused by chronic inflammation of
the proximal nail fold.

Figure 24-24
Median nail dystrophy.

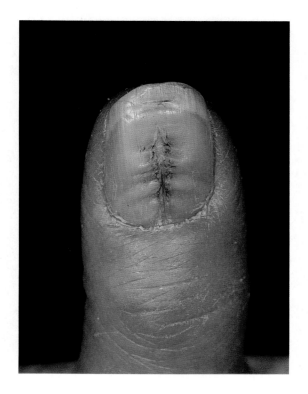

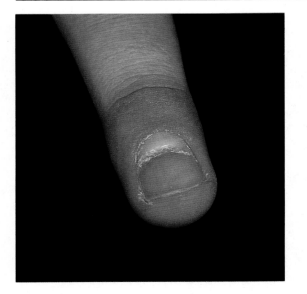

Figure 24-25
Beau's lines. A transverse depression of the nail plate occurring several weeks after certain illnesses.

The Nail and Internal Disease

Beau's lines. Beau's lines are transverse depressions of all of the nails, which appear at the base of the lunula weeks after a stress that temporarily interrupts nail formation (Figures 13-10 and 24-25). The lines progress distally with normal nail growth and eventually disappear at the free edge. They develop in response to many diseases, such as syphilis, uncontrolled diabetes mellitus, myocarditis, peripheral vascular disease, zinc deficiency, and those with high fevers, such as scarlet fever, measles, mumps, and pneumonia.[11]

Yellow nail syndrome. The spontaneous appearance of yellow nails occurs before, during, or after certain respiratory diseases or diseases associated with lymphedema. Patients note that nail growth slows and appears to stop. The nail plate may become excessively curved and turn dark yellow. The surface remains smooth or acquires transverse ridges indicating variations in the growth rate; nails grow at less than one-half the normal rate. Partial or total separation of the nail plate may occur. The diseases reported to be associated with

Figure 24-26
Finger clubbing. The nail is enlarged and curved.

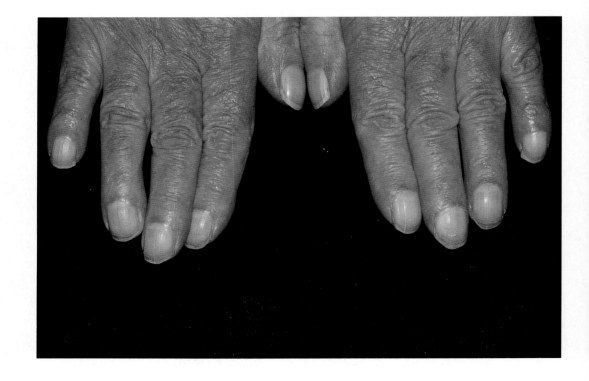

the yellow-nail syndrome are edema of the lower extremities, facial edema, pleural effusion, and upper and lower chronic respiratory disease.[12] There is no treatment, but the nails may spontaneously improve.

Spoon nails. Lateral elevation and central depression of the nail plate causes the nail to be spoon shaped; this is called koilonychia. Spoon nails are seen in normal children and may persist a lifetime without any associated abnormalities. The spontaneous onset of spoon nails has been reported to occur with iron deficiency anemia and in 50% of patients with idiopathic hemochromatosis.[13] The nail reverts to normal when the anemia is corrected.

Finger clubbing. Finger clubbing (Hippocratic nails) is a distinct feature associated with a number of diseases, but it may occur as a normal variant. The distal phalanges of the fingers and toes are enlarged to a rounded bulbous shape. The nail enlarges and becomes curved, hard, and thickened (Figure 24-26). The angle made by the proximal nail fold and nail plate (Lovibond's angle) increases and approaches or exceeds 180 degrees. The proximal nail fold feels as though it is floating on the underlying tissue. Clubbing is associated with a variety of lung diseases, cardiovascular disease, cirrhosis, colitis, and thyroid disease. The changes are permanent.

Terry's nails. Patients whose nails appear white but retain a normal pink color at the distal 1 or 2 mm (Figure 24-27) may have cirrhosis with hypoalbuminemia. However, many patients with this distinctive finding are normal.

Congenital Anomalies

Numerous congenital syndromes involve nail changes. All of the most widely understood have autosomal dominant inheritance patterns.

In pachyonchia congenita, there are yellow, very thick nail beds with elevated nails, palmar and plantar hyperkeratosis, and white keratotic thickening of the tongue, among other signs. Some patients have erupted teeth at birth. In nail-patella syndrome, there are defective short nails and small or absent patella, in addition to other signs.

Figure 24-27
Terry's nails. The nail bed is white with only a narrow zone of pink at the distal end.

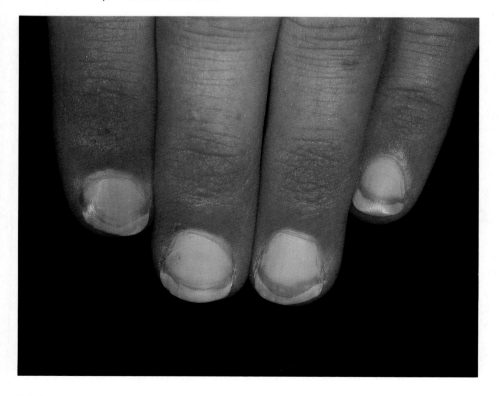

TABLE 24-1

COLOR CHANGES OF NAILS

Etiology	Pattern of color change
Brown nails	
Antimalarial drugs	Diffuse blue, brown
Cancer chemotherapeutic agents; (doxorubicin; daunorubicin)	Transverse black bands
Hyperbilirubinemia	Diffuse brown
Junctional nevi	Longitudinal brown bands
Malnutrition	Diffuse brown or black bands
Melanocyte stimulating hormone over-secretion	Longitudinal brown bands
Addison's disease	
Cushing's disease (after adrenalectomy)	
Pituitary tumor	
Melanoma	Longitudinal bands, may increase in width
Normal finding in more than 90% of blacks	Longitudinal brown bands
Photographic developer	Diffuse brown
Green nails	
Pseudomonas	Green streaks and patches
Yellow nails	
Yellow-nail syndrome	Diffuse yellow

TABLE 24-2

WHITE NAIL OR NAIL BED CHANGES

Disease	Clinical appearance
Anemia	Diffuse white
Arsenic	Mees' lines: transverse white lines
Cirrhosis	Terry's nails: most of nail, zone of pink at distal end (Figure 24-27)
Congenital leukonychia (autosomal dominant; variety of patterns)	Syndrome of leukonychia: knuckle pads, deafness; isolated finding: partial white
Darier's disease	Longitudinal white streaks
Half-and-half nail	Proximal white, distal pink; azotemia
High fevers (some diseases)	Transverse white lines
Hypoalbuminemia	Muehrcke's lines: stationary paired transverse bands
Hypocalcemia	Variable white
Malnutrition	Diffuse white
Pellagra	Diffuse milky white
Punctate leukonychia	Common white spots
Tinea and yeast	Variable patterns
Thallium toxicity (rat poison)	Variable white
Trauma	Repeated manicure: transverse striations
Zinc deficiency	Diffuse white

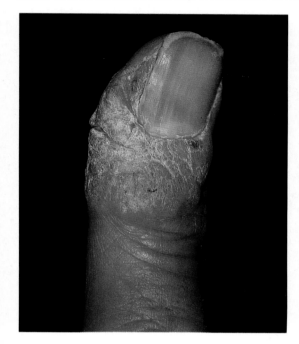

Figure 24-28
Periungual wart.

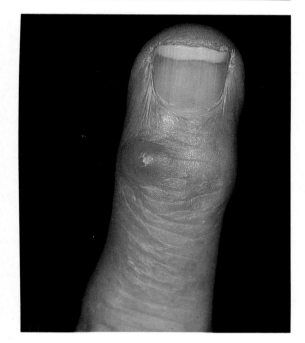

Figure 24-29
Digital mucous cyst.

Color Changes

Changes in nail color may result from a color change in the nail plate or the nail bed. A recent article[14] lists approximately 200 entities associated with nail pigmentation. Some of these are listed in Tables 24-1 and 24-2.

Tumors

A limited number of tumors have been reported to occur around and under the nails.

Warts. The most common periungual growth is the periungual wart. It is discussed in the chapter dealing with virus infections. Warts are most common in children who bite their nails. Warts of the lateral nail fold and on the fingertip may extend deeply under the nail (Figure 24-28). A longitudinal nail groove may result from warts situated over the nail matrix. Warts are epidermal growths, but if massive they can erode the underlying bony matrix by displacement.

Digital mucous cysts. These structures occur on the dorsal surface of the distal phalanx of middle-aged and elderly patients (Figure 24-29). A longitudinal nail groove results from cysts located at the proximal nail fold. These cysts contain a clear viscous jelly-like substance that exudes if the cyst is incised.

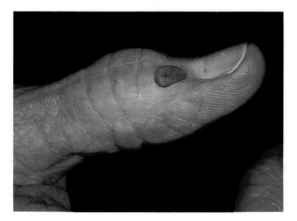

Figure 24-30
Digital mucous cyst. A clear, sometimes blood tinged, viscous jelly-like substance exudes when the cyst is incised.

Simple surgical removal leads to frequent recurrence with failure rates ranging from 25% to 100%.[15] Injection with triamcinolone (10 mg/ml) deep into the cyst is also associated with a high recurrence rate. The highest rate of cure has been reported with the simple technique of repeated punctures and expression of the cyst contents.[16] Cysts that resisted multiple needlings were usually reduced to small asymptomatic nodules. Without anesthesia, the cyst is punctured with a medium-sized hypodermic needle (26-gauge) to a depth of 3 to 5 mm. The clear contents, sometimes tinged with blood (Figure 24-30), are squeezed out by fingertip pressure. The patient is given a supply of needles to repeat the procedure at home if the cyst recurs. Epstein[16] reported that from one to ten or more needlings resulted in a cure or an asymptomatic lesion in 95% of patients.

Pyogenic granuloma. Pyogenic granuloma occasionally occurs in the lateral nail fold. This benign mass of vascular tissue is removed with thorough desiccation and curettage (Figure 24-31). Recurrences are common if any residual tissue is left. Periungual malignant melanoma can mimic pyogenic granuloma.

Nevi and melanoma. Junction nevi can appear in the nail matrix and produce a brown pigmented band. Brown longitudinal bands are common in blacks (see Figure 24-4) but rare in whites. Melanoma of the nail region, or melanomic whitlow, although rare, is a distinctive lesion. Most are classified as acral-lentiginous melanomas. The growth is usually painless and slow-growing and can occur anywhere around or under the nail.[17] The lesion may begin as a pigmented band that increases in width. There has not been enough experience to make specific recommendations concerning the management of pigmented bands in whites. The spontaneous appearance of such a band is noteworthy to most physicians, who will promptly require a biopsy. A pigmented subungual lesion is more frequently malignant than benign and should therefore be biopsied.

Other rare tumors that occur in the nail area are Bowen's disease (nail bed), enchondromas, epidermal cysts, fibroma (tuberous sclerosis), glomus, keratoacanthoma, and squamous cell carcinoma.[18] Their appearance in and around the nails is similar to their appearance in other regions.

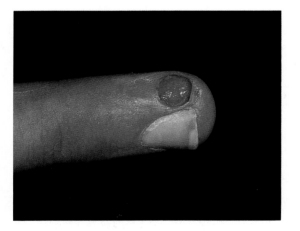

Figure 24-31
Pyogenic granuloma. A pedunculated nodule with a smooth glistening surface. The surface frequently becomes crusted, eroded, or ulcerated. Minor trauma may produce considerable bleeding.

REFERENCES

1. Peachey RDG, Pye RJ, Harman RRM: Treatment of psoriatic nail dystrophy with intradermal steroid injections. Br J Dermatol **95**:75, 1976.
2. Zaias N, Ackerman BA: The nail in Darier-White disease. Arch Dermatol **107**:193, 1973.
3. Chapel TA, Adcock M: Pseudomonas chromonychia. Cutis **27**:601, 1981.
4. Zaias N: The nail in health and disease. New York, 1980, Spectrum Publication, Inc.
5. Zaias N: Onychomycosis. Arch Dermatol **105**:273, 1972.
6. Davies RR, Everall JD, Hamilton E: Mycological and clinical evaluation of griseofulvin for chronic onychomycosis. Br Med J **3**:464, 1967.
7. South DA, Farber EM: Urea ointment in the nonsurgical avulsion of nail dystrophies: a reappraisal. Cutis **25**:609, 1980.
8. Danial III CR, Scher RK: Nail changes secondary to systemic drugs or ingestants. J Am Acad Dermatol **10**:250, 1984.
9. Siegle RJ, Harkness J, Swanson NA: Phenol alcohol technique for permanent matricectomy. Arch Dermatol **120**:348, 1984.
10. Mitchell JC: A clinical study of leukonychia. Br J Derm **65**:121, 1953.
11. Sweren RJ, Burnett JW: Multiple Beau's lines. Cutis **29**:41, 1982.
12. Venincie PY, Dicken CH: Yellow nail syndrome: report of five cases. J Am Acad Dermatol **10**:187, 1984.
13. Chevrant-Breton J, Simon M, Bourel M, et al: Cutaneous manifestations of idiopathic hemochromatosis. Arch Dermatol **113**:161, 1977.
14. Daniel, III CR, Osment LS: Nail pigmentation abnormalities: their importance and proper examination. Cutis **30**:348, 1982.
15. Goldman JA, Goldman L, Jaffee MS, et al: Digital mucinous pseudocysts. Arthritis Rheum **20**:997, 1977.
16. Epstein E: A simple technique for managing digital mucous cysts. Arch Dermatol **115**:1315, 1979.
17. Mihm MD Jr, Fitzpatrick TB: Early detection of malignant melanoma. Cancer **37**:597, 1976.
18. Mikhail GR: Subungual epidermoid carcinoma. J Am Acad Dermatol **11**:291, 1984.

ADDITIONAL READING

Baran R, Dawber RP, editors: Diseases of the nails and their management. London, 1984, Blackwell Scientific Publications.

Chapter Twenty-Five

Cutaneous Manifestations of Internal Disease

Cutaneous manifestations of diabetes mellitus
- Necrobiosis lipoidica diabeticorum
- Granuloma annulare
- Nonclostridial gas gangrene

Pyoderma gangrenosum
Acanthosis nigricans
Xanthoma and xanthelasma
von Recklinghausen's neurofibromatosis
Tuberous sclerosis
Glucagonoma syndrome
Pseudoxanthoma elasticum
Eruptions of pregnancy

Certain cutaneous diseases are frequently associated with internal disease. The skin disease itself may be inconsequential, but its presence should prompt one to investigate possible related internal disorders. A selected group of such diseases is discussed in this chapter. Pigmentary skin changes associated with internal diseases are also discussed in the chapter dealing with disorders of pigmentation. A comprehensive list of skin diseases associated with internal malignancy is shown in Table 25-1.[1-3]

Cutaneous Manifestations of Diabetes Mellitus

Approximately 30% of patients with diabetes mellitus develop a skin disorder sometime during the course of disease. These are listed in Table 25-2. Diabetic bullae are described in the chapter on bullous diseases.

TABLE 25-1

CUTANEOUS LESIONS AND INTERNAL MALIGNANCY

Syndrome	Clinical presentation	Malignancy
Ataxia telangiectasia	Cerebellar ataxia, telangiectasia (pinna, bulbar conjunctiva, etc.)	Reticulum cell sarcoma, Hodgkin's, gastric
Alopecia mucinosa	Patch of follicular papules and boggy infiltrate, face, trunk, scalp	Mycosis fungoides
Amyloidosis	Macroglossia; smooth tongue; shiny, translucent, waxy papules on eyelids, nasolabial folds, lips, and intertriginous areas; "pinch purpura"—skin bleeds with trauma	Multiple myeloma
Acanthosis nigricans	Adult onset in absence of obesity, endocrinopathy, and family history; hyperkeratotic, hyperpigmented skin folds in flexural areas (neck, axillae, antecubital fossa, breast, groin)	Abdominal cancer, other adenocarcinomas
Bazex's syndrome (acrokeratosis para neoplastica)	Three stages: 1. psoriasiform lesions, tips of fingers and toes; 2. keratoderma, hands and feet; 3. lesions extend locally and new lesions appear on knees, legs, thighs, arms	Carcinoma of esophagus, tongue, lower lip, upper lobes of the lungs
Bloom's syndrome	Erythema face ("butterfly area"), stunted growth	Acute leukemia
Carcinoid syndrome	Episodes of flushing (face, neck, chest), dyspnea, asthma, diarrhea, murmur of pulmonary stenosis and insufficiency	Serotonin-containing tumor of appendix, small intestine, bronchus, etc.
Cowden's syndrome (multiple hamartoma syndrome)	Warty papules on face, hands, mouth	Breast, thyroid
Dermatomyositis (adult)	Heliotrope erythema eyelids, bluish-red plaques on knuckles	Breast, gastrointestinal, genitourinary, lung, ovary
Erythema gyratum repens	Rapidly moving waxy bands of erythema with a serpiginous outline and "wood grain" pattern	Breast, lung, stomach, bladder, prostate
Gardner's syndrome	Epidermal cysts, cutaneous osteomas and fibromas, polyps in small and large intestine	Adenocarcinoma of colon
Glucagonoma syndrome	Migratory necrolytic erythema in intertriginous and dependent areas, elevated serum glucagon levels	Glucagon secreting alpha cell tumor of the pancreas
Hypertrichosis lanuginosa (acquired)	Long hair on face and trunk	Bronchus, gall bladder, rectum
Ichthyosis (acquired)	Generalized scaling, prominent on extremities, spares the flexural area	Hodgkin's disease; other lymphoproliferative malignancies; cancer of lung, breast, cervix
Kaposi's sacroma	Red papular and nodular neoplasms most common on lower legs	Internal organ Kaposi's sarcoma, high incidence of other cancers

Continued.

TABLE 25-1, cont'd

CUTANEOUS LESIONS AND INTERNAL MALIGNANCY

Syndrome	Clinical presentation	Malignancy
Leser-Trélat sign	Sudden appearance (3-6 months) and rapid increase in size and number of seborrheic keratoses	Colon, breast
Melanosis (generalized)	Generalized cutaneous melanosis	Metastatic melanoma
Metastases to the skin	Metastasis to any cutaneous site	Variety of tumors
Paget's disease (breast)	Eczematous crusted lesion of nipple, areola	Breast
Paget's disease (extra-mammary)	Eroded scaling plaques of vulva, scrotum, axilla, perianal, groin	Cervical cancer and adenocarcinoma of anus and rectum
Palmoplantar kerato-derma (tylosis)	Skin thickening of palms and soles	Gastrointestinal carci-nomas
Peutz-Jeghers syn-drome	Pigmented macules on lips and oral mucosa; polyposis of small intestine	Adenocarcinoma of stomach, duodenum, colon
Sipple's syndrome	Multiple mucosal neuromas	Medullary carcinoma of thyroid, C cell neo-plasia, pheochromocy-toma
Torre's syndrome	Multiple sebaceous adenomas	Visceral carcinomas
Urticaria pigmentosa (disseminated macu-lopapular form)	Brown-red macules and papules that contain mast cells and urti-cate when traumatized	Hematologic malig-nancies
von Hippel–Lindau	Angiomas of skin, angiomatosis of cerebellum or medulla	Hypernephroma, pheo-chromocytoma
von Recklinghausen's neurofibromatosis	Café-au-lait spots, white macules, multiple cutaneous neuromas, internal neuromas	Malignant neurilemoma, astrocytoma, pheo-chromocytoma
Wiskott-Aldrich syn-drome	Eczematous lesions in atopic der-matitis distribution	Reticuloendothelial malignancy

TABLE 25-2

CUTANEOUS MANIFESTATIONS OF DIABETES MELLITUS

Candidia infections (mouth, genital)	Granuloma annulare
Carotenodermia (yellow skin)	Localized
Diabetic bullae	Generalized
Diabetic dermopathy (shin spots)	Insulin lipodystrophy
Erythema (face, lower legs, feet)	Necrobiosis lipoidica diabeticorum
External otitis	Yellow nails
Foot ulcers	Xanthomas
Gas gangrene (nonclostridial)	

Necrobiosis lipoidica diabeticorum

Necrobiosis lipoidica diabeticorum (NLD) is a disease of unknown origin, but more than 50% of the patients with NLD are generally insulin-dependent.[4] Most patients with diabetes do not develop NLD. The skin lesions may appear years before the onset of diabetes. The disease may occur at any age, but most commonly begins in the third and fourth decade. Most of the patients are females and in most cases the lesions are confined to the anterior surfaces of the lower legs (Figure 25-1).

The eruption begins as an oval violaceous patch and expands slowly. The advancing border is red and the central area turns yellow-brown. The central area atrophies and has a waxy surface and telangiectasias become prominent (Figure 25-2). Ulceration is possible, particularly after trauma. In many instances the clinical presentation is so characteristic that biopsy is not required.

Treatment. There is no effective treatment, but recent reports suggest that ulceration can be controlled with oral medication. Topical and intralesional steroids arrest inflammation, but promote further atrophy. Systemic steroids arrest inflammation, but aggravate diabetes. A number of changes are seen in the microvasculature in the dermis of plaques of NLD; recently, treatment has been used to inhibit those changes. Use of low-dose aspirin and dipyridamole to inhibit platelet aggregation has been successful in healing ulcers in plaques of NLD.[5,6] The recommended treatment is aspirin (2 to 8 mg/kg/day), which for the average patient is 325 gm (1

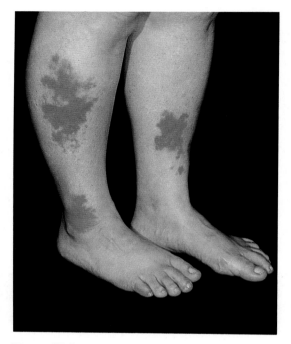

Figure 25-1
Necrobiosis lipoidica diabeticorum. Erythematous violaceous plaques on the anterior surfaces of the lower legs.

Figure 25-2
Necrobiosis lipoidica diabeticorum. The central area is waxy yellow with prominent telangiectasia.

tablet) 2 or 3 times a day and dipyridamole (Persantine) (2 to 3 mg/kg/day), which for the average patient is 150 to 200 mg daily in divided doses. Effective control of ulceration with platelet-inhibition therapy requires a minimum of 3 to 7 months. Recommended treatment schedules should be followed because of evidence that higher doses can decrease treatment effectiveness.

Granuloma annulare

There are conflicting reports about the association of granuloma annulare and diabetes mellitus.[7,8] Most patients with the localized form do not have clinical or laboratory evidence of diabetes. The association between disseminated granuloma annulare and diabetes has been established, but the frequency is unknown.[9]

Granuloma annulare is characterized by a ring of small, firm, flesh-colored or red papules (Figure 25-3). The localized form, most common in young women, is most frequently found on the lateral or dorsal surfaces of the hands and feet. The disease begins with an asymptomatic flesh-colored papule that undergoes central involution. A ring of papules slowly (over months) increases in diameter to 0.5 to 5 cm (Figure 25-4). The duration of disease is highly variable. Many lesions undergo spontaneous involution without scarring whereas others last for years.

Disseminated granuloma annulare occurs in adults as numerous flesh-colored or erythematous papules, some of which form annular rings. The papules may be accentuated in sun-exposed areas. The course is variable; many lesions persist for years.

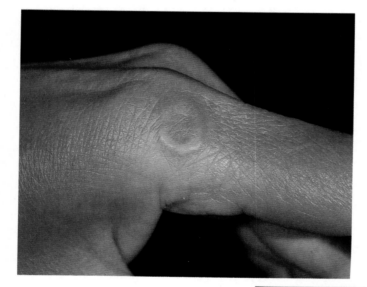

Figure 25-3
Granuloma annulare. A ring of flesh-colored papules.

Figure 25-4
Granuloma annulare is often symmetrically distributed.

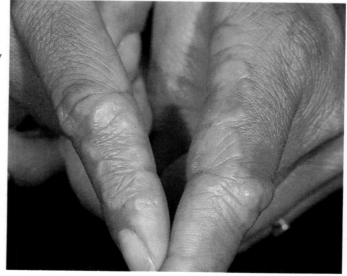

Diagnosis. The clinical presentation is characteristic and biopsy may not be required. The histology shows collagen degeneration, a feature similar to that seen in necrobiosis lipoidica diabeticorum.

Treatment. Localized lesions are asymptomatic and are best left untreated. Those patients troubled by appearance may be treated with intralesional injections of triamcinolone acetonide (2.5 to 5.0 mg/ml). Inject the solution only into the elevated border. Disseminated granuloma annulare has been reported to respond to low-dose chlorambucil[10] and dapsone.[11]

Nonclostridial gas gangrene

Nonclostridial organisms (anaerobic streptococci, *Bacteroides* species, enterococcus, and other anaerobic and facultative bacteria) may contaminate devitalized tissue, causing necrotizing gas-producing infections of subcutaneous tissues. This occurs with a greater frequency in diabetics.[12] The infected area becomes swollen, but pain is minimal. The disease progresses rapidly, infecting fat, muscle, and bone. Gas may be detected by roentgenogram. The skin over the surface may develop a green-black blister. Surgical treatment is required immediately. All necrotic muscle and bone must be removed. Specimens for Gram stain and culture are taken and the wound is left exposed. Appropriate antibiotics are started immediately after a Gram stain.

Pyoderma Gangrenosum

Pyoderma gangrenosum, not to be confused with ecthyma gangrenosum, is a poorly understood ulcerating skin disease which, in approximately 50% of cases, occurs in association with ulcerative colitis.[13] One to ten percent of patients with ulcerative colitis have pyoderma gangrenosum. Pyoderma gangrenosum has been reported to occur in patients with Crohn's disease, rheumatoid arthritis, and hematologic and lymphoreticular malignancies.[14,15] The remaining patients have no other associated disease in most cases. Arthralgia commonly occurs in patients with pyoderma gangrenosum.[16]

The disease begins as a tender erythematous macule or nodule. Lesions are frequently located on the lower legs, but they may occur anywhere on the skin. Pustules or vesicles appear and the surrounding skin becomes dusky red and indurated (Figure 25-5). The indurated plaque enlarges, vesiculation may become more prominent, and central portions of the plaque may ulcerate (Figure 25-6). The fully evolved lesion is generally less than 10 cm, but it may *also* be enormous (Figure 25-7). Lesions tend to be enduring and heal with scarring.

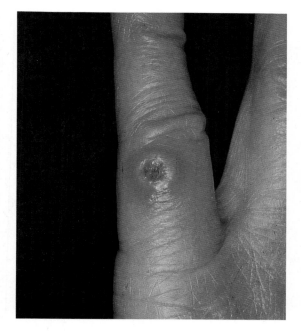

Figure 25-5
Pyoderma gangrenosum. An early lesion with a dusky red indurated border.

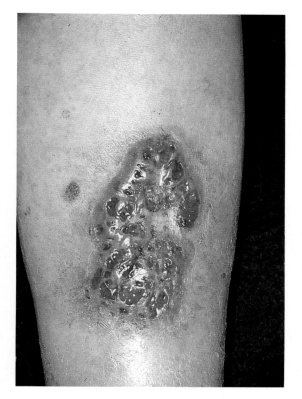

Figure 25-6
Pyoderma gangrenosum. The indurated plaque is ulcerating in several areas.

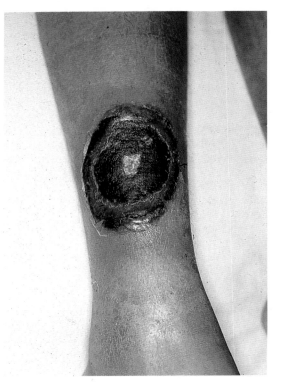

Figure 25-7
*Pyoderma gangrenosum. A fully evolved lesion,
the entire surface of which is ulcerated.*

The diagnosis is made by clinical appearance; a biopsy is of little value, simply showing nonspecific inflammation.

Treatment. Trauma must be avoided. The small early lesion may be aborted with an intralesional injection of triamcinolone acetonide (Kenalog, 5 mg/ml). If multiple lesions are present, a short course of systemic steroids may be administered. Fully evolved lesions may be treated with decreasing doses of prednisone. Dosages of 40 to 80 mg are required for initial control.[17] The ulcer is treated locally with silver nitrate (⅛%) or Burow's wet compresses applied several times each day. The following drugs have been reported effective: dapsone (300 to 400 mg/day),[18] minocycline (300 mg/day),[19] clofazimine (300 mg/day),[20,21] topical sodium cromoglycate,[22] methylprednisolone sodium succinate (1 gm in 1 hour each day for 5 days).[23]

Acanthosis Nigricans

Acanthosis nigricans is a nonspecific process that may accompany a number of different entities. In all cases the disease develops in a similar manner with symmetric, brown thickening of the skin. In time the skin may become quite thickened as the surface becomes warty or papillomatous (Figure 25-8). The most common site of involvement is the axillae, but the changes may be observed in other

Figure 25-8
*Acanthosis nigricans. The skin is brown
and thickened and has a papillomatous
surface.*

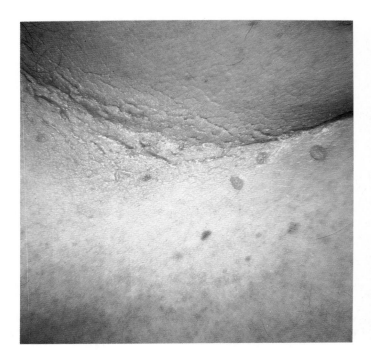

areas, such as the flexural areas of the neck and groin, the belt line, over the dorsal surfaces of the fingers, in the mouth, and around the areolae of the breasts and umbilicus. The majority of cases are idiopathic and associated with obesity; this process is referred to as pseudoacanthosis nigricans. Acanthosis nigricans may occur as an autosomal dominant trait evident at birth or beginning during childhood or puberty; it may also occur in patients treated with prolonged high-dose nicotinic acid.[24]

A number of syndromes have been reported in which benign acanthosis nigricans is associated with abnormal glucose tolerance tests and insulin resistance. The two best known are the type A and type B syndromes. The type A syndrome usually occurs in young black women. They have accelerated growth and excessive androgen production with hirsutism and virilization.

The type B syndrome occurs in older women with signs of autoimmune disease. They frequently have positive antinuclear and anti-DNA antibodies, leukopenia, alopecia, and arthralgia.

Lipoatrophy characterized by partial or total absence of adipose tissue with type V hyperlipidemia is another of the distinctive syndromes associated with acanthosis nigricans and insulin resistance.[25]

The cases of greatest concern are those originating in nonobese adults patients. These patients must be evaluated for internal malignancy, such as an adenocarcinoma of the stomach, or an endocrine disorder.[26] In approximately one-third of patients, the skin lesions precede the clinical manifestations of cancer. Many endocrine disorders are associated with acanthosis nigricans, such as Cushing's syndrome, diabetes, and Stein-Leventhal syndrome.[27] The skin changes may improve with treatment of the cancer of endocrine disorder, but rarely clear completely. There is no effective treatment.

Xanthoma and Xanthelasma

Xanthoma[28-30] are lipid deposits in the skin and tendons that occur secondary to a lipid abnormality. These localized deposits are yellow and frequently very firm (Figure 25-9). Although certain types of xanthoma are characteristic of certain lipid abnormalities, none is absolutely specific; further investigation is always required (Figure 25-10). Classification is based on their clinical appearance and location (Table 25-3).

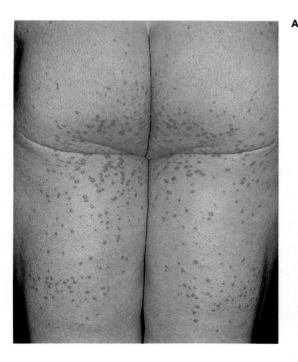

A

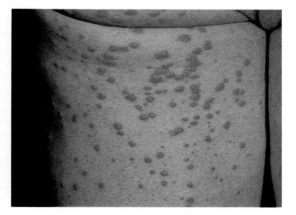

B

Figure 25-9
Eruptive xanthomas.

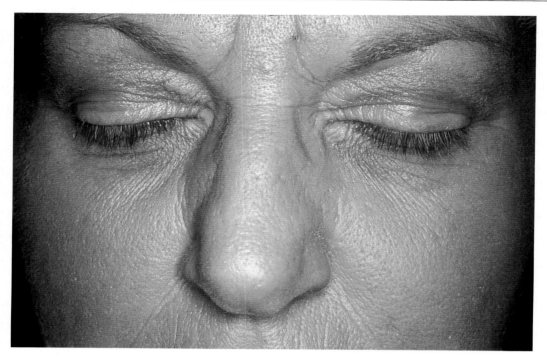

Figure 25-10
Plain xanthomas in a patient with biliary cirrhosis.

TABLE 25-3

XANTHOMAS

Type	Clinical characteristics	Associated lipid abnormality
Xanthelasma	Inner or outer canthus; plane or papular	No lipid abnormality; increased frequency of apo E-ND phenotype and hyperapobetalipoproteinemia; type II*
Eruptive	Crops of discrete yellow papules on an erythematous base on buttocks, extensor aspects of elbows and knees; lesion clear when triglycerides return to normal	Indicative of hypertriglyceridemia and seen with types I, II, IV, and rarely III and diabetes mellitus
Plane	Palms and palmar creases, eyelids, face, neck, chest	Biliary cirrhosis, type III; reported in types II, IV
Tuberous	Lipid deposits in dermis and subcutaneous tissue; plaque-like or nodular; frequently found on the elbows or knees	Hypertriglyceridemia (familial or acquired); types II, III; biliary cirrhosis
Tendinous	Nodules involving the elbows, knees, Achilles tendon, and dorsum of hands and feet	Indicates hypercholesterolemia; type II, occasionally III

*There are five types of familial hyperlipidemia.

---

von Recklinghausen's Neurofibromatosis

Neurofibromatosis is an autosomal dominant disease characterized by the presence of café-au-lait spots, multiple neurofibromas, and Lisch nodules (pigmented iris hamartomas); there are several other less common features. It is an autosomal dominant disease that occurs in approximately 1 of every 3,000 births and affects both sexes with equal frequency and severity. Neurofibromatosis is one of the most common mutations in humans; at least one-half the cases represent new mutations.

Clinical manifestations

Café-au-lait spots. The clinical characteristics of café-au-lait spots have been described elsewhere; see the chapter on light and pigmentation. The diagnosis of neurofibromatosis is likely when the number and size of café-au-lait spots are greater than 6 and 1.5 cm or larger in adults and greater than 5 and 0.5 cm or larger in children 5 and under.[31] The spots are present in virtually every patient with neurofibromatosis and are usually present at birth, but may take months to appear. Their size and number increase with age. Intertriginous freckling, a pathognomonic sign, may occur in the axillae, inframammary region, and groin (Figures 18-20 and 25-11).

Neurofibromas. Tumors are usually not present in childhood, but begin to appear at puberty. Both number and size increase as the patient ages. Some patients have only a few small tumors, whereas others develop hundreds over the entire body surface, including the palms and soles (Figure 25-12). There are three different types of cutaneous tumors. The most common is sessile or pedunculated. Early tumors are soft, dome-shaped papules or nodules that have a distinctive violaceous hue. Digital pressure on the soft tumor causes invagination or "button-holing." When the soft tumors attain a certain size, they bend and hang down, or become pendulous. The plexiform neuroma is an elongated tumor that occurs along the course of peripheral nerves.

Elephantiasis neuromatosa is a term used to describe a diffuse tumor of nerve trunks that extends into surrounding tissues causing gross deformity. This form of neuroma produced the facial deformity in Joseph Merrick of London, England, the man who was described in the play and movie *The Elephant Man.* Most tumors are benign, but malignant degeneration to a neurofibrosarcoma or malignant schwannoma has been reported in approximately 2% of cases;[32] it is rare before age 40.

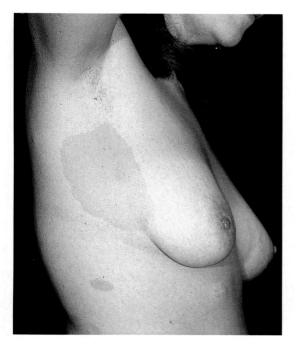

Figure 25-11
Neurofibromatosis. Café-au-lait spots vary in size and have a smooth border.

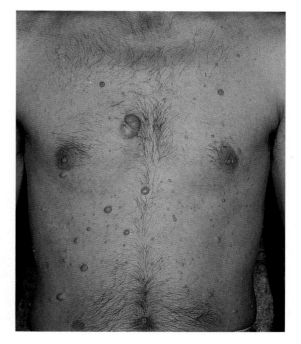

Figure 25-12
Neurofibromatosis. Adult patient with hundreds of neurofibromas.

TABLE 25-4

SYSTEMIC MANIFESTATIONS OF NEUROFIBROMATOSIS

Central nervous system tumors
    Optic gliomas
    Astrocytomas, acoustic neuromas,
      meningiomas, neurilemomas
Constipation
Headache
Intellectual handicap
Kyphoscoliosis
Macrocephaly

Malignant disease
    Neurofibrosarcoma
    Malignant schwannoma
    Neuroblastoma
    Wilms' tumors
    Rhabdomyosarcoma
    Leukemia
Pheochromocytomas
Premature or delayed puberty
Pseudarthrosis (tibia, radius)
Seizures
Speech impediment
Short stature

From Riccardi VM: Von Recklinghausen neurofibromatosis. N Engl J Med **305:**1617, 1981. Reprinted by permission of the New England Journal of Medicine.

Lisch nodules. Lisch nodules are pigmented iris hamartomas and are present in over 90% of patients with neurofibromatosis who are 6 years of age or older.[33] They increase in number with age and are asymptomatic.

Systemic manifestations. A number of systemic abnormalities can occur in neurofibromatosis[34] and these are listed in Table 25-4.

Genetic counseling. The patient's offspring, both male and female, have a 50% chance of inheriting this autosomal dominant disease. The penetrance is virtually 100%, but the expressivity is extremely variable.

Management. Cutaneous tumors may be excised. The patient must be followed closely to detect malignant degeneration of neurofibromas. Genetic counseling is of utmost importance. Periodic complete evaluations are required to detect the numerous possible internal manifestations.

Tuberous Sclerosis

Tuberous sclerosis (epiloia) is an autosomal dominant disease characterized by skin lesions (adenoma sebaceum, shagreen patch, white macules, or periungual fibromas), seizures, and mental retardation; there are several other less common features. The incidence is approximately 5 to 7 per 100,000. At least one-half the cases represent new mutations.

Clinical manifestations

Adenoma sebaceum. Adenoma sebaceum is the most common cutaneous manifestation of tuberous sclerosis.[35] The lesions consist of smooth, firm, 1 to 5 mm yellow-pink papules with fine telangiectasia (Figure 25-13). Their color and location suggest an origin from sebaceous glands, but these growths are benign hamartomas composed of fibrous and vascular tissue (angiofibromas). The angiofibromas are located on the nasolabial folds, cheeks, and chin and occasionally on the forehead, scalp, and ears. The number varies from a few inconspicuous lesions to dense clusters of papules. They are rare at birth, but may begin to appear by age 2 to 3.

Shagreen patch. The shagreen patch is a highly characteristic feature of tuberous sclerosis, being found in up to 80% of patients; it occurs in early childhood and may be the first sign of disease. The lesion varies in size from 1 to 10 cm. There is usually one lesion, but several may be present. They are soft, flesh-colored to yellow plaques with an irregular surface that has been likened to pigskin (Figure 25-14). The lesion consists of dermal connective tissue and appears most commonly in the lumbosacral region.

Hypopigmented macules and white tufts of hair. Hypopigmented macules (oval, ash leaf shaped, or stippled) that are concentrated on the arms, legs, and trunk are the earliest signs of tuberous sclerosis (Figure 25-15).[36,37] They are present in between 40% and 90% of patients with the disease and number from 1 to 32 in affected individuals.[38,39] The white macules are present at birth and increase in number and size throughout life. The Wood's light can be used to accentuate the white macules and is particularly useful when examining patients with light skin. A biopsy shows melanocytes, thus excluding the diagnosis of vitiligo. Hypo-

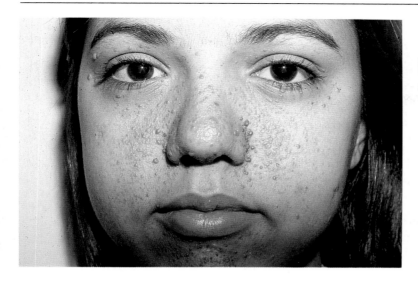

Figure 25-13
Tuberous sclerosis. Adenoma sebaceum.

Figure 25-14
Tuberous sclerosis. Shagreen patch is most commonly found in the lumbosacral region.

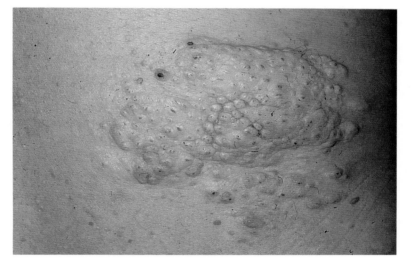

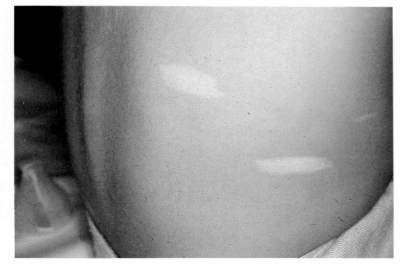

Figure 25-15
Tuberous sclerosis. Hypopigmented macules.

pigmented macules, present at birth, are not invariably associated with tuberous sclerosis, but their presence is an indication for further study. It is essential that the diagnosis be established as soon as possible so that parents can obtain genetic counseling. A tuft of white hair with no depigmentation of the scalp skin underlying the white tuft has recently been reported as an early sign of tuberous sclerosis.[40]

Periungual fibromas. Periungual fibromas appear at or after puberty in approximately 50% of cases. They are smooth, flesh-colored, conical projections that emerge from the nail folds of the toenail and fingernail (Figure 25-16).

Systemic manifestations. Mental retardation occurs in over 50% of cases. Sclerotic patches (tubers) consisting of astrocytes and giant cells are scattered throughout the cortical gray matter. Calcium is deposited in tubers and may be detected shortly after birth by computed tomography (CT) scan or roentgenogram.[41] Brain lesions cause seizures in over 75% of patients. Benign tumors consisting of vascular fibrous tissue, fat and smooth muscle are found in numerous organs, including the kidneys, liver, and gastrointestinal tract. Gray or yellow retinal plaques occur in 50% of cases.

Genetic counseling. The patient's offspring, both male and female, have a 50% chance of inheriting this autosomal dominant disease. The penetrance is high, but expressivity is variable. Patients with normal parents acquire the disease from a new mutation.

Management. Evidence for tuberous sclerosis must be sought in infants with white macules, white hair tufts, or other cutaneous signs. The diagnosis may be established by demonstrating brain calcifications that may occur in early infancy. A positive CT scan is often obtainable before the calcifications are present on skull radiographs and even before the pathognomonic cutaneous findings appear.[41] Facial angiofibromas may be surgically removed for cosmetic purposes by electrosurgery, cryosurgery, laser, or dermabrasion.

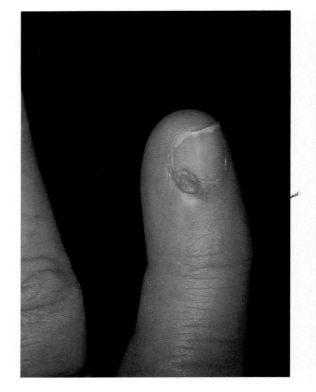

Figure 25-16
Tuberous sclerosis. Periungual fibromas.

Glucagonoma Syndrome

The glucagonoma syndrome (necrolytic migratory erythema)[42-44] is characterized by considerably elevated serum glucagon levels and a dermatitis referred to as necrolytic migratory erythema. Most patients are women, with ages varying from 20 to 71. Reported glucagon levels in patients with the glucagonoma syndrome have ranged from 380 to 6,750 pg/ml (normal, 100 to 200 pg/ml). A glucagon secreting islet-cell pancreatic tumor is most frequently located in the tail of the pancreas. It is very difficult to histologically determine whether these tumors are benign or malignant. Metastasis occurred in 62% of patients with glucagonoma syndrome; the liver is the most common site. Patients with the glucagonoma syndrome also have a number of other disorders, such as glossodynia (beefy, sore tongue), angular cheilitis, diabetes or abnormal glucose tolerance test results, weight loss, normochromic normocytic anemia, elevated sedimentation rate (30 to 100 mm/hour), and hypocholestrolemia.

The dermatitis referred to as necrolytic migratory erythema begins as an erythematous area, progresses to superficial blisters, and gradually spreads ("migrates"), with central crusting and then healing, followed by hyperpigmentation 7 to 14 days after the initial erythema (Figure 25-17). The pattern is most evident on the perineum, lower legs, ankles, and feet. The process is most severe in areas of trauma and pressure areas (Figure 25-18). The early histologic changes consist of cell death in the superficial epidermis; thus the designation "necrolytic." The eruption clears shortly after resection of the tumor.

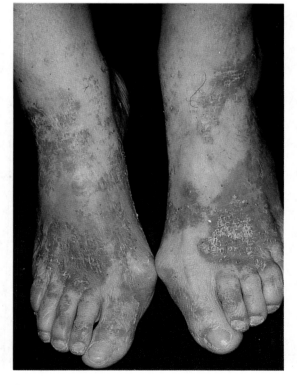

Figure 25-17
Glucagonoma syndrome. A gradually spreading irregular border. Central erythema, crusting, and hyperpigmentation are evident.

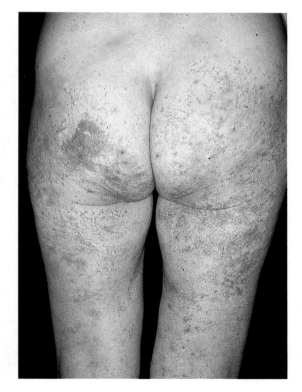

Figure 25-18
Glucagonoma syndrome. The dermatitis is accentuated on the pressure areas of the buttocks.

Pseudoxanthoma Elasticum

Pseudoxanthoma elasticum (PXE) is an inherited defect of elastic tissue. There is both autosomal dominant and autosomal recessive inheritance (Table 25-5).[45] The syndrome is characterized by flexurally distributed yellowish papules, vascular complications, such as hypertension and intermittent claudication, and retinal damage (angioid streaks). The skin lesions have a xanthomatous quality; thus the designation pseudoxanthoma. Degenerated and calcified elastic fibers are found internally and in the skin. The skin lesions consist of numerous tiny, yellowish papules arranged in lines in flexural areas such as the neck and axillae (Figure 25-19). The appearance has been compared to the skin of a plucked chicken. The skin may be lax and hang in folds. Degenerative changes in the elastic fibers of the media and intima of the blood vessels result in vascular complications, such as angina, coronary artery disease, claudication, and gastrointestinal bleeding.

Degeneration of the elastic portion of Bruch's membrane, a homogeneous layer located adjacent to the pigment layer of the retina, results in angioid streaks. Rents occur in Bruch's membrane, followed by a proliferation of the pigment epithelium over the rents. Deep brown streaks simulating blood vessels radiate in a spoke-like pattern (Figure 25-20) directly beyond the optic disc. After the patient reaches the age of 20, retinal changes may first be observed with the ophthalmoscope. Loss of central vision and blindness may occur in the dominant type I form.

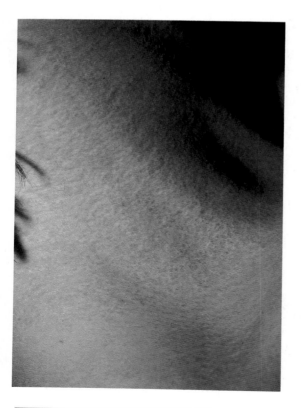

Figure 25-19
Pseudoxanthoma elasticum. Yellowish papules are found in flexural areas such as the neck and axillae.

TABLE 25-5

CLINICAL MANIFESTATIONS OF PSEUDOXANTHOMA ELASTICUM

	Recessive type I	Recessive type II (very rare)	Dominant type 1	Dominant type 2
Skin disease (yellowish papules)	Flexural in 77% of cases	Entire skin	Flexural in 100% of cases	Flexural in 24% of cases
Vascular complications	20% of cases mild	None	75% of cases angina, coronary artery disease, claudication	7.8% of cases minimal
Degenerative choroidoretinopathy	35% of cases mild	None	75% of cases early blindness	8% of cases mild
Hematemesis	16% of cases	None	8% of cases	3.8% of cases

Derived from Pope FM: Two types of autosomal recessive pseudoxanthoma elasticum. Arch Dermatol **110:**209, 1974.

Figure 25-20
Pseudoxanthoma elasticum. Angioid streaks.

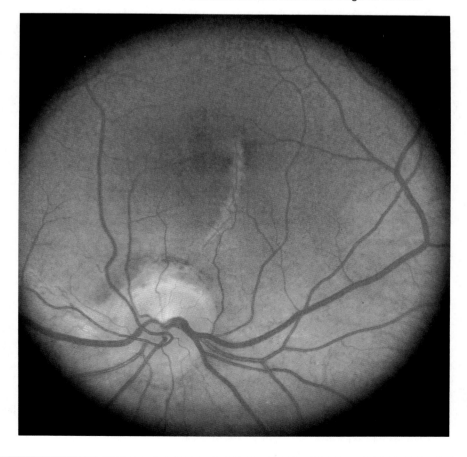

Eruptions of Pregnancy

A group of eruptions is unique to pregnant women; some are well defined. The papular eruptions are the most common, but their status is confused by the variety of terms assigned to entities that appear to be closely related.

Three groups of diseases can be identified based on primary lesions. No primary lesion, only itching and excoriations, indicates pruritus gravidarum. Pruritic papules, alone or concurrent with urticarial papules and plaques, indicate pruritic urticarial papules and plaques of pregnancy, prurigo gestationis, toxemic rash of pregnancy, or papular dermatitis of pregnancy. Vesicles and bullae arising from normal skin or from an urticarial base indicate herpes gestationis or impetigo herpetiformis.

The major concern in eruptions of pregnancy is the degree of discomfort produced and the potential for maternal and fetal morbidity and mortality. The majority of eruptions occurring during pregnancy are papular and nonspecific and clear after the mother delivers the child. The child is normal and not affected by the disease. Itching is common during pregnancy; other than causing discomfort, it is benign and clears shortly after delivery.

The classification of the papular eruptions is confusing.[46] Of the many diseases listed here, the only one that has been carefully studied is pruritic urticarial papules and plaques of pregnancy (PUPPP). It was thoroughly described in 1979[47] and most observers have discovered that the majority of papular eruptions of pregnancy conform to this well-defined category. Literature descriptions of other diseases varied slightly from PUPPP regarding the time of onset and distribution; therefore, unless further clarification is forthcoming, the papular eruptions of pregnancy will be referred to as PUPPP.

A papular eruption referred to as papular dermatitis of pregnancy associated with a 27% fetal mortality rate and elevated urinary chorionic gonadotropin has been reported, but only a few cases have been documented in the world literature.[48] The vesicular and bullous diseases of pregnancy are rare, but very important. Rapid diagnosis and treatment may prevent potential serious complications.

One case of autoimmune progesterone dermatitis of pregnancy and two cases of prurigo annularis have been reported in the medical literature; these diseases will not be covered in this chapter.

Pruritus gravidarum. Pruritus gravidarum (PG) is a condition of late pregnancy characterized by generalized itching without any primary lesion. It clears at delivery, may recur with successive pregnancies, and is benign. Pruritus occurs in about 20% of pregnant women and may be caused by the same diseases affecting nonpregnant women (e.g., urticaria, drug eruptions, scabies, atopic dermatitis, neurodermatitis, and pediculosis). About 1% of pregnant women have generalized itching in the last trimester of pregnancy, but have no lesions other than excoriations.

Pruritus gravidarum results from bile salt accumulation in the skin.[49] Physiologic concentrations of estrogens and progestins are thought to interfere with hepatic excretion of bile salts and cause cholestasis in genetically predisposed women. A few patients, particularly those with itching early in pregnancy, will become jaundiced and develop hepatomegaly with laboratory evidence of hepatic cholestasis. Obstetric cholestasis has been associated with an increased incidence of premature labor, low fetal birth weight, and postpartum hemorrhage. PG clears spontaneously shortly after delivery, but may recur with subsequent pregnancies.

Mild itching is controlled with antipruritic lotions, such as calamine, and oatmeal baths. Antihistamines do not control the pruritus caused by skin bile salt accumulation, but their sedative properties do offer some relief. Diphenhydramine and chlorpheniramine may be safely used during pregnancy. Severe cases are treated with the bile salt-sequestering ion-exchange resin cholestyramine, which binds bile acid in the intestine. Cholestyramine is distasteful and causes nausea, bloating, and constipation.

Pruritic urticarial papules and plaques of pregnancy. PUPPP[46,47,50-52] is most frequently seen in primigravidas and begins late in the third trimester of pregnancy and occasionally after delivery. The eruption, appearing suddenly, frequently begins on the abdomen (Figure 25-21) and anterior thighs and in a few days may spread symmetrically to involve the buttocks, proximal arms, and backs of the hands (Figure 25-22). The initial lesions may be confined to striae. The face is not involved. Itching is moderate to intense but excoriations are rarely seen. The lesions begin as red papules, which increase in number and may become confluent, forming edematous urticarial plaques or erythema multiforme–like target lesions. In other cases the in-

Figure 25-21 (opposite, top)
Pruritic urticarial papules and plaques of pregnancy. The pregnant abdomen is often the initial site of involvement. Initial lesions may be confined to striae.

Figure 25-22 (opposite, bottom)
Pruritic urticarial papules and plaques of pregnancy—the fully evolved eruption.

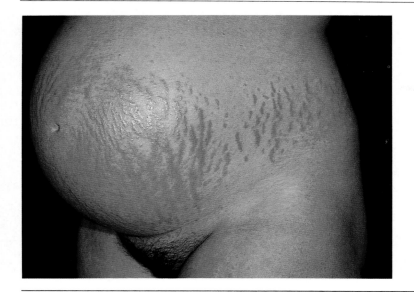

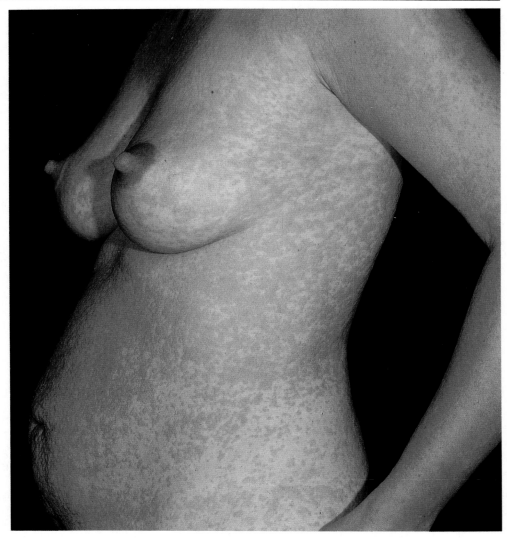

volved sites acquire broad areas of erythema and the papules remain discrete. Papulovesicles were reported in one case. Unlike urticaria, the eruption remains fixed and increases in intensity, clearing in most cases before or within 1 week after delivery.

The eruption may not appear with subsequent pregnancies. There have been no fetal or maternal complications. Infants do not develop the eruption. The biopsy reveals a nonspecific perivascular lymphohistiocytic infiltrate. Eosinophils have also been noted in most biopsies. There are no laboratory abnormalities and direct immunofluorescence of lesional and perilesional skin shows negative results.

Treatment is supportive. The expectant mother can be assured that pruritus will quickly terminate before or after delivery. Itching can be relieved with Group V topical steroids, cool wet compresses, oatmeal baths, and diphenhydramine. Prednisone (40 mg/day) may be required if pruritus becomes intolerable.[51]

Herpes gestationis. This rare blistering disease of pregnancy is probably a variant of bullous pemphagoid and is described in the chapter on bullous diseases.

Impetigo herpetiformis. Impetigo herpetiformis is an extremely rare disease in which pustular lesions resemble pustular psoriasis; the disease may represent pustular psoriasis triggered by pregnancy. Superficial pustules appear at the advancing margin of mildly pruritic erythematous patches that originate in intertriginous areas. The lesions progress to involve wide areas of the skin. The fragile pustules rupture, leaving erosions which, after accumulating serum and crust, look like impetigo. Hypocalcemia secondary to hypoparathyroidism is observed in some patients. Without systemic steroids, the disease may be fatal for mother and fetus.

REFERENCES

1. Haynes HH, Curth HO: Cutaneous manifestations associated with malignant internal disease. In Dermatology in general medicine, second edition. New York, 1979, McGraw-Hill.
2. Johnson M-L: Cutaneous lesions associated with malignancy. In Cecil's textbook of medicine, fifteenth edition. Philadelphia, 1979, WB Saunders Co.
3. Menon PA: Dermatologic aspects of internal malignancies: a review. J Assoc Military Dermatologists 8: 22, 1982.
4. Muller SA, Winkelmann RK: Necrobiosis lipoidica diabeticorum: the clinical and pathological investigation of 171 cases. Arch Dermatol 93:272, 1966.
5. Rhodes EL: Fibrinoclytic agents in the treatment of necrobiosis lipoidica. Angiology 29:60, 1978.
6. Eldor A, Diaz EG, Naparstek E: Treatment of diabetic necrobiosis with aspirin and dipyridamole. N Engl J Med 297:1033, 1977.
7. Muhlbauer J: Granuloma annulare. J Am Acad Dermatol 3:217, 1980.
8. Huntley AC: The cutaneous manifestations of diabetes mellitus. J Am Acad Dermatol 7:427, 1982.
9. Haim S, Friedman-Birnbaum R, Shafrir A: Generalized granuloma annulare: relationship to diabetes mellitus as revealed in 8 cases. Br J Dermatol 83:302, 1970.
10. Kossard S, Winkelmann RK: Low-dose chlorambucil in the treatment of generalized granuloma annulare. Dermatologica 158:443, 1979.
11. Saied N, Schwartz RA, Estes SA: Treatment of generalized annulare with dapsone. Arch Dermatol 116: 1345, 1980.
12. Feingold DS: Gangrenous and crepitant cellulitis. J Am Acad Dermatol 6:289, 1982.
13. Perry HO: Pyoderma gangrenosum. South Med J 62: 879, 1969.
14. Hickman JG, Lazarus GS: Pyoderma gangrenosum: a reappraisal of associated systemic diseases. Br J Dermatol 102:235, 1980.
15. Perry HO, Winkelmann RK: Bullous pyoderma gangrenosum and leukemia. Arch Dermatol 106:901, 1972.
16. Holt PJ, Davies MG, Saunders KC, et al: Pyoderma gangrenosum: clinical and laboratory findings in 15 patients with special reference to polyarthritis. Medicine 59:114, 1980.
17. Braun, III, M: Pyoderma gangrenosum. Dermatology p 28, December 1982.
18. Malkinson FD: Pyoderma gangrenosum. Dialogues in Dermatology 10(1): April 1982.
19. Lynch WS, Bergfeld WF: Pyoderma gangrenosum responsive to minocycline hydrochloride. Cutis 21: 535, 1978.
20. Kark EC, Davis BR, Pomeranz JR: Pyoderma gangrenosum treated with clofazimine. J Am Acad Dermatol 4:152, 1981.
21. Kark EC, Davis BR: Clofazimine treatment of pyoderma gangrenosum. J Am Acad Dermatol 5:346, 1981.
22. DeCock KM, Thorne MG: The treatment of pyoderma gangrenosum with sodium cromoglycate. Br J Dermatol 102:231, 1980.

23. Johnson RB, Lazarus GS: Pulse therapy: therapeutic efficacy in the treatment of pyoderma gangrenosum. Arch Dermatol **118**:76, 1982.

24. Pedro S: Drug induced acanthosis nigricans. N Engl J Med **291**:422, 1974.

25. Plourde PV, Marks JG Jr, Hammond JM: Acanthosis nigricans and insulin resistance. J Am Acad Dermatol **10**:887, 1984.

26. Curth HO, Hilberg AW, Machacek GF: The site and histology of the cancer associated with acanthosis nigricans. Cancer **15**:433, 1962.

27. Winkelmann RK, Scheen SR Jr, Underdahl LO: Acanthosis nigricans and endocrine disease. JAMA **174**:1145, 1960.

28. Pedace FJ, Winkelman RK: Xanthelasma palpebrarum. JAMA **193**:121, 1965.

29. Frederickson DS, Goldstein JF, Brow MS: The familial hyperlipoproteinemias. In The metabolic basis of inherited disease, fourth edition. New York, 1978, McGraw-Hill Book Co.

30. Douste-Blazy P, Marcel YL, Cohen L, et al: Increased frequency of apo-E-ND phenotype and hyperapobetalipoproteinemia in normolipidemic subjects with xanthelasma of the eyelids. Ann Intern Med **96**:164, 1982.

31. Crowe FW, Schull WJ, Neel JV: A clinical, pathologica, and genetic study of multiple neurofibromatosis. Adv Neurol **29**:33, 1981.

32. Hope DG, Mulvihill JJ: Malignancy in neurofibromatosis. Adv Neurol **29**:33, 1981.

33. Lewis RA, Riccardi VM: Von Recklinghausen neurofibromatosis: incidence of iris hamartomata. Ophthalmology **88**:348, 1981.

34. Riccardi VM: Von Recklinghausen neurofibromatosis. N Engl J Med **305**:1617, 1981.

35. Nickel WR, Reed WB: Tuberous sclerosis. Arch Dermatol **85**:209, 1962.

36. Soter NA, Fitzpatrick TB: Abnormalities of pigmentation. In Dermatology in general medicine, second edition. New York, 1979, McGraw-Hill Book Co.

37. Hurwitz S, Braverman IM: White spots in tuberous sclerosis. J Pediatr **77**:587, 1970.

38. Roth JC, Epstein CJ: Infantile spasms and hypopigmented macules: early manifestations of tuberous sclerosis. Arch Neurol **20**:547, 1971.

39. Fois A, Pindinelli CA, Berardi R: Early signs of tuberous sclerosis in infancy and childhood. Helv Paediatr Acta **28**:313, 1973.

40. McWilliam RC, Stephenson JBP: Depigmented hair: the earliest sign of tuberous sclerosis. Arch Dis Child **53**:961, 1978.

41. Burkhart CG, El-Shaar A: Computerized axial tomography in the early diagnosis of tuberous sclerosis. J Am Acad Dermatol **4**:59, 1981.

42. Binnick AN, Spencer SK, Dennison WL Jr, et al: Glucagonoma syndrome. Arch Deramtol **113**:749, 1977.

43. Leichter S: Clinical and metabolic aspects of glucagonoma. Medicine **59**:100, 1980.

44. Goodenberger DM, Lawley TJ, Strober W, et al: Necrolytic migratory erythema without glucagonoma: report of two cases. Arch Dermatol **115**:1429, 1979.

45. Pope FM: Two types of autosomal recessive pseudoxanthoma elasticum. Arch Dermatol **110**:209, 1974.

46. Holmes RC, Black MM: The specific dermatoses of pregnancy. J Am Acad Dermatol **8**:405,1983.

47. Lawley TJ, Hertz KC, Wade TR, et al: Pruritic urticarial papules and plaques of pregnancy. JAMA **241**:1696, 1979.

48. Spangler AS, Emerson K: Estrogen levels and estrogen therapy in papular dermatitis of pregnancy. Am J Obstet Gynecol **110**:534, 1971.

49. Winton GB, Lewis CW: Dermatosis of pregnancy. J Am Acad Dermatol **6**:977, 1982.

50. Yancey KB, Hall RP, Lawley TJ: Pruritic urticarial papules and plaques of pregnancy: clinical experience in twenty-five patients. J Am Acad Dermatol **10**:473, 1984.

51. Callen JP, Hanno R: Pruritic urticarial papules and plaques of pregnancy (PUPPP): a clinicopathologic study. J Am Acad Dermatol **5**:401, 1981.

52. Holmes RC, Black MM: The specific dermatoses of pregnancy: a reappraisal with special emphasis on a proposed simplified clinical classification. Clin Exp Dermatol **7**:65, 1982.

ADDITIONAL READINGS

Braverman IM: Skin signs of systemic disease. Philadelphia, 1981, WB Saunders Co.

Callen JP: Cutaneous aspects of internal disease. Chicago, 1980, Year Book Medical Publishers, Inc.

Chapter Twenty-Six

Dermatologic Surgical Procedures

Basic dermatologic surgical procedures
   Skin biopsy
   Electrodesiccation and curettage
   Blunt dissection
   Cryosurgery
Mohs' chemosurgery
Dermabrasion
Dermal implants
   Bovine dermal collagen implants
   Fibrel

Basic Dermatologic Surgical Procedures

Punch biopsy, shave biopsy, electrodesiccation and curettage, blunt dissection, and simple excision and suture closure are the basic techniques that should be learned by physicians who treat skin disease. One should be familiar with the more sophisticated techniques, such as dermabrasion and Mohs' chemosurgery, so that referral to physicians who perform these techniques can be made at the proper time. The instruments used for most basic dermatologic surgical procedures are shown in Figure 26-1.

Skin biopsy

A skin biopsy is a simple office procedure. Several techniques are practiced and each has specific advantages (Table 26-1).

Choice of site. Generally, biopsies should not be taken from lesions below the knee if other sites are available. Specimens from this area are sometimes difficult for the pathologist to interpret, particularly for older patients in whom mild inflammation and pigmentation produced by stasis may be present. On the face, particularly in the elderly, the arteries are superficial at the following three locations: the temple lateral to the eyebrow (the temporal artery), the nasolabial fold as it intersects the alae (angular artery), and the supraorbital notch at the medial end of the brow (the supraorbital artery). Arteries may be injured by a deep punch biopsy at these sites.

Selection of lesion for biopsy. As a general rule, one should biopsy lesions that are fresh but well developed. Very early lesions may not have developed diagnostic histologic features and older lesions may be excoriated or crusted. However, it is important to biopsy very early lesions for diagnosis

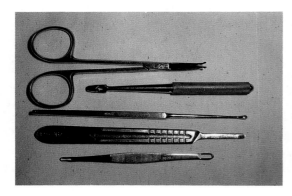

Figure 26-1
Instruments used for basic dermatologic surgical procedures. From top to bottom: curved probe-tipped scissors. 3-mm dermal punch, #1 curet, blunt dissector, Schamburg comedo expressor.

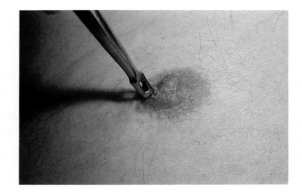

Figure 26-2
The dermal punch is rotated back and forth while gently advancing it through the dermis into the subcutaneous tissue.

TABLE 26-1

DERMATOLOGIC BIOPSY TECHNIQUES

Type of biopsy	Indications
Punch	Most superficial inflammatory and bullous diseases; benign and malignant tumors except malignant melanoma
Shave	Superficial benign and malignant tumors (e.g., seborrheic keratosis, warts, dome-shaped nevi, and nonmelanoma malignancies)
Excision	Deep inflammatory diseases (e.g., erythema nodosum); malignant melanoma

of vesiculobullous diseases, such as pemphigus and dermatitis herpetiformis. Chronic diseases such as discoid lupus erythematosus may not develop diagnostic features for weeks; older lesions should be biopsied in these cases.

Punch biopsy. A full thickness of skin can easily be obtained with a cylindrical dermal punch biopsy tool. Dermal punch biopsy instruments are available in 2- to 6-mm widths. The 3-mm punch is adequate for most lesions. The face may be biopsied with a 2-mm punch to minimize scarring.

The resulting wound has smooth round edges and heals with a slightly depressed scar. The procedure is adequate for the diagnosis of most inflammatory skin diseases and tumors. If possible, lesions suspected of being malignant melanoma should be removed completely intact with an excisional biopsy. Suturing round or oval defects produced by the punch has been advocated by some authors, but this technique does not lead to satisfactory approximation of the margins. Healing by sec-

ond intention is slow but cosmetically acceptable.

The technique is as follows: Prepare the biopsy site with an alcohol pad; sterile technique is not required. Induce local anesthesia with 1% lidocaine with epinephrine. Epinephrine is avoided for biopsy of the digits. Inject around and under but not directly into the lesion.

Rotate the punch back and forth between the thumb and forefinger while at the same time pushing it vertically into the tissue. Resistance is felt while the instrument penetrates through the dermis, but ceases as the punch sinks quickly upon entry into the subcutaneous tissue (Figure 26-2).

Withdraw the punch and gently support the cylindrical piece of tissue with smooth-tipped forceps; with scissors cut the specimen deep to include subcutaneous tissue. Forceps with teeth may crush the specimen (Figure 26-3).

Immediately transfer the tissue to preservative and control bleeding with Monsel's solution, a ferric subsulfate solution (Figure 26-4).

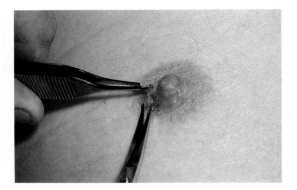

Figure 26-3
The cylindrical piece of tissue is gently supported with forceps and cut deep to include subcutaneous tissue.

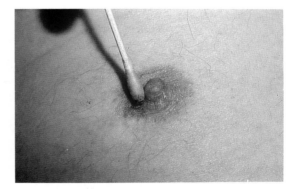

Figure 26-4
Bleeding is controlled with Monsel's solution.

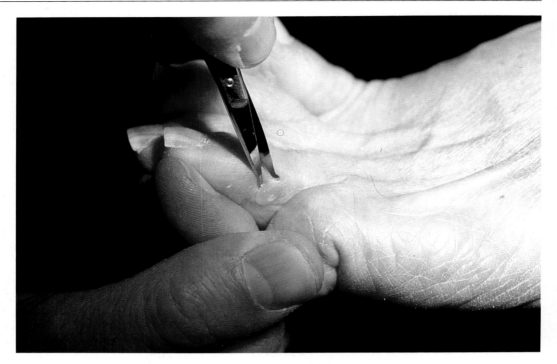

Figure 26-5
Scissor excision of a corn.

Shave biopsy and shave excision. Shave biopsy and shave excision are useful for elevated lesions and when a full thickness of tissue is unimportant. The technique, therefore, is not useful for most inflammatory skin diseases. Shave excision of nevi produces excellent cosmetic results. Any pigmented lesions suspected of being a melanoma must be totally removed by excisional biopsy.

The technique is as follows: Elevate the lesion from the surrounding skin by infiltration with lidocaine. Lay the flat surface of a #15 surgical blade against the skin next to the lesion. With long strokes smoothly draw the blade through the lesion; back-and-forth sawing motions produce a jagged surface. Several strokes may be required around the periphery of larger lesions. The last attachment of skin may be more easily severed with scissors than with a scalpel blade. Control bleeding with Monsel's solution (ferric subsulfate solution).

Simple scissor excision. Firm lesions that resist curettage may be removed by simple scissor excision. Polypoid and dome-shaped nevi, firm seborrheic keratosis, and corns are removed by resting the curved section of a curved probe-pointed scissors on the skin surface and cutting about the border while slowly advancing the tip of the scissors toward the center of the lesion. The resulting defect is smooth and remains in the same plane as the skin surface (Figures 26-5 to 26-7).

Figure 26-6 (opposite, top)
Chondrodermatitis nodularis chronica helicis before scissor excision.

Figure 26-7 (opposite, bottom)
The lesion in Figure 26-6 was excised and healed with a white smooth scar. Another lesion appeared anterior to the first and was excised by scissor excision. Note the exposed cartilage.

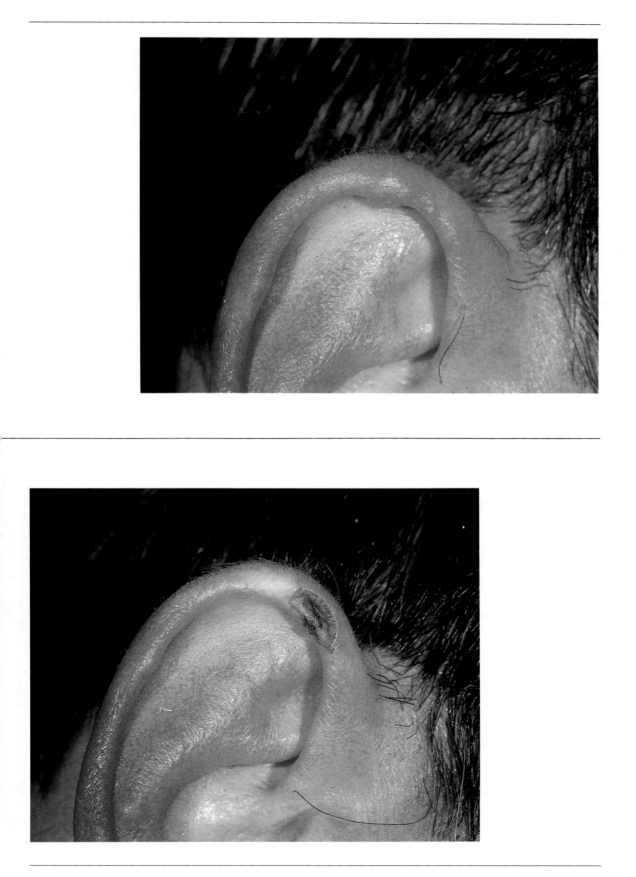

Electrodesiccation and curettage

Electrodesiccation and curettage (D and C) is an invaluable technique for removing a variety of superficial skin lesions, such as seborrheic keratosis, basal cell carcinoma, squamous cell carcinoma, pyogenic granuloma, granulation tissue, and genital warts. The required instruments are an electrodesiccation unit and a set of sharp dermal curettes. Electrodesiccation without curettage is sufficient for spider angioma, small digitate, filiform, and genital warts and small skin tags around the neck and axillae. The curette may be used without electrodesiccation to remove soft seborrheic and actinic keratosis and filiform warts.

Many inexpensive office electrosurgical units can be used for electrodesiccation, fulguration, and coagulation. Electrodesiccation and fulguration are accomplished without the use of an indifferent electrode. The effects are superficial; electrodesiccation and fulguration are the techniques of choice for most dermatologic applications. Coagulation produces greater tissue destruction and requires the use of an indifferent electrode. Examples of commonly used office electrosurgical units are the Electricator, Hyfrecator, Bantam Bovie, and the Ritter coagulator.

Fulguration. The surface to be treated should be dry and relatively free of blood. The pointed electrode is held slightly away from the tissue surface and a "sparking" occurs, resulting in superficial dehydration. The tissues in the immediate surrounding area are charred.

Desiccation. The pointed electrode contacts the skin surface or is inserted slightly into the tissue. The resulting tissue char is essentially that produced by fulguration.

Electrocoagulation. The bipolar setting is required. The active electrode (needle, small ball) is placed in contact with the tissue. Tissue necrosis tends to be more extensive than with fulguration or desiccation.

Curettage. A dermal curette has a round or oval sharp surface. Curettes are available in diameters ranging from 1 to 7 mm. The smaller-diameter instruments are most useful for the majority of minor dermatologic procedures. The instrument is used to remove soft tumors, such as seborrheic keratosis, or tissues that have been softened by electrosurgery.

The procedure is as follows: Local anesthesia is induced with lidocaine delivered with a needle or, for soft lesions such as warts and seborrheic keratosis, with a jet injector.

The skin around the lesion is supported by the surgeon's fingers. With several smooth firm strokes (Figure 26-8), the curette is drawn through the tissue. The surgeon may actually feel the consistency of the tumor with the curette. This ability is very helpful when curetting nodular basal cell carcinoma, which has a firm, gelatin-like consistency. The dermis at the base of the tumor is very firm and resists curettage. The interface between tumor and dermis is not as distinct in the elderly patient with actinically damaged dermal connective tissue. Bleeding is controlled with Monsel's solution (ferric subsulfate).

Electrodesiccation and curettage of basal cell carcinoma. The technique for electrodesiccation and curettage[1,2] of nodular basal cell carcinoma (BCC) is as follows: Induce local anesthesia with lidocaine and epinephrine. Support the surrounding tissue with the finger, and curette the soft friable tumor until firm dermis is reached. The soft-textured tumor offers little resistance to the curette and more than 90% of the tumor mass can be quickly removed. Electrodesiccate or coagulate the entire surface and border by slowly drawing the probe back and forth until a soft uniform char has been created at the base. Remove the charred tissue with the curette and repeat the desiccation and curettage two more times or until a normal tissue plane is observed and developed throughout. Desiccate and curette at least 0.5 cm beyond the visible borders of the lesion to ensure that microscopic extensions of the tumor are destroyed. Active bleeding from the base may indicate residual tumor. Tumor-free dermis oozes blood in a uniform manner.

Bleeding is controlled with Monsel's solution. The wound may be left exposed to the air or covered with a Band-Aid or light dressing. Daily soap and water washing is encouraged. Hydrogen peroxide may be applied once or twice daily. Antibiotic ointments are unnecessary; the ointment base may prolong healing. The patient returns in 7 to 10 days and the adherent crust, if present, is removed.

Postoperative care. For large surgical defects that are allowed to heal by secondary intention, infection is prevented and crust formation is discouraged by the following methods: paint the surgical site daily with a thin film of 2% merbromin (Mercurochrome) solution with a cotton swab; clean the skin surrounding the wound with hydrogen peroxide and dry thoroughly; cover the area with a dry gauze. Gauze is unnecessary when oozing terminates.

Figure 26-8
*Curettage of an inflamed seborrheic keratosis
with a #1 curette.*

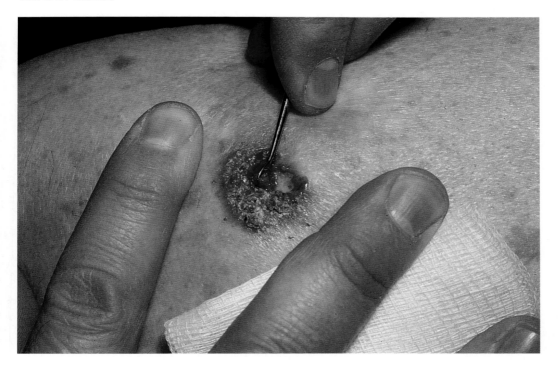

Blunt dissection

Blunt dissection is a simple surgical procedures for removing epidermal tumors, such as warts[3,4] and keratoacanthomas,[5] which is fast, effective, and usually nonscarring. In many instances it is superior to both electrodesiccation and curettage and excision because normal tissue is not disturbed.

Blunt dissectors are available commercially or may be homemade by altering the blade end of a Bard-Parker handle by flattening it with a grinding wheel and bending the tip about 30 degrees. A Schamberg acne expressor may also be used as a blunt dissecting instrument.

The technique is as follows: The patient may be premedicated with analgesics for lesions where postoperative pain is anticipated, such as with large plantar or periungual warts. The procedure is rela-tively painless when performed on areas other than the palms and soles.

Local anesthesia is induced with 2% lidocaine with epinephrine delivered with a needle or jet injector. Plain lidocaine is used for the fingers and toes. The jet injector is less painful than a needle for inducing anesthesia for plantar warts. The jet injector is positioned over the wart and the lidocaine is delivered directly into the substance of the wart. The first shot is painful, but the pain lasts for only an instant. Subsequent shots with the injector or with a needle can be made through the anesthetized skin.

A plane of dissection is established by inserting the tip of a blunt-tipped scissors between the wart and normal skin and cutting the skin circumferentially (Figure 26-9).

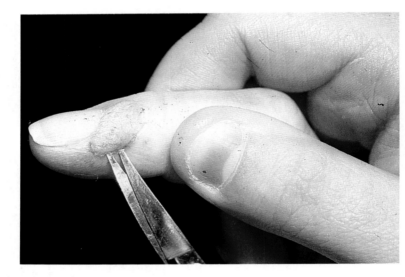

Figure 26-9
Blunt dissection. A plane of dissection is established by cutting circumferentially around the lesion with probe-tipped curved scissors.

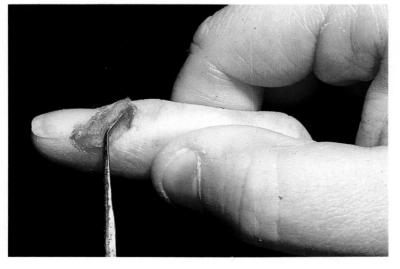

Figure 26-10
Blunt dissection. The blunt dissector is inserted in the plane of cleavage and firmly pressed against the lesion with several short firm strokes.

The blunt dissector is inserted in the plane of cleavage and the intact lesion can be separated easily with short firm strokes from the surrounding and underlying normal tissue (Figure 26-10). At the conclusion of this gross dissection, the blunt dissector is firmly drawn back and forth over the exposed surface of the bed to assure that no tissue fragments remain (Figure 26-11).

Bleeding is controlled with Monsel's solution. A Band-Aid is placed on the wound and the patient is advised to change it daily for 3 to 4 days. Thereafter, the wound is left exposed. Caution the patient that moderate to intense pain may occur for 30 minutes to 2 hours after blunt dissection of periungual and plantar warts. Removal of a large periungual wart is illustrated in Figures 26-12 and 26-13.

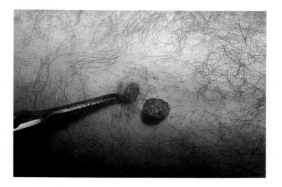

Figure 26-11
The blunt dissector is drawn firmly back and forth over the exposed surface to remove remaining fragments of tissue.

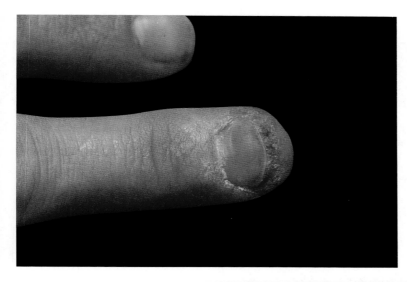

Figure 26-12
A large periungual wart is located at the tip of the finger.

Figure 26-13
Blunt dissection of the wart shown in Figure 26-12. The nail has been removed. A large wart is blunt dissected intact from the nail bed.

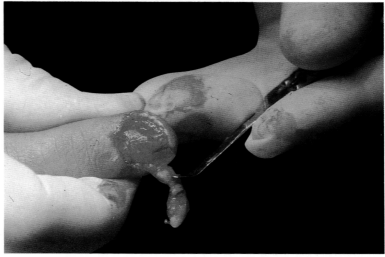

Cryosurgery

Small superficial nonmalignant lesions may be quickly and effectively treated by freezing with liquid nitrogen. Cryosurgery for malignant lesions requires sophisticated equipment with thermocouples that measure the depth of freeze. Cryosurgery is often used to treat seborrheic keratosis, actinic keratosis, warts, and lentigo. Severe pain may result from freezing thick areas, such as the palms and soles, or areas that are anatomically confined, such as the area around the nails. Lesions located on these areas are best treated by other methods. The superficial portions of dermatofibromas[6] and sebaceous hyperplasia can be destroyed by freezing and will reepithelialize in the plane of normal skin.

Maximum tissue destruction occurs with rapid freezing and slow thawing. Repeated freeze-thaw cycles increase cell damage.[7] Epithelial cells, melanocytes, and nerve tissue are more susceptible to cold injury than the connective tissue of the dermis and vessels.

Liquid nitrogen is available in most cities and can be stored in the office in 1- to 2-gallon tanks for approximately 10 days. A large cotton swab, for instance, a rectal swab, is used to administer the nitrogen. Nitrogen is conserved if the swab is dipped into the large tank. Pouring nitrogen into a small thermos is wasteful.

The technique is as follows: Prepare a large cotton-tipped swab by winding the tip to a point. Dip the applicator into the nitrogen tank and apply the tip immediately to the center of the lesion. A white hard area of freeze will rapidly propogate in all directions. Pain is moderate to intense during freezing. Remove the swab after a 1-mm rim of freeze surrounding the lesion has been established. Larger lesions such as seborrheic keratosis may be frozen in sections (Figure 26-14).

The depth of freeze is about 1.5 times the lateral spread.[8] Freezing from the center of a large lesion would result in too great a depth of freeze. The end point of 1-mm freeze for small lesions corresponds to a thaw time of about 20 to 40 seconds and is adequate for epidermal lesions such as warts and actinic keratosis. Longer freeze-thaw times will result in destruction of portions of the dermis. It is better to undertreat a benign lesion than to freeze too vigorously and destroy excessive amounts of normal tissue.

Postcryosurgery. Eythema and edema occur within minutes of thawing. Superficial freezing causes separation at the dermoepidermal junction and can produce a vesicle or bullae. Bullae are apt to occur on the arms and hands (Figure 26-15). They can be large and hemorrhagic. They resolve within a few days, but sometimes require drainage if discomfort occurs.

Complications. Scarring is minimal with superficial freezing. The cosmetic results are equal or better than those obtained with desiccation and curettage.

The nerves are superficial on the lateral aspects of the digits,[9] angle of the jaw, and ulnar fossa of the elbow. Cryosurgery should be avoided in these areas to prevent nerve damage.

Melanocytes are very sensitive to cold injury and healing with hypopigmentation is common. For dark-complexioned individuals, cryosurgery should be used with caution.

Figure 26-14 (opposite, top)
Cryosurgery of a small wart. The nitrogen-soaked cotton-tipped applicator is applied to the surface until a 1-mm rim of frozen tissue has been established.

Figure 26-15 (opposite, bottom)
Hemorrhagic bullae can occur 24 to 48 hours after cryosurgery. This is most likely to occur on the arms and hands.

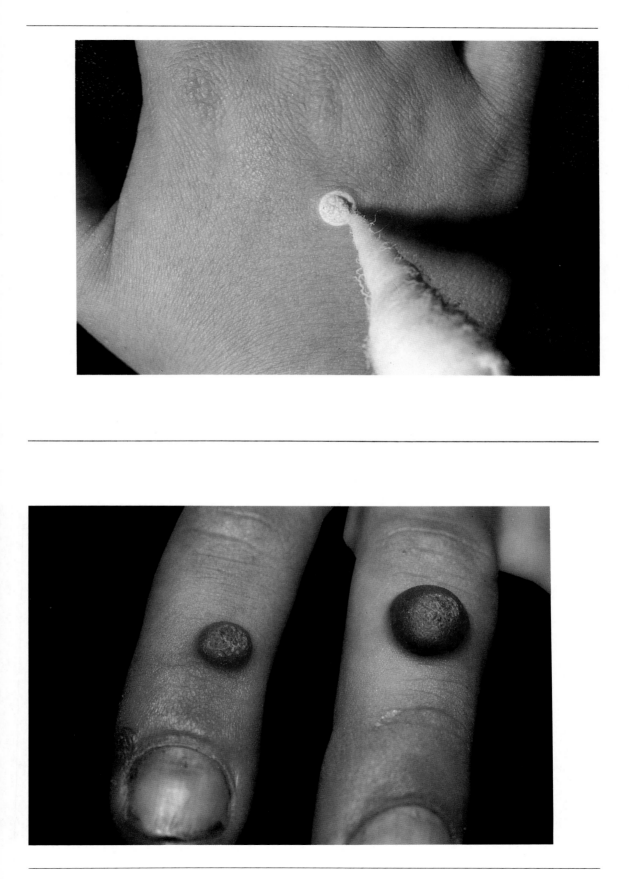

Mohs' Chemosurgery

Rather than increase in a sphere-shaped mass, certain skin tumors, such as basal cell carcinoma, transmit random finger-like projections into the surrounding connective tissue. These microscopic tumor strands may go undetected with standard desiccation and curettage or excision techniques, resulting in recurrence. In the past multiple procedures have been performed on unfortunate patients who, after a series of unsuccessful procedures, acquired a diffuse mass of substantial proportions.

In 1941 Frederick Mohs described a microscopically guided method of tracing and removing basal cell epitheliomas.[10]

The technique is as follows (Figure 26-16): The clinically apparent area is removed with a curette. Zinc chloride paste, a fixative, is applied and allowed to penetrate into the tissue. Since a chemical was used during the procedures, the technique was named chemosurgery. At the present time the fixation step is omitted in most instances; thus the designation "fresh tissue technique."[11,12]

A thin horizontal layer of tissue is removed with a scalpel and divided into more convenient smaller specimens for frozen section. Two adjacent edges of tissue are dyed red and blue to provide spatial orientation. A diagram of the section is prepared and the number and color coding are indicated on the map. Specimens are mounted in a cryostat and then sectioned. Cut sections are stained and microscopically examined.

The location of the tumor cells is indicated on a map and the above steps are repeated only on areas with tumor until a cancer-free plane is reached.

Zinc chloride paste fixation is rarely used today. The defect created by the "fresh tissue technique" can heal by secondary intention or can be closed primarily. Cure rates of 94% to 99%[13] have been achieved (Figures 26-17 to 26-19).

The advantages of the microscopically controlled technique are preservation of maximal amounts of normal tissue around the cancer while providing great reliability in determining adequate margins of excision. The disadvantages are that it is time-consuming, requiring hours or several days to perform.

The indications for Mohs' chemosurgery[14] are listed in Table 26-2.

Figure 26-16
Microscopically guided excision of cutaneous tumors—Mohs' chemosurgery.

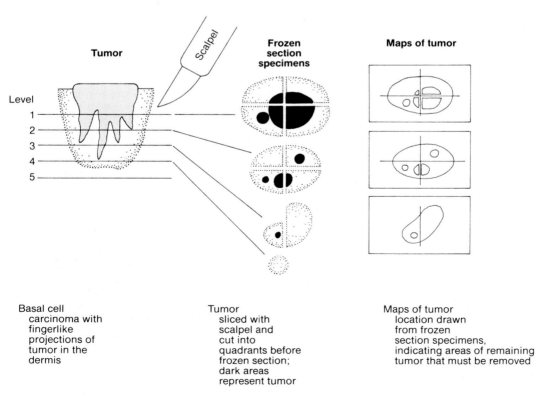

Basal cell
  carcinoma with
  fingerlike
  projections of
  tumor in the
  dermis

Tumor
  sliced with
  scalpel and
  cut into
  quadrants before
  frozen section;
  dark areas
  represent tumor

Maps of tumor
  location drawn
  from frozen
  section specimens,
  indicating areas of remaining
  tumor that must be removed

TABLE 26-2

INDICATIONS FOR MOHS' CHEMOSURGERY

1. Extensive recurrent skin cancers that have failed to respond to aggressive standard conventional surgical techniques or radiation
2. Unusually large primary skin cancers of long duration
3. Poorly differentiated squamous cell carcinoma
4. Morpheaform or fibrotic basal cell carcinoma
5. Tumors with poorly demarcated clinical borders
6. Tumors on the face in locations where deeper invasion of the skin along natural skin planes is possible or the extent of the tumor is difficult to define, such as eyelids, nasal alae, nasolabial folds, and circumauricular areas
7. Areas where maximum conservation of tumor-free tissue is important for preservation of function, such as penis or finger

Derived from Albright SD III: Treatment of skin cancer using multiple modalities. J Am Acad Dermatol 7:143, 1982.

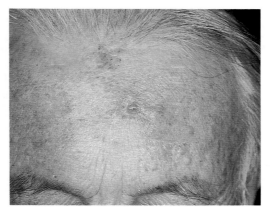

Figure 26-17
Sclerosing basal cell carcinoma. A small nodule is surrounded by an ill-defined erythematous area of induration.

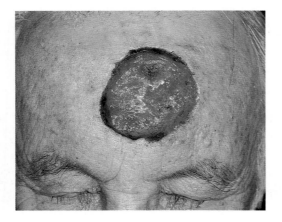

Figure 26-18
Mohs' chemosurgery reveals the extent of the tumor shown in Figure 26-17, which clinically appeared to be rather small.

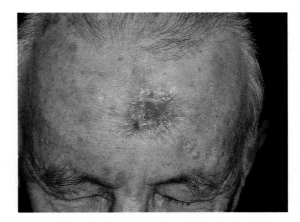

Figure 26-19
Six weeks after Mohs' chemosurgery. The defect is healing by secondary intention.

Dermabrasion

Dermabrasion is a technique primarily used for removing pitted acne scars. Patients to be treated by dermabrasion must be carefully selected by physicians experienced in the technique. A wire brush is spun at high speeds and drawn over the skin surface so that the entire epidermis and upper dermis is removed. Residual portions of the skin adnexa (sweat ducts and hair follicles) proliferate and reepithelialize the smooth-planed surface. Dermabrasion is generally limited to the face, where adnexal structures are abundant (Figures 26-20 to 26-22). Postoperatively, the patient experiences a deep warmth and throbbing sensation. A crust forms and begins to peel. The length of time for complete reepithelialization varies with the depth of dermabrasion and the patient's age, but it generally requires 7 to 21 days. Direct sun exposure is avoided for several weeks after the procedure. Complications include hypopigmentation and hypertrophic scarring.

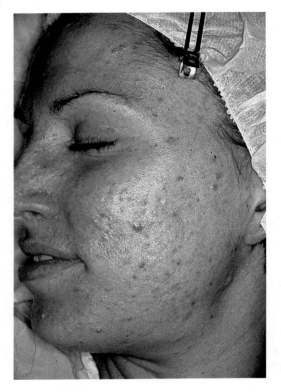

Figure 26-20
Pitted acne scars before dermabrasion. (Courtesy June Robinson, M.D., Northwestern University.)

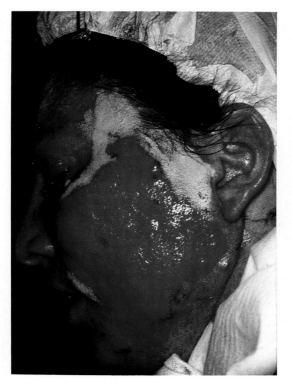

Figure 26-21
Immediately after facial dermabrasion of the cheeks. Trichloroacetic acid peeling (white color) was used on the edges to blend in the skin tone. (Courtesy June Robinson, M.D., Northwestern University.)

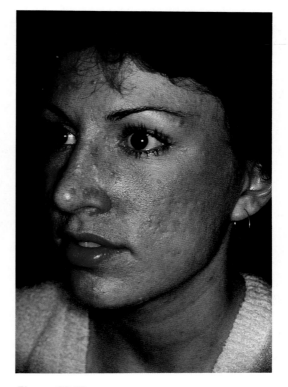

Figure 26-22
Same patient as in Figures 26-20 and 26-21 6 months after dermabrasion. (Courtesy June Robinson, M.D., Northwestern University.)

Dermal Implants

Bovine dermal collagen implants

A new processing technique has been developed to render bovine collagen nonantigenic and suitable for augmenting scars in humans. Lidocaine-dispersed collagen (Zyderm) is supplied in preloaded syringes for intradermal injection. It is indicated in the dermal augmentation of a variety of deficiencies, including acne scars, frown lines, nasolabial folds, depressed skin grafts, and many other soft tissue defects.[15] Soft distensible lesions with smooth margins are the most amenable to correction, whereas "ice-pick" acne, adherent hard fibrosed acne scars and tiny punched lesions do not respond as well (Figures 26-23 and 26-24).

A 0.1 ml test injection is inserted into the volar forearm and observed for a untoward response after 72 hours and also at the end of 4-weeks. About 2% of patients have adverse test reactions and cannot receive Zyderm. Scar augmentation is accomplished by introducing into the plane of deformity sufficient material to deliberately overcorrect the lesion by 1.5 to 2.0 times the initial depth of deformity. Unlike silicone injections, Zyderm implants have not resulted in instances of overcorrection. Several sessions may be necessary to obtain the desired correction. Leakage of collagen through pores and small sinus tracts created during the inflammatory acne process may limit the ability of Zyderm to augment certain scarred areas. Zyderm implantation is contraindicated in patients with a personal or immediate family history of autoimmune disease.

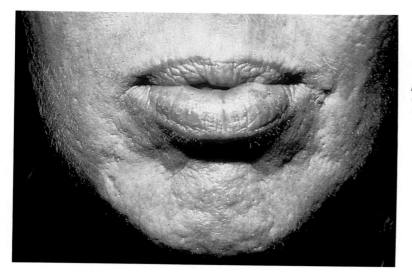

Figure 26-23
Multiple shallow scars are present on the cheeks. (Courtesy Collagen Corporation.)

Figure 26-24
Patient shown in Figure 26-23 after bovine dermal collagen implants (Zyderm). (Courtesy Collagen Corporation.)

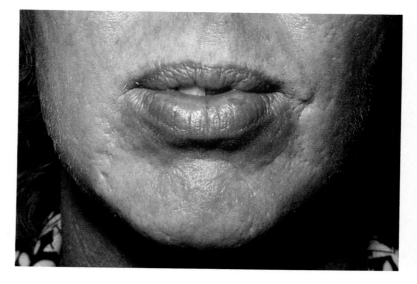

Fibrel

A new, experimental device for elevating cutaneous scars and wrinkles is currently under investigation. This device, Fibrel, which utilizes the patient's plasma as a component, may produce a more permanent correction than methods now available because the body's own collagen is stimulated to form at the injection site.

The components of Fibrel include absorbable gelatin powder, to form a matrix for retaining the factors necessary for clot formation, and aminocaproic acid, a fibrinolytic inhibitor. Just before use, Fibrel is mixed with a patient's plasma, which provides supplemental fibrinogen and other clotting factors. The material is injected through a special needle that undermines the scar just prior to implantation. Tissue injury initiates the process of coagulation and wound healing, which leads to the formation of new collagen. When injected beneath a cutaneous depression, Fibrel will elevate the depression and maintain the effect until it is replaced by the body's own collagen.

REFERENCES

1. Whelan CS, Deckers PJ: Electrocoagulation for skin cancer: an old oncologic tool revisited. Cancer **47:** 2280, 1981.
2. Salasche SJ: Curettage and electrodesiccation in the treatment of midfacial basal cell epithelioma. J Am Acad Dermatol **8:**496, 1983.
3. Pringle WM, Helms BC: Treatment of plantar warts by blunt dissection. Arch Dermatol **108:**79, 1973.
4. Habif TP, Graf FA: Extirpation of subungual and periungual warts by blunt dissection. J Dermatol Surg Oncol **7:**553, 1981.
5. Habif TP: Extirpation of keratoacanthomas by blunt dissection. J Dermatol Surg Oncol **6:**652, 1980.
6. Spiller WF, Spiller RF: Cryosurgery in dermatologic office practice. South Med J **68:**157, 1975.
7. Farrant J, Walter CA: The cryobiological basis for cryosurgery. J Dermatol Surg Oncol **3:**403, 1977.
8. Torre D: Understanding the relationship between lateral spread of freeze and depth of freeze. J Dermatol Surg Oncol **5:**51, 1979.
9. Elton RF: Complications of cutaneous cryosurgery. J Am Acad Dermatol **8:**513, 1983.
10. Mohs FE: Chemosurgery: a microscopically controlled method of cancer excision. Arch Surg **42:**279, 1941.
11. Tromovitch TA, Stegman SJ: Microscopic-controlled excision of cutaneous tumors: chemosurgery, fresh tissue technique. Cancer **41:**653, 1978.
12. Amonette RA: Mohn's technique: chemosurgery and fresh tissue surgery. In Epstein E, Epstein E Jr, editors. Techniques in skin surgery. Philadelphia, 1979, Lea & Febiger.
13. Mohs FE: Chemosurgery: microscopically controlled surgery for skin cancer. Springfield, Ill, 1978, Charles C Thomas, Publisher.
14. Albright SD: Treatment of skin cancer using multiple modalities. J Am Acad Dermatol **7:**143, 1982.
15. Tromovitch TA, Stegman SJ, Glogau RG: Zyderm collagen: implantation technics. J Am Acad Dermatol **10:** 273, 1984.

Index

Deer tick, 312
Deet; *see* Diethyltoluamide
Demeclocycline as cause of phototoxic reactions, 394
Demulen
  composition of, 107
  effect of, on acne, 106
Depo-Medrol; *see* Methylprednisolone acetate
Dermabrasion, 558-559
  acne scars before and after, 558-559
  for scars, 110
Dermacentor andersoni, 312, 315
Dermacentor variabilis, 312, 315
Dermal implants, 560-561
  bovine collagen, 560
Dermal nerves and vasculature, 11
Dermatitis; *see also* Eczema
  associated with swimming, 322-323
  atopic; *see* Atopic dermatitis
  caterpillar; *see* Caterpillar dermatitis
  contact; *see* Contact dermatitis
    allergic, 28; *see also* Contact dermatitis
  hand, 36-44
    allergic contact, 40
      causes of, 40
      physical findings in, 40
      treatment of, 40
    atopic, 39, 77-78
    differential diagnosis of, 37
    and eczema, 31-53
    irritant contact, 37-39
      clinical presentation of, 37
      inflammatory stages of, 37, 39
      instructions for patients with, 39
      pathophysiology of, 37
      patients at risk for, 39
      treatment of, 39
  metal, 62-63
  peridigital, 52
  perioral, 121
  rhus, 59-61
  schistosome cercarial, 322
  sea urchin, 322
  seborrheic; *see* Stasis dermatitis
  shoe, 61-62
  stasis; *see* Stasis dermatitis
  sweaty sock, 52
Dermatitis herpetiformis, 328-330
  classical, immunofluorescent tests for, 327
  clinical presentation of, 328-329
  gluten-sensitive enteropathy in, 329
  linear, 328-330
  lymphoma in, 329-330
  treatment of, 329-330
Dermatofibroma, 412
  treatment of, 412
Dermatologic surgical procedures; *see* Surgical procedures, dermatological
Dermatology formula cream, 13
Dermatomyositis, 356-358
  childhood, 358
  cutaneous lesions in, 527
  diagnosis of, 358
  erythema with, 356

Dermatomyositis—cont'd
  with neoplasia, 357
  overlap syndromes in, 358
  possible malignancy in, evaluation of, 358
  treatment of, 358
Dermatone areas, 267, 268
Dermatophilus congolensis as cause of pitted keratolysis, 178
Dermatophyte fungal infections; *see* Fungal infections, dermatophyte
Dermatophyte Test Medium, 209
Dermatosis, bullous, of childhood; *see* Bullous dermatosis of childhood
Dermatosis papulosa nigra, 409
Dermis, anatomy of, 11
Dermographism, 95-96
Dermopathy, diabetic, 400
Desenex; *see* Undecylenic acid
Desiccation, 550
Desonide, potency of, 16
Desoximetasone
  potency of, 16
  for psoriasis of scalp, 138
Desquam-X; *see* Benzoyl peroxide
Dexchlorpheniramine maleate, dosage for, 99
Diabetes mellitus, cutaneous manifestations of, 526, 528, 529-531
Diabetic, bullae in, 330
  treatment of, 330
Diabetic dermopathy, 400
Diagnosis
  anatomy and principles of, 1-10
  of skin disease, 1-10
Dial soap for furunculosis, 172
Diaper candidiasis, 234
  treatment of, 234
Dicloxacillin
  for acute eczema, 33
  for ecthyma, 162
  for furunculosis, 172
  for impetigo, 162
  for sycosis barbae, 166
Diethyltoluamide for repelling insects, 318
Diflorasone diacetate, potency of, 16
Digital fibrokeratoma, acquired, 410, 411
Digits, pustular psoriasis of, 132, 133
Dimetane; *see* Brompheniramine maleate
Dinitrochlorobenzene
  for alopecia areata, 503
  for plantar warts, 248
DIP joint disease, 134
Diphenhydramine HCl
  for acute eczema, 33
  dosage for, 99
  for eruptions of pregnancy, 542, 544
  for insect stings, 317
  for urticaria, 100
Diprolene; *see* Betamethasone dipropionate
Diprosone; *see* Betamethasone dipropionate
Dissection, blunt; *see* Blunt dissection
Dithranol; *see* Anthralin
DNCB; *see* Dinitrochlorobenzene
Dome paste bandage for edema, 48